AGING ISSUES, HEALTH AND FINANCIAL ALTERNATIVES

SKIN AGING, FREE RADICALS AND ANTIOXIDANTS

AGING ISSUES, HEALTH AND FINANCIAL ALTERNATIVES

Additional books in this series can be found on Nova's website under the Series tab.

Additional E-books in this series can be found on Nova's website under the E-book tab.

AGING ISSUES, HEALTH AND FINANCIAL ALTERNATIVES

SKIN AGING, FREE RADICALS AND ANTIOXIDANTS

BORUT POLJSAK
EDITOR

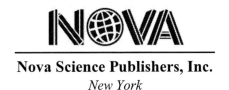

Nova Science Publishers, Inc.
New York

Copyright © 2012 by Nova Science Publishers, Inc.

All rights reserved. No part of this book may be reproduced, stored in a retrieval system or transmitted in any form or by any means: electronic, electrostatic, magnetic, tape, mechanical photocopying, recording or otherwise without the written permission of the Publisher.

For permission to use material from this book please contact us:
Telephone 631-231-7269; Fax 631-231-8175
Web Site: http://www.novapublishers.com

NOTICE TO THE READER

The Publisher has taken reasonable care in the preparation of this book, but makes no expressed or implied warranty of any kind and assumes no responsibility for any errors or omissions. No liability is assumed for incidental or consequential damages in connection with or arising out of information contained in this book. The Publisher shall not be liable for any special, consequential, or exemplary damages resulting, in whole or in part, from the readers' use of, or reliance upon, this material. Any parts of this book based on government reports are so indicated and copyright is claimed for those parts to the extent applicable to compilations of such works.

Independent verification should be sought for any data, advice or recommendations contained in this book. In addition, no responsibility is assumed by the publisher for any injury and/or damage to persons or property arising from any methods, products, instructions, ideas or otherwise contained in this publication.

This publication is designed to provide accurate and authoritative information with regard to the subject matter covered herein. It is sold with the clear understanding that the Publisher is not engaged in rendering legal or any other professional services. If legal or any other expert assistance is required, the services of a competent person should be sought. FROM A DECLARATION OF PARTICIPANTS JOINTLY ADOPTED BY A COMMITTEE OF THE AMERICAN BAR ASSOCIATION AND A COMMITTEE OF PUBLISHERS.

Additional color graphics may be available in the e-book version of this book.

Library of Congress Cataloging-in-Publication Data

Poljsak, Borut.
  Skin aging, free radicals, and antioxidants / Borut Poljsak.
     p. ; cm.
  Includes bibliographical references and index.
  ISBN 978-1-61324-718-1 (hardcover)
  1. Skin--Aging. 2. Antioxidants--Therapeutic use. 3. Free radicals. I. Title.
  [DNLM: 1. Skin Aging. 2. Antioxidants--therapeutic use. 3. Free Radicals. 4. Oxidative Stress. WR 102]
  QP88.5.P65 2011
  612.7'9--dc23
                              2011017276

Published by Nova Science Publishers, Inc. † New York

Contents

Preface		**vii**
Part I	The Consequence: Aging Process	
Chapter 1	Introduction and Description of the Problem	**1**
Chapter 2	What Is Aging?	**7**
Part II	The Cause: Free radicals, Reactive Oxygen Species (ROS) and Oxidative Stress	
Chapter 3	The Role of Oxidative Stress on the General Aging Process	**19**
Chapter 4	Basic Information about the Skin	**31**
Chapter 5	General Overview of Skin Aging: The Role of Extrinsic (External) and Intrinsic (Free Radical Mediated Internal) Factors	**39**
Chapter 6	Mechanisms of Skin UV and Photoaging	**67**
Chapter 7	Skin, Free Radicals and Antioxidants	**113**
Chapter 7.1.	General Overview of Antioxidative Protection	**115**
Part III	The Act: Measures to Decrease Oxidative Stress	
Chapter 7.2.	Antioxidant Prevention of Damage Induced by Extrinsic Factors (Environmental Pollutants)	**167**
Part III	Decreasing Oxidative Stress Caused by Endogenous (Intrinsic) Factors—The Use of Antioxidants	
Chapter 7.3.	Can Antioxidants as Dietary Supplements Offer Appropriate Protection against ROS-Induced Damage?	**175**
Part III	Decreasing the Formation of Endogenous Oxidative Stress—Preventing the Formation of Free Radicals	
Chapter 7.4.	Methodology for the Detection of Oxidative State in Biological Systems	**191**

Chapter 8	Alternative Methods to Decrease Oxidative Stress and Retard the Aging Process	**199**
Chapter 9	The Role of Telomeres in Skin Aging	**259**
Chapter 10	Hormones and Skin Aging	**263**
Chapter 11	Topical Treatment of Skin Aging	**271**
Chapter 12	Skin Curative Approaches	**289**
Conclusion		**295**
References		**311**
Index		**387**

Preface

This book describes mechanisms of skin damage generation and examines the potential impact of free radicals, reactive oxygen species (ROS) and oxidative damage on the skin-aging process. It also evaluates methods to decrease skin oxidative stress, oxidative damage, and skin aging. The identification of free radical reactions as promoters of the skin-aging process implies that interventions aimed at limiting or inhibiting free radical reactions should be able to reduce the rate of formation of aging-related changes with a consequent reduction of the aging rate. This book highlights how aging of the skin happens, as well as what the causes are and the best ways to prevent and treat it.

Part I. The Consequence: Aging Process

Chapter 1

Introduction and Description of the Problem

We're all dying of the same insidious disease, it's called human aging. But there are ways to retard and even reverse the aging process to live a longer, more youthful life. Getting older does not have to mean growing older.

- Dr. Ronald Klatz, President of the American Academy of Anti-Aging Medicine

Skin is the most easily observed organ of the human body. It is an important indicator of our health (pale, sweaty, red, cyanotic) as well as our age (wrinkles) and emotions (blushing, sweating, frowning). Skin isimportant meansofcommunication and judging each other justby seeing the 4% to 5% of the skin that covers the face. Our western society is "youth-obsessed," and there is a strong desire for everlasting beauty. The proportion of individualswho are55 years or older is continuously increasing, predicted to be 31% in the USA in the year 2030 (US Census Bureau).

Aging of the population, in particular the "baby boomers," has resulted in increased interest in methods of reversal of skin damage and aging. An increasing part of the elderly population feels disturbed about age-dependent signs of skin aging and wish therapeutic interventions to hide the signs of aged skin. Novel cosmetic procedures and treatments fulfill some of the expectations but not all of them. Everybody wants to stay young, and there is nothing wrong with this trend. However, most of us do not do anything at the stage of aging prevention. On the other hand, when the signs of skin age appear, we are willing to invest much more money into expensive surgical procedures in order to obtain younger appearance. Such an approach is ratherinappropriate. Instead of investing in theprevention of increased and accelerated aging by adopting an appropriate lifestyle and eating habits, people are seeking for an"easier" and more expensive cure. Non-invasive treatments are in high demand, and our knowledge of mechanisms of skin damage and aging, protection of the skin, and repair of photodamage are becoming more sophisticated and complex. In recent years, there has been an increasing interest in reversing the effects ofage-related changes to restore a youthful appearance and improvethe individual's self-perception. As we all know, prevention is better, more secure and more efficient than a cure.

Appearanceof the skin is primarily determined by its surface texture,color, and physiologic properties such as elasticity, sweat,scent, and sebum production. The skinreveals to others the information of our biological age, and its appearance summates our lifetime exposure to skin-aging compounds (free radicals, UVlight, unhealthy lifestyle, etc.). There are so many different products that are available on the market that claim to be able to help us to regain our youthful appearance.Unfortunately, many of these products fall well short of being able to truly provide what they promise. People constantly look for "magic bullets"— single products, creams and procedures that can improve the appearance of their skin and bodies. Although they are claimed and promised by cosmetic industry, such "magic bullets" do not exist and do not work in reality and will never be produced. We should not forget that producersmay claim that their products can do miracles, without any scientific study that would prove it. The only goal of some of the anti-aging products is to be sold in huge amounts in order to providehuge profits to the producers. By 2010, the anti-aging market is expected to account for over $16.5 billion in sales (Choi and Berson, 2006).

Aging in general is an extremely complex, multifactorial process and represents the gradual deterioration in functions that occurs after maturity and leads to disability and death. In essence, aging is progressive accumulation through life of a variety of random molecular defects that build up within the cells and tissues.For this reason, only one "magic bullet" will never be able to prevent or reverse the complex and multicausal process of aging. Harman (2002) defines aging as "the progressive accumulation ofdiverse deleterious changes in cells and tissues with advancingage that increase the risk of disease and death" (Harman, 2001). Thisdefinition illustrates two widely recognized and equally importantaspects of the aging process: *1*) aging is characterized as aprogressive decline in biological functions with time, and *2*)aging results in a decreased resistance to multiple forms ofstress, as well as an increased susceptibility to numerous diseases (Kregel, 2006).

These defects start to arise very early in life, probably *in utero*, but in the early years, both the fraction of affected cells and the average burden of damage per affected cell are low (Kirkwood and Mathers, 2009). It is believed that the signs of aging relevant to the outlook start to appear after maturity—the time of optimal health, strength and appearance. Throughout the adult life, and especially after puberty, all physiological functions gradually decline. There is diminished capacity for protein synthesis, a decline in immune function, a loss of muscle mass and strength, and a decrease in bone mineral density as well as a decrease in enzymatic and non-enzymatic antioxidative protection, together with a decline in cell repair processes. The quality of skin and hair also declines significantly. Greying of the hair is a result of melanocyte loss from the hair bulb with increasing age. Wrinkle formation is a result of accumulated damage and decreased synthesis of collagen.

Through a variety of studies, longevity experts are now identifying key factors that contribute to long lifespans, including genetics, lifestyle choices and exercise habits. For the past two decades, research directed toward the basic understanding of biological aging mechanisms has given us new insights into the molecular bases and biological events that contribute to age-related deterioration. But there was too little research and investmentinto the possible aging interventions. Researchers estimate that 25 percent of aging variances can be attributed to good genes, and the remaining 75 percent to environmental factors such as lifestyle, exercise and diet. This indicates that aging interventions could significantly alter the process of aging.

The precise biological and cellular mechanisms responsible for primary and secondary aging are not known, but according to Fontana and Klein (2007), they are likely to involve a constellation of complex and interrelated factors, including (1) oxidative stress–induced protein and DNA damage in conjunction with inadequate DNA damage repair, as well as genetic instability of mitochondrial and nuclear genomes; (2) noninfectious chronic inflammation caused by increased adipokine and cytokine production; (3) alterations in fatty acid metabolism, including excessive free fatty acid release into plasma with subsequent tissue insulin resistance; (4) accumulation of cellular "garbage," such as advanced glycation end products, amyloid, and proteins that interfere with normal cell function; (5) sympathetic nerve system and angiotensin system activation as well as alterations in neuroendocrine systems; and (6) loss of post-mitotic cells, resulting in a decreased number of neurons and muscle cells as well as deterioration in structure and function of cells in all tissues and organs.

However, chronological aging is not necessarily the same asbiological aging. Youmay notice that some people age better than others; they feel and look younger than their (ex) schoolmates of the same age. Evidence is accumulating that the aging process evolves at different rates among individuals of the same age. Besides, any given subject shows a variable senescence among her/his organs, and among each of the constituent tissues, cells and molecules (Quatresooz et al., 2010). Age is usually measured in full years and in months for young children. Roughly 100,000 people worldwide die each day of age-related causes (de Grey, 2007). Chronological aging, referring to how old a person is, is arguably the most straightforward definition of aging, but as we said, chronological age is not the same as biological age. Chronological age is a crude index of a probable length of a remaining life of a person and chronological skin aging comprises those changes in the skin that occur as a result of passage of time alone. These changes occur as the result of cumulative endogenous damage from the continuous formation of reactive oxygen species (ROS) due to the oxidative cellular metabolism. Biological age can be regarded as a more accurate estimation of one's position in time relative to one's potential lifespan. There are major differences between life expectancy and lifespan. Life expectancy is a statistical projection of the length a human being is expected to live based on probabilities and assumptions of genetic predispositions, living conditions, medical discoveries and advances, natural disasters, and other environmental factors. Lifespan, however, is defined as the characteristic observed age of death of a group's very oldest individuals (Vitetta and Anton, 2007). Maximum lifespan, defined as the average lifespan of the longest-lived decile of a cohort (Holloszy, 2000), is often used as a standard for evaluating the aging process, because valid biomarkers of physiological aging have not been identified (Johnson, 2006). In general, an average human lifespan increased due to improvements in nutrition, sanitation, healthcare quality over the past century. But not the maximum lifespan. Hair graying, recession of hair from the forehead and lip height were influenced mainly by genetic factors, whereas environmental factors influenced hair thinning. These findings indicate that women who look young for their ages have large lips, avoid sun-exposure and possess genetic factors that protect against the development of gray hair and skin wrinkles. Findings also demonstrate that perceived age is a better biomarker of skin, hair and facial aging than chronological age (Gunn et al., 2009).

This perspective is problematicdue to the fact that chronological age does not correlate perfectly with functional age, i.e., two people may be of the same chronological age but differ in their mental and physical capacities. When our biological age is higher than our real age, we will feel older than we really are. This stage should be estimated early, and approaches of reverse accelerated aging should be adopted. It is never too late, but the sooner you start, the better your results will be. There are many factors that have a major influence on our biological age. The most important is our lifestyle (e.g., quality and quantity of sleep, number of sunburns that caused blistering, tobacco use on a regular basis or being around people who smoke, alcohol intake, satisfaction with our lives, how many close friends and relatives (and pets)we have, how many personal incidents and financial situations thatcaused stresswe were exposed to, etc.); body characteristics (e.g., resting heart rate, average blood pressure (systolic/diastolic), total and HDL cholesterol level, allergies, etc.); eating habits (e.g., eating breakfast, number of servings of high-fiber grains, servings of fruits and vegetables per day, servings of nuts and legumes, servings of red meat, fish, etc.); sport activities (e.g., how oftenwe do aerobic exercise, strength-training exercise, etc.).

If we eat well, exercise and have meaningful social interactions in life, our biological ages could besmaller than our chronological age. Although the chronological age of a person is fixed, the biological age of a person is not. Our biological age is how healthy our bodiesareand how much damage our cells have accumulated rather than how old we are in calendar years. If our chronological age is 40, our arteries could be 30or even 50 years old. Research suggests that biological age is a more accurate evaluation of your age, and the good news is that biological age can actually bedecreased if we pursue healthy lifestyle choices. Successful aging means "absence of diseases and disabilities, maintenance of high levels of physical and cognitive abilities, preservation of the social and productive activities."To date, dietary restriction is the only scientifically proved paradigm shown to affect both average and maximum lifespans. It should be noted that the increase of maximum life extension, not average lifespan, is considered a more reliable indicator of biological aging intervention (Yu, 1995).

There arenumerous factors in life that can cause people to feel older or younger than they really are.Those that cause us to age at a faster rate than others include lack of a healthy diet or exercise anda range of stress factors and risks that may occur in one's life. The secret to living longer, feeling well and looking better involves various factors, including consideration of our attitudes towards certain things and being mindful of diet and activity levels. Elderly population increases, the prevalence of aging-related diseases increases and methods that provide health benefits to control aging and prolong health span will become appreciated. There are many possible interventions on the skin-aging process. I believe that free radical-mediated damage is the major cause of the skin-aging process. A lot of chapters in this book analyze free radical formation, oxidative stress and their impact on skin aging as well as the strategies to decrease the oxidative stress in skin cells.

Skin aging is a highly complex mechanism, involving multiple mechanisms at different levels. The research investigated hundreds of diseases of human skin but little research has been done in the field of skin aging. The research gradually reveals how and why our skin ages and what opportunities there arefor intervention. Although the fundamental mechanisms of skin aging are still poorly understood, a growing body of evidence points towards reactive oxygen species (ROS) as one of the primary determinants of aging. Evidence suggests that an important theme linking several different kinds of damage is the action of reactive oxygen species, which are generated as by-products of the body's essential use of oxygen to produce energy (Martin et al., 1996; von Zglinicky et al., 2001). The damage that contributes to eventual aging accumulates in our bodies throughout the life-course, beginning in the womb. For years, people have attempted to hide, reverse or control changes in their skin, such as wrinkling, roughness, mottling, blotching and dryness. For many people, skin aging is one of the worst aspects of getting older. It may not seem to matter that much from a health perspective, but for many of us, our appearance has a great impact on our confidence and self-esteem. Youmay notice that some people age better than others, and this has a lot to do with having inherited good genes, but remember: you can prevent premature skin aging, and it is never too late to start taking the necessary steps to obtain a younger looking skin. While some signs of skin aging are inevitable, there is a lot you can do to look your best at any age. Nevertheless, humans live relatively longer, and sooner or later older people's skin becomes more susceptible to skin diseases and malformations.

Numerous lines of evidence indicate that environmental factors, including diet and lifestyle, are the most important in determining aging process. Considering this, the book focuses on interventions highlighted in Table 1.

Additionally, this book will highlight how skin aging happens—the causes for it and the best ways to prevent, retard and treat it. Ways to promote successful and healthy skin aging as well as specific strategies for prevention or delay of unwanted age-associated changes will also be discussed. Since the (skin) aging process is accompanied by enhanced oxidative stress and damage, the goal of this book is to describe mechanisms of free radical generation, examine the potential impact of ROS and oxidative damage on the skin-aging process, and evaluate methods to decrease skin oxidative stress, oxidative damage, and the signs of skin aging. The identification of free radical reactions as promoters of the skin-aging process implies that interventions aimed at limiting or inhibiting these factors should be able to reduce the rate of formation of aging-related changes with a consequent reduction of the aging rate. The concept of the book is divided into three parts. In Part I, a general overview of the aging process will be presented for a better understanding of skin aging. For many decades, the field of gerontological researchfocused only on understanding how physiological functions decline with the increasing age, and almost no research was dedicated to methodsof aging intervention. In Part II, the mechanisms of oxidative stress as the main reason of aging will be elucidated, and Part III will focus on how elevated oxidative stress can be decreased. The reduction of oxidative stress can be achieved on three levels: i) by lowering exposure to environmental pollutantse.g., how to avoid excessive exogenous free radical formation and exposure; ii) by increasing levels of antioxidants in order to scavenge ROS before they can cause any damage; or iii) by employing primary preventive strategies for lowering the generation of oxidative stress by stabilizing mitochondrial energy production and efficiency—reducing the amount of ROS formed per amount of O_2 consumed necessary in producing a given quantity of ATP. Additionally, the process of oxidative stress damage repair is discussed.

However, the solution of aging prevention or retardation is not so simple. If free radical formation were totally eliminated, the consequences would lead to improper functioning of our cells. For example, the production of too much superoxide is bad, but the complete elimination is even worse. It is the balance that must be obtained for proper functioning, cell proliferation and normal aging. In order to reach this balance, the level of oxidative stress should be determined first. How to measure it will be discussed in the chapter dedicated to methods for the detection of oxidative stress in biological samples. Any therapeutic attempts aimed to reverse the aging process must face this paradox regarding the balance between ROS formation and antioxidant protection.

Table 1. Some of the factors discussed in this book that influence the aging process

Nutritional regimen	*Dietary components*
	Vitamin and antioxidant supplements
	Caloric restriction
	Others
Physical modification	*Physical exercise*
	Reduction of body metabolism and temperature
Environmental factors	*Pollutants like UVradiation, pesticides, additives and others*

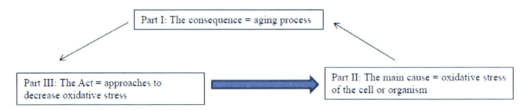

Figure 1. Cause, consequence and the methods to combat the process of aging.

Chapter 2

What Is Aging?

Aging Theories

The process of aging or senescence is complex; it may derive from a variety of different mechanisms and is caused by a variety of different factors. There are many theories trying to explain the aging process, each from its own point of view. Traditionally, theories explaining senescence have generally been divided into programmed and stochastic theories of aging. Two principal theories of aging have been developed (Gilca et al., 2007): theories of "accidental" aging produced by "errors" represented by random deleterious mechanisms that induce progressive damage of various levels; and theories of "programmed" aging induced by a collection of by-products of gene action selected to enhance reproductive fitness (Beckman and Ames, 1998). The wear-and-tear theories describe aging as an accumulation of damage and garbage that eventually overwhelms our ability to function.The programmed theories propose a clock in our bodies that controls not only our process of development but also triggers our self-destruction.Even if there are no genes that specifically evolved to induce senescence, scientists estimated that allelic variation or mutation at up to 7,000 relevant genes might modulate patterns of aging man (Martin, 1987). Certain polymorphisms (antagonistic pleiotropy) might underline common or "public" mechanisms of aging, while rare mutations lead to uncommon or "private" mechanisms of aging (Corder et al., 1993; Sherrington et al., 1995). These theories of aging are not mutually exclusive, especially, when oxidative stress is considered (Gilca et al., 2007).

Since extensive research on the relation between polymorphisms likely to be responsible for the common mechanisms of aging and resistance to the oxidative stress has been neglected in almost all scientific studies, the paucity of data does not allow us to conclude yet that the oxidative theory supports the theory of programmed aging (Gilca et al., 2007). However, the most recent studies support the idea that oxidative stress is a significant marker of senescence being established in different species. Resistance to oxidative stress is a common trait of long-lived genetic variations of non-mammalian and mammalian organisms (Martin et al., 1996; Mooijaart et al., 2004). In recent years, accumulating evidence strongly suggests that oxidative stress underlies aging processes.Denham Harman first proposed the free radical theory of aging in the 1950s, and in the 1970s, extended the idea to implicate mitochondrial production of reactive oxygen species(Harman, 1972). According to the free radical theory of aging (Harman, 1956; Harman, 1972; Beckman and Ames, 1998), enhanced and unopposed metabolism-driven oxidative stress plays a major role in diverse chronic age-related diseases. The free-radical theory of aging states that organisms age because cells accumulate free radical damage over time. The notion that free radical destruction of macromolecules is a basis of aging and age-related diseases has considerable experimental support (Reiter, 1995). It was subsequently discovered that reactiveoxygen species (ROS), some of which are not free radicals becausethey do not have an unpaired electron in their outer shells,contribute to the accumulation of oxidative damage to cellularconstituents. Consistent with free radical theory of aging (Harman, 1956), aged mammals contain high quantities of oxidized lipids and proteins as well as damaged/mutated DNA, particularly the mitochondrial genome. In support of a mitochondrial theory of aging, evidencesuggests that mitochondrial DNA damage increases with aging(Hagen et al., 2004; Hamilton et al., 2001). Thus, a more modern version of this tenet is the"oxidative stress theory" of aging, which holds that increasesin ROS accompany aging and lead to functional alterations, pathologicalconditions, and even death (Hagen, 2003).

It was observed that oxygen consumption, mitochondrial ATP production and free-radical production are linked processes (Sohal, 2002), since energy metabolism is one major determinant of endogenous oxidative stress. As already mentioned, in 1956, Harman first proposed that normal aging results from random deleterious damage to tissues by free radicals (Hartman, 1956) and then focused on mitochondria as generators of free radicals (Hartman, 1972). Halliwell and Gutteridge later suggested to rename this free radical theory of aging as the "oxidative damage theory of aging" (Halliwell and Gutteridge, 2007), since aging and diseases are caused not only by free radicals, but also by other reactive oxygen and nitrogen species. "Oxidative mitochondrial decay is a major contributor to aging," according to Ames (2004). Increases in mitochondrial energy production at the cellular level might have beneficial and/or deleterious effects. Increased regeneration of reducing agents (NADH, NADPH and $FADH_2$) and ATP can improve the recycling of antioxidants and assist the antioxidant defense system. On the other hand, enhanced mitochondrial function could increase the production of superoxide free radicals, thereby aggravating oxidative stress and further burdening the antioxidant defense system.

Mitochondrial Theory of Aging

The theory that links oxygen consumption, metabolism, ATP and ROS formation is the mitochondrial theory of aging, which hypothesizesthat mitochondria are the critical component in the control of aging. The number of mitochondria in a cell is determined by the cell's specific function and energy needs. Cells such as heart muscle cells have many mitochondria. Heart cells, for example, have thousands of mitochondria, while skin cells have only one mitochondria each. According to the mitochondrial theory of aging, the accumulation of damage to mitochondrial components should affect mitochondrial functions.An accumulation of damage decreases the cell's ability to generate ATP, so that cells, tissues, and individuals function less well. There is now considerable evidence that mitochondria are altered in the tissues of aging individuals and that the damage to mitochondrial DNA (mtDNA) increases 1,000-fold with age.

The phagocytic lysosome system for removing mitochondria is also considerably altered in the cells of aging organisms. Thus, damaged mitochondria play an important role in apoptosis and aging. The theory expands on the idea that the mitochondria are the major source of toxic oxidants, which have the potential of reacting with and destroying cell constituents and which accumulate with age. The result of this destructive activity is an inefficient cell and a body that more readily displays signs of age (e.g., wrinkled skin, cells that produce low energy level). The mutation rate of mitochondrial DNA is ten-times higher than that of nuclear DNA. However, the role of the mitochondria in skin aging has not been significantly investigated. The study of Yang et al. (1994) investigated a specific deletion of mitochondrial DNA in human aging skin. The study revealed thatnone of the individuals below the age of 60 years were found to bear specific type of mtDNA deletion. The incidence of deletions increased with advancing age (time trend), and the incidence was significantly higher in UVR-exposed skin than in non-exposed skin (Yang et al., 1994). This indicated an additional exogenous source of ROS thatsignificantly affects skin aging. A similar study was done by Greco et al. (2003). Human dermal fibroblasts from 51 donors aged 1 to 103 showed a clear reduction in mitochondrial processes with age (protein synthesis, respiration rate and coupling to respiration for ATP production). In the skin cells, particularly from donors over the age of 40, metabolic functions decline as a function of age (Hourigan, 2010).

Mitochondrial DNA (mtDNA) is a naked double-stranded circular genetic element continuously exposed to the matrix that contains great amounts of ROS. Moreover, mtDNA is replicated much faster than nuclear DNA lacking proofreading and efficient DNA repair mechanisms (Yang et al., 1994). This is important for UVradiation-induced skin damage, which can directly penetrate the skin and damage DNA but cannot be efficiently repaired. Thus, mtDNA is vulnerable to attack by various ROS and free radicals. Mitochondria are vulnerable to oxidative stress, and damaged mitochondria can cause an energy crisis in the cell, leading to senescence and tissue aging. An accumulation of damage decreases the cell's ability to generate ATP, so that cells, tissues, and individuals function less well. The gradual loss of energy experienced with age is paralleled by a decrease in the ratio of mitochondria per cell, as well as the health and energy-producing efficiency of the remaining mitochondria. The mitochondrial damage theory has been recently reviewed by Wilkes and Rennie (2009). Age-related functional deficits have been observed in some, but not all, studies of aging mitochondria, lending support to the mitochondrial damage theory. Given that mitochondrial DNA exists in the inner matrix and this is in close proximity to the inner membrane where electrons can form unstable compounds, mitochondria DNA has a relatively high chance of getting damaged by unstable compounds. This damage is hypothesized to play a critical role in the aging process according to the mitochondrial theory of aging. For example, muscle mitochondrial oxidative enzymes are diminished with time, resulting in a reduction in fatty acid oxidation (Rasmussen et al., 2003) and ATP production (Trounce et al., 1989; Petersen et al., 2003).

A major effect of mitochondrial dysfunction is said to be an appropriately high generation of ROS and proton leakage, resulting in a diminution of ATP production in relation to electron input from mitochondrial metabolism. Leaked ROS and protons cause damage to a wide range of macromolecules, including enzymes, nucleic acids and membrane lipids within and beyond mitochondria, and thus are consistent also with the inflammation theory of aging as being proximal events triggering the production of pro-inflammatorycytokines. The age-related increases in the levels of both oxidative damage and mutational load of mtDNA predicted by the mitochondrial theory of aging have beendescribed in multiple species and organ systems (Golden et al., 2006). However, whether this damage affects mitochondrial function or significantly modulates the physiology of aging has remained controversial (Jacobs, 2003; Pak et al., 2003). As already mentioned, free radicals can damage the mitochondrial inner membrane, creating a positive feedback-loop for increased free-radical creation. Induction of ROS generates mtDNA mutations, in turn leading to a defective respiratory chain. Defective respiratory chain generates even more ROS and generates a vicious cycle. This vicious cycle creates even more damage to mtDNA. Mitochondria develop a peculiar type of mutation called the common deletion, in which a particular 477 base pair section of DNA is deleted. This increase in the common deletion up to levels of 32-fold (Berneburg et al., 2004), independent of the inducing agent (e.g., UVR), may represent the first evidence for the presence of such vicious cycle in general and in human skin in particular.

The frequency of the common deletion in the mitochondria of human skin cells does not correlate with chronological age, but rather with sun exposure and photoaging (Berneburg et al., 2004). Additionally, Berneburg et al. (2005) reported that creatine supplementation normalizes mutagenesis of mitochondrial DNA as well as functional consequences. The observations that induction of the common deletion in human skin fibroblasts is paralleled by a measurable decrease of oxygen consumption, mitochondrial membrane potential, and ATP content, as well as an increase in MMP-1, suggest on the link not only between mtDNA and cellular energy metabolism but also between mtDNA mutagenesis, energy metabolism, and a fibroblast gene expression profile which correlate with the premature skin aging (Krutmann, 2010).

On the other hand, the "vicious cycle" theory, which states that free radical damage to mitochondrial DNA leads to mitochondria that produce more superoxide, has been questioned by some scientists since the most damaged mitochondria are degraded by fagocytosis, whereas the more defective mitochondria (which produce less ATP as well as less superoxide) remain to reproduce themselves (de Grey, 2005). But the efficiency of lysosomes to consume malfunctioning mitochondria also declines with age, resulting in more mitochondria producing higher levels of superoxide. Mitochondria of older organisms are fewer in number, larger in size and less efficient (produce less energy and more superoxide).

It is proposed that electrons leaking from the electron transportchain (ETC) produce ROS and that these molecules can then damageETC components and mitochondrial DNA, leading to further increasesin intracellular ROS levels and a decline in mitochondrial function(Wallace, 2005).

Free radicals could also be involved in signaling responses, which subsequentlystimulate pathways related to cell senescence and death, and in pro-inflammatory gene expression. This inflammatory cascade is exaggeratedduring aging and has been linked with much age-associated pathologies,such as cancer, various cardiovascular diseases, arthritis,and several neurodegenerative diseases (Chung et al., 2006).

In recent years, oxidative stress has been implicated in a wide variety of degenerative processes, diseases and syndromes, including the following: mutagenesis, cell transformation and cancer; atherosclerosis, arteriosclerosis, heart attacks, strokes and ischemia/reperfusion injury; chronic inflammatory diseases, such as rheumatoid arthritis, lupus erythematosus and psoriatic arthritis; acute inflammatory problems, such as wound healing; photooxidative stresses to the eye, such as cataract; central-nervous-system disorders, such as certain forms of familial amyotrophic lateral sclerosis, certain glutathione peroxidase-linked adolescent seizures, Parkinson's disease and Alzheimer's dementia; and a wide variety of age-related disorders, perhaps even including factors underlying the aging process itself (Davies, 2005).

One of the central themes of the oxidative stress hypothesisis that ROS represent the primary causal factor underlying aging-associateddeclines in physiological function. Several lines of directand indirect evidence generated over the past two decades havedemonstrated a positive relationship between increased *in vivo*oxidative stress and biological aging. While the majority ofthese correlative studies have supported the oxidativestress hypothesis of aging, one controversial aspect of thehypothesis has been the lack of data clearly demonstrating acause-and-effect relationship between the accumulation of oxidation-mediatedcellular damage and aging (Kregel and Zhang, 2007).

Nevertheless, it was demonstrated that normal metabolism is associated with unavoidable mild oxidative stress (for more information on the oxidative stress, see next chapter), resulting in biomolecular damage that cannot be totally repaired or removed by cellular degradative systems, including lysosomes, proteasomes, and cytosolic and mitochondrial proteases.

Oxidative stress, being merely a biochemical process, generally does not exhibit any specific clinical symptoms or clinical signs at the beginning. Therefore, it is not diagnosed until unavoidable damage to the patient occurs and the consequences manifest as a sign of a disease thatcould last for decades (Figure 2).

Under normal aerobic conditions, approximately 1% to 4% of the oxygen metabolized by mitochondria is converted to the superoxide ion that can be converted subsequently to hydrogen peroxide, hydroxyl radical and eventually other reactive species, including other peroxides and singlet oxygen, which can, in turn, generate free radicals capable of damaging structural proteins and DNA (Figure 3).

Certain metal ions found in the body, such as copper and iron, may participate in the process of free radical formation. Apart from the free radical theory, aging is explained by many other theories (see the table below).

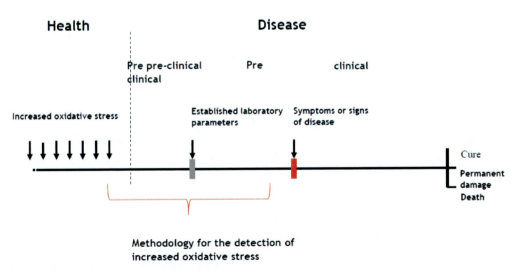

Figure 2. Recognition of the risk of diseases in the "pre-preclinical" stage should be aimed in order to implement relevant therapies, to predict disease complications and, hence, to reduce healthcare costs and to maintain the quality of life.

**Table 2. Human diseases most frequently associated
(as a cause or consequence) with the oxidative stress**

Clinical conditions associated with the oxidative stress	
Alzheimer's disease (dementia)	*Heart Failure*
Arthritis	*Arterial hypertension*
Atherosclerosis	*Chronic Inflammatory Bowel Disease*
Cancer	*Macular degeneration*
Cataract	*Multiple Sclerosis*
Chronic Obstructive Pulmonary Disease	*Parkinson's disease*
Diabetes	*Reperfusion injuries*
Coronary artery disease	*Others*

Theories of aging have become significantly more important because of discoveries that indicate that aging is not universal or inevitable and that, therefore, suggest that major medical intervention in aging is possible. Disciplines ranging from physiology and geneticsto epidemiology and demography have developed a large numberof theories that attempt to explain why we age (Medvedev, 1990), although definitivemechanisms to explain the process across species remain equivocal.

Detailed descriptions of different theories of aging are beyond the scope of this chapter. Brief descriptions of other aging theories arefound below (Wikipedia.org):

Telomere Theory

Telomeres (structures at the ends of chromosomes) have experimentally been shown to shorten with each successive cell division. Shortened telomeres activate a mechanism that prevents further cell multiplication. This may be an important mechanism of aging in certain tissues. Cellular senescence is the phenomenon by which normal diploid cells lose the ability to divide, normally after about 50 cell divisions *in vitro*. This phenomenon is also known as "replicative senescence," the "Hayflick phenomenon" or the Hayflick limit, in honor of Dr. Leonard Hayflick, who was the first to publish this information in 1965. Telomere shortening hypothesis says nothing about the aging of nondividing cells, such as neurons and muscle, and cannot explain the aging process in all the cells of any single organism. Nevertheless, telomere shortening is important for skin-aging process, and further discussion on the role of telomeres can be found in the chapter entitled,"The role of telomeres in skin aging."

Reproductive-Cell Cycle Theory

The idea that aging is regulated by reproductive hormones that act in an antagonistic pleiotropic manner via cell cycle signaling, promoting growth and development early in life in order to achieve reproduction, but that later in life, in a futile attempt to maintain reproduction, become dysregulated and drive senescence (dyosis).

Wear-and-Tear Theory

The very general idea that changes associated with aging are the result of chance damage that accumulates over time.

Somatic Mutation Theory

The biological theory that aging results from damage to the genetic integrity of the body's cells.

Error Accumulation Theory

The idea that aging results from chance events that escape proofreading mechanisms, which gradually damage the genetic code.

Evolutionary Theories

These are by far the most theoretical; however, their usefulness is somewhat limited as they do not provide readily testable biochemically based interventions.

Accumulative-Waste Theory

The biological theory of aging that points to a build-up of cell waste products that presumably interferes with metabolism.

Garbage Catastrophe Theory of Aging

Increasing evidence suggests an important role of oxidant-induced damage in the progress of senescent changes, providing support for the free radical theory of aging proposed by Harman in 1956. However, considering that biological organisms continuously renew their structures, it is not clear why oxidative damage should accumulate with age (at least in normal diploid cells, which still divide). The author of the theory (Terman, 2001) believes that the process of aging may derive from imperfect clearance of oxidatively damaged, relatively indigestible material, the accumulation of which further hinders cellular catabolic and anabolic functions. From this perspective, it might be predicted that: (i) suppression of oxidative damage would enhance longevity; (ii) accumulation of incompletely digested material (e.g., lipofuscin pigment) would interfere with cellular functions and increase probability of death; (iii) rejuvenation during reproduction is mainly provided by dilution of undigested material associated with intensive growth of the developing organism; and (iv) age-related damage starts to accumulate substantially when development is complete and mainly affects post-mitotic cells and extracellular matrix, not proliferating cells.

Mitochondria and lysosomes of post-mitotic cells suffer the most remarkable age-related alterations of all cellular organelles. Many mitochondria undergo enlargement and structural disorganization, while lysosomes, which are normally responsible for mitochondrial turnover, gradually accumulate an undegradable, polymeric, autofluorescent material called lipofuscin, or age pigment. These changes occur not only due to continuous oxidative stress (causing oxidation of mitochondrial constituents and autophagocytosed material), but also because of the inherent inability of cells to completely remove oxidatively damaged structures (biological "garbage") (Brunk and Terman, 2002). Interrelated mitochondrial and lysosomal damage irreversibly leads to functional decay and death of post-mitotic cells.

Autoimmune Theory

The idea that aging results from an increase in auto-antibodies that attack the body's tissues. A number of diseases associated with aging, such as atrophic gastritis and Hashimoto's thyroiditis, are probably autoimmune in this way. While inflammation is very much evident in old mammals, even SCID mice (mice that lack both T and B lymphocytes) in specific pathogen-free colonies still undergo senescence.

Aging-Clock Theory

The theory that aging results from a pre-programmed sequence, as in a clock, built into the operation of the nervous or endocrine system of the body. In rapidly dividing cells, the shortening of the telomeres would provide such a clock. This idea is in direct contradiction with the evolutionary-based theory of aging.

Cross-Linkage Theory

The idea that aging results from the accumulation of cross-linked compounds that interfere with normal cell function.

Reliability Theory of Aging and Longevity

A general theory about systems failure. It allows researchers to predict the age-related failure kinetics for a system of a given architecture (reliability structure) and given reliability of its components. Reliability theory predicts that even those systems that are entirely composed of non-aging elements (with a constant failure rate) will nevertheless deteriorate (fail more often) with age if these systems are redundant in irreplaceable elements. Aging, therefore, is a direct consequence of system redundancy.

Mitohormesis

It has been known since the 1930s that restricting calories while maintaining adequate amounts of other nutrients can extend lifespan in laboratory animals. Michael Ristow's group has provided evidence for the theory that this effect is due to increased formation of free radicals within the mitochondria causing a secondary induction of increased antioxidant defense capacity(Schulz et al., 2007).

Disengagement Theory

This is the idea that separation of older people from active roles in society can have an aging effect.

Activity Theory

This theory implies that the more active elderly people are, the more likely they are to be satisfied with life and the higher will be their metabolism and ambition.

Misrepair-Accumulation Theory and Others

Many of the theories overlap, e.g., ROS can cause DNAdamage (free radical theory) and also accelerate telomere shortening (telomere theory), since telomere loss is mostly due to the effect of oxidative stress. Another example is telomere shortening accelerated by oxidative stress in vascular endothelial cells (Kurz et al., 2004). Additionally, systemic inflammatory responses can influence metabolic hormones, some of which regulate telomere activity (Bayne and Liu, 2005). None of the theories entirely explains the aging process, which I believe is too complex to be covered by only one theory. According to Arking (2006), there is no reason to expect that there is only one biological mechanism responsible for aging in all of the different species and kingdoms of living organisms. We should not forget that the main problem this book is dealing with is the explanation of the correlation between aging and oxidative stress, which is caused mainly due to oxygen metabolism. On the other hand, there are anaerobic organisms, which were the first organisms on our planet, and they still live in regions where oxygen is not present. And yet, they also age and finally die. The aging process of anaerobes is a bit different from the one of aerobic organisms and will not be further dealt with in this book. For further reading on the biology of aging, see the excellent book by Arking (2006).Different aging theories could be used to explain to a certain extent the aging process of our skin. Several biological skin-aging mechanisms have been proposed, like photoaging, oxidative stress-induced damage, telomere shortening, neurological and physical stress, hormonal interactions, etc. All of them will be discussed later in the following chapters. Most probably, each mechanism plays its role in skin aging,and the entire mechanism acts in a synergistic way to contribute to the final unattractive features of our skin, such as wrinkling, uneven pigmentation and sagging. Currently, each mechanism is under intense research and untilnow the contribution of each mechanism to skin aging has been hard to predict.

Part II. The Cause: Free radicals, Reactive Oxygen Species (ROS) and Oxidative Stress

Chapter 3

The Role of Oxidative Stress on the General Aging Process

No matter where we live or how careful we are, we can't avoid endogenous free radical formation due to the normal metabolism and exposure to environmental toxins—oxidants. They are in the air we breathe, the food we eat and the water we drink all over the planet. Free radical reactions have been implicated in the action of many environmental pollutants. Free radicals are unstable chemicals produced when our cells create energy from food and oxygen and when we are exposed to pollutants or toxins such as cigarette smoke, alcohol, ionizing and UVradiation, pesticides, ozone, etc. The most important endogenous sources of oxidant agents in aging are mitochondrial—electron transport chain, nitric oxide synthase reaction— and non-mitochondrial—Fenton reaction, microsomal cytochrome P450 enzymes, peroxisomal beta-oxidation and respiratory burst of phagocytic cells (Gilca et al., 2007). Free radicals help our bodies to generate energy and fight infections, but when we have too many free radicals, they attack healthy cells causing them to age prematurely. Free radical damage (or oxidation) has been linked to the formation of every degenerative disease known, including cancer, cardiovascular disease, cataracts and the aging process itself. Oxidative stress is the term referring to the imbalance between generating of reactive oxygen species (ROS) and the activity of the antioxidant defense (Halliwell and Gutterigde, 1999). Oxidative stress in a physiologicalsetting can be defined as an excessive bioavailability of ROS,which is the net result of an imbalance between production anddestruction of ROS (with the latter being influenced by antioxidantdefenses). ROS are, due to their high reactivity, prone to cause damage and are thereby also potentially toxic, mutagenic and carcinogenic (Nordberg and Arner, 2001). Oxidative stress is the direct consequence of an increased generation of free radicals and/or reduced physiological activity of antioxidant defenses against free radicals. All forms of life maintain a reducing environment within their cells. This reducing environment is preserved by enzymes that maintain the reduced state through a constant input of metabolic energy. Disturbances in this normal redox state can cause toxic effects through the production of peroxides and free radicals that damage all components of the cell. Severe oxidative stress can cause cell damage and death. Oxidative stress is proportional to the concentration of free radicals, which depends on both processes (formation and quenching). The degree of oxidative stress experienced by a cell will be a function of the activity of free radical generating reactions on the one hand and the activity of the free radical scavenging system on the other (Tijskens Pol, personal communication). Human skin is naked and is constantly directly exposed to the air, solar radiation, other environmental pollutants or other mechanical and chemical insults, which are capable of inducing the generation of free radicals as well as ROS of our own metabolism. According to Dr. Mauro Carratelli, "Free radicals are only a part of all the chemical species responsible of oxidative stress. Oxidative stress is induced by other agents. indeed, like hydrogen peroxide or hypochlorous acid, which are not free radicals. Therefore all chemical species—radical and not radical species—which are responsible of oxidative stress have been grouped in a unique large family of 'reactive' or oxidant chemical species." Reactive oxygen species are formed and degraded by all aerobic organisms, leading to either physiological concentrations required for normal cell function or excessive quantities that result in a state of oxidative stress. Oxidative stress is also thought to be involved in the process of aging, by inducing damage to mitochondrial DNA and through other mechanisms (Nordberg and Arner, 2001). At the cellular level, oxidative stress generated by ROS andROS-modified molecules can influence a wide range of cellularfunctions. The direct consequence of oxidative stress is damageto various intracellular constituents (Figure 3). For example, when lipidperoxidation occurs, changes in cellular membrane permeabilityand even membrane leakage may occur (Shafer, 2000). Oxidativedamage to both nuclear and mitochondrial DNA has detrimentaleffects, leading to uncontrolled cell proliferation or acceleratedcell death (Evans et al., 2004). As would be expected, protein oxidation hasmany important physiological consequences that affect normalcellular functions (Lopez et al., 2002). There is evidence that oxidative stress-mediatedprotein aggregation may be the primary cause of neuronaldeath in several forms of aging-related neurodegenerative diseases(Goswami, 2006). Furthermore, redox modification of transcriptional factors,as discussed in the further sections, leads to the activationor inactivation of signaling pathways, which will subsequentlyproduce changes in gene expression profiles (Martindale et al., 2002), includingthose affecting cellular proliferation, differentiation, senescenceand death (Kregel and Zhang, 2007).

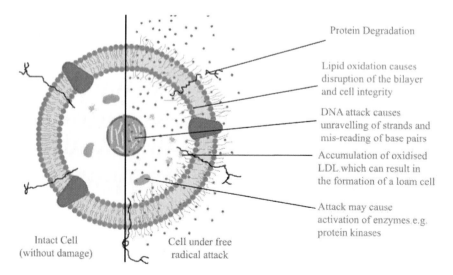

Figure 3. Simplified overview of free radical attack on cellular macromolecules (source: http://ourworld.compuserve.com/homepages/randox).

Although the skin possesses an elaborate antioxidant defense system to deal with UV-induced oxidative stress and immunotoxicity, excessive and chronic exposure to UV light or cigarette smoke can overwhelm the cutaneous antioxidant and immune response capacity, leading to oxidative damage and immunotoxicity, premature skin aging, and skin cancer.

ROS and Free Radicals

A free radical is a chemical species possessing an unpaired electron (Cheeseman and Slater, 1993). It can also be considered a fragment of a molecule. As such, free radicals can be formed in three ways: (1) homolytic cleavage of a covalent bond of a normal molecule, with each fragment retaining one of the paired electrons; (2) loss of a single electron from a normal molecule; and (3) addition of a single electron to a normal molecule. The addition of an electron, involving electron transfer, is far more common in biological systems (Cheeseman and Slater, 1993) than homolytic fission, which generally requires a high-energyinput. A free radical can be either positively or negatively charged or electrically neutral.

Beneficial Role of ROS

Oxidant agents, including reactive oxygen species (ROS), and reactive nitrogen species (RNS) are recognized to play a dual role as both malefic and beneficial species, being sometimes compared with fire, which is dangerous, but nonetheless useful to humans (de Magalhaes and Church, 2006). ROS along with reactive nitrogen species (RNS) are well recognized for playing a dual role as both deleterious and beneficial species. The "two-faced" character of ROS is substantiated by growing body of evidence that ROS within cells act as secondary messengers in intracellular signaling cascades, which induce and maintain the oncogenic phenotype of cancer cells; however, ROS can also induce cellular senescence and apoptosis and can, therefore, function as anti-tumorigenic species. ROS and RNS have many crucial biological functions as signaling molecules of growth, apoptosis, neurotransmission, etc. The beneficial physiological cellular use of ROS is now being demonstrated in different areas, including intracellular signaling and redox regulation. For several transcription factors, ROS function as physiological mediators of transcription control (Nordberg and Arner, 2001). Nitric oxide was identified as a signaling molecule as early as 1987 (Palmer et al., 1987), and is now well known as a regulator of transcription factor activities and other determinants of gene expression. Hydrogen peroxide and superoxide have similar intracellular effects (Kimata and Hirata, 1999). ROS can directly affect conformation and/or activities of all sulfhydryl-containing molecules, such as proteins or GSH, by oxidation of their thiol moiety. Among many other enzymes and membrane receptors, this type of redox regulation affects many proteins important in signal transduction and carcinogenesis, such as protein kinase C, Ca^{2+}-ATPase, collagenase, and tyrosine kinase (Dalton et al., 1999). Well-known examples of redox-sensitive transcription factors are nuclear factor-kB (NF-kB) and activator protein-1 (AP-1). By selective dimerization of AP-1 family members (Jun/Jun or Fos/Jun partners) and diverse binding specificities with the promoter regions of genes, the AP-1 transcription factor regulates gene expression important in cell injury, repair, proliferation, and differentiation.

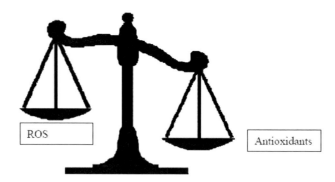

Table 3. Balance between free radical formation and antioxidative protection

FREE RADICAL STATUS	PROTECTIVE SYSTEM
Free radical generation Free radical damage	• Free radical protection (antioxidants, scavenging enzymes, metal chelators) • Damage repair • Elimination of damage (DNA base excision, elimination of damaged proteins, etc.)

Thus, increased antioxidative protection might not be always beneficial for the cell, besides an increase in cellular reducents might impact redox regulation and signal transduction. To control these reactive species with "two faces," cells evolved complex and critical regulatory mechanisms which become disrupted with age (Gilca et al., 2007). Senescence is just one example of pathophysiological implications of redox dysregulations (Valkoet al., 2007). The initiation of aging is marked by a shift from redox regulation to redox dysregulation (Humphries et al, 2006). Why this shift takes place is yet not clear.

The (im) Balance between ROS Production and Antioxidative Defense

A number of factors influence the antioxidant defense systems in our bodies. Metabolic processes that produce antioxidants are controlled and influenced by an individual's genetic make-up and environmental factors (such as diet, smoking and pollution) to which the body is exposed. Unfortunately, modern lifestyles, which include high environmental pollution, stress, poor quality foods and unbalanced diets, result in greater exposure to free radicals.

Causes of increased free-radical production include:

- endogenous
  - inflammation
  - increased respiration
  - elevation in O_2 concentration
  - increased mitochondrial leakage
  - others
- exogenous

- environment (pollution, pesticides, radiation, etc.)
- lifestyle
- strenuous excercise
- smoking
- nutrition (processed food, food additives, etc.)
- diseases and chronic illnesses
- chronic inflammation
- psychological and emotional stress
- others

Causes of decreased antioxidant defense:

- reduced activity of endogenous antioxidative enzymes
- reduced biokinetics of antioxidant metabolism
- reduced intake of antioxidants from food
- reduced bioabsorbtion of antioxidants from food
- others

Risk factors for increased oxidative stress include age, physiological status (pregnancy, lactation, menopause), overweight/obesity, abnormal caloric intake, mineral and vitamin deficiency in the diet, alcohol abuse, cigarette smoke, inadequate exercise, psycho-emotional stress, significant exposure to UV radiation, significant exposure to electromagnetic radiation, significant exposure to environmental pollutants, current intake of estrogen-progesterone combination (especially as a contraceptive pill), current chemotherapy, current radiotherapy, current dialysis, current cortisone treatments, and so on.

Oxidative stress is caused mainly by:

- mutation or reduced activity of enzymes (catalase, SOD, glutathione peroxidase)
- decreased intake of exogenous antioxidants from food
- increased intake of dietary compounds prone to increase initiation rates:
  - increased metal ion intake (e.g., Fe, Cu, Cr)
  - polyunsaturated lipids
  - easiliy peroxidized amino acids (e.g., lysine)
- increased $^3O_2$ concentration
- increased physical activity of an untrained individual
- psychical stress
- ROS from the environment (ionizing radiation, air pollution, smoking) chronic inflammation

The imposed oxidative damage potential is opposed by the antioxidant defense capacity of the system. The opposed processes should be in dynamic equilibrium with each other. Excess generation of free radicals may overwhelm natural cellular antioxidant defenses, leading to oxidation and further cellular functional impairment. In reality, the oxidative damage potential is greater, and thus there is a constant small amount of toxic free radical formation, which escapes the defense of the cell. A certain amount of oxidized proteins and nucleic acids exists at all times in cells, which reflects the occurrence of oxidative events.

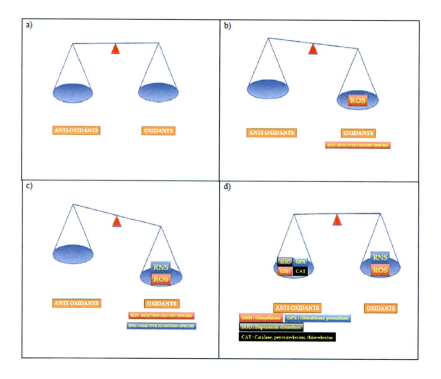

Figure 4. With age, the production of free radicals increases, while the endogenous defense mechanisms decrease. This imbalance leads to the progressive damage of cellular structures, presumably resulting in the aging phenotype. a) balance between antioxidants and ROS; b) increased oxidative stress due to ROS formation; c) increased oxidative stress due to ROS and RNS formation; d) enzymatic and non-enzymatic antioxidants can neutralize ROS and RNS and decrease oxidative stress and restore the balance.

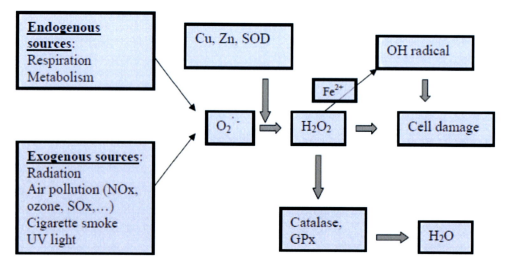

Figure 5. Cellular generation of reactive oxygen species and antioxidant defense system.

Table 4. The major ROS molecules and their metabolism (Nordberg and Arner, 2001)

ROS molecule	Main source	Enzymatic defense system	Products
Superoxide O_2^-	-Leakage of electrons from electron transport chain -Activated phagocytes -Xanthine oxidase -Flavoenzymes	Superoxide dismutase (SOD) Superoxide reductase (in some bacteria)	$H_2O_2 + O_2$ H_2O_2
Hydrogen peroxide (H_2O_2)	From O_2^- via SOD NADPH-oxidase (neutrophils)	Glutathione peroxidase Catalases	H_2O_2 + GSSG $H_2O + O_2$
Hydroxyl radical	From O_2^- and H_2O_2 via transition metals (Fe, Cu and Cr)		
Nitric oxide (NO)	Nitric oxide syntheses	Glutathione/TrxR	GSNO

The amount of oxidized macromolecules in the cell could thus be the sum of the rate of the formation less the rate of repair processes. When estimating oxidative stress according to Tijskens (personal communication), "The rate with which antioxidants scavenge free radicals has almost no effect on remaining damage (no repair). But the level of antioxidants has a marked effect. That would mean that intake of many antioxidants has a severe effect, but that the electronic strength of the antioxidants has almost no effect."

Table 4 lists the most common intracellular forms of ROS, together with their main cellular sources of production, as well as the relevant enzymatic antioxidant systems scavenging these ROS molecules.

$$O_2 + e^- \rightarrow O_2^{\bullet-} \qquad \text{superoxide anion} \qquad (1)$$

$$O_2^{\bullet-} + e^- + 2H^+ \rightarrow H_2O_2 \qquad \text{hydrogen peroxide} \qquad (2)$$

$$H_2O_2 + e^- + H^+ \rightarrow H_2O + OH^{\bullet} \qquad \text{hydroxyl radical} \qquad (3)$$

$$OH^{\bullet} + e^- + H^+ \rightarrow H_2O \qquad \text{water} \qquad (4)$$

Sum:

$$O_2 + 4e^- + 4H^+ \rightarrow 2H_2O \qquad (5)$$

Scheme 1. The step-wise reduction of molecular oxygen via one electron transfer, producing and also connecting the ROS molecules listed in Table 4.

The three major forms of ROS in terms of pathways of formation and their cellular effects will now be discussed briefly.

Major Forms of ROS in Biological Systems

With the exception of unusual circumstances, such as the influence of ionizing radiation, free radicals are generally produced in cells by electron transfer reactions. These can be mediated by the action of enzymes, or non-enzymatically, often through redox chemistry of metal ions (Halliwell and Gutteridge, 1999). Free-radical production in cells can be either accidental or deliberate (Halliwell and Gutteridge, 1999).

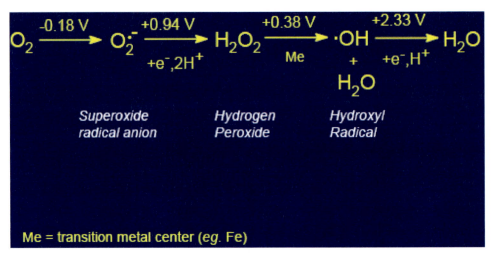

Figure 6. Oxygen, free radicals and reactive oxygen species formation (figure from Rafael Radi: Formation and Properties of Reactive Oxygen and Nitrogen Species, Techniques in Free Radical Biology, FEBS Practical Course, Debrecen, Hungary, 2010).

Superoxide ($O_2^{\cdot -}$)

The superoxide anion created from molecular oxygen by the addition of an electron is, in spite of being a free radical, not highly reactive. It lacks the ability to penetrate lipid membranes and is, therefore, enclosed in the compartment where it was produced. The formation of superoxide takes place spontaneously, especially in the electron-rich aerobic environment in the vicinity of the inner mitochondrial membrane with the respiratory chain (Nordberg and Arner, 2001). Two molecules of superoxide rapidly dismutate to hydrogen peroxide and molecular oxygen, and this reaction is further accelerated by superoxide dismutase (SOD). Superoxide can act either as an oxidizing or reducing agent; it can oxidize sulphur, ascorbic acid or NADPH, and can reduce cytochrome C and metal ions. Under physiological conditions, the daily yield of $O_2^{\cdot -}$ may reach 3×10^7 per mitochondrion, although its scavenging ability by Mn-SOD and other enzymes brings it to a steady-state *in vivo* concentration of 10 pmol/l (Sigler, 1999). This, in turn, results in the generation of an estimated 10,000 DNA lesions per genome per day (Shackelford, 1999). $O_2^{\cdot -}$ has been shown to inhibit antioxidant enzymes, such as glutathione peroxidase, and partially catalase (Sigler, 1999).

Hydrogen Peroxide (H₂O₂)

H₂O₂ is not a free radical, but it is nonetheless highly important because of its ability to penetrate biological membranes. It plays a radical-forming role as an intermediate in the production of more reactive ROS molecules (Nordberg and Arner, 2001), most importantly, in the formation of OH˙ via oxidation of transition metals.

$$H_2O_2 + Cr(V)/Fe(II)/Cu(I) \rightarrow OH^\cdot + OH^- + Cr(VI)/Fe(III)/Cu(II)$$

Another important function of H₂O₂ is that of an intracellular signaling molecule (Rhee, 1999). Numerous enzymes (peroxidases) use hydrogen peroxide as a substrate in oxidation reactions involving the synthesis of complex organic molecules. H₂O₂ is noteworthy because it readily permeates membranes and is, therefore, not compartmentalized in the cell (Halliwell and Gutteridge, 1999). Once H₂O₂ is produced by the above-mentioned mechanisms, it is removed by at least three antioxidant enzyme systems: catalases, glutathione peroxidases, and peroxiredoxins (Nordberg and Arner, 2001).

The reactivity of H₂O₂ is not due to its inherent activity per se, but requires the presence of a metal reductant to form a highly reactive hydroxyl radical, which is the strongest oxidizing agent known and reacts with organic molecules at diffusion-limited rates (Halliwell and Gutteridge, 1984).

At natural or acidic pH, hydrogen peroxide exists predominantly as fully protonated H₂O₂. Therefore, its molecule carries no charge and can freely penetrate membranes and diffuse throughout the cell. This long-range action is increased by its ability to form adducts with various cell constituents. In cells under physiological conditions, H2O2 levels are maintained at a low level (1 to 100 nmol/l) through the action of catalase and glutathione peroxidase (Sigler, 1999).

Hydroxyl Radical (OH˙)

Due to its strong reactivity with biomolecules, OH˙ is probably capable of doing more damage to biological systems than any other ROS (Halliwell, 1987). The radical is formed from H₂O₂ in a reaction catalyzed by metal ions (e.g., Cr(V), Fe(II)), often found in complexes with different proteins or other molecules (Nordberg and Arner, 2001). This is known as the Fenton reaction:

$$Metal^{(n)} + H_2O_2 \rightarrow Metal^{(n+1)} + HO^\cdot + HO^-$$
(Fenton reaction) (6)

$$H_2O_2 + {}^\cdot O_2^- \xrightarrow{Metal^{(n-1)}} O_2 + HO^\cdot + HO^-$$
(Haber-Weiss reaction) (7)

Superoxide, ascorbic acid and α-tocopherol also play an important role as reducing agents in Reaction 6 in which the metal ions are recycled. The Reaction 7 is the Haber-Weiss reaction, which supports the notion that transition metals play an important role in the formation of hydroxyl radicals. H₂O₂ is produced by a wide variety of intracellular events, particularly in normal oxidative transport in mitochondria, and is normally present in most cells at a concentration of about 10^{-8} M (Forman and Boveris, 1982). OH˙ is an extremely strong oxidant, with a redox potential of approximately + 1.35 V, making it capable of degrading most biological molecules, including DNA (Keyer and Imlay, 1996). The number of different DNA modifications that OH˙ is capable of producing appears to be over 100 (Hutchinson, 1985).

It is clear that any increase in the levels of superoxide anion, hydrogen peroxide or the redox active metals (e.g., iron, chromium, cupper) is likely to lead to the formation of high levels of the hydroxyl radical by the chemical mechanisms listed above. Therefore, the valence state and bioavailability of redox active metal is a key determinant in its ability to participate in the generation of reactive oxygen species.

Reactions of activated oxygen with organic substrates are complex even *in vitro* with homogenous solutions, but in biological systems, there are even more complications due to the surface properties of membranes, electrical charges, binding properties of macromolecules, and compartmentalization of enzymes, substrates and catalysts. Thus, various sites even within a single cell differ in the nature and extent of their reactions to ROS.

It can be concluded that primary source of free radicals is the mitochondrial electron transport, and there are two secondary sources. One is endogenous secondary source (e.g., inflammation process) and the other is exogenous secondary source (e.g., smoking, stress, pollution, food, etc).

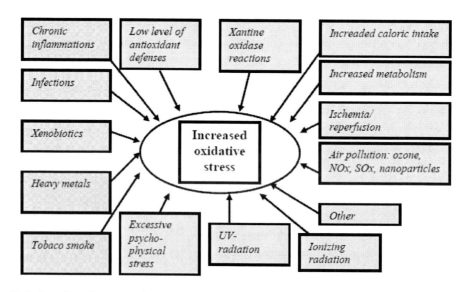

Figure 7. Endogenic and exogenic free-radical triggering factors related to the aging process.

ROS as a Cause of the Oxidative Damage

ROS are, due to their high reactivity, prone to cause damage and are thereby also potentially toxic, mutagenic and carcinogenic (Nordberg and Arner, 2001). The targets of

ROS damage include all major groups of biomolecules, summarized in the following chapters.

DNA

ROS have been proven to be mutagenic (Marnett, 2000), an effect that should be derived from chemical modification of DNA. A number of alterations (e.g., cleavage of DNA, DNA-protein cross-links, oxidation of purine, etc.) are due to reactions with ROS, especially OH$^·$. If the DNA repair systems are not able to immediately regenerate intact DNA, a mutation will result from erroneous base pairing during replication. This mechanism may partly explain the high prevalence of cancer in individuals exposed to oxidative stress (Marnett, 2000). The fact that apoptosis in some cases is mediated by ROS (Kamata and Hirata, 1999) may in part be due to the ROS-derived damage to DNA but is also related to increased mitochondrial permeability, released cytochrome c, increased intracellular Ca^{2+}, and other effects (Nordberg and Arner, 2001).

The principal cause of single-strand breaks is oxidation of sugar moiety by the hydroxyl radical. *In vitro*, neither H_2O_2 alone nor $O_2^·$, cause strand breaks under physiological conditions, and therefore their toxicity *in vivo* is most likely the result of Fenton reactions with a metal catalyst (McKersie, 1996). Cross-linking to proteins is another consequence of hydroxyl radical attack on either DNA or its associated proteins (Oleinck et al., 1986). Although DNA protein cross-links are about one order of magnitude less abundant than single-strand breaks, they are not as readily repaired and may be lethal if replication or transcription precedes the repair (McKersie, 1996).

Eukaryotic DNA packaged into chromatin is significantly more resistant to oxidative damage than naked DNA, underscoring the role of DNA packaging as a protective mechanism as well as playing a key role in compartmentalization and gene regulation (Santoro and Thiele, 1997).

OH$^·$ can add on to guanine at positions C4, C5 and C8 in the purine ring. Addition to C-8 produces a C-8 OH adduct radical that can be reduced to 8-hydroxy-7,8-dihydroguanine, oxidized to 8-hydroxyguanine, or undergo opening of the imidazole ring, followed by one-electron reduction and protonation, to give 2,6-diamino-4-hydroxy-5-formamidopyrimidine, abbreviated as FAPyG (Halliwell and Gutterigde, 1999). The number of different DNA modifications that OH$^·$ is capable of producing appears to be over 100 (Hutchinson, 1985).

Today, many normal physiological processes, such as phagocytosis, are known to involve the formation of OH$^·$ radicals. In addition, many toxic agents seem to generate OH$^·$: tetrachloride, chloroform, paraquat, ethanol, nitrogen dioxide, ozone, sulphur dioxide, cigarette smoke, cadmium, arsenic, mercury, lead, tetracyclines, radiation, etc. (Halliwell and Gutteridge, 1999). Their toxicity is apparently due to the subsequent reactions of the OH$^·$.

Lipids

With multiple double bonds, polyunsaturated fatty acids (PUFAs) are excellent targets for the radical attack. They are particularly susceptible to hydrogen abstraction due to the presence of double bonds. Such oxidation is also essential for the generation of atherosclerotic plaques (Frei, 1999; Stadtman and Berlett, 1998). The peroxidation of lipids involves three distinct steps: initiation, propagation and termination. Once the hydroxyl radical initiates the peroxidation reaction by abstracting a single H atom, it creates a carbon radical product, which is capable of reacting with ground-state oxygen in a chain reaction. The basis of the hydroxyl radical extreme reactivity in lipid system is that at very low concentrations, it initiates a chain reaction involving triplet oxygen, the most abundant form of oxygen in a cell (Halliwell and Gutteridge, 1999).

Proteins

Proteins—whether structural or free cytoplasmic ones—are probably the main target of externally induced ROS in animal and in bacterial cells (Sigler et al., 1999). Oxidative attack on proteins results in site-specific amino acid modifications, fragmentation of the peptide chain, aggregation of cross-linked reaction products, altered electrical charge and increased susceptibility to proteolysis (McKersie, 1996). The amino acids in a peptide differ in their susceptibility for attack, and the various forms of activated oxygen differ in their potential reactivity. Primary, secondary, and tertiary protein structures alter the relative susceptibility of certain aminoacids (McKersie, 1996). ROS have been shown to react with several amino acids residues *in vitro*, generating modified and less active enzymes to denaturated, nonfunctioning proteins (Stadtman and Berlett, 1998). Among the most susceptible parts are sulfur or selenium-containing residues. General antioxidant systems such as thioredoxin (TRx) and GSH protect proteins from ROS-mediated modifications. In biopsies from individuals with histologically confirmed solar elastosis, an accumulation of oxidatively modified proteins was found specifically in the upper dermis (Sander et al., 2002). Protein oxidation in photoaged skin is most likely due to UV irradiation.

Chapter 4

Basic Information about the Skin

In order to understand skin-aging process and approaches to decrease or prevent it, it is important to introduce basic information about the anatomy and physiology of the skin.

Skin is the largest organ of the body, accounting for 12% to 16% body weight (at least six pounds (2.7 kg)for the average adult);it covers 18 to 20 square feet (about twosquare meters) and has the largest surface area of any organ and is the most vulnerable to environmental insults. The approximate chemical composition of the skin is: water 70.0%, protein 25.5%, lipids 2.0%, trace minerals 0.5%, other 2.0%. Over the lifetime, over 40 kg of squames are shed, equating to about three to five million squames each day. The skin replaces itself about every 28 days and continuously produces a horny protective cover of hardened proteins (keratinization) while shedding the outermost layer of dead cells (exfoliation).

Skin itself is a complex organ made up of multiple cell types with a high-energydemand. For example, suprabasal layers of the epidermis and cells with the roots of the hair follicle have high metabolic activity associated with the synthesis of keratin and the cornified envelopes (Hourigan, 2010). Skin is made up of two layers that cover a third fatty layer. The outer layer is called the epidermis; it is a tough protective layer that contains melanin (which protects against the rays of the sun and gives the skin its color). The epidermis has no blood vessels. Epidermis is a visible part of the skin; it is only as thick as a piece of paper. The thickness of the skin varies from one region of the body to another. It is thickest over the back and thinnest over the scalp or wrist. Most of the variances in thickness are accounted for by the differences in thickness of the dermis. Epidermis has many functions, e.g., it protects the skin from the external damage and maintains hydration of the internal tissues. Most functions are performed by the stratum corneum (SC), the outer layer of the epidermis. The uppermost layer of epidermis (stratus corneum) represents the final stage and consists of dead anucleate cells (corneocytes) embedded in a keratin- and lipid-rich matrix, forming a barrier. These cells are constantly shed and are a major contributor to household dust (Halliwell and Gutteridge, 2007). Individual cells (squames) are shed continuously (desquamated) from the skin surface in a highly coordinated process requiring multiple protease activation in the uppermost epidermal layer. The outer layer or epidermis is made primarily of keratinocytes (keratinocytes comprise 90% of the epidermal population) but has several other minor cell populations, like melanocytes and immune cells (Langerhans cells). Melanocytes are specialized cells that are located in the basal layer of the epidermis. They synthesize and transfer melanin pigments to surrounding keratinocytes, thus protecting from UV carcinogenic effects (Dumas et al., 1994; Bykov et al., 2000; Seiberg, 2001). Melanocytes are derived from neural crest cells and migrate to the epidermal compartment near the eighth week of gestational age. Melanocyte proliferation is normally regulated by keratinocytes via cell-cell adhesion receptors. These receptors are lost in a vertical growth phase melanomas. Langerhans cells are a third cell type in the epidermis and have a primary function of antigen presentation. In the skin, Langerhans cells (professional antigen presenting cells) form a network of cells interspersed between keratinocytes in the epidermis. Langerhans cells act as a "surveillance system," detecting and transmitting foreign antigens for recognition by the adaptive immune system. These cells reside in the skin for an extended time and respond to different stimuli, such as ultraviolet light or topical steroids, that cause them to migrate out of the skin.

Keratinocytes produce keratin, the special protective protein. Keratinocytes are sometimes called by different names in different layers of the epidermis (basal cells, granular cells, stratus corneum). Where epidermis meets dermis is a layer of actively dividing cells. Cells from this layer (keratinocytes) migrate upwards in the epidermis and undergo differentiation, in the process of keratinization, sometimes called cornification. Keratinocyte proliferates in the basal layer, differentiates and, as the keratinocytes mature and move towards the skin surface, give rise to the stratified epithelium. New keratinocytes are constantly being produced by the division of basal cells into daughter cells. The bottom layer is formed of basal keratinocytes abutting the basement membrane. The epidermis contains mostly keratinocytes that egress to the skin surface as they differentiate progressively to form enucleated corneocytes that comprise the outer part of the epidermis, the stratum corneum (SC). The SC contains neither viable cells nor nerve endings. Rather, it is composed of core and envelope proteins embedded in a lipophilic matrix (Elias, Feingold, 1992). When keratinocytes die, they leave their proteins as a protective layer in the outermost part of the epidermis. A total of 15 to 20 layers of so-called ''cornified envelopes'' turns over in approximately two weeks by desquamating the outer layer. If dead skin cells fall off faster than new cells are formed, then the skin becomes thin, eroded, or anthropic. If new cells are formed faster than dead cells are sloughed off, then the stratum corneum piles up and appears as scales or thickened skin. The SC plays an important role as the skin barrier, limiting the penetration of exogenous compounds into the body. Moreover, it limits the evaporation of water across the skin, the so-called transepidermal water loss, thus preventing the body from drying out. Perturbation of the skin barrier is involved in several dermatological pathologies (Elias, Feingold, 1992; Ghadially et al., 1995; Mao-Qiang et al., 1996; Weber and Packer, 2001). The skin barrier is linked to the lipids of the inter-corneocyte space. Intercellular lipids consist of an organized mixture of ceramides, sterols and fatty acids (Bonté, 1999; Bonté et al., 1997), especially linoleic acid (Elias, 1996). The lipids in intercellular membranes form short- and long-periodicity lamellar phases (Bonté et al., 1997). As pointed out, the SC plays an important role as the skin barrier. Both proteins and lipids cooperate in maintaining the barrier function. Homeostasis of lipids has especially been shown to be crucial for functionality. Disturbance of the lipid ratios results in a reduction in barrier function and an increase in the water flux across the skin, the already mentioned transepidermal water loss (Ghadially et al., 1996). For further information, see also the chapter on skin moisturizing.

The second layer (located under the epidermis) is called the dermis; it contains nerve endings, sweat glands, oil glands, and hair follicles. Dermis is the thicker layer that gives skin much of its substance and mass. The primary function of the dermis is to sustain and support the epidermis. The dermis is a more complex structure and is composed of two layers, the more superficial papillary dermis and the deeper reticular dermis. The papillary dermis is thinner, consisting of loose connective tissue containing capillaries, elastic fibers, reticular fibers, and some collagen. The reticular layer contains fibroblasts, mast cells, nerve endings, lymphatics, and epidermal appendages. The extracellular matrix in the dermis consists of type I and type II collagen, elastin, proteoglycans and fibronectin. Type I collagen is the most abundant structural protein in skin connective tissue. It accounts for about 85% of total dermal protein. Type III collagen interacts with type II collagen and is present at approximately one-tenth the level of type I collagen. Types I and III collagens are synthesized by fibroblasts in the dermis, as precursor protein (procollagens). Dermal fibroblasts make precursor molecules called procollagen, which is converted into collagen. There are two important regulators of collagen production: transforming growth factor (TGF)-β, a cytokine that promotes collagen production, and activator protein (AP)-1, a transcription factor that inhibits collagen production and upregulates collagen breakdown by upregulating enzymes matrix metalloproteinases (MMPs) (Kang et al., 1997; Massague, 1998). Collagen is a group of naturally occurring proteins. It is the main protein of connective tissue.Collagen is the most abundant protein in the body; it makes up to 70% of the dry weight of human skin and is a critical component of the vascular and osteomuscular system. It is primarily composed of glycine, proline and hydroxyproline. It is one of the strongest proteins in nature and gives skin its strength and durability. As we age, it is believed that collagen begins to deteriorate and causes the skin to become thinner and eventually sag. Collagen fibrils are important for the strength and resilience of skin, and alteration in their number and structure are thought to be responsible for wrinkle formation. Collagen in skin undergoes continuous skin remodeling and turnover, with TGF-βand AP-1 playing important roles. Matrix metalloproteinases are zinc-dependent endopeptidases and show proteolitic activity in their ability to degrade matrix proteins such as collagen and elastin. Each MMP degrades different dermal matrix proteins (MMP-1 cleaves collagen types I, II and III; MMP-9 cleaves collagen type IV and V and gelatin). Both UVB and UVA irradiation induce MMP. While UVA acts indirectly by the generation of ROS, UVB also induce ROS, but its main mechanism of action is by direct interaction with DNA. The half-life of skin collagen is estimated to be several years, and degradation of collagen fibers requires the action of collagenases. Three mammalian collagenases exist, MMP-1, MMP-8, and MMP-13, which have the capacity to initiate cleavage of mature collagen (Rittie et al., 2006). In particular, collagen fibrils are important for the strength and resilience of skin.

Elastin is similar to collagen but is a more stretchable protein that maintains the skin's elasticity. It provides the matrix that holds individual skin cells in place. Elastin is a protein in connective tissue that is elastic and allows many tissues in the body to resume their shapes after stretching or contracting. Elastin helps skin to return to its original position when it is poked or pinched. Elastic fibers in the dermis form an amorphous matrix of elastin and intertwining bundles of microfibrils, which measure 10 to 14 nm in diameter. The oxytalan fibers are rich in microfibrils and are orientated perpendicularly to the basal lamina of the epidermis.Elastin is composed of the protein fibrillin and amino acids such as glycine, valine, alanine, and proline. Elastin also contains two unique amino acids, desmosine and isodesmosine. The two proteins together permit the skin to stretch and then regain its original shape. With age, the skin's elastin breaks down, and the lack of elastin causes wrinkles.

The dermis contains multiple cell types, embedded in a fibrous network of connective tissue containing proteoglycans, elastin and collagen. The dermis is largely composed of an intra- and extracellular matrix. Prominent cell types in this compartment are fibroblasts, endothelial cells, and transient immune system cells. Dermal fibroblasts synthesize a complex extracellular matrix containing collagenous and elastic fibers and proteoglycans. Blood capillaries reach the upper part of the dermis.

We should also mention the microbe layer of the skin. Human skin is covered with microbes. The total number of microbes on the skin surface is typically within the range of 10^4-10^6 cells/cm^2. Skin microflora plays a role in both maintenance of health and development of skin diseases (Ouwehand et al., 2010).

Under dermis is a fatty layer of subcutaneous tissue (the word subcutaneous means "under the skin").

Hair, Nails and Glands of the Skin

Early in fetal life, the single-cell-thick ectoderm and underlying mesoderm begin to proliferate and differentiate. The specialized structures formed by the skin, including teeth, hair, hair follicles, fingernails, toenails, sebaceous glands, sweat glands, apocrine glands, and mammary glands, also begin to appear during this period in development. Teeth, hair, and hair follicles are formed by the epidermis and dermis, while fingernails and toenails are formed by the epidermis alone. Epidermal appendages include sebaceous glands, sweat glands, apocrine glands, mammary glands, and hair follicles.

The normal function of the sweat gland is to produce sweat, which cools the body by evaporation. The thermoregulatory center in the hypothalamus controls sweat gland activity through sympathetic nerve fibers that innervate the sweat glands. Sweat excretion is triggered when core body temperature reaches or exceeds a set point. The excess heat is lost by evaporation of water from the skin surface. Sweat is rich in transitional metal ions capable of catalyzing free-radical reactions and promoting bacterial growth (Jasin, 1993).

Sebaceous Glands

The sebaceous glands produce a large amount of a complex liquid called sebum. Apocrine glands secrete a milky fluid. Apocrine secretions are odorless, but when certain bacteria grow and decompose the secretions, personal problems could arise.

Sebum is used as a vehicle for odors involved in sexual and social attraction. Sebum protects the skin also by interfering with skin microbial biocenosis since it possesses fungistatic and bacteriostatic properties (Pierard-Franchimont et al., 2010). The sebum amount is altered with aging and varies according to the age, gender and climacteric period.

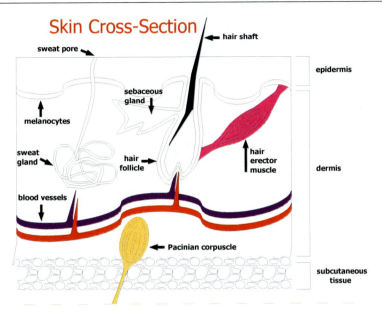

Figure 8. Skin cross section. Skin is a multilayered tissue with an outer stratum corneum (10 to 20 μm), a living epidermis (50 to 100 μm), a dermis (1 to 3 mm) and hypodermis composed primarily of adipocytes.

Also, sebaceous glands get bigger but produce less sebum, and the number of sweat glands decreases with aging. Both of these changes lead to skin dryness. The human sebaceous gland undergoes both extrinsic and intrinsic aging (morphological changes in the sebaceous gland activity). The highly androgen-dependent sebum secretion in neonates reaches its maximum in young adults. The number of sebaceous glands remains unchanged throughout life, but sebum production tends to decrease after menopause in women and after the eighth decade in men. The age-dependent decrease in androgen leads to a slower cell turnover in the sebaceous glands, resulting in hyperplasia of the facial sebaceous glands (Rocquet and Bonte, 2002). UV may contribute to this process, too. The dryness of the aging skin is caused by the decreased circulation as well as decreases in sweat and oil secretion by glands and changed structure of epidermis.

Hair

As keratinocytes multiply and make the keratin of stratum corneum, some epidermal cells specialize to make the keratin of hair and nails. Hair is a filament of keratin consisting of a root and a shaft formed in a specialized follicle in the epidermis. The human body, apart from its glabrous skin, is covered with folliclesthat produce thick terminal and fine vellum hair. Aging of hair manifests as decrease of melanocyte function or graying and decrease in hair production or alopecia. There is circumstantial evidence that oxidative stress may be a pivotal mechanism contributing to hair graying and hair loss (Trüeb, 2009). Arck et al. (2006) reported that intriguingly, the continuous melanin synthesis in the growing (anagen) hair follicle generates high oxidative stress. They, therefore, hypothesized that hair bulb melanocytes are especially susceptible to free-radical-induced aging. Authors tested this hypothesis by subjecting human scalp skin anagen hair follicles from graying individuals to macroscopic and immunohistomorphometric analysis and organ culture. It was found that there was evidence of melanocyte apoptosis and increased oxidative stress in the pigmentary unit of graying hair follicles.

Nails

Nail is a horn-like envelope covering the dorsal aspect of the terminal phalanges of fingers and toes. Nails are epidermal specializations that are homologous with the claws of lower animals.

Melanin

Sunlight induces the synthesis of melanin, which has a broad absorbance spectrum that ranges through the UVB, UVA and visible ranges. Melanin, the pigment deposited by melanocytes, is the first line of defense against DNA damage at the surface of the skin. The UV light causes the melanocytes to begin working harder to provide more melanin as sunscreen. The increased pigmentation results in an acquired darkening we popularly refer as tan. Melanine is made in melanocytes, which then transfer it to keratinocytes and to hair. Each melanocyte has long projections of dendrites, which reach many surrounding keratinocytes and act to pass the pigment particles (melanosomes) into the keratinocytes. As the keratinocytes migrate upward, they carry the pigment particles with them. Melanocytes are also present in the lowest layers of the hair bulb cells and pass pigment on to color the hair itself. Although human beings generally possess a similar concentration of melanocytes in their skin, the melanocytes in some individuals and ethnic groups more frequently or less frequently express the melanin-producing genes, thereby conferring a greater or lesser concentration of skin melanin. Melanine is formed as part of the process of metabolizing an amino acidcalled tyrosine. The most common form of biological melanin is eumelanin, a brown-black polymer of dihydroxyindole carboxylic acid, and their reduced forms. Another common form of melanin is pheomelanin, a red-brown polymer of benzothiazine units largely responsible for red hair and freckles. Eumelanin is found in hair, areola, and skin, and colors hair grey, black, yellow, and brown. In humans, it is more abundant in people with dark skin. Eumelanin is protective against photodamage (Halliwell and Gutteridge, 2007) but this is not always true of pheomelanin. The photochemical properties of melanin make it an excellent photoprotectant. It absorbs harmful UV radiation and transforms the energy into harmless amounts of heat. Pheomelanin and eumelanin have different free radical quenching properties. Red or yellow pheomelanin is less effective free radical scavenger since UV-exposed pheomelanin is degraded with a net formation of superoxide (Kollias et al., 1991). Decreased protection and increased damage of pheomelanin in the epidermis may partly underlie the markedly increased risk of skin cancer associated with red-haired people (Brash et al., 2010).

People whose ancestors lived for long periods in the regions of the globe near the equator generally have larger quantities of eumelanin in their skins. This makes their skins brown or black and protects them against high levels of exposure to the sun, which more frequently results in melanomas in lighter skinned people.

Darker skin has more protective melanin pigment, and the incidence of skin cancer is lower in dark-skinned people. Nevertheless, skin cancers do occur with this group, and unfortunately they are often detected at a later, more dangerous stage. The risk of UV radiation-related health effects on the eye and immune system is independent of skin type.

Since the epidermis permits some transmission of light, we are also able to see the bright red of oxygenated hemoglobin and the bluish-red of reduced hemoglobin in the superficial blood vessels in the dermis of the skin.

The skin has a wide variety of functions, including biologic, social, cosmetic, communicative, and sensory, among others. The skin must be strong enough to be protective, yet sensitive enough to give us many important messages from our environment by a variety of nerve endings that react to heat and cold, touch, pressure, vibration, tissue injury, etc. First, the skin is an important barrier from pathogens and damage between the internal and external environment, Second, the skin is important in heat regulation: the skin contains a blood supply far greater than its requirements, which allows precise control of energy loss by radiation, convection and conduction. Skin acts as a water-resistant barrier so essential nutrients aren't washed out of the body. It is believed that the skin assumed the protective role once performed by the cell wall in unicellular organisms since the skin is the limiting membrane or outer envelope that defines the boundaries of the organism. Maintenance and repair of the layers of protection and physical barriers depend upon continual replacement and repair by the living cells. Knowledge of the anatomy, physiology and function of the skin and the mechanisms of the disease and aging permits the development of new approaches to treat skin diseases and to implement appropriate preventive methods to delay the skin-aging process. More about this topic is presented in the further chapters.

Chapter 5

General Overview of Skin Aging: The Role of Extrinsic (External) and Intrinsic (Free Radical Mediated Internal) Factors

Human skin, like all other organs, undergoes chronological and biological aging. Aging of the skin is a composite of actinic damage, chronological aging, and internal influences. In addition, unlike other organs, skin is in direct contact with the environment and, therefore, undergoes aging as a consequence of environmental damage (Fisher et al.,2002). Factors contributing to premature aging are dependent on age, sex, pigmentation, smoking, sun exposure history, alcohol consumption and other environmental, genetic and lifestyle factors—some of them will be presented in the following chapters (Ernster et al., 1995; Frances, 1998; Grady and Ernster, 1992; Kadunce et al., 1991).Age-related physiological changes in elderly skin include clinical, histological, and biochemical changes, as well as changes in neurosensory perception, barrier function, wound healing and higher incidence of benign and cancerous diseases (Rasche and Elsner, 2010). Skin aging appears to be the result of two types of aging, intrinsic and extrinsic aging. Intrinsic structural changes occur as a natural consequence of aging and are genetically determined. Intrinsic aging is the rate of aging that occurs with the passage of time. Extrinsic aging, on the other hand, is the skin's response to external damage and is controllable to a very large degree by the lifestyle choices we make every day. In this book, evidence for the fact that also intrinsic aging can be modified by appropriate lifestyle and nutrition is presented. The rate of aging is significantly different among different populations, as well as among different anatomical sites, even within a single individual. The intrinsic rate of skin aging in any individual can also be dramatically influenced by personal and environmental factors, particularly the amount of exposure to ultraviolet light. Photodamage, which considerably accelerates the visible aging of skin, also greatly increases the risk of cutaneous neoplasm (Farage et al., 2008). Damage to human skin due to ultraviolet light from the sun (photoaging) and damage occurring as a consequence of the passage of time (chronologic or natural aging) were considered to be distinct entities. The findings of the study performed by Varani et al. (2000) indicate that naturally aged, sun-protected skin and photoaged skin share important molecular features, including connective tissue damage, elevated matrix metalloproteinaselevels, and reduced collagen production. The intrinsic (genetically determined) and the extrinsic (UV and toxic exposure mediated) skin-aging processes are thus overlapped and are strongly related to the increased generation of free radicals in the skin. Oxidative stress is believed to underlie changes associated with both photoaging and natural aging. Although the skin possesses extremely efficient antioxidant activities, during aging, ROS levels rise and antioxidant activities decline. The ROS are necessary in multiple MAP kinase pathways, and the induction of AP-1, in turn, upregulates expression of matrix-metalloproteinases providing a plausible mechanism for the increased collagen degradation in aged human skin (Callaghan and Wilhelm, 2008). Oxidative stress is thus considered of primary importance in driving the skin-aging process. Extrinsic skin aging develops due to several factors: ionizing radiation, severe physical and psychological stress, alcohol intake, poor nutrition, overeating, environmental pollution, and exposure to UV radiation. It is estimated that among all these environmental factors, UV radiation contributes up to 80%. UV radiation is the most important environmental factor in the development of skin cancer and skin aging. Visible aging of the skin starts at about age 25, as the natural regenerative process begins to slow down. The skin replaces old cells more slowly, and there is a slower turnover of the surface skin and slower wound healing. The number, affinity and rate of internalization of epidermal growth factor (EGF) receptors are different in young and old fibroblasts, explaining the loss of responsiveness to EGF with age and the impaired wound healing in the elderly (Reenstra et al., 1993). After age 45, a thinning of the skin begins, due in part to hormonal changes. This thinning makes the skin more fragile and vulnerable to damage by abrasion and more sensitive to irritating environmental factors and allergens. Thin, wrinkled skin is very often attributed to a lack of collagen. The dermis and overlying epidermis of aging skin are profoundly altered (Schmid et al., 2002). Slower protein synthesis is one of the most common events observed during aging. The synthesis of both structural proteins, such as collagen, and enzymes that repair and maintain the normal metabolic functions of the cell, is slowed down. This leads to the inefficient removal of damaged molecules and decreased intra-and intercellular signaling pathways (Rocquet and Bonté, 2002). In aged skin, there is elevation of AP-1 as compared to a young skin (Chung et al., 2000). In aged human skin, MMP activity is increased, which leads to increased levels of degraded collagen (Fisher et al., 2002). Synthesis of types I and III procollagen is reduced in aged skin (Varani et al., 2000). There is progressive disappearance of elastic tissue in the dermis due to reduction in elastin gene expression after the age of 40 to 50. Additionally, decreased proliferative capacity of skin cells and decreased matrix synthesis contribute to intrinsic skin-aging process. Telomere shortening and Hayflick phenomenon affect the skin of the oldest population. The coils of collagen and elastin suffer cuts and cross-linking damage and as a result, the skin loses much of its strength and elasticity. The moisture-holding proteoglycans and glycosaminoglycans decrease in abundance, making the skin become dryer and looser. Proteoglycans make up a major part of the extracellular matrix, the material between cells that provides structural support. Proteoglycans are heavily glycosylated glycoproteins. This means that they are proteins with chains of polysaccharides, a kind of carbohydrate, attached. The specific type of polysaccharides attached to proteoglycans are called glycosaminoglycans (GAGs). The skin loses fat, so it looks less plump and smooth. The number of blood vessels in aged skin decreases, and the skin loses its youthful color and glow (http://www.skinbiology.com/skinhealth&aging.html). Since blood circulation in the dermic layer slows down, the delivery of nutrients and oxygen to skin cells is decreased. Skin atrophy is marked only after the fifth decade of human life and shows a plethora of histomorphologic changes including epidermal thinning, flattening of the dermal-epidermal junction, loss of melanocytes, and immunocompetent Langerhans cells (Bhattacharyya, 2010). There are also dermal changes such as reduced fibroblast population and sebaceous glands. There are typical ultrastructural changes in microvasculature of elderly people. Two of the most noticeable changes as skin ages are alterations to pigment production (e.g., age spots) and the formation of wrinkles. Altered melanocyte function and reorganized, cross-linked highly structured collagen matrices directly drive these visible aging changes respectively, but the primary cause of both is excessive lifetime exposure to the sunlight (Jenkins et al., 2009). The major histological features of sun-protected, intrinsically aged skin include a thin epidermis, significant flattening of the dermal-epidermal junction (this results in a reduced exchange of nutrients and metabolites between these two parts), thinning of the dermis and subcutaneous adipose layer and reduced numbers of keratinocytes, fibroblasts, Langerhans cells, mast cells and melanocytes. The dermis appears hypocellular with fewer fibroblasts and mast cells and loss of dermal volume. The major cutaneous changes in chronologically aged skin are observed in the dermoepidermal junction, which displays flattening of the rete ridges leading to reduced surface contact between the epidermis and dermis and, as a result, reduced exchange of nutrients and metabolites between these compartments (Yaar, 2006). There is a decrease in the number of dermal blood vessels and a decrease in the density of Pacinian and Meissner's corpuscles, responsible for pressure and light touch perception (Yaar and Gilchrest, 2003). The repair ability of the skin is decreased. Increased matrix metalloproteinase (MMP) activity and decreased collagen synthesis are typical changes thatoccur both in an intrinsically and extrinsically aged skin (Jenkins et al., 2009). Physiological changes of aged skin include changes in skin biochemistry, neurosensory perception, permeability, vascularisation, response to injury, repair capacity and increased incidence of particular skin diseases (Farage et al., 2010). As already discussed, the MMPs in the skin are responsible for breaking down macromolecules of the skin extracellular matrix (ECM), which ensures the skin's three-dimensional integrity. The balance between MMPs and MMP inhibitors is perturbed by environmental factors, such as light. This leads to collapse of the EMC and the visible effects of UV damage: wrinkling, loss of elasticity. Since some of the MMPs, a family of at least 16 enzymes that digest matrix macromolecules, are activated by UV irradiation (Thibodeau, 2000), type 1 MMPs (interstitial collagenase) and type 9 MMP (gelatinase) break down skin collagen fibers, particularly during photodamage (Fisher et al., 1996; Fisher et al., 1997). MMP-2 (gelatinase) acts on collagen types I, IV, and VII. Gelatin, elastin and fibronectin are all substrates for MMP-2, whose activity increases with age (Mauviel, 1993; Ashcroftet al., 1997). MMP-1 degrades collagen, which accounts for at least 70% of the dry weight of the dermis (Rocquet and Bonte, 2002). Thus, metalloproteinases 1, 3 and 9 (MMP-1, 3 and 9) in the epidermis are activated by UVB, while UVA stimulates MMP-1 in vivo and MMP-2 and 3 in vitro. Besides chronological aging, actinic aging, also called photodamage, causes premature skin aging: thinning of the dermis, a loss of collagen content and protein organization and a breakdown of the ECM (Fenske and Lober, 1986; Bolognia, 1993). There is also a depressed sensory and autonomic innervation of epidermis and dermis.

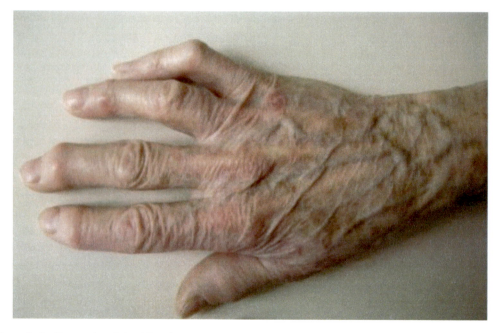

Figure 9. Senile atrophy of the skin (picture provided by: assistant professor Mateja Dolenc-Voljč, MD).

The signs of intrinsic aging are:

- Fine wrinkles,
- Thin and transparent skin,
- Loss of underlying fat, leading to hollowed cheeks and eye sockets as well as noticeable loss of firmness on the hands and neck; bones shrink away from the skin due to bone loss, which causes sagging skin,
- Dry skin that may itch,
- Inability to sweat sufficiently to cool the skin,
- Graying hair that eventually turns white,
- Hair loss,
- Unwanted hair,
- Nail plate thins, the half moons disappear, and ridges develop.

Biomarkers of the intrinsic skin aging include hyaluronic acid depolymerization, a reduced melanogenesis and estrogen-dependent collagen synthesis, lowered ATP generation and wound repair capabilities, impaired antioxidant defense and increased lipofuscin generation (Ionescu, 2005). Biomarkers of the extrinsic skin-aging process include products of lipid peroxidation, collagenase activation, glycation/oxidation of proteins (AGE products), activation of p53 transcription factors, low DNA repair capacity and cumulative DNA damage/mutations leading to skin cancer, etc. (Ionescu, 2005). Lipofuscin, or age pigment, accumulates in cells within the lysosomal vacuoles, especially in fibroblasts. Lipofuscin can also accelerate aging and senescence under mild hyperoxia (Von Zglinicki et al., 1995). The accumulation of lipofuscin may also be involved in spot formation (age spots).

To sum up, intrinsic aging is influenced by internal physiological factors alone and extrinsic aging by many external factors. Intrinsic aging is also called *chronologic aging*, and extrinsic aging is most often referred to as *photoaging*. Intrinsic aging includes qualitative and quantitative changes and includes diminished or defective synthesis of collagen and elastin in the dermis mostly due to free radical formation during metabolism. Age-associated accumulation of mitochondrial deficits due to oxidative damage is likely to be a major contributor to cellular, tissue, and organismal intrinsic aging (Shigenega et al., 1994). Classically, chronologic aging includes those cutaneous changes that occur in non-sun-exposed areas, such as the buttocks, and are observed in both men and women. A clinical example would be soft tissue sagging due to elastic fiber degeneration (Bologna, 1995).

The problem of intrinsic skin-aging research is in the fact that most information relating to intrinsic aging process comes from tissues other than skin. Nevertheless, intrinsic aging is based on general biological processes that apply more or less to all proliferating cells and terminally differentiated cells as well (Blatt et al., 2010) and is caused primarily by the build-up of damage due to free radical reactions as a by-product of cellular metabolism and by ROS-induced damage to critical cellular macromolecules. The next chapter will provide some detailed information about this process.

Metabolism, Reactive Oxygen Species (ROS) and the Oxidative Stress as Triggers of Intrinsic Skin Aging

Intrinsic aging depends on time. Generation of reactive oxygen species (ROS) is believed to play a major role also in chronologic and biologic skin aging. The problem of intrinsic factors contributing to skin aging is the fact that some of them (e.g., free radicals) are an essential part of metabolism we cannot live without. The changes in our skin cells occur partially as the result of cumulative endogenous damage due to the continuous formation of reactive oxygen species (ROS), which are generated by oxidative cellular metabolism. Despite a strong antioxidant defense system, damage generated by ROS affects cellular constituents such as membranes, enzymes, and DNA.

In order to understand basic principles of intrinsic skin aging, the biochemistry of free radical formation is briefly presented.

There is no doubt that oxygen (O_2) is essential for life (Balantine, 1982; Gilbert, 1981). Humans and other aerobes need O_2 because they evolved electron transport chains and other enzyme systems utilizing O_2 and can tolerate its toxic by-products by antioxidant defenses. The predecessors of the anaerobic bacteria that exist today followed the "blind" evolutionary path of restricting themselves to environments devoid of O_2. It could be argued that the evolution of multi-cellular aerobes and antioxidant defense mechanisms are intimately related (Hohmann and Mager, 1997).

Even present-day aerobes suffer oxidative damage. Free radicals, formed in living organisms, include hydroxyl ($OH^\cdot$), superoxide ($O_2^{\cdot-}$), nitric oxide ($NO^\cdot$), thyl ($RS^\cdot$) and peroxyl ($RO_2^\cdot$). Peroxynitrite ($ONOO^-$), hypochlorous acid ($HOCl$), hydrogen peroxide (H_2O_2), singlet oxygen ($^1O_2$) and ozone (O_3), are not free radicals but can easily lead to free radical reactions in living organisms. The term reactive oxygen species (ROS) is often used to include not only free radicals but also the non-radicals ($^1O_2$, $ONOO^-$, H_2O_2, O_3).Reactive oxygen species are reactive molecules that contain the oxygen atom.

The essence of metabolic energy production is that food is oxidized: in the process, the electrons are accepted by electron carriers, such as nicotinamide dinucleotide (NAD^+) and flavins (flavin mononucleotide FMN and flavin adenine dinucleotide FAD). The resulting reduced nicotinamide adenine dinucleotide (NADH) and reduced flavins ($FMNH_2$ and $FADH_2$) can be re-oxidized in mitochondria, producing large amounts of ATP (revised in Halliwell and Gutteridge, 1999).

There are two main sources of reactive oxygen species: mitochondrial sources (which play the principal role in aging) and non-mitochondrial sources (which have different, sometimes specific, roles especially in the pathogenesis of age-related diseases). Mitochondrial sources are represented by the electron transport chain (Figure 10) and the nitric oxide synthase reaction.

The rate of mitochondrial respiration is responsible for the rate of generation of reactive oxygen species; this characteristic is consistent with the observation that the higher metabolic rates an organism has, the shorter maximum lifespan it presents (Sohal, 1976), with some exceptions to this rule. Fenton reaction is an example of the non-mitochondrial source of ROS. The H_2O_2 degrading Fenton reaction is catalyzed by the free iron bivalent ions and leads to the generation of $OH^.$. It should be taken into account that the body's content of iron increases with age(Koster and Sluiter, 1995; Vercellotti, 1996). Sources of H_2O_2 could be mitochondria superoxide dismutase reaction, peroxisomes (acyl-CoA oxidase reaction) and amyloid β of senile plaques (superoxide dismutase-like reactions) (Rottkamp et al., 2001). Sources of superoxide (O_2^-) are mitochondria, microsomesthatcontain the cytochrome P450 enzymes, the respiratory burst of phagocytic cells and others. Fenton's reaction is described in detail in the chapter "The role of macro and micro nutrients."Most estimates suggest that the majority of intracellular ROS production is derived from mitochondria. The mitochondrion is an essential organelle, playing a central role in much of the metabolism. The site of oxidative phosphorilation, mitochondria provides the majority of energy in the form of ATP, which fuels cellular processes. An electron transport chain (ETC) in mitochondria couples a chemical reaction between an electron donor (such as NADH) and an electron acceptor (such as O_2) to the transfer of H^+ ions across a membrane, through a set of mediating biochemical reactions. These H^+ ions are used to produce adenosine triphosphate (ATP), the main energy intermediate in living organisms, as they move back across the membrane. Electron transport chains are used for extracting energy from sunlight (photosynthesis) and from redox reactions such as the oxidation of food. The basic mechanism that transforms food into the energetic ATP is the same in all aerobic organisms. It includes the process of mitochondrial oxidative phosphorylation. All eukaryotic organisms (and most prokaryotic ones) digest food molecules and extract energy from food using almost identical metabolic processes. A by-product of cell respiration in mitochondria is the formation of reactive oxygen species due to electron leakage in the electron transport chain during oxidative phosphorylation. The site of oxidative phosphorylation in mitochondria provides the majority of energy in the form of ATP, which fuels cellular processes (Figure 10a).

General Overview of Skin Aging 45

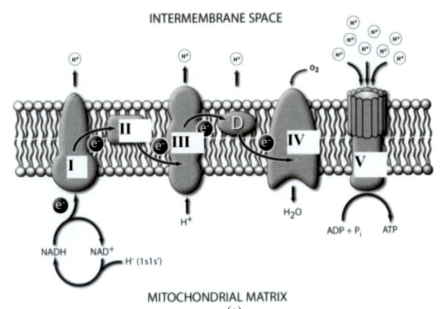

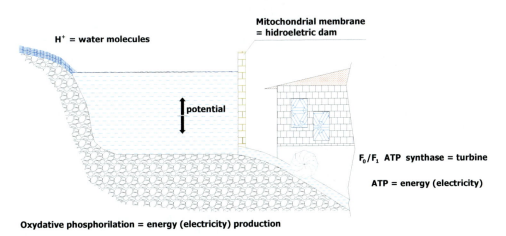

Figure 10. Schematic diagram of the electron transport chain in the mitochondria (a) and comparison of oxidative phosphorilation with the hydroelectric (nuclear and thermal) (b) power plant.

Dr. de Grey, in his book entitled *Ending Aging* (2007), made a good comparison of oxidative phosphorilation process with the hydroelectric powerplant (Figure 10b). Mitochondria generate most of their cellular power using almost identical principles to the one used by hydroelectric dams (de Grey, 2007). Using a series of preliminary biochemical reactions, energy from food in the form of electrons is transferred to a carrier molecule NAD^+. These electrons are used to run series of "pumps" electron transport chain that fills up "reservoir" of protons held back by mitochondrial "dam"—the mitochondrial inner membrane (de Grey, 2007). The build up of protons behind the "dam" creates an electrochemical force that sends them "down hill" to the other side of the mitochondrial inner membrane, just as water behind a dam is drawn downward by gravity. And just as a hydroelectric dam exploits the flow of water to run a turbine, the inner membrane contains a quite literal turbine of its own called "Complex V" or "F_0/F_1 ATP synthase" that is driven by the flow of protons. The rushing of protons through the Complex V turbine causes it to spin, and this motion is harnessed to the addition of phosphate ions to a carrier molecule adenosine diphosphate (ADP), transforming it to ATP. But while hydroelectric dams are environmentally benign, mitochondria are in one key aspect more like conventional power sources. Just like coal or nuclear power plants, mitochondria create toxic wastes during the conversion of energy from one form into another (de Grey, 2007).

The production of mitochondrial superoxide radicals occurs primarily at two discrete points in the electron transport chain, namely, at complex I (NADH dehydrogenase) and complex III (ubiquinone–cytochrome$c$ reductase). Under normal metabolic conditions, complex III is the main site of ROS production (Turrens, 1997). With respect to human aging, the Achilles' heel of this elegant system lies in the formation of the free radical semiquinone anion species (·Q-) that occurs as an intermediate in the regeneration of coenzyme Q. Once formed, ·Q- can readily and non-enzymatically transfer electrons to molecular oxygen with the subsequent generation of a superoxide radical. The generation of ROS, therefore, becomes predominantly a function of metabolic rate and, as such, the rate of living can be indirectly translated to a corresponding rate of oxidative stress (Finkel and Holbrook, 2000). But there are some exceptions that will be described later. Analyses of the control of activity of the oxidative phosphorylation-electron transport chain suggest that the system appears to be primarily pull regulated, rather than push regulated (Speakman, 2003): putting in more NADH at the front end does not drive up respiration, but restricting the availability of ADP shuts it down. When there is an abundant, non-limiting amount of ADP available, mitochondria are said to be operating in state 3 respiration. When ADP is absent, there can be no production of ATP, and the proton transduction mechanism becomes backed up, which is called state 4 respiration. Since the proton-motive force declines in state 3 compared to state 4 respiration, free-radical production would be expected to be considerably elevated in state 4 compared to state 3. This effect is interesting because it is actually the exact opposite of the postulated link between energy metabolism and free-radical production (aging) (Speakman, 2003). The flux through the electron transport chain is relevant to the aging process because it is related to the rate of the production of ROS. Small reductions in metabolic flux through the electron transport chain occur at the cost of increased upstream substrate levels (Mazat et al., 2001). This increased concentration of reduced upstream substrates allows a larger generation of ROS.Aerobic metabolism requires constant removal of excess electrons through the reduction of oxygen. The need for oxygen as an electron acceptor is the sole reason that we breathe air. Inevitable by-products of this process are O_2^-, H_2O_2 and $HO·$. This happens mainly by complexes I and III (Speakman, 2003) of the electron transport chain, the most important sources of endogenous free radicals. About 1,012 oxygen molecules are processed by each human cell daily, and the leakage of partially reduced oxygen molecules is about 1% to 5%, yielding about $2 \times 1,010$ superoxide and hydrogen peroxide molecules per cell per day (Floyd, 1995). Based on the amount of oxygen damaged and altered nucleotides detected in human urine, it has been estimated that approximately 2×10^4 oxidative DNA lesions occur per human genome every day (Ames et al., 1993). Assuming that the repair of each excised adduct involves replacing one to five nucleotides, then oxygen-induced damage to DNA results in the replacement of 2×10^5 nucleotides per human cell per day (Friedberg et al., 1995).Each human cell receives 10.000

ROS hits per day, which equals seventrillion insults per second per person. Estimates of how much oxygen reacts directly to generate free radicals vary (Speakman, 2003). However, typically cited values are around 1.5% to 5% of the total consumed oxygen (Beckman and Ames, 1998b; Casteilla et al., 2001). These estimates have been questioned by Hansford et al. (1997) and Staniek and Nohl (1999, 2000), whosuggested that H_2O_2 production rates were less than 1% of consumed O_2. Yet, even if we accept a conservative value of 0.15%, this still represents a substantial amount of free radicals (Speakman, 2003). As it was already mentioned, the rate of generation of H_2O_2 is dependent on the state of the mitochondria as determined by the concentration of ADP, substrates and oxygen (Kaul and Forman, 2000). A step increase in electron-transfer chain activity produces a linear increase in ATP production but an exponential increase in ROS formation. The cells can produce the same amount of ATP for less ROS by having a greater number of mitochondria running at a lower rate of electron-transfer chain activity. Heart cells, for example, have thousands of mitochondria, while skin cells have less mitochondria each. Whether skin cells because of this fact suffer more ROS-induced damage has not yet been established. Also, the skin cells are constantly exposed to ROS and oxidative stress from exogenous and endogenous sources. It has been found that in aged rat skin, the oxidized lipid phosphatidylcholine hydroperoxide (PCOOH) increases from 3.46 ±1.02 μmol/PC mol at sixmonths to 7.14 ±1.63 μmol/PC mol at 24 months. The free 7-hydro-peroxycholesterol (ChOOH) content also increased from 22.83 ±3.97 at sixmonths to 42.58 ± 16.59 μmol/ free Ch mol at 24 months. The TBARS (ThioBarbituric Acid Reactive Substances, harmful substances formed by lipid peroxidation, and detected by the TBARS assay, using thiobarbituric acid as a reagent) content increases from 4.71 ± 1.53 nmol/ mg protein at sixmonths to 11.10 ± 2.05 nmol/ mg protein at 30 months. The oxidized DNA in rat skin also increases with age and reaches the level of 2.04 ± 0.27 8-oxoG/ 10^5 dG at 30 months of age compared to 1.67 ± 0.16 8-oxoG/ 10^5 dG at sixmonths of age. Results suggest that chronic accumulation of oxidative damage occurs also in skin cells with age (Sivonova et al., 2007; Tahara et al., 2001; Lasch et al., 1997). High levels of ROS can inflictdirect damage on macromolecules such as lipids, nucleic acidsand proteins (Figure 11). It seems that oxidative damage is the major cause of DNA damage. Reducing free radical production in the first place is far more efficient than trying to neutralize free radicals after they have been produced. The energy demand of skin cells comes from three sources: mitochondrial oxidative phosphorylation, glycolysis and creatine/phosphocreatine system. All three major energy sources are affected by intrinsic and extrinsic skin aging and offer potential entry points for intervention strategies to decelerate the skin-aging process (Blatt et al., 2010). The study conducted by Hagen et al. (2002) revealed that feeding acetyl-L-carnitine (ALCAR) and lipoic acid (LA) to old rats significantly improves metabolic function while decreasing oxidative stress. ALCAR+LA partially reversed the age-related decline in average mitochondrial membrane potential and significantly increased hepatocellular O(2) consumption, indicating that mitochondrial-supported cellular metabolism was markedly improved by this feeding regimen. ALCAR+LA also increased ambulatory activity in both young and old rats; moreover, the improvement was significantly greater in old versus young animals and also greater when compared with old rats fed ALCAR or LA alone.

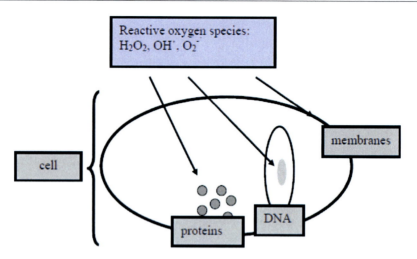

Figure 11. ROS are capable of generating cellular damage at a number of levels, including lipid peroxidation, oxidation of proteins, as well as DNA and membrane damage.

Due to impaired mitochondria with age, less energy is produced by mitochondrial oxidative phosphorylation, although the number of mitochondria does not change with age. Higher energy demand needs higher energy production via non-mitochondrial pathways, such as glycolysis. With advancing age, energy production is mostly anaerobic. Primary keratinocytes derived from old donors show a higher glucose uptake and the increased lactate production, which indicates a suboptimal utilization of glucose and a shift in metabolism towards an increased glycolysis (Blatt et al., 2010). Glucose metabolism and its side-products are discussed in a further section on advanced glycosylation end products (AGE's).

Normal human dermal fibroblasts have a limited lifespan in vitro and stop proliferation after a fixed number of cell divisions. This process by which cells stop proliferation is called senescence. Senescence is also characterized by a decrease in the total cell number. ROS is the major damaging factor of human skin. It is not yet clear if aging causes mitochondrial damage and defects or if mitochondrial defects cause aging. The loss in mitochondrial functions can cause premature senescence of the skin cells. This has been demonstrated in human fibroblast's reduction in the level of oxidative phosphorylation, which caused a reduction in cell proliferation and premature senescence (Stöckl et al., 2006). Besides the well-established influence of ROS on proliferation and senescence, a reduction in the level of oxidative phosphorylation is causally related to reduced cell proliferation and the induction of premature senescence. Changes that occur with senescence can effect mitochondrial respiration. Using the human fibroblast model of in vitro senescence, Zwersche et al. (2003) analyzed age-dependent changes in the cellular carbohydrate metabolism. Authors show that senescent fibroblasts enter into a metabolic imbalance, associated with a strong reduction in the levels of ribonucleotide triphosphates, including ATP, which are required for nucleotide biosynthesis and hence proliferation. ATP depletion in senescent fibroblasts is due to dysregulation of glycolytic enzymesand finally leads to a drastic increase in cellular AMP, which is shown to induce premature senescence (Zwerschke et al., 2003). With increasing passage number, senescent fibroblasts show a loss in membrane potential (Mammone et al., 2006) and a decline in ATP production (Zwersche et al., 2003).

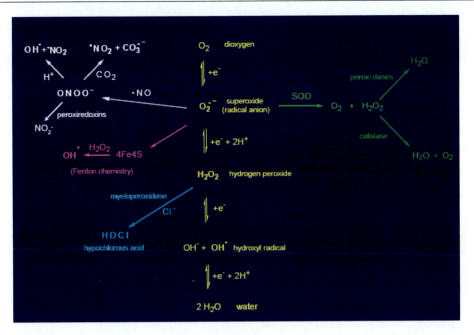

Figure 12. Radicals, oxidants and their catabolism in biological systems (figure from Rafael Radi: Formation and Properties of Reactive Oxygen and Nitrogen Species, Techniques in Free Radical Biology, FEBS Practical Course, Debrecen, Hungary, 2010).

Intrinsic aging is mainly caused by free radical generation from the normal metabolic process: NADPH oxidases, generation of hydrogen peroxide as a by-product of fatty acid metabolism, oxidative burst of phagocytes, activity of cytosolic enzymes such as cyclooxigenases, etc. However, a vast majority of endogenous ROS formation can be attributed to impaired mitochondrial respiration, and oxidants generated by mitochondria are supposed to be the major source of the oxidative lesions that accumulate with age (Shigenaga et al., 1994). Mostly, skin tissues engage in, and derive energy, using aerobic glycolysis. Despite the presence of oxygen, there is preferential conversion of glucose to lactate via the glycolytic cycle (Krebs, 1972; Philpott and Kealey, 1991). This results in the production of substantial amounts of lactate, which is carried to the liver by the bloodstream and converted back to glucose (the Cory cycle). Skin tissues have a strong preference for the metabolism of glucose rather than fatty acids or ketone bodies, though alternative citric acid cycle intermediates such as glutamine are also actively utilized (Williams et al., 1993). Interestingly, of the relatively small amount of oxygen that is metabolized by skin, the majority is supplied to the epidermis and upper dermis by diffusion from the atmosphere (Stucker et al., 2000). As the majority of ATP is generated by glycolysis in skin, the mitochondria may be less important for the ATP generation, but nevertheless, they have a pivotal role in aging effects (Wallace, 1992; Jenkins et al., 2009).

Extrinsic Factors Important for Skin Aging

Living organisms are constantly exposed to xenobiotics, which can enter our bodies by ingestion, inhalation or contact with the skin. In order of importance, the skin is the second most frequent route by which chemicals can enter the body. Skin is constantly exposed to many xenobiotics. A xenobiotic is a chemical thatis found in an organism but thatis not normally produced or expected to be present in it. Skin as the outermost barrier of the body must constantly withstand direct exposure to environmental pollutants and occupational hazards. Most frequent xenobiotics are: O2, air pollutants (ozone, NOx, SO2), deodorants, applied chemicals (creams, lotions, soaps, shower gels, shampoos, oils), water-born toxins (chlorine, metal ions, e.g., chromium(VI)), microorganisms (bacteria, viruses and fungi), radiation (ionizing and non-ionizing), agents excreted in sweat. Additionally, pro-oxidant dermatotoxic chemicals comprise metal salts, phenols, quinones, primary amines, azo-compounds, hydroperoxides, peroxides, alkylating agents, polyhalogenated and polycyclic aromatic hydrocarbons, some pesticides, and organic solvents (Fuchs,2001).

The skin's barrier has a difficult dual function. First, it must protect the body against invasion from xenobiotics, microorganisms and against losing fluid and drying out. However, this barrier must still be open and permeable enough to allow an exchange of warmth, air and fluids. It also must act as the sensory organ for our delicate sense of touch. The skin regulates the body temperature by evaporating water.

The main extrinsic factor of skin aging is sun exposure or photoaging and smoking, which accounts for 90% of premature aging skin.

Extrinsic skin aging is closely related to (Ionescu, 2005):

- the photoaging process induced by sunlight or artificial UVexposure, which exerts a major impact on skin appearance through an obvious free radical generation in the skin
- toxic environmental exposure via smoking, industrial exhausts, heavy metals, detergents, all known as potent free radical inducers
- chronic infection/inflammatory states associated with an increased free radical attack (superoxide, peroxinitrite, hypochlorite)
- sleep deficiency and stress.

Other external factors are:

- air pollution
- wind
- heat
- cold
- personal care products (PCP)
- sleeping patterns
- gravity
- radiation
- bad habits and poor diet: the body is designed to heal and repair itself with the aid of proper nutrition. The body requires two vital materials to complete this: energy and raw material. Inappropriate nutrition has excess of refined carbohydrates, fats, food additives, alcohol, low water intake and high alcohol consumption.

Skin aging results in cumulative or synergistic effect of specific intrinsic and extrinsic factors, each of them being independent from others.

The photochemical effects of UV radiation can be exacerbated by chemical agents, including birth control pills, tetracycline, sulphathiazole, cyclamates, antidepressants, coal tar distillates found in antidandruff shampoos, lime oil, and some cosmetics.

Briefly, we will introduce selected external factors affecting skin aging mostly through the stimulation of oxidative stress formation.

Air Pollution

Skin is in constant contact with environmental air. Polluted air usually contains a mixture of toxins, and interactions between them could act in a synergistic effect. The three traffic-related pollutants causing most concern include the primary pollutants NO_2 and particulate matter (PM) of <10 nm, and the secondary pollutant O_3. Although the properties of these pollutants vary markedly, they all have one common feature, which is that they can cause oxidative stress to the skin. There is some evidence that increased antioxidant intake may protect against the effects of air pollution.

Ozone

The skin can be directly exposed to tropospheric O3. The lowest ozone concentration to cause measurable oxidative stress in the stratum corneum was 1 ppm, a concentration that is about double the maxima encountered in heavily polluted metropoles (Weber and Packer, 2001). The decrease of vitamin E and increase of protein oxidation was shown in in vivo studies, where O3 effects on cutaneous tissues have been investigated (Valacchi, 2010 and references there).

Frequently, at times when O3 concentrations are high, the ground levels may also be exposed to increased UV radiation (Mustafa, 1990), which is known to be an important oxidative stress in itself (Scharffetter-Kochanek et al., 1997). It was, therefore, hypothesized that O3 and solar UV radiation may synergize in terms of oxidative challenge to the skin, especially the stratum corneum. The data from different studies demonstrate that O3 and UV radiation exhibit additive effects in terms of oxidative damage to the skin barrier. Topical exposure to tropospheric O3 may induce oxidative stress in the skin. Most of the O3 reacts within the stratum corneum. It depletes hydrophilic and lipophilic antioxidants dose dependently (Weber and Packer, 2001).

Cigarette Smoke

Smoking tobacco is the most preventable cause of morbidity and is responsible for more than three million deaths a year worldwide. In addition to a strong association with a number of systemic diseases, smoking is also associated with many dermatological conditions, including poor wound healing, premature skin aging, squamous cell carcinoma, melanoma, oral cancer, acne, psoriasis, and hair loss (Morita, 2007). Tobacco smoking is one of the numerous factors contributing to premature skin aging (Smith and Fenske, 1996)."Smoker's face" or "cigarette skin" is characteristic, implying increased facial wrinkling and an ashen and gray skin appearance (Boyd et al., 1999; Smith and Fenske, 1996). Smoking can decrease the moisture content of the facial stratum corneum, which, in turn, contributes to facial wrinkling. Pushing the lips during smoking with contraction of facial muscles as well as squinting because of the irritation of smoke may enhance the formation of wrinkles (Schroeder et al., 2006). Degradation of the elastic fibers by ROS and repeated mechanical solicitations by some muscle contractions play a putative role in the formation of the smoker's wrinkles.

Also, epidemiological studies have showed that heavy smoking causes premature skin aging (Yin et al., 2001). In vitro studies indicate that tobacco smoke extract impairs the production of collagen and increases the production of tropoelastin and matrix metalloproteinases (MMP), which degrade matrix proteins, and also cause an abnormal production of elastosis material. Smoking increases MMP levels, which leads to the degradation of collagen, elastic fibers, and proteoglycans, suggesting an imbalance between biosynthesis and degradation in dermal connective tissue metabolism. Matrix metalloproteinases (MMPs) and specific tissue inhibitors of matrix metalloproteinase (TIMPs) play an important role in physiological as well as in inflammatory processes, particularly in prolonged skin inflammation or photoaging (Maillard et al., 1995; Kahari and Saarialho-Kere, 1997). These enzymes are produced by fibroblasts, keratinocytes, mast cells, endothelial cells, and leukocytes. MMPs are not constitutively expressed in skin but are induced in response to cytokines and growth factors. Reactive oxygen species are also involved in tobacco smoke-induced premature skin aging (Morita, 2007). Already in 1971, Daniell's study investigated smoking and "tobacco wrinkles" formation. Smoking cigarettes ages skin faster than anything else apart from sun damage. The study of Jin et al. (2001) revealed that sun exposure, age and pack year independently contributed to facial wrinkle formation. The Chief Medical Officer of the UK recently highlighted the link between smoking and skin damage, saying that smoking adds between 10and20 years to person's natural age. Smokers look older than non-smokers of the same age. During the last 20 years, at least five studies have examinedthe association between cigarette smoking and facial wrinkling.Although there are methodological concerns with each of thesestudies, the data are consistent with the conclusion that smokingcauses skin wrinkling that could make smokers appear unattractiveand prematurely old (Grady and Ernster, 1995).

Maternal smoking during pregnancy and lactation was identified a risk factor for development of atopic dermatitis in the offspring (Schaefer et al., 1997).

Smoking also reduces facial stratum corneum moisture as well as vitamin A levels, which is important in reducing the extent of collagen damage (Baumann, 2002).

Additionally, cigarette smoking has been shown to decreasecapillary and arteriolar blood flow in the skin, perhaps damagingconnective tissue components that are important for maintainingthe integrity of the skin.

The study of Lahmann et al. (2001) compared the concentrations of mRNA for matrix metalloproteinase 1 (MMP-1) in the buttock skin of smokers and non-smokers with quantitative real-time polymerase chain reactions.MMP-1 degrades collagen, which accounts for at least 70% of the dry weight of dermis. The study reported significantly more MMP-1 mRNA in the skin of smokers than non-smokers. The study suggests that smoking-induced MMP-1 might be important in the skin-aging effects of tobacco smoking. Additionally, tobacco smoke and UVA cause wrinkle formation independently of each other. The study of Jin et al. (2001) proposed that both factors cause aging of human skin through additive induction of MMP-1 expression.

There is a relationship between smoking, gray hair and baldness. The mechanisms by which smoking causes hair loss are multifactorial and are probably related to effects of cigarette smoke on the microvasculature of the dermal hair papilla, smoke genotoxicants causing damage to DNA of the hair follicle, smoke-induced imbalance in the follicular protease/antiprotease systems controlling tissue remodeling during the hair growth cycle, pro-oxidant effects of smoking leading to the release of pro-inflammatory cytokines resulting in follicular micro-inflammation and fibrosis and finally increased hydroxylation of estradiol as well as inhibition of the enzyme aromatase creating a relative hypo-estrogenic state (Trüeb, 2003). The study of D'Agostini et al. (2007) revealed that high-dose environmental cigarette smoke induces apoptosis-related alopecia in mice, and oral administration of L-cystine/vitamin B6 is an effective preventive treatment. After three months exposure to a mixture of side-stream and mainstream cigarette smoke, most mice developed areas of alopecia and grey hair, while no such lesions occurred either in sham-exposed mice or in smoke-exposed mice receiving the chemopreventive agent N-acetylcysteine with drinking water. Smoke-exposed mice had extensive atrophy of the epidermis, reduced thickness of the subcutaneous tissue, and scarcity of hair follicles (D'Agostini et al., 2000).

Thus, in vitro and in vivo evidence indicates that smoking tobacco leads to accelerated aging of the skin. These findings might be useful to motivate those patients who are more concerned about their appearance than the potential internal damage associated with smoking to stop smoking. The association of smoking and facial wrinkling may be important evidence to convince youngpersons not to begin smoking and older smokers to quit. The traditional public health approach, warning that smoking can cause later health problems, such as lung cancer and emphysema, often does not influence younger people. Many young people shrug off these warnings due to feelings of invincibility or lack of concern about the future. Americans are highly motivated toavoid or eliminate facial wrinkles. Campaigns that promote life without tobacco smoke should inform smokers about all these facts.

Alcohol and Caffeine

Caffeineis a bitter, white crystalline xanthine alkaloid that is a psychoactive stimulant. Ethanol (C_2H_5OH) is the type of alcohol found in alcoholic beverages, and in common speech, the word alcohol refers specifically to ethanol. Alcohol and caffeine are diuretics. An excess amount of either or both substances can result in dry skin because they cause individuals to urinate more often. This, in turn, results in a depletion of the water from the body. After a glass of coffee or wine, it is important to drink another glass of water to rehydrate the body.

On the other hand, one decade ago, scientists began noticing the effects of caffeine on the ATR protein, which plays a large role in cell replication. Previous studies already showed that coffee and tea drinkers in several countries tended to develop fewer skin cancers.

Administration of caffeine was shown in earlier studies to enhance UVB-induced apoptosis and inhibit UVB-induced carcinogenesis in hairless SKH-1 mice (Lu et al., 2008).

Exposure to Cold

The climate to which our skin is exposed might have great influence on the health of our skin. In winter time, winter xerosis or "winter itch" is primarily the result of low temperature and humidity (Blank, 1953). Epidemiological evidence indicates that exposure to low temperatures is associated with visible signs of skin aging, e.g., type I and II rosacea to the appearance of spider veins (Giacomani and Rein, 2010). Cold winds and low temperatures contribute to aging skin additionally by making skin dry but also heated rooms can be very drying to skin. Air conditioning in summer and heating in winter removes moisture from the air. For this reason a good skin moisturizer should be used in extreme weather conditions to prevent the loss of water from the skin. Winter skin care should consist of a cleanser that is thick and rich in texture.

Personal Care Products (PCP)

PCP are generally applied to human skin and mainly produce local exposure, although skin penetration or use in the oral cavity, on the face, lips, eyes and mucosa may also produce human systemic exposure. In the EU, U.S. and Japan, the safety of PCP is regulated under cosmetic and/or drug regulations. Ultraviolet filters have important benefits by protecting the consumer against adverse effects of UV radiation; these substances undergo a stringent safety evaluation under current international regulations prior to their marketing. Concerns were also raised about the safety of solid nanoparticles in PCP, mainly TiO2 and ZnO in sunscreens. However, current evidence suggests that these particles are non-toxic, do not penetrate into or through normal or compromised human skin and, therefore, pose no risk to human health (Nohynek et al., 2010).

Repeated Movements

Young's modules (elasticity modules) of the skin, a ratio between stress and deformation, increases linearly with age. This is in agreement with data indicating that skin becomes more rigid and less able to stretch in response to stress with age. This has to be correlated with the increased cross-linking of collagen, the disorganization of the fibril network and the large amount of free water in the dermis. Facial expressions are produced by 43 unique facial muscles, which can combine to produce over 100.000 facial movements and provide infinite variation on each emotional expression (Hillebrand, 2010). However, muscle contraction forces the skin to repetitively fold alone the same groove. With time, this repeated mechanical stress causes that groove or temporary wrinkle to etch in as a permanent or persistent wrinkle (Kligman et al., 1985). Repetitive facial movements actually lead to fine lines and wrinkles. Each time we use a facial muscle, a groove forms beneath the surface of the skin, which is why we see lines form with each facial expression. The facial skin responds to every movement of the underlying muscles in smiling, frowning, and physical movement, and such movement produces temporary but repeated wrinkling of the same portion of the face. This repeated temporary wrinkling has been suggested to play an important role in the formation of permanent wrinkles. Expression lines occur as a result of repeated fraction exerted by facial muscles that ultimately leads to the formation of deep creases over forehead and between the eyebrows (Yaar, 2006) and in nasolabial folds and periorbital areas (Puizina-Ivic, 2008). As skin ages and loses its elasticity, the skin stops springing back to its line-free state, and these grooves become permanently etched on the face as fine lines and wrinkles. While fine lines are due to the gradual breakdown of collagen and elastin fibers, and they are exacerbated by sun damage, very deep wrinkles are associated with the muscle below the skin surface. UV-induced skin damage is not the cause, but an accelerator of facial wrinkling when combined with repeated mechanical stress (Hillebrand, 2010). Muscles contract more with age to compensate for the loss of volume. The persistent facial wrinkling is thus depending on both the cumulative amount of mechanical stress in combination with the decline in skin elasticity caused byage and sun exposure. The loss of skin mechanical properties is significantly faster on sun-exposed vs. sun-protected skin sites (Jemed et al., 2001).

The American Academy of Dermatology (AAD) claims that "repetitive facial movement—like squinting—overworks facial muscles, forming a groove beneath the skin's surface. This groove eventually becomes a wrinkle. Keep those eyes wide: Wear reading glasses if you need them. And get savvy about sunglasses, which can protect skin around the eyes from sun damage and keep you from squinting.

Factors that contribute to wrinkling include changes in muscles, the loss of subcutaneous fat tissue, gravitational forces, and the loss of substance of facial bones and cartilage (Yaar, 2006). Longitudinal studies confirmed that persistent wrinkles evolve directly from temporary wrinkles (Hillebrand and Demirli, 2009). An image-based method was developed that showed that subjects' unique pattern of persistent facial wrinkling observed with a neutral expression at eightyears was predicted by the pattern of temporary wrinkling observed with a smiling expression at baseline (Hillebrand, 2001; Miyamoto and Hillebrand, 2002).

Sleeping Positions

Repeated folding of the skin during sleeping in the same position on the side of the face contributes to appearance of "sleeping lines." Histologically, thick connective tissue strands containing muscle cells are present beneath the wrinkle (Pierard et al., 2003). The deterioration of neuromuscular control contributes to wrinkle formation (Dayan et al., 1988). Resting your face on the pillow in the same way every night for years on also leads to wrinkles.

Called sleep lines, these wrinkles eventually become etched on the surface of the skin and no longer disappear when the head is not resting on the pillow. Women, who tend to sleep on their sides, are most likely to see these lines appear on their chin and cheeks. Men tend to notice these lines on the forehead since they usually sleep with the face pressed down on the pillow. People who sleep on their backs do not develop these wrinkles since their skin does not lie crumpled against the pillow.

The American Academy of Dermatology (AAD) cautions that sleeping in certain positions night after night leads to "sleep lines"—wrinkles that become etched into the surface of the skin and do not disappear once you are up. Sleeping on your side increases wrinkles on cheeks and chin, while sleeping facedown gives you a furrowed brow. To reduce wrinkle formation, the AAD says, sleep on your back.

Gravity

Gravitaional aging should also be mentioned. Skin of any part of the body is subjected to intrinsic and extrinsic mechanical forces. Among them, earth gravitation influences skin folding and sagging during aging.

The constant gravitational force also acts on the facial skin, resulting in an altered distribution of fat and sagging. Skin becomes lax, and soft tissue support is diminished. Gravitational effects with advanced years play an important role and contribute to advanced sagging.

The force of gravity that continuously acts on the body influences the skin affecting the distribution of facial soft tissues resulting in sagging and loose skin (Yaar, 2006). This factor is particularly prominent in the upper and lower eyelids, on the cheeks, and in the neck region.

Radiation

Radiation is energy in the form of waves or moving subatomic particles. Radiation can be classified as *ionizing* or *non-ionizing radiation*, depending on its effect on atomic matter. When the energy of a photon exceeds the energy needed to displace an electron from a molecule, it may cause the ionization of that molecule. Most of the biological effects of ionizing radiation are mediated by ROS. These ROS can either be generated primarily via radiolysis of water, or they may be formed by secondary reactions. A significant degree of the initial damage done to cells by ionizing radiation is due to free radical formation, particularly OH^-. Non-ionizing radiation refers to any type of electromagnetic radiation that does not carry enough energy per quantum to ionize atoms or molecules but has sufficient energy for excitation, the movement of an electron to a higher energy state. Visible and UVlight are insufficient to ionize most biomolecules. Nevertheless, human exposure to ultraviolet radiation has important public health implications. Exposure of the human skin to UV radiation leads to depletion of coutaneous antioxidants, regulation of gene expression and ultimately to the development of skin diseases. UVA and UVB radiation are known to cause several biological effects via different mechanisms, among which ROS play an importantrole.

UV Radiation and Sun Exposure

Prolonged human exposure to solar UV radiation may result in acute and chronic health effects on the skin, eye and immune system (WHO, 2010). Sunburn (erythema) is the best-known acute effect of excessive UV- radiation exposure. The difference between sunburn and suntan is only quantitative. In both cases, skin damage is formed. Melanin production is the defense reaction triggered by skin damage, but melanin cannot totally prevent skin damage from occurring. Over the longer term, UV radiation induces degenerative changes in cells of the skin, fibrous tissue and blood vessels, leading to premature skin aging, photodermatoses and actinic keratoses. Photodermatoses are skin diseases where the skin lesions are caused by light. Such lesions may be itching papules, whealing of the skin, fierce reddening and peeling, etc. Another long-term effect is an inflammatory reaction of the eye. In the most serious cases, skin cancer and cataracts can occur.

The various forms of energy, or radiation, are classified according to wavelength, measured in nanometers (nm). One nanometer is a millionth of a millimeter. The shorter the wavelength, the more energetic is the radiation. In order of decreasing energy, the principal forms of radiation are gamma rays, X rays, ultraviolet (UV) radiation, visible light, infrared (IR) radiation, microwaves and radio waves. Various types of light differ in their wavelengths, frequencies and energies; higher energy waves have higher frequencies and shorter wavelengths. Pigments inside the retina of our eyes absorb wavelengths of light between 400nm-700nm, collectively referred to as "visible light." Stratospheric oxygen and ozone molecules absorb 97% to 99% of the sun's high frequency. The ultraviolet region of the electromagnetic spectrum is subdivided into three bands termed UVA, UVB and UVC. The subdivisions are arbitrary and differ somewhat depending on the discipline involved (Diffey, 1991). Environmental photo biologists normally define the wavelength regions as: UVA, 400 to 320 nm; UVB, 320 to 290 nm; and UVC, 290 to 200 nm. The division between UVB and UVC is chosen as 290 nm since ultraviolet radiation (UVR) at shorter wavelengths is unlikely to be present in terrestrial sunlight, except at high altitudes (Henderson, 1977).

UVC can form oxidants by photolysis of H2O; UVA and UVB generate oxidants through photodynamic action such as dissociation of H2O2. It is believed that direct absorbtion of energy by DNA and the formation of thymidine dimmers is more significant to skin carcinogenesis than the formation of free radicals. The deep wrinkles, age spots, and leathery skin indicate premature aging caused by years of unprotected exposure to the sun. Dermal thinning, loss of dermal collagen and decreased lipid production are complicated by the effects of life-long sun exposure. These changes manifest as wrinkling, loss of elasticity, dryness and textural changes that characterize mature skin (for more information on skin sun damage, see chapter on skin UV and photoaging). The intensity of solar UV reaching the earth's atmosphere would probably be lethal to most living organisms on the earth's surface without the shielding afforded by ozone layer in the atmosphere. Solar UV undergoes absorption and scattering as it passes through the earth's atmosphere with absorption by molecular oxygen and ozone being the most important processes. The ozone layer prevents almost all UV of wavelengths lambda < 290 nm and a substantial fraction (in excess of 90% of the total energy) from 290 to 315 nm from reaching the earth's surface (WHO, Ultraviolet radiation, Environmental health criteria: 160). Terrestrial life is dependent on radiant energy from the sun. Before the beginning of this century, the sun was essentially the only source of UVR, but with the advent of artificial sources the opportunity for additional exposure has increased (IARC, 2010). Everyone is exposed to UV radiation from the sun, and an increasing number of people are exposed to artificial sources used in industry, commerce and recreation. Emissions from the sun include visible light, heat and UV radiation. Approximately 5% of solar terrestrial radiation is ultraviolet radiation (UVR), and solar radiation is the major source of human exposure to UVR. Ultraviolet radiation is a form of electromagnetic energy. Generally, the shorter the wavelength, the more biologically damaging UV radiation can be if it reaches the Earth in sufficient quantities. UVA is the least damaging (longest wavelength) form of UV radiation and reaches the Earth in greatest quantity. Most UVA rays pass right through the ozone layer in the stratosphere. UVB radiation can be very harmful. Fortunately, most of the Sun's UVB radiation is absorbed by ozone in the stratosphere.

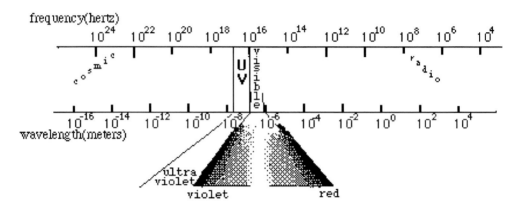

Figure 13. UV specter.

UVB is typically the most destructive form of UV radiation because it has enough energy to cause photochemical damage to cellular DNA, yet not enough to be completely absorbed by the atmosphere. UVB is needed by humans for synthesis of vitamin D; however, harmful effects can include erythema (sunburn), cataracts, and development of skin cancer. Most solar UVB is blocked by ozone in the atmosphere, and there is concern that reductions in atmospheric ozone could increase the prevalence of skin cancer. Individuals working outdoors are at the greatest risk of UVB effects.

UVA is the most commonly encountered type of UV light. UVA exposure has an initial pigment-darkening effect (tanning) followed by erythema if the exposure is excessive. Atmospheric ozone absorbs very little of this part of the UV spectrum. UVA is also needed by humans for synthesis of vitamin D; however, overexposure to UVA has been associated with toughening of the skin, suppression of the immune system, and cataract formation. UVA light is often called black light. Most phototherapy and tanning booths use UVA lamps.

UVC radiation is potentially the most damaging because it is very energetic. Fortunately, all UVC is absorbed by oxygen and ozone in the stratosphere and never reaches the Earth's surface.

In order to understand and avoid the damaging effects of UVR, it is important in the first place to understand the environmental factors that influence the UV level. According to World Health Organization they are (WHO, 2010):

- Sun height—the higher the sun in the sky, the higher the UV radiation level. Thus, UV radiation varies with time of day and time of year, with maximum levels occurring when the sun is at its maximum elevation, at around midday (solar noon) during the summer months.
- Latitude—the closer the equator, the higher the UV radiation levels.

- Cloud cover—UV radiation levels are highest under cloudless skies. Even with cloud cover, UV radiation levels can be high due to the scattering of UV radiation by water molecules and fine particles in the atmosphere.
- Altitude—at higher altitudes, a thinner atmosphere filters less UV radiation. With every 1,000-meter increase in altitude, UV levels increase by 10% to 12%.
- Ozone—ozone absorbs some of the UV radiation that would otherwise reach the Earth's surface. Ozone levels vary over the year and even across the day.
- Ground reflection—UV radiation is reflected or scattered to varying extents by different surfaces, e.g., snow can reflect as much as 80% of UV radiation, dry beach sand about 15%, and sea foam about 25%.

People are largely unaware of the degree of these changes. At noon, when the sun is overhead, the level of UV at a wavelength of 300 nm is ten times greater than at either three hours before (9 am) or three hours after noon (3 pm). An untanned person with fair skin may receive a mild sunburn in as little as 25 minutes at noon (depending on the time of year and the latitude) but would have to lie in the sun for at least two hours to receive the same dose after 3 pm (WHO, Ultraviolet radiation, Environmental health criteria: 160). The global biologically effective UV falling on a horizontal surface occurs primarily during the midday hours, about 50% during the four hours centered on noontime zenith (Sliney, 1987).

Infrared Radiation (IR)

Most research regarding extrinsic skin aging was dedicated to UV radiation. Until recently, it has become evident that also other parts of the solar electromagnetic spectrum (e.g., IR) could induce skin damage and influence the increased skin-aging process (Schroeder and Krutmann, 2010). Solar radiation is divided into three bands: ultraviolet (UV), visible light and infrared radiation (760 to 4000 nm). IR is further subdivided into IR-A (λ=760 to 1440 nm), IR-B (λ= 1440 to 3000 nm) and IR-C (λ=3000 nm to 1mm). While the proton energy of IR is lower than that of UV, the total amount of solar energy reaching humans' skin contains approximately 54% IR, while UV only accounts for 5% to 7% (Kochevar et al., 2007). Most of the IR lies within IR-A band (approximately 30% of total solar energy), which deeply penetrates human skin, while IR-B and IR-C only penetrate the upper skin layer (Kochevar et al., 1999). In comparison, IR-A penetrates better than UV into the skin, with approximately 50% reaching the dermis (Kochevar et al., 2007; Cobarg, 1995). Molecular mechanisms of damaging effect of IR-A on the skin is attributed to the induction of matrix mtalloproteinase-1, as well as ROS generation (Schroeder et al., 2004). After IR-A irradiation, the cellular ROS are increased in irradiated cells and a disturbance of the cellular glutathione occurs (Schroeder et al., 2004) leading to a shift of the GSH/GSSG equilibrium towards the oxidized forms. Since there are no chemical or physical UV filters available thathave shown to provide IRA protection, the use of antioxidants seems to be promising.

Metal Ions

Many metal ions are necessary for normal cell metabolism, but in higher concentrations, they might represent a health risk. Increased rates of ROS generation have often been suggested as contributors of toxicity during exposure to high levels of metal ions, e.g., iron, copper, lead, cobalt, mercury, nickel, chromium, selenium and arsenic but not manganese and zinc. These transition metal ions are redox active and can play an important role in ROS production in the cell. Reduced forms of redox active metal ions participate in the Fenton reaction where hydroxyl radical is generated from hydrogen peroxide. Furthermore, the Haber-Weiss reaction, which involves the oxidized forms of redox active metal ions and superoxide anion, generates the reduced form of metal ion, which can be coupled to Fenton chemistry to generate hydroxyl radical.

Fenton reaction:

$$\text{Metal}^{(n+1)} + H_2O_2 \rightarrow \text{Metal}^{(n+1)+} + HO^{\cdot} + H_2O$$

Haber-Weiss reaction

$$\text{Metal}^{(n+1)+} + 2O_2^{\cdot -} \rightarrow \text{Metal}^{(n+1)} + O_2$$

Redox cycling is a characteristic of transition metals (Klein et al., 1991), and Fenton-like production of ROS appear to be involved for iron-, copper-, chromium-, and vanadium-mediated tissue damage (Fuchs, 2001). Thus, it is clear that any increase in the levels of superoxide anion, hydrogen peroxide or the redox active metal ions are likely to lead to the formation of high levels of hydroxyl radical by the chemical mechanisms listed above. Therefore, the valence state and bioavailability of redox active metal ions are key determinants in its ability to participate in the generation of reactive oxygen species.

Metal Ions and Skin

Skin manifestations of metal toxicity mainly comprise irritant contact dermatitis (ICD) and allergic contact dermatitis (ACD) (Fuchs, 2001). Metal ions are important causes of human allergies, and the majority of metals induce allergicreactions in the skin. Through their chelating abilities, mercury (II), palladium (II), platinum (II), and gold (III) may directly from protein adducts and thus alter self-proteins (Schuppe et al., 1998). In particular, nickel (II), cobalt (II), chromium (III,VI), mercury (I,II), gold (III), platinum(II), and palladium (II) cause ACD in human skin. In rare cases, immediate contact urticarial(ICU), systemic allergic reactions (SAR), or granulomatous reactions to metals (e.g.,aluminium, beryllium) have been observed. At least nickel, cadmium, lead, chromium,beryllium, and arsenic are proven or putative human carcinogens and a possible role ofoxidative damage in metal-induced carcinogenesis is emerging (Klein et al., 1991; Kasprzak, 1991; Standeven and Wetterhahn, 1991; Kasprzak, 1995).

Metal-mediated formation of free radicals causes various modifications to DNA bases, enhanced lipid peroxidation, and altered calcium and sulfhydryl homeostasis. Lipid peroxides, formed by the attack of radicals on polyunsaturated fatty acid residues of phospholipids, can further react with redox metals finally producing mutagenic and carcinogenic malondialdehyde, 4-hydroxynonenal and other exocyclic DNA adducts (etheno and/or propano adducts). Whilst iron (Fe), copper (Cu), chromium (Cr), vanadium (V) and cobalt (Co) undergo redox-cycling reactions, for a second group of metals, mercury (Hg), cadmium (Cd) and nickel (Ni), the primary route for their toxicity is depletion of glutathione and bonding to sulfhydryl groups of proteins. Arsenic (As) is thought to bind directly to critical thiols; however, other mechanisms, involving formation of hydrogen peroxide under physiological conditions, have been proposed. The unifying factor in determining toxicity and carcinogenicity for all these metals is the generation of reactive oxygen and nitrogen species. Common mechanisms involving the Fenton reaction, generation of the superoxide radical and the hydroxyl radical appear to be involved for iron, copper, chromium, vanadium and cobalt primarily associated with mitochondria, microsomes and peroxisomes. The carcinogenic effect of these metals has been related to activation of mainly redox-sensitive transcription factors, involving NF-kappaB, AP-1 and p53. Antioxidants (both enzymatic and non-enzymatic) provide protection against deleterious metal-mediated free radical attacks. e.g., vitamin E and melatonin can prevent the majority of metal-mediated (iron, copper, cadmium) damage both in vitro systems and in metal-loaded animals (Valko et al., 2005).

Age-related changes in fibroblasts due to the metal-catalyzed oxidation of proteins lead to an exponential increase in the concentration of protein carbonyl groups in tissue samples taken from people aged 10 to 80 years (Rockuet and Bonte, 2002). Oxidative damage to proteins may be most important in aging because oxidized proteins become inactive and can accumulate in the cell, thereby triggering programmed cell death. ROS increase the carbonyl content of proteins by forming aldehydes and ketones from certain aminoacid residues (Berlett and Stadtman, 1997; Stadtman and Berlett, 1997).

Iron Chelators

Iron plays a critical role in oxidative reactions as a catalyst in the Fenton reaction so that cellular levels of free iron need to be kept low. Because cutaneous iron catalyses ROS generation, it is thought to play a key role in photoaging. Iron is essential to almost all forms of life. However, excess iron is potentially toxic as its catalytic activity induces the generation of ROS. Iron-catalyzed ROS generation is involved in numerous pathological conditions, including cutaneous damage. When skin is directly exposed to UVR, cutaneous intracellular catalytic iron levels increase because of the release of iron from iron-binding proteins such as ferritin. Consequently, the subsequent ROS generation may overwhelm cutaneous defense systems such as the cellular iron sequestration and ROS scavenging capacity. The harmful role of excess cutaneous iron implies that there may be a potential for topical iron chelator treatments (Kitazawa et al., 2006). The intracellular storage protein, ferritin may, therefore, play a critical role in cellular antioxidant defense. UVA radiation (and other oxidant stress) leads to high levels of expression of the heme oxygenase 1 gene (HO1) (Keyse and Tyrrell, 1989), which, in turn, leads to the catabolism of heme and release of free iron. The increased ferritin levels that result appear to be directly responsible for a UVA-mediated adaptive response involving the protection of human fibroblast membranes against subsequent UVA radiation damage (Vileet al.,1994).

Ferritin thus constitutes the major storage site for nonmetabolized intracellular iron and, therefore, plays a critical role in regulating the availability of iron to catalyze certain harmful reactions such as the Fenton reaction and peroxidation of lipids. This inducible response, HO-1, is seen in human skin fibroblasts but not in epidermal keratinocytes (Applegate et al., 1991).

However, high HO activity is always notable in the keratinocytes (150% to 300% higher than in matching dermal fibroblasts) presumably due to the constitutively high level of HO-2 mRNA present, which is also linked to 3.0 times higher levels of the protective protein ferritin in the epidermis. As dermal fibroblasts are shielded from UV radiation to a considerable extent by the overlying epidermis with its stratum corneum, the adaptive response mediated by HO-1 is perhaps more appropriate and metabolically economic for fibroblasts, whereas keratinocytes require the constitutive pathway that appears to involve HO-2. To sum up, in both epidermal and dermal skin cells, both the constitutive and inducible pathway of HO are closely linked to the intracellular levels of the iron storage protective protein, ferritin (Laurent-Applegate and Schwarzkopf, 2001).

Applegate and Frenk (1995) reported that skin cells derived from chronically sun-exposed areas have higher cellular levels of ferritin (Applegate and Frenk, 1995). In this respect, authors observed that the epidermal keratinocytes have up to six fold higher levels of ferritin than the underlying dermal fibroblasts. Thus, the keratinocyte, as clearly the primary target for oxidative stress generated by solar UV irradiation, would benefit from the continuous protection provided by the high levels of ferritin (Laurent-Applegate and Schwarzkopf, 2001).

Iron-catalyzed ROS generation is involved in numerous pathological conditions, including cutaneous damage. When skin is directly exposed to UVR, cutaneous intracellular catalytic iron levels increase because of the release of iron from iron-binding proteins such as ferritin. Consequently, the subsequent ROS generation may overwhelm cutaneous defense systems such as the cellular iron sequestration and ROS scavenging capacity. The harmful role of excess cutaneous iron implies that there may be a potential for topical iron chelator treatments (Kitazawa et al., 2006).

Because cutaneous iron catalyzes ROS generation, sequestering iron by chelating agents is thought to be an effective approach toward preventing photoaging. N-(4-pyridoxylmethylene)-l-serine (PYSer) was designed as an antioxidant to suppress iron-catalyzed ROS generation by its iron-sequestering activity. In the study by Kitazawa et al.(2005), PYSer showed protective effects against skin damage in hairless mice irradiated with ultraviolet B (UVB). Topical application of PYSer to the skin significantly delayed and/or decreased the visible wrinkle formation induced by chronic UVB irradiation. A histological study indicated that UVB-induced epidermal hypertrophy and lymphocytic infiltration were suppressed by PYSer. These results indicate that PYSer is a promising antioxidant for the prevention of chronic skin photoaging by its iron-sequestering activity.

It was reported that also melanin from the skin might serve a protective role other than photoprotection (Liu et al., 2004). Melanin is able to effectively ligate metal ions through its carboxylate and phenolic hydroxyl groups, in many cases much more efficiently than the powerful chelating ligand ethylenediaminetetraacetate (EDTA). It may thus serve to sequester potentially toxic metal ions, protecting the rest of the cell. Topical application of iron chelators were also reported to reduce erythema, epidermal and dermal hypertrophy, wrinkle formation, tumor appearance. It has been proposed that iron chelators can be useful agents against damaging effects of both short- and long-term UV exposure.

Organic Solvents

"Organic solvents are commonly used for cleaning, degreasing, and extraction and are ubiquitous environmental pollutants. Solvents can be divided into families according to the chemical structure and the attached functional groups. The basic structures are aliphatic, alicyclic, and aromatic. The functional groups include halogens, alcohols, ketons, glycols, esters, ethers, carboxylic acids, amines, and amides.

"Solvents that are soluble in both lipid and water phase are readily absorbed through the skin. A few solvents are known to cause allergic contact dermatitis (e.g., aldehydes, amines, glycolethers), and in rare cases chemical scleroderma in susceptible patients. However, the majority of organic solvents are primary skin irritants as a result of skin defatting, which is related to their lipophilicity, or act through denaturation of proteins or perturbation of membranes. Defatting the epidermis results in disruption of the skin barrier function and is associated with an increased transepidermal water loss, finally leading to irritant contact dermatitis" (Fuchs, 2001).

A direct correlation between antioxidant levels and skin reactivity to irritants was found, which suggested that oxidative stress plays a general role in the pathophysiology of acute ICD (Winyard andBlake, 1997). Most organic solvents are believed to trigger skin inflammation by defatting the epidermis.

Disturbed epidermal lipid composition can result in increased production and release of pro-oxidant cytokines from keratinocytes, such as TNF-α. Thus formation of ROS is a late event in the inflammatory cascade triggered by organic solvents. Besides, several studies have shown depletion of low-molecular-weight antioxidants and increased production of ROS in the inflammatory phase of ACD (Sarnstrand et al., 1999; Miyachi et al., 1985; Sharkey et al., 1991).

Synergistic/Antagonistic Effect

There might form a synergistic effect when we are exposed to two or more environmental pollutants. An antagonistic effect between environmental pollutants and the skin antioxidant level could be formed as well. Research demonstrates that UVA combined with environmental pollutants (including cigarette smoke) significantly increases the risk of skin cancer. Similarly synergistic effect was demonstrated between environmental pollutants and UV: e.g., when ozone exposure precedes UV exposure, there is enhancement of UV-induced depletion of protective vitamin E from the skin's stratum corneum (Burke and Wei, 2009).

It should be taken into consideration the fact that skin is constantly exposed to several environmental pollutants each day and the possible additive effect among them should be evaluated in order to find strategies to prevent exogenous oxidative stress exposure.

Twin Studies Related to Skin Aging

Environmental factors, which could damage skin or accelerate the skin-aging process, were presented. What about the genetic impact on skin aging? Some studies on twins could help us to answer this question.

Twins have identical DNA, but they experience different lives. Different habits and life experiences over the years should affect the way they look like. Research published by Martires et al. (2009) found highly correlated photodamage scores among both monozygotic (identical) and dizygotic (fraternal) twins. Examination of monozygotic, as well as dizygotic twins, allows a unique opportunity to control forgenetic differences. The recent study of twins provides an opportunityto control for genetic susceptibility in order to elucidateenvironmental influences on skin aging (Kathryn et al., 2009). The study found the relationships between smoking, weight, sunscreen use, skin cancer, and photodamagein these twin pairs. Results may help to motivate the reduction of riskybehaviors. Kathryn and colleagues studied 65 pairs of twins attending the 2002 annual Twin Days Festival in Twinsburg, Ohio. A total of 130 individuals completed surveys collecting information about skin type, history of skin cancer, smoking and drinking habits and weight. Clinicians assigned each participant a photodamage score, graded by such characteristics as wrinkling and change in pigmentation. Photodamage scores were highly correlated among both monozygotic (identical) and dizygotic (fraternal) twins. Other factors associated with higher levels of photodamage included a history of skin cancer, heavier weight and smoking, whereas alcohol consumption was associated with lower photodamage scores. Sunscreen use, for example, was negatively correlated with the extent of an individual's photodamage, as was alcohol consumption. However, cigarette smoke was positively correlated with photodamage—more cigarettes smoked or a history of smoking was associated with an aged appearance of skin. Also Doshi et al. (2007) and Antell and Taczanowski (1999) reported a significant difference in facial aging between twins with smoking differences. Rexbie et al. (2006) investigated 1,826 Danish twin sets over the age of 70 and reported that smoking 20 cigarettes per day per year for 20 years increased perceived age by one year. For women, this number was increased to 20 cigarettes per day for 40 years. Guyuron (2009) reported that approximately tenyears of smoking difference lead to a 2.5 years older appearance.

Several studies have identified an inverse relationship between BMI and facial wrinkling (Rowe and Guyuron, 2010). Self-reported weight was found to correlate with the photodamage score, but the relationship changed as participants got older. In individuals younger than 45, excess fat seemed to correlate with higher levels of photodamage. According to the researchers, this finding is contradictory to previous Danish research that reported the higher the body mass index the lower the levels of facial aging. According to the study, the relationships between self-reported weight, lipid intake and levels of photodamage to the skin are complicated. A number of animal studies have suggested that higher fat intake could increase skin sensitivity to UV damage; but, in contrast, some lipids may potentially have antioxidative and, therefore, protective effects.

In addition, in individuals older than 45, the relationship was reversed, and higher weight was correlated with reduced photodamage. The researchers suggested that although excess fat might make skin more susceptible to UV damage, it could also mask the appearance of wrinkles in older age (Martires et al.,2009). Nevertheless, Leung and Harvey (2002) found that sun exposure alone did not have a significant effect on the perceived age. In their study, it was reported that 30 years of sun exposure for fivehours per day only produced 1.5 years of perceived difference. Also Guinot et al. (2002) found that photodamage did not contribute considerably to the age score. On the contrary, sun exposure was correlated with increased perceived age in the study of Rexbye et al. (2006), and additionally Guyuron et al. (2009) reported that the increase in sun exposure as well as the participation in outdoor activities both significantly increased perceived age, and the use of sunscreen significantly decreased perceived age. Additionally, several studies reported that face wrinkling is significantly negatively correlated with BMI (Guinot et al., 2002; Purba et al., 2001). Guyuron et al. (2009) showed that the influence of BMI on wrinkling is dependent on the age of twin set. If twins were younger than 40 years of age, a four-point increase in BMI was associated with a perceived older appearance. On the other hand, with a four-point increase in BMI in twins older than 40 years of age, there was an association with the perceived younger appearance. Eight-point higher body mass index was associated with an older appearance in twins younger than age 55 but was associated with a younger appearance after age 55.

A study of what causes aging in identical twins published in the journal *Plastic and Reconstructive Surgery* examined how a lifetime of good or bad habits made twins look younger or older compared to their once identical counterparts (Guyuron et al., 2009). External social factors have been found to significantly alter biological aging. Being divorced or taking antidepressants made people appear older, suggesting that a stressful life can take a toll on your appearance. Also, Osler et al. (2007) reported that twins that were divorced, widowed, or never married had higher depression scores and smoked more than their married counterparts. The study of Guyuron et al. (2009) found that the use of antidepressants led to an increase in perceived age. Additionally, in the analysis of twins, women who were divorced were perceived to be approximately 1.7 years older than those who were either single or married. What is more, the longer the twins smoked, the older they appeared. Increased sun exposure was associated with an older appearance and accelerated with age, as was a history of outdoor activities and lack of sunscreen use. Twins who used hormone replacement therapy had a younger appearance. Facial rhytids were more evident in twins with a history of skin cancer and in those who smoked. Dark and patchy skin discoloration was less prevalent in twins with a higher body mass index and more common in twins with a history of smoking and those with sun exposure. Hair quantity was better with a higher body mass index although worse with a history of skin cancer and better with the use of hormones. Twin studies offer statistical evidence to support the role of some of the known factors that govern facial aging.

Discriminating between the levels of involvement of both aging processes, intrinsic and extrinsic, is problematic since both processes continually occur and could interact between each other. Intrinsic changes of the face include those of the skin, subcutaneous tissue, dermal appendages, facial musculature, as well as the facial skeleton. The process of extrinsic facial aging causes progressive damage at both the molecular and cellular level and, unlike intrinsic aging, most extrinsic factors exert their effects at the skin level only (Rowe and Guyuron, 2010). Both intrinsic and extrinsic aging share many of the features and possible mechanisms. In both photoaging and chronological aging of the skin, the involvement of elevated free radical production and elevated concentrations of degraded collagen are present. Furthermore, both mechanisms of aging have been theorized to occur as a result of oxidative damage (Sohal and Weindruch, 1996). Reactive oxygen and nitrogen species are responsible for endogenous and exogenous skin aging and damage. ROS oxidize lipids and proteins, initiate the generation of proinflammatory cytokines *in vitro*, damage DNA, downregulate the immune response, induce apoptosis and play a critical role in altering the structure of the skin.

During both intrinsic and extrinsic aging free radical formation and consequently free radical-induced damage appears. Additionally, cellular energy levels decline during intrinsic and extrinsic aging as well, and consequently the capacity of the skin to counteract stress and induction of repair mechanisms declines with aging. Decreased compensation of environmental stress and insufficient repair, in turn, accelerate skin aging, which consequently leads to further decline of cellular energy levels in the skin (Blatt et al., 2010).

Intrinsic and extrinsic aging depends on genetic predisposition, living environment and lifestyle. While there is not much an individual can do about genes or environmental pollution, there is much one can do about their lifestyle by implementing methods that positively influence the aging velocity, so that significant improvement of skin aging could be achieved. More on this topic is discussed later in the book. For example: the study conducted by Rexbye et al. (2006)evaluated influence of environmental factors on facial aging(Rexbye et al., 2006). Results revealed statistically significant determinants of facial aging associated with high-perceived age for men were smoking, sun exposure and low body mass index (BMI), while for women they were low BMI and low social class. The number of children (men) and marital status and depression symptomatology score (women) were borderline significantly associated with facial aging. This study confirms previous findings of a negative influence of sun exposure, smoking and a low BMI on facial aging. Furthermore, this study indicates that high social status, low depression score and being married are associated with a younger look, but the strength of the associations varies between genders.

Another study by Guinot et al. (2002) determined whether certain lifestyle habits known to have effects on skin aging were related to the discrepancies between chronological age and the skin age score. Significant effects were identified for phototype, body mass index, menopausal status, degree of lifetime sun exposure, and number of years of cigarette smoking. However, these factors accounted for only 10% of the discrepancies. Moreover, most skin characteristics used reflected changes understood to represent intrinsic aging rather than photodamage or other extrinsic factors. The study concludes that factors related to the rate of intrinsic aging seem to play a larger role than previously suspected.

Certain measures can be taken to prevent extrinsic and intrinsic premature aging. Many of the internal and external causes of aging skin are determined by the health and lifestyle decisionsonemakes every day. Making unhealthy choices can cause prematurely aging skin, and this makes you look older too early. In further chapters, lifestyle decisions thathave beneficial effects on skin aging are additionally discussed, as well as bad habitsthatshould be avoided.

Chapter 6

Mechanisms of Skin UV and Photoaging

Wear a sunscreen every day of your life, or live a shady life as possible.

Prof. Albert Kligman

Because UV and photoaging playvery important roles in skin aging, this chapter describes their damaging effects on skin in a more detailed way. Unlike chronological aging, which depends on the passage of time per se, photoaging depends primarily on the degree of sun exposure and skin pigment. Individuals who have outdoor lifestyles, live in sunny climates, and are lightly pigmented will experience the greatest degree of UVR skin penetration and thus suffer from the effects of the photoaging (Fisher et al., 2002).

What are the clinical signs of skin aging and photoaging:

The term "photoaging" (also known as "Dermatoheliosis") was first coined in 1986, and describes the effects of chronic ultraviolet (UV) light exposure on skin (Kligman and Kligman, 1986). Photoaging refers to the physiologic and pathological changes that occur specifically inaged tissue that has experienced chronic sun exposure over time. Human skin aging resulting from UV irradiation is a cumulative process that occurs based on the degree of sun exposure and the level of skin pigment. Many of the skin changes commonly associated with aging, changes in pigmentation, sallowness, and deep wrinkling, are caused mainly by sun exposure. Clinical signs of photoaging include wrinkles; mottled pigmentation; rough skin, and loss of skin tone; dryness; irregular, dark/light pigmentation; sallowness; either deep furrows or severe atrophy; telangiectases; premalignant lesions; laxity; and a leathery appearance (Yaar, Eller, and Gilchrest, 2002). Other signs include elastosis (a coarse, yellow, cobblestoned effect of the skin) and actinic purpura (easy bruising related to vascular wall fragility in the dermis) (Gilchrest, 1990). Sun-exposed areas of the skin, such as the face, neck, upper chest, hands, and forearms, are the sites where these changes occur most often (Rosi Helfrich et al., 2008).Chronologic skin aging, on the other hand, is characterized by laxity and fine wrinkling, as well as development of benign growths such as seborrheic keratoses and angiomas but is not associated with increased pigmentation or the deep wrinkles that characterize photoaging (Yaar et al., 2002). Seborrheic keratoses are regarded as the best biomarker of intrinsic skin aging since its appearance is independent of sun exposure. While intrinsically aged skin does not show vascular damage, photodamaged skin does.

Studies in humans and in the skh-1 (albino and hairless) mouse model for skin aging have shown that acute and chronic UVB irradiation greatly increases skin vascularization and angiogenesis (Bielenber et al., 1998; Yano et al., 2002).

Skin Exposure to UVR

The sun is the main source of UVR and the main contributor to the photoaging. In order to understand sun's effects on the skin, a brief introduction on basic characteristics of UV light and its environmental exposure will be presented again. Solar radiation reaching the Earth's surface includes wavelengths in the range 290 to 4000 nm and is divided into three bands: UV radiation (290 to 400 nm), visible light (400 to 760 nm) and IR (760 to 4000 nm). UV radiation (100 to 400 nm) comprises only 5% of the terrestrial solar radiation. Sun's ultraviolet radiation is divided into categories based on the wavelength.

- UVC - 100 to 290 nm
- UVB - 290 to 320 nm
- UVA - 320 to 400 nm

  - UVC Radiation. UVC radiation is almost completely absorbed by the ozone layer and does not affect the skin. UVC radiation can be found in artificial sources such as mercury arc lamps and germicidal lamps.
  - UVB Radiation. UVB affects the outer layer of skin, the epidermis, and is the primary agent responsible for sunburns. It is the most intense between the hours of 10:00 am and 2:00 pm, when the sunlight is brightest. It is also more intense in the summer months, accounting for 70% of a person's yearly UVB dose. UVB does not penetrate glass.
  - UVA Radiation. UVA was once thought to have a minor effect on skin damage, but now studies are showing that UVA is a major contributor to skin damage. UVA penetrates deeper into the skin and works more efficiently. The intensity of UVA radiation is more constant than UVB without the variations during the day and throughout the year. UVA is also not filtered by glass.

According to Laurent-Applegate and Schwarzkopf (2001) "the UVA has greater penetration (e.g., about 20% at 365 nm). Whereas UVB is much more damaging to the skin than UVA if equal exposures are carried out; the deeper penetration of UVA and its greater abundance in sunlight (about 95% UVA, 5% UVB) suggest that it can also be a significant contributor to damage (Halliwell and Gutteridge, 2007). As the photons in the UVA waveband are less energetic, significantly more photons are needed to cause the same damage as that induced by the shorter wavelengths in the UVB region. It is important to remember that UVA photons are present in sunlight in much higher quantities than those of UVB and that these longer wavelengths have the potential to penetrate into the dermis to a far greater extent than UVB because of its less energetic potential" (Laurent-Applegate and Schwarzkopf, 2001). All the time during human history, people tried to avoid direct sun exposure. During evolution, poor skin lost some of endogenous sun protection. The skin was less protected by hairs and melanine. Already in the middle age, it was known the damaging effect of sun, which caused "farmer's skin," and pale skin was appreciated. In the last decades, this trend changed. Dark skin complexion was propagated as a sign of "healthy skin." The exposure of human skin to environmental and artificial ultraviolet irradiation has increased significantly in the last 50 years. This is not only due to an increased solar UV irradiation as a consequence of the stratospheric ozone depletion, but also the result of an inappropriate social behavior with the use of tanning parlors being very popular. Besides this, leisure activities and living style with travelling to equatorial regions also add to the individual annual UV load. Total UVR load depends on time of exposure, duration and intensity of exposure. Since the population in industrialized countries shows an increasing total lifespan, in parallel the cumulative lifetime dose of solar and artificial UV irradiation is dramatically augmented (Grether-Beck et al., 2005).

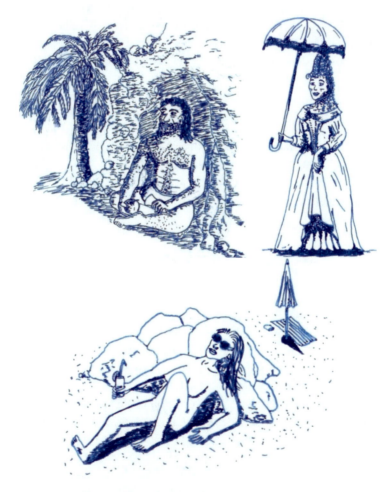

Figure 14. Sun exposure during human history (picture made by Florian Probst).

While there is no standard measure, sun exposure can be generally classified as intermittent or chronic, and the effects may be considered acute or cumulative. Intermittent sun exposure is obtained sporadically, usually during recreational activities, and particularly by indoor workers who have only weekends or vacations to be outdoors and whose skin has not adapted to the sun. Chronic sun exposure is incurred by consistent, repetitive sun exposure during outdoor work or recreation. Acute sun exposure is obtained over a short time period on skin that has not adapted to the sun (National Cancer Institute).UV-induced extrinsic aging is visible on chronically UV-exposed skin areas in persons frequently engaged in outdoor activities. Exposed skin surface is irradiated differently depending on cultural and social behavior, clothing, the position of the sun in the sky and the relative position of the body. Exposure to UVB of the most exposed skin surfaces, such as nose, tops of the ears and forehead, relative to that of the lesser exposed areas, such as underneath the chin, normally ranges over an order of magnitude. Ground reflectance plays a major role in exposure to UVB of the eyes and shaded skin surfaces, particularly with highly reflective surfaces such as snow (IARC, 2010). The cumulative annual exposure dose of solar UVR varies widely among individuals in a given population, depending to a large extent on occupation and extent of outdoor activities (IARC, 2010). For example, it has been estimated that indoor workers in mid-latitudes (40 to 60 oN) receive an annual exposure dose of solar UVR to the face of about 40 to 160 times the MED, depending upon propensity for outdoor activities, whereas the annual solar exposure dose for outdoor workers is typically around 250 times the MED. Because few actual measurements have been reported of personal exposures, these estimates should be considered to be very approximate and subject to differences in cultural and social behavior, clothing, occupation and outdoor activities. Cumulative annual outdoor exposures may be augmented by exposures to artificial sources of UVR. For example, the use of cosmetic tanning appliances increased in popularity in the 1980s. The majority of users are young women, and the median annual exposure dose is probably 20 to 30 times the "minimal erythema dose" (MED). Currently, used appliances emit primarily UVA radiation; prior to the 1980s, tanning lamps emitted higher proportions of UVB and UVC (IARC, 2010).

Ozone Depletion and UVR

The quality and quantity of ultraviolet radiation at the Earth's surface depend on the energy output of the Sun and the transmission properties of the atmosphere. From a biological viewpoint, UVB radiation is by far the most significant part of the terrestrial ultraviolet spectrum, and the levels of radiation in this waveband reaching the surface of the Earth are largely controlled by ozone, a gas which comprises approximately one molecule out of every two million in the atmosphere (Diffey, 1991). Ozone layer in the stratosphere is also the major barrier to UVC (and largely to UVB). Depletion of this layer may result in more UVB reaching the Earth's surface, with the corresponding increase in photochemical damage to living organisms. It has been estimated that each 5% depletion of stratospheric ozone will raise UVB flux at ground level by 10%. Up to 10% of UVB light falling on the skin can penetrate the epidermis to reach the dermis. In 1974, Molina and Rowland (Molina and Rowland, 1974) first warned that chlorofluorocarbons (CFCs) and other gases released by human activities could alter the natural balance of creative and destructive processes and lead to depletion of the stratospheric ozone layer. Substantial reductions of up to 50% in the ozone column observed in the austral spring over Antarctica and first reported in 1985 (Farmanet al.,1985) are continuing (SORG, 1990). Coupled with this, there has been a statistically significant downward trend in wintertime total ozone over the northern hemisphere of about

2% to 3% per decade for the past 30 years, although summertime ozone levels have remained approximately constant (Frederick, 1990). In its report in June 1990, the UK Stratospheric Ozone Review Group concluded that there are serious limitations in our understanding and ability to quantify ozone depletion at the present levels of contaminant release and in our ability to predict the effects on stratospheric ozone of any further increases (SORG, 1990).The atmosphere has a profound effect on the irradiance thatreaches the surface of the earth. In January (in the northern hemisphere) or July (in the southern hemisphere), when the solar elevation is low, direct UV travels a longer path through the atmosphere, and a large amount of scattering occurs. In addition, much of the resultant scattered UV propagates downwards to the earth's surface at angles to the horizontal that are larger than the solar elevation, hence travelling a shorter and less absorptive path. This results in large ratios of scattered to direct UV. During the summer, the ratio of diffuse to direct UV is smaller (International programme on chemical safety, Environmental Health Criteria,,160).

Factors Affecting Terrestrial UVR

As already mentioned, the spectral irradiance of UVR at the Earth's surface is modified by temporal, geographical and meteorological factors (Frederick et al., 1989).

According to Diffey (1991) the following factors contribute significantly to terrestrial UVR intensity:

- *Time of day.* About 20% to 30% of total daily UVR is received one hour either side of midday in summer, with 75% between 9 am and 3 pm.
- *Season.* In temperate regions, the biologically damaging UVR reaching the Earth's surface shows strong seasonal dependence. However, seasonal variation is much less nearer the equator.
- *Geographical latitude.* Annual UVR flux decreases with increasing distance from the equator.
- *Clouds.* Clouds reduce solar irradiance at the Earth's surface, although changes in the ultraviolet region are not as great as those of total intensity, since water in clouds attenuates solar infrared much more than UVR. The risk of overexposure may be increased under these conditions because the warning sensation of heat is diminished. Light clouds scattered over a blue sky make little difference to UVR intensity unless directly covering the sun, whilst complete light cloud cover reduces terrestrial UVR to about one-half of that from a clear sky. Even with heavy cloud cover, the scattered ultraviolet component of sunlight (often called skylight) is seldom less than 10% of that under clear sky (Paltridge and Barton,, 1978). However, very heavy storm clouds can virtually eliminate terrestrial UVR, even in summertime (Diffey, 1988).
- *Surface reflection.* Reflection of UVR from ground surfaces, including the sea, is normally low (<7%). However, gypsum sand reflects about 25% of incident UVB and fresh snow about 30% (Doda and Green, 1980, 1981), although other authors (McCullough, 1970; Blumthaler and Ambach, 1985) have reported that the UVB reflectance of fresh snow exceeds 80%.

- *Altitude.* In general, each 1 km increase in altitude increases the ultraviolet flux by about 6% (Cutchis, 1980). Conversely, places on the Earth's surface below sea level are relatively poorer in UVB content than nearby sites at sea level. This is strikingly apparent around the Dead Sea in Israel, 400 m below sea level (Kushelevsky and Slifkin, 1975).

UVR and Its Penetration to the Skin

UV incident on human skin can follow one of three courses: it can undergo absorption, reflection, or scattering. The first step in a photochemical reaction is the absorption of a single photon by a molecule and the production of an excited state in which one electron of the absorbing molecule is raised to a higher energy level. Such radiative transition can only occur efficiently when the photon energy of the radiation is close to the energy difference of theatom in the initial and final state (energy level). The photochemistry that may then occur will, therefore, depend upon the molecular structure and the wavelength of UV as well as the specific reaction conditions. The primary products generated by UV absorption are generally reactive species. Reflection not only occurs at the surface of the stratum corneum but at all interfaces changing in refractive index. Scattering occurs because of the different structural elements, such as hair follicles and sebaceous glands, and also by cellular components, such as mitochondria and ribosomes. The remaining UV can penetrate into deeper skin layers (International programme on chemical safety, *Environmental Health Criteria*, 160).

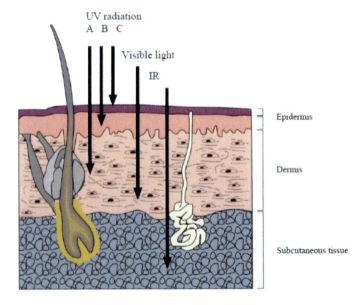

Figure 15. Wavelength-dependent penetration of UV radiation into human skin. UVB acts mostly on epidermis, where it can damage DNA in keratinocytes and melanocytes. In contrast, UVA radiation has the ability to penetrate more deeply and can exert direct effects on both the epidermal and dermal layer and affect keratinocytes in the epidermis and fibroblasts in the dermis. UVA is also 10 to 100 times more abundant in the sunlight. The initiation of skin tumors probably requires penetration of UV to the actively dividing basal layer of the epidermis in order for acute damage to become fixed as mutations.

UV penetrates into the dermis exposing a variety of cells and structures, depending in part on the thickness of the human stratum corneum and epidermis. The depth of penetration is wavelength dependent—the longer the wavelength the deeper the penetration (Brulset al.,1984).

Damaging Effect of UVR

"Studies in hairless mice demonstrated the carcinogenicity of exposures to UVR in the wavelength ranges 315 to 400 nm (UVA), 280 to 315 nm (UVB) and ¾ 280 nm (UVC), UVB radiation being the most effective, followed by UVC and UVA. UVB radiation is three to four orders of magnitude more effective than UVA. Nevertheless, both short-wavelength UVA (315 to 340 nm) and long-wavelength UVA (340 to 400 nm) induced skin cancer in hairless mice. The carcinogenic effectiveness of the latter waveband is known only as an average value over the entire range; the uncertainty of this average is about one order of magnitude. In none of the experiments involving UVC was it possible to exclude completely a contribution of UVB, but the size of the effects observed indicate that they cannot be due to UVB alone" (IARC, 2010).UVB is three to four times more effective than UVA in producing erythema. In humans, pigmentation protects against erythema and histopathological changes. People with a poor ability to tan, who burn easily and have light eye and hair color are at a higher risk of developing melanoma, basal-cell and squamous-cell carcinomas (IARC, 2010). UVB most commonly causes damage in the form of cyclobutane pyrimidine dimmers. UVA, on the other hand, primarily causes DNA damage indirectly by the production of short-lived ROS such as singlet oxygen, superoxide and H_2O_2 via endogenous photosensitizers. UVA radiation generates more phosphodiester bond breaks in DNA than would be expected by the total amount of energy directly absorbed by the DNA. Therefore, most likely there is indirect damage to DNA accomplished by endogenous photosensitizers such as riboflavin, nicotinamide coenzymes, and rare RNA bases (Laurent-Applegate and Schwarzkopf, 2001).

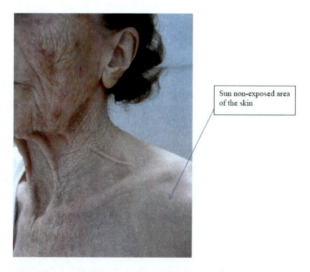

Figure 16. Picture shows the difference between wrinkle formation and pigmentation on the sun-exposed (face, neck) and non-exposed areas (picture provided by Ana Benedicic, MD, MSc).

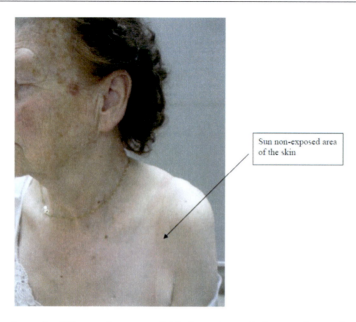

Figure 17. Picture shows the difference between wrinkle formation and pigmentation on the sun-exposed (face, neck) and non-exposed areas as well as the beginning epithelioma in front of the ear (picture provided by Ana Benedicic, MD, MSc).

Skin Response to Acute and Chronic UV Radiation

Skin pigmentation is induced both by UVB and UVA rays. According to Diffey (1991), the normal responses of the skin to UVR can be classed under two headings: acute effects and chronic effects. An acute effect is one of rapid onset and generally of short duration, as opposed to a chronic effect, which is often of gradual onset and long duration. These effects should be distinguished from acute and chronic exposure conditions, which refer to the length of the UVR exposure. The acute reactions considered will be sunburn, tanning and vitamin D production. Photoaging and skin cancer will be discussed as those chronic reactions produced by prolonged or repeated UVR exposure (Diffey, 1991). Exposure to ultraviolet (UV) radiation increases skin pigmentation and usually results in an even darkening of the skin. However, it may also occasionally lead to the development of hyperpigmented lesions due to a local overproduction of pigment.

Skin Antioxidant Defense

Although the skin possesses an elaborate antioxidant defense system to deal with UV-induced oxidative stress and immunotoxicity, excessive and chronic exposure to UV light can overwhelm the cutaneous antioxidant and immune response capacity, leading to oxidative damage and immunotoxicity, premature skin aging, and skin cancer (see also the chapter on endogenous and exogenous skin antioxidants). Photoaged skin has significantly reduced concentrations of antioxidant enzymes in the stratum corneum and the epidermis, while the concentration of oxidized proteins in the upper dermis is increased. Acute exposure to UV irradiation depletes the catalase activity in the skin and increases protein oxidation (Sander et al., 2002). More on the antioxidant protection of the skin can be read in the following chapters.

DNA Damage

DNA is constantly exposed to DNA-damaging agents. Environmental DNA-damaging agents include UV light and ionizing radiation, as well as a variety of chemicals encountered in foodstuffs, or as air- and water-borne agents. Endogenous damaging agents include metabolites that can act as alkylating agents and the ROS that arise during respiration.

Since there arealways less antioxidants available to neutralize all oxidizing agents involved in free radical formation and damage, a third line of defense evolved—damage repair mechanisms. Defense mechanisms are available to cope with constant free radical-induced damage in our cells. Among them are DNA repair systems to replace damaged DNA bases and antioxidants to neutralize free radicals. Damaged cells are eliminated by apoptosis and non-functional proteins are turned-over by proteases. But DNA repair capacity has been found to decrease with age. For example, decrease in the level of proteins that participate in nucleotide excision repair was reported to occur for aged dermal fibroblasts (Goukassian et al., 2000). Oxidation of DNA can produce different types of DNA damage: strand breaks, sister chromatide exchange, DNA-protein cross-links, sugar damage, abasic sites, and base modifications. Cell death, chromosome changes, mutation and morphological transformations are observed after UV exposure of prokaryotic and eukaryotic cells. Numerous types of UV-induced DNA damage have now been recognized that include stand breaks (single and double), cyclobutane-type pyrimidine dimers, 6-4 pyo photoproducts and the corresponding Dewar isomer, thymine glycols, 8-hydroxy guanine, and many more. Additionally, the specific lesions in DNA thatcan be induced by UVA radiation include pyrimidine dimmers, single-strand breaks (both not thought to be the critical lesions in UVA radiation-induced cellular lethality), and, perhaps more importantly, DNA protein cross-links (Peak et al., 1987; Rosenstein and Ducore, 1983; Peak et al.,1988; Peak et al.,1985). Solar UV causes formation of ROS, which can oxidize guanine in DNA to form 8-hydroxy-7,8-dihydroguanine (8-OHdG). The frequency of this characteristic mutation in human skin increases with cumulative sun exposure and could be used as internal dosimeter of cumulative sun exposure (Yarosh, 2010). OH$^.$ can add on to guanine at positions 4, 5 and 8 in the purine ring. Addition to C-8 produces a C-8 OH adduct radical that can be reduced to 8-hydroxy-7,8-dihydroguanine, oxidized to 8-hydroxyguanine, or undergo opening of the imidazole ring, followed by one-electron reduction and protonation, to give 2,6-diamino-4-hydroxy-5-formamidopyrimidine, abbreviated as FAPyG (Halliwell and Gutterigde, 1999). Photoexcitation of cytosine and guanine may lead to the formation in relatively minor yields of 6-hydroxy-5,6-dihydrocytosine and 8-oxo-7,8-dihydroguanine, respectively. A second mechanism that requires the participation of endogenous photosensitizers together with oxygen is at the origin of most of the DNA damage generated by the UVA (320 to 400 nm) and visible light. Singlet oxygen, which arises from a type II mechanism, is likely to be mostly involved in the formation of 8-oxo-7,8-dihydroguanine that was observed within both isolated and cellular DNA.

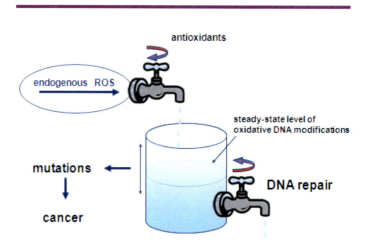

Figure 18. Basal "steady state" levels of oxidative DNA modifications are observed in all cells.

However, it may be expected that the latter oxidized purine lesion together with DNA strand breaks and pyrimidine base oxidation products are also generated with a lower efficiency through Fenton type reactions (Cadet et al., 1997). The number of different DNA modifications that OH˙ is capable of producing appears to be over 100 (Hutchinson, 1985), see Figure 19. In addition, DNA-protein cross-links are produced during UV exposure. Larger scale genetic alterations include chromosome breakage, sister chromatid exchanges and chromatid aberrations. Although partial UV action spectra are now available for many of these lesions, the most studied have been the different types of pyrimidine dimers (International programme on chemical safety, Environmental Health Criteria, 160).

Photoproducts

Solar UVR induces a variety of photoproducts in DNA, including cyclobutane-type pyrimidine dimers, pyrimidine-pyrimidone (6-4) photoproducts, thymine glycols, cytosine damage, purine damage, DNA strand breaks and DNA-protein cross-links (Patrick and Rahn, 1976). Substantial information on biological consequences is available only for the first two classes. Both are potentially cytotoxic and can lead to mutations in cultured cells, and there is evidence that cyclobutane-type pyrimidine dimers may be precarcinogenic lesions (IARC, 2010).

Pyrimidine dimers can cause CC → TTtandem double–base transition mutations in DNA. Mutations in tumor suppression gene p53 appear to be early events in skin cancer development, and double transition mutations are much more common in mutated p53 genes from skin cancers than in cancers from internal organs, consistent with the role of sunlight (Halliwell and Gutteridge, 2007).

Single-base modifications can also occur via sensitized reactions, including Type 1 and Type II processes.

The cyclobutane pyrimidine dimer (CPD) is formed ten times more frequently than 8-OHdG, and is caused by direct absorbtion of UV photons without any ROS intermediate, which could be quenched by antioxidants. A second type of base fusion, a 6-4 photoproduct, is similarly formed about one-sixth frequently as CPD (Yarosh, 2010). The UV-induced cyclobutane pyrimidine photoproducts cause distortions in the DNA helix and halt DNA polymerase II transcription of DNA.

The absorbtion of UVB by thymine or cytosine creates excited states that can react with water to form pyrimidine hydrates or with an adjacent pyrimidine to produce cross-links (Halliwell and Gutteridge, 2007). Cytosine within dimers undergoes accelerated deamination to uracil. Thymidine dimers, presumably arising from nucleotide excision repair, have been detected in increasing amounts (Le Curieux and Hemminki, 2001; Kotova et al., 2005) in urine after subjects were exposed to sunlight.

ROS induced by sun radiation have been proven to be mutagenic (Marnett, 2000), an effect that should be derived from chemical modification of DNA. A number of alterations (e.g., cleavage of DNA, DNA-protein cross links, oxidation of purine, etc.) are due to reactions with ROS, especially $OH^{\cdot}$.

If the DNA repair systems are not able to immediately regenerate intact DNA, a mutation will result from erroneous base pairing during replication. This mechanism may partly explain the high prevalence of cancer in individuals exposed to oxidative stress (Marnett, 2000) or sun radiation. The principal cause of single-strand breaks is oxidation of sugar moiety by the hydroxyl radical.

However, *in vitro*, neither H_2O_2 alone nor $O_2^{\cdot-}$, cause strand breaks under physiological conditions, and therefore, their toxicity*in vivo* is most likely the result of Fenton reactions with a metal catalyst (McKersie, 1996).

Cross-linking to proteins is another consequence of hydroxyl radical attack on either DNA or its associated proteins (Oleinck et al., 1986). Although DNA protein cross-links are about one order of magnitude less abundant that single-strand breaks, they are not as readily repaired and may be lethal if replication or transcription precedes the repair (McKersie, 1996).

For readers interested in this topic, we suggest an excellent review by Diffey (1991): *Solar ultraviolet radiation effects on biological systems*. DNA molecule is constantly "bombarded" by ROS originating from endogenous processes as well as from environmental agents and from radiation sources. Damaged DNA is being constantly repaired by many cellular repair systems.

If the frequency of damaging events exceeds the repair capacity, damaged DNA is not repaired in time, and damaged DNA can pass to daughter cells and thus trigger tumor initiation and progression process. DNA is the most critical target for damage by UVA, UVB and UVC radiations.

To produce any change, UV must be absorbed by the biomolecule. This involves absorption of a single photon by the molecule and the production of an excited state in which one electron of the absorbing molecule is raised to a higher energy level. The primary products caused by UV exposure are generally direct DNA oxidation or reactive species or free radicals generation, which form extremely quickly but which can produce effects that can last for hours, days or even years.

While a considerable amount of knowledge is available concerning the interaction of UV with nucleic acids, controversy exists as to which lesion constitutes the most important type of pre-mutagenic damage (International programme on chemical safety, 1994).

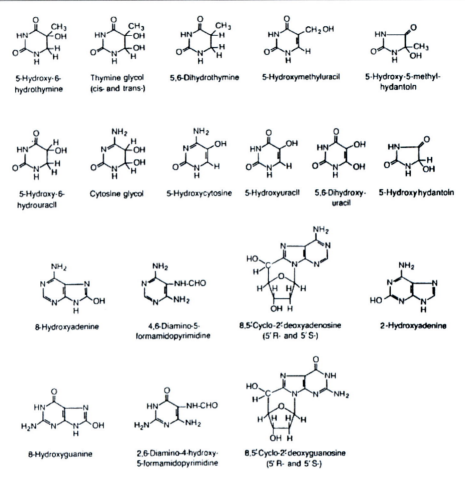

Figure 19. Chemical structures of some of the oxidation products of DNA. These modified bases can be formed when an OH radical attacks DNA (Helbock et al., 1999).

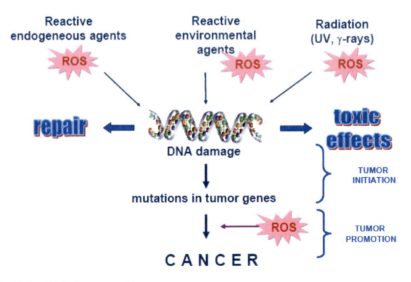

Figure 20. Oxidative DNA damage and its consequences.

DNA Repair

The aging and survival of endothelial cells are linked to molecular mechanisms that control cell proliferation, quiescence, apoptosis and senescence.

Despite the fact that biological species, including man, are exposed to potentially harmful levels of solar UVR, mechanisms have evolved to protect cells and to repair damaged molecules (Figure 21). The cell component most vulnerable to injury is nuclear DNA. Measurable DNA damage is induced in human skin cells *in vivo* after exposure to UVA, UVB and UVC radiation, including doses in the range commonly experienced by humans. A number of different DNA repair mechanisms have been established (Freifelder, 1987), the best known being photoreactivation, excision repair, postreplication repair and sos repair. Most of the DNA damage after a single exposure is repaired within 24 h. The majority of DNA lesions are repaired by BER (Base Excision Repair), NER (Nucleotide Excision Repair), and MMR (Mismatch Repair) (Norbury and Hickson, 2001). BER involves the concerted effort of several repair proteins that recognize and excise specific DNA damages, eventually replacing the damaged moiety with a normal nucleotide. The NER process involves damage recognition, local opening of the DNA duplex around the lesion, dual incision of the damaged DNA strand, gap repair synthesis, and strand ligation. The most significant of lesions repaired by NER are pyrimidine dimers (cyclobutane pyrimidine dimers and 6-4 photoproducts) caused by the UV component of sunlight. The MMR system is responsible for the post-replicative repair of mismatches and small single-stranded DNA loops, and it is critically involved in preventing recombination between homologous DNA sequences.

Even under normal physiological conditions, it has been reported that DNA base modifications can exist as high as 1 in 130,000 bases in nuclear DNA and 1 in 8,000 for mitochondrial DNA (Ames, 1983). Here again, it is in the interest of the organism to have efficient repair systems for the DNA. As already mentioned, there are several repair mechanisms that include also direct repair of altered DNA bases by GSH transferases and peroxidases, and DNA methylases (Ketterer and Meyer, 1989; Thomas et al., 1990). In addition, there is excision repair of damaged DNA where endonucleases and glycosolases have been identified in eukaryotic cells that have been previously described in prokaryotes with the induction of SOS genes (Wallace, 1988; Johnson and Demple, 1988; Helland et al., 1986). The nuclear enzyme poly(ADP-ribose) polymerase 1 (PARP 1) participates in the regulation of both DNA repair and transcription. Moderation of PARP following DNA damage has also been proposed to protect skin cells from UV-induced acute and chronic photodamage (Farkas et al., 2002).

Changing Gene Expression in an Epigenetic-Like Manner

Small degrees of oxidative damage in a cell can switch gene expression in an epigenetic-like manner. Cutler reported (2003) that there appears to be no correlation in rate of accumulation of oxidative damage and rate of physiological aging. He believes that the same processes that were involved in changing gene expression during normal differentiation and development are the ones involved in the dysdifferentiation process (Dysdifferentiation hypothesis of aging), so no mutations are required and the process of aging is largely epigenetic in nature. Cutler additionally observed that aging rate of an organism is predicted to correlate positively with the rate of dysdifferentiation occurring, which, in turn, is positively related to the oxidativestress status of the cell.

Photoreactivation

Photoreactivation is an extremely specific light-dependant repair process. It exists for repair of pyrimidine dimers in situ. This repair process begins with a photoreactivating enzyme binding to UV-induced pyrimidine dimers in the dark. If this complex is exposed to optical radiation between about 330 and 600 nm, the active enzyme separates from the dimer and a repaired DNA segment results. Repair proceeds via photolyase, which has been shown to be present almost ubiquitously throughout the animal world from *E coli* to non-placental mammals. Recent evidence suggests that photoreactivation may be less important in human cells (Liet al.,1993). Photoreactivation as a DNA repair process is used by plants, fish, reptiles, and amphibians but is not present in humans or other mammals (Yarosh, 2010).

Apoptosis

Apoptosis is a cellular end point of the stress response. Apoptosis removes damaged cells from UV-irradiated tissues. If the cell damage cannot be repaired before the next cell division, the cell rather decides to "commit a suicide" than to spread mutations to its daughter cells. Activation of apoptosis is associated with generation of reactive oxygen species. Superoxide is produced by mitochondria isolated from apoptotic cells due to a switch from the normal 4-electron reduction of O_2 to a 1-electron reduction when cytochrome c is released from mitochondria. Apoptosis is stimulated through release of mitochondrial cytochrome c, which results in activation of death protease (caspase-3) and increased free radical generation due to uncoupled respiration (Cai and Jones, 1998; Cai et al., 1998). The increased oxidant generation stimulates a mitochondrial permeability transition that causes further release of cytochrome c from mitochondria and activates a second apoptosis inducing factor (AIF). The proapoptotic protein bax is elevated in basal cell carcinoma as well as other skin cancers (Delehedde et al., 1999); in absence of other changes, this should limit growth. The fact that growth is not successfully limited may result partly from an elevation of bcl-2, which can block apoptosis (Balin and Allen, 2003). The antiapoptotic activity of bcl-2 stems partly from its ability to upregulate an antioxidant pathway in cells (Hockenbery et al., 1993). Mutations in the anti-tumor p53 gene have also been reported to occur frequently in basal cell carcinoma and may also permit survival of tumor cells by preventing the normal stimulation of apoptosis by p53 (Ballin and Allen, 2003). Oxidative damage is a cellular stress that can cause senescence like growth arrest or even apoptosis (Rocquet and Bonte, 2002). Antioxidant treatment could sometimes possess anti-apoptotic properties, and for this reason, antioxidants should be consumed before exposure to the factors that increase oxidative stress and not after. The genes that control apoptosis in the epidermis, such as the bcl-2 gene, are disregulated during aging. The decreased efficiency of apoptosis may contribute to chronological aging and extrinsic skin aging (Rocquet and Bonte, 2002). Differentiation, proliferation, and cell death are coordinated tightly within the epidermis. Alterations within keratinocytes that disrupt these processes are believed to contribute to the development of nonmelanoma skin cancers. Only epidermal stem cells escape cellular senescence. It appears that epidermal terminal differentiation, apoptosis and cell senescence are all triggered by stimuli. Nevertheless, keratinocytes will undergo classical epidermal differentiation or will irreversibly enter into senescence or apoptosis, depending on their statesand on the nature and strength of the stimuli. The differentiation, apoptosis and senescence of keratinocytes share some molecular pathways. Epidermal differentiation and apoptosis lead to cell death and the removal of cells by transglutaminase activation and proteolysis.

Mitochondrial Damage

Besides oxidation of nuclear DNA, UVR can induce also oxidative damage to mtDNA. It has been suggested that sunlight passing through the skin can even cause DNA damage in white cells circulating through skin capillaries (Yang et al., 2004), but the greatest damage is within the skin cells, including the damage to dermal mitochondrial DNA (Wang et al., 2004). Singlet oxygen produced by UVA light has been shown to cause strand breaks in the mitochondrial DNA, which has resulted in mtDNA deletions. Mitochondrial DNA is believed to be the most critical target of endogenous ROS production since it lies in the inner mitochondrial membrane, in close proximity to the electron transport chain where the most free radicals are formed. Besides, mtDNA has a high mutation rate due to its lack of histones and decreased capacity of repair. Mitochondria contain their own genome, a maternally inherited, circular, double-stranded DNA of 16,569 bp encoding 22 tRNAs, two rRNAs, and 13 polipeptides, all of which are subunits in the electron transport chin (Anderson et al., 1981, 1999; Giles et al., 1980). The remainder of the proteins that function in the mitochondria are encoded in the nucleus and imported into the mitochondrion (Norman et al., 2010).

In the past, it was believed that mitochondria lack DNA repair capacity but this is not true. However, it is true that mitochondria do not remove UV-induced DNA damage, which might be important in photodamage and skin cancer formation. Besides, there is evidence that mtDNA oxidative damage increases with damage and DNA repair declines with age (Anderson and Bohr, 2000). There have been observed greater accumulation of mtDNA found in sun-exposed skin compared to protected skin (Berneburg et al.,1999; Birch-Machin et al., 1998). The most frequent mutation is a 4,977-base pair deletion also called the common deletion, which is increased in photoaged skin. It is thought that strand breaks in mtDNA caused by UVR are mediated by ROS, particularly by superoxide. Mutations of mitochondrial DNA may be useful as a marker of cumulative ultraviolet radiation exposure.

In cultured fibroblasts, during aging, typical changes of mitochondrial ultra structure can be observed: loss of branched mitochondria in old cells, enlargement of mitochondria, matrix vacuolization, shortened cristae, loss of dense granules (Goldstein et al., 1984). Similar changes in mitochondrial ultra structure as seen in aged fibroblasts are also seen in photoaged keratinocytesthatwere chronically exposed to low levels of UVB irradiation (Feldman et al., 1990). Mitochondria toward the upper regions of the epidermis were swollen and had fragmented cristae; mitochondria in the lower areas of the epidermis usually contained smaller and less dense inclusions and intact or partially disrupted cristae. Besides intrinsic aging effect on the mitochondrial capacity of aged skin cells, a substantial decline of the mitochondrial membrane potential can be observed following UV irradiation of keratinocytes in vitro (Li andYu, 1994).

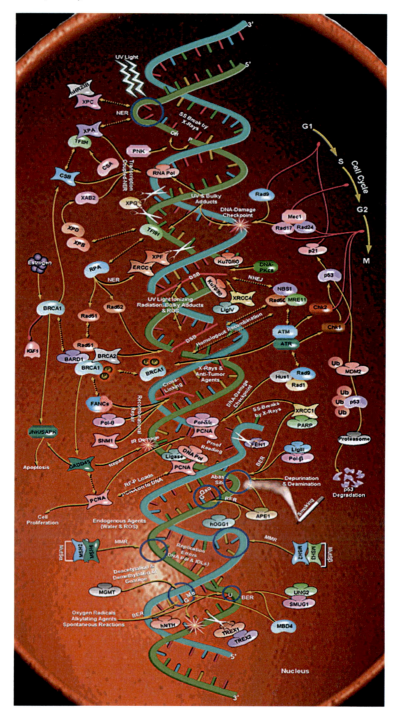

Figure 21. The complex system of DNA Repair Mechanisms (source: SABiosciences, a QIAGEN company. http://www.sabiosciences.com/). A number of different DNA repair mechanisms constantly remove and repair damage caused to DNA by endogenous and exogenous sources.

Protein Damage

UVR can generate damage also to proteins. The UVA-generated reactive oxygen species cause cross-linking of proteins (e.g., collagen), oxidation of sulfydryl groups causing disulfide cross-links, oxidative inactivation of certain enzymes causing functional impairment of cells (fibroblasts, keratinocytes, melanocytes, Langerhans cells) and liberation of proteases, collagenase and elastase. Merker et al. (2000) demonstrated that aged fibroblasts accumulate increased oxidized proteins upon oxidative stress and are less efficient in removing oxidized proteins. Besides, several key enzymes are oxidatively inactivated by mixed function oxidases during aging. These inactivated enzymes accumulate but only after the age of 60 (Oliver et al., 1987).

The majority of UV-induced protein damage appears to be mediated by $^1O_2$, which reacts preferentially with Trp, His, Tyr, Met, Cys and cystine side chains. Direct photooxidation reactions (particularly with short-wavelength UV) and radicals can also be formed via triplet excited states of some of these side chains. The initial products of $^1O_2$-mediated reactions are endoperoxides with the aromatic residues, and zwitterions with the sulfur-containing residues. These intermediates undergo a variety of further reactions, which can result in radical formation and ring-opening reactions; these result in significant yields of protein cross-links and aggregates but little protein fragmentation (Pattison and Davies, 2006).

Lipid Damage

Unsaturated lipids react with ROS generated from UVR and form lipid peroxyl (LOO˙) and alkoxyl radicals (LO˙), which tend to initiate chain-propagating, autocatalytic reactions. These lipid peroxidation end-products (malondialdehyde (MDA) or 4-hydroxynonanol (4-HNE)), induce cellular stress responses. UVlight also leads to oxidation of PUFA side chain and cholesterol in skin lipids (Whiteman et al., 2004) and generation of aldehydes such as acrolein and HNE from peroxides can damage proteins and DNA (Bates et al., 1985). Products of lipid peroxidation can activate UCPs and promote feedback downregulation of mitochondrial ROS production (Jarmuszkiewicz and Woyda-Płoszczyca, 2008).

Damage to Elastin and Collagen and Wrinkle Formation

Wrinkling in the skin is caused by habitual photoaging, facial expressions, aging, smoking, poor hydration, and various other factors (Anderson, 2006). The effects of aging on the dermal layer are significant. Not only does the dermal layer thin but also less collagen is produced, and the elastin fibers that provide elasticity wear out. These changes in the scaffolding of the skin cause the skin to wrinkle and sag.Photoaged skincan be associated with either increased epidermal thickness or pronounced epidermal atrophy. The most pronounced histological change is the accumulation of elastin-containingmaterial just below the dermal-epidermal junction, known as solar elastosis (Lavker, 1995). Collagen, which composes over 90% of the skin's total proteins, becomes disorganized (Bernstein et al., 1996). While elastin levels are increased in photoaged skin, levels of types I and III collagen precursors and cross-links are reduced (Braverman and Fonferko, 1982; Talwar et al., 1995). It is likely that such changes in collagen precursors lead to reduced levels and/or altered organization of fibrillar collagen and thus may contribute to the wrinkled appearance of photodamaged human skin.The Glogau classification system was developed to objectively measure the severity of photoaging and especially wrinkles. Four types of skin depressions can be defined according to their depth: folds, permanent wrinkles, reducible wrinkles and skin micro-relief.When UV rays from the sun penetrate the skin, they damage elastic fibers. As the elastin weakens, skin becomes less elastic and loses its ability to snap back after being stretched.Photoaged skin contains elastic material in the reticular dermis, and the fibrillin deposits in the reticular dermis are enlarged. Elastic fibers have a central core of hydrophobic cross-linked elastin surrounded by fibrillin-rich microfibrils. The papillary dermal microfibrillin-rich microfibril network is truncated and depleted in photoaged skin.

There are fewer fibrillin-rich microfibrils in wrinkled photoaged skin, probably due to inflammatory cell proteinases (neutrophil elastase) or activation of matrix metalloproteinase (Tsuji et al., 2001). Cross-linking causing decreased elasticity could also be involved in wrinkle formation (Watson et al., 1999).Wrinkles form especially in parts of skin that get stretched and move a lot (like around eyes, mouth and nose). Anti-aging skin care products should focus on wrinkles prevention also as anti-sun damage products in order to prevent elastin and collagen damage. A decrease in the overall ROS load by efficient sunscreens or other protective agents may represent promising strategies to prevent or at least minimize ROS-induced photoaging.

For example, the study of Seo et al. (2001) on photoaged skin has shown that UV irradiation increases the tropoelastin mRNA in keratinocytes and fibroblasts (Seo et al., 2001). Selective inhibition of skin fibroblast elastase could be one way to fight wrinkle formation following cumulative ultraviolet B irradiation (Tsukahara et al., 2001). Lysozyme may alter the elastic fibers in the surface, preventing further degradation and the accumulation of altered elastic fibers.

Table 5. Glogau Classification of Photoaging

Group	Classification	Typical Age	Description	Skin Characteristics
I	Mild	28 to 35	No wrinkles	Early Photoaging: mild pigment changes, no keratosis, minimal wrinkles, minimal or no makeup
II	Moderate	35 to 50	Wrinkles in motion	Early to Moderate Photoaging: Early brown spots visible, keratosis palpable but not visible, parallel smile lines begin to appear, wears some foundation
III	Advanced	50 to 65	Wrinkles at rest	Advanced Photoaging: Obvious discolorations, visible capillaries (telangiectasias), visible keratosis, wears heavier foundation always
IV	Severe	60 to 75	Only wrinkles	Severe Photoaging: Yellow-gray skin color, prior skin malignancies, wrinkles throughout— no normal skin, cannot wear makeup because it cakes and cracks

Source: Baumann, 2002; Glogau, 1994.

Why UV Radiation Accelerates the Aging Process?

As already mentioned, UV radiation can cause significant DNA damage and especially to mtDNA. In a study byBerneburg et al. (2004), it was confirmed that repetitive exposure to UVA light leads to an approximately 40% increase in the level of the common deletion in skin tissue. Even 16 months after cessation of UV exposure, accumulated damage was increased in some individuals by 32-fold (Berneburg et al., 2004).The causative role of oxidative stress for the increased frequency of mitochondrial DNA aberrations was demonstrated also in a variety of other experimental models and in human studies (Blatt et al., 2010). Also, a causative link between mtDNA mutations and aging phenotypes in mammals was evidenced in knock-out mice. Age-related phenotypes such as reduced subcutaneous fat, weight loss, alopecia, reduced fertility and heart enlargement were observed besides increased amount of point mutations and increased amount of deleted mtDNA (Trifunovic et al., 2004). Increased formation of oxidative stress due to endogenous or exogenous sources (e.g., UVR) causes mtDNA lesions in human cells and detrimental changes in mitochondrial respiration. Blatt et al. (2010) explain that due to a negative feedback loop, damaged mtDNA is a cause and a consequence of aging as well. Any lack of mitochondrial function impairs cellular ATP synthesis, thus reducing the "fuel supply" for repair mechanisms. It does further stimulate the formation of ROS as byproducts of an impaired mitochondrial respiration. More ROS are produced, more damage accumulates in neighboring mitochondrial complexes, membranes and mtDNA, progressive decline in the energy-generating capacity of the cell is observed, what further accelerates the aging process. Due to impaired ATP formation, the switch to anaerobic pathway such as glycolysis occurs, but also glycolysis additionally increases the formation of oxidative stress by the formation of reactive glycolytic intermediates, which favor the formation of advanced glycation end products (AGEs). Thus even a single sunburn period could, in theory, start the above-described chain reaction leading to accelerated aging process in the skin cell (Figure 22).

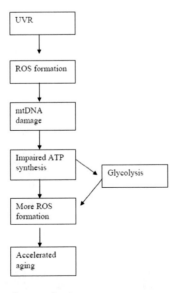

Figure 22. Oxidative stress formation from endogenous or exogenous sources can trigger the chain reaction, which leads to accelerated aging process in the cell.

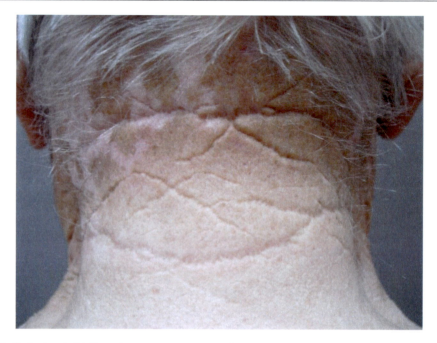

Figure 23. Cutis rhomboidalis nuchae as a consequence of sun exposure (picture provided by Ana Benedicic, MD, MSc).

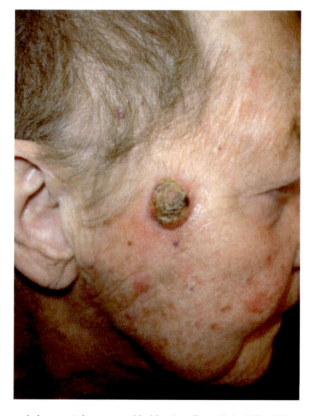

Figure 24. Epithelioma cutis buccae (picture provided by Ana Benedicic, MD, MSc).

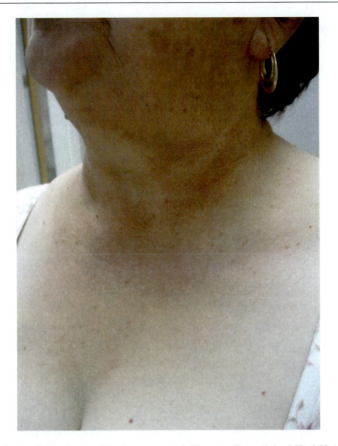

Figure 25. Erythrosis interfollicularis colli (picture provided by Ana Benedicic, MD, MSc).

"ROS and RNS are constitutively produced also by endogenous sources in most cell types, including epidermal keratinocytes and dermal fibroblasts (Fuchs, 1992;Darr and Fridovich, 1994). In addition to stimulated ROS/RNS production by resident epidermal and dermal cells, these species as well as reactive halogen species (RHS) can be produced and released into skin by invading macrophages as well as polymorphonuclear and eosinophilic leukocytes. Several chemical agents can induce ROS generation in skin, either directly or mediated by proinflammatory cytokines. ROS, which are an ubiquitous component of inflammation, may exacerbate inflammation through generation of cytokines, thus initiating a positive feedback cycle. These ROS potentially regulate levels and activity of phosphorylated proteins and protein kinases within the keratinocytes (Coquette et al., 2000) and could be modulated by enzymatic and low-molecular-weight antioxidants" (Fuch et al., 2001).

UVR and ROS Formation: $^1O_2$, $O_2^{-\cdot}$ and $OH^\cdot$, $H2O2$

UVR can increase the ROS formation in the skin cells. Oxidativestress is believed to underlie changes associated with both photoaging and natural aging. According to Pattison and Davies (2006), UV radiation can mediate damage via two different mechanisms: (a) direct absorption of the incident light by the cellular components, resulting in excited state formation and subsequent chemical reaction, and (b) photosensitization mechanisms, where the light is absorbed by endogenous (or exogenous) sensitizers that are excited to their triplet states. The excited photosensitizers can induce cellular damage by two mechanisms: (a) electron transfer and hydrogen abstraction processes to yield free radicals (Type I); or (b) energy transfer with O2 to yield the reactive excited state, singlet oxygen (Type II) (Pattison and Davies,2006).

The primary mechanism by which UV radiation initiates molecular responses in human skin is via photochemical generation of ROS mainly formation of superoxide anion (O_2^-), hydrogen peroxide (H2O2), hydroxyl radical (OH·), and singlet oxygen ($^1O_2$) (Hanson and Clegg, 2002). The main DNA product generated by (1)O2 is 8-oxo-Gua; this is a common lesion in DNA and is formed by a range of other oxidants in addition to UV. UV light does not deposit sufficient energy inwater molecules to fragment them, in contrast to X-rays and γ-rays. However, in the presence of H_2O_2 (formed during normal metabolism),UVB forms hydroxyl radical OH·.

H2O2 + UV → OH· + OH⁻

In vitro, ex vivo and solution-phase studies have found that ROS, such as singletoxygen (1O2), H2O2, superoxide (O_2^-) and nitric oxide,are generated after absorption of UV radiation by chromophoresthat are also found in keratinocytes (urocanic acid,riboflavin, reduced form of nicotinamide adenine dinucleotide–reduced nicotinamide adenine dinuclcotidc phosphatc[NADH/NADPH], tryptophan) (PeakandPeak, 1986; Peak andPeak, 1989; Cunningham et al., 1985; Hanson et al., 1997, 1998; Jurkiewicz and Buettner, 1996).

UVA radiation produces cellular modifications that considerably overlap those induced by oxidative damage (Tyrrell, 1991;McCormick et al., 1976). UVA radiation constitutes an oxidant stress that involves the generation of active species including singlet oxygen and hydroxyl radicals. Hydrogen peroxide can be generated by UVA irradiation of tryptophan (McCormick et al., 1976), and superoxide can be produced by UVA irradiation of NADH and NADPH (Cunningham et al., 1985). The skin-damaging effects of UVA appear to result from type II, oxygen-mediated photodynamic reactions in which UVA or near-UV radiation in the presence of certain photosensitizing chromophores (e.g., riboflavin, porphyrins, nicotinamide adenine dinucleotide phosphate (NADPH), etc.) leads to the formation of reactive oxygen species (1O2, O2.-, .OH) (Dalle Carbonare and Pathak, 1992).

Iron-free porphyrins also generate singlet oxygen upon exposure to UVA radiation. Also, other small molecules have the potential to generate active oxygen intermediates upon UVA exposure (Tyrell, 1992). For example, the photochemical degradation of tryptophan by wavelengthsthatinclude the more energetic portion of the UVA spectrum is able to generate hydrogen peroxide and N-formyl kynurenin (McCormicket al.,1976). Although the level of hydrogen peroxide generated*in vivo*by such a pathway would appear to be in the low micromolar range, it could nevertheless be crucial to biological processes since iron complexes (such as citrate) that are present in the cytoplasm will react with hydrogen peroxide to generate the highly reactive hydroxyl radical in a superoxide driven Fenton reaction (see Gutteridge, 1985; Imlay et al.,1988). Since the reaction is driven by the continual reduction of ferric iron to the ferrous state by superoxide anions, a cellular source of superoxide anions is also required. In this context, it should be noted that both hydrogen peroxide and hydroxyl radical are generated by UVA irradiation of NADH and NADPH (Czochralskaet al.,1984; Cunninghamet al.,1985). However, it is not at all clear whether this is really the key source of superoxide anions or whether the main source is as a consequence of normal cellular metabolism. Iron liberation and photodamaged skin contribute to oxidative damage and activation of transcription factors (Halliwell and Gutteridge, 2007). Indeed, chronic exposure of hairless mice to low levels of UVB increases non-hem iron content of the skin; increases in iron with age and sun exposure are also observed in human skin. Topical application of certain iron ion chelatorsto skin of hairless mice appeared to delay the onset of UVB-induced damage (Halliwell and Gutteridge, 2007). Naturally occurring iron complexes can react in vivo with hydrogen peroxide in the presence of superoxide anion in the Haber–Weiss reaction, which produces the potentially lethal hydroxyl radical. For further reading, see the chapter on iron as a macronutrient. See also the chapter on Fenton reaction and metals and the paragraph on Iron chelators.

NOS formation: $NO^{\cdot}$ and $ONOO^{-}$

Levels of cytokines and iNOS also increase after UVR exposure, causingexcess $NO^{\cdot}$ production and ONOO- generation.

Molecular Mechanisms by Which UVR Causes Photoaging

In previous paragraphs, evidence was given that UV radiation generates reactive oxygen species and ROS can further oxidize cellular components. UV irradiation also directly or indirectly initiates and activates a complex cascade of biochemical reactions in human skin. Besides,the UV light-induced ROS interfere with signaling pathways. On a molecular level, UV radiation from the sun attacks keratinocytes and fibroblasts, resulting in the activation of cell surface receptors, which initiate signal transduction cascades. This, in turn, leads to a variety of molecular changes, which causes a breakdown of collagen in the extracellular matrix and a shutdown of new collagen synthesis (Fisher and Cutis, 2005). UV-induced liberation of ROS in human skin is responsible for stimulation of numerous signal transduction pathways via activation of cell surface cytokine and growth factor receptors. UVA or UVB induce activation (sometimes via peroxides or singlet O2 as signaling molecules) of a wide range of transcription factors in skin cells, including AP-1 and NF-κB (Halliwell and Gutteridge, 2007). This can increase production of matrix metalloproteinases that can degrade collagen and other connective tissue components. For example, the UV light-induced ROS induce the transcription factor activator protein-1 (AP-1). AP-1 induces upregulation of matrix metalloproteinases (MMPs) like collagenase-1 (MMP-1), stromelysin-1 (MMP-3), and gelatinase A (MMP-2), which specifically degrade connective tissue such as collagen and elastin and indirectly inhibit the collagen synthesis in the skin (Rasche and Elstner, 2010).As indicated by their name, these zinc-dependent endopeptidases show proteoplytic activity in their ability to degrade matrix proteins such as collagen and elastin (Krutmann and Gilchrest, 2006).Destruction of collagen is a hallmark of photoaging. The major enzyme responsible for collagen 1 digestion is matrix metalloproteinase-1 (MMP-1) (Dong et al., 2008). Skin fibroblasts produce MMP-1 in response to UVB irradiation, and keratinocytes play a major role through an indirect paracrine mechanism involving the release of epidermal cytokine after UVB-irradiation (Fagot et al., 2002). MMPs are produced in response to UVB irradiation in vivo and are considered to be involved in the changes in connective tissue that occur in photoaging (Brinckmann et al., 1995). They are associated with a variety of normal and pathological conditions that involve degradation and remodeling of the matrix (Smutzer, 2002; Mac Cawley and Matrisian, 2001; Mac Cawley and Matrisian, 2000; Greenwald et al., 1999). UV rays and aging lead to excess proteolytic activity that disturbs the skin's three-dimensional integrity (Rocquet and Bonte, 2002). These proteinases are important for breaking down the extracellular matrix during chronic wound repair, in which there is re-epithelialization by keratinocyte migration. Thus, MMPs are continuously involved in the remodeling of the skin after chronic aggression.Photodamage also results in the accumulation of abnormal elastin in the superficial dermis, and several MMPs have been implicated in this process (Rocquet and Bonte, 2002). ROS activate cytoplasmic signal transduction pathways in resident fibroblasts that are related to growth, differentiation, senescence, and connective tissue degradation (Scharffetter-Kochanek et al., 2000). As well as causing permanent genetic changes involving protooncogenes and tumor suppressor genes, ROS activate cytoplasmic signal transduction pathways that are related to growth differentiation, senescence, transformation and tissue degradation (Scharffetter-Kochanek et al., 1997). The study of Kang et al. (2003) revealed that UVA/UVB irradiation of skin causes generation of H_2O_2 within 15 minutes. AP-1, which leads to increased collagen breakdown, becomes elevated and remains elevated within 24hours following UV irradiation (Fisher et al., 1996). Decreased procollagen synthesis within eight hours of UV irradiation was demonstrated (Quan et al., 2002). Consequently, increased collagen breakdown was demonstrated (Fisher et al., 1997). It is hypothesized that dermal breakdown is followed by repair that, like all wound repair, is imperfect. Imperfect repair yields a deficit in the structural integrity of the dermis, a solar scar. Dermal degradation followed by imperfect repair is repeated with each intermittent exposure to ultraviolet irradiation, leading to accumulation of solar scarring and ultimately visible photoaging (Fisher and Voorhees, 1998). While it may seem that the signs of photoaging appear overnight, they actually lie invisible beneath the surface of the skin for years (Figure 37). Clinical signs of photoaging include dryness; irregular, dark/light pigmentation; sallowness; either deep furrows or severe atrophy; telangiectases; premalignant lesions; laxity; and a leathery appearance (Yaar, Eller, and Gilchrest, 2002). Other signs include elastosis (a coarse, yellow, cobblestoned effect of the skin) and actinic purpura (easy bruising related to vascular wall fragility in the dermis) (Gilchrest, 1990). UV exposure of the skin causes oxidative stress, leading to inflammatory reactions, such as erythema, sunburn, and chronic reactions. Most problematic chronic reactions include premature skin aging and skin cancer. (Oresajo et al., 2010).The amount of photoaging that develops depends on: 1) a person's skin color and 2) their history of long-term or intense sun exposure. People with fair skin who have a history of sun exposure develop more signs of photoaging than those with dark skin.

Photoaging is a complex biochemical condition, but its hallmark is the destruction of dermal collagen. This has been attributed to the direct activation of fibroblast matrix metalloproteinases by solar UV. Yarosh et al. (2008) reported that unirradiated fibroblasts increase metalloproteinase production and digest collagen when exposed to cell culture media from irradiated keratinocytes. Enhanced DNA repair in the keratinocytes ameliorates this response. This suggests that soluble factors induced by DNA damage in UV-exposed epidermal keratinocytes signal collagen degradation by fibroblasts in the dermis (Yarosh, 2008).

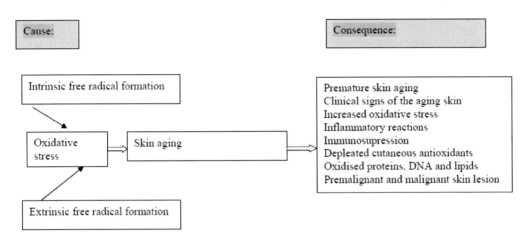

Figure 26. Causes and consequences of skin aging.

It should be remembered that solar radiation includes not only UVR but also visible and infrared radiation. Visible light is thought to be unimportant in photoaging (Kligman,,1986), but studies have confirmed that infrared radiation can certainly damage the dermal matrix (Kligman and Kligman, 1984). It could be concluded that photoaging plays a significant role in skin-aging process. Certain damaging effects on the skin could be preventedby appropriate preventive approaches that are discussed in next chapters.

The next paragraph will shortly introduce UVR as a main cause of DNA damage responsible for the skin cancer formation.

Skin Cancer

Ultraviolet radiation (UVR) is an essential risk factor for the development of premalignant skin lesions as well as of melanoma and non-melanoma skin cancer. Skin cancer is a malignant growth on the skin, which can have many causes. Skin cancer generally develops in the epidermis (the outermost layer of skin), so a tumor is usually clearly visible, which makes it easier to detect. There are various types of skin cancer. One main class is formed by the cutaneous melanocytes—melanoma. The other main types are basal cell carcinomas and squamous cell carcinomas, cancers of the epithelial cells. These carcinomas of the skin (basal cell and squamous cell carcinomas) are sometimes, collectively, called "non-melanoma skin cancers."

The target organ of UV radiation is the skin. Sun exposure is the major known environmental factor associated with the development of skin cancer of all types. While exposure to ultraviolet radiation is the risk factor most closely linked to the development of skin cancer, other environmental factors (such as ionizing radiation, chronic arsenic ingestion, and immunosuppression) and genetic factors (such as family history, skin type, and genetic syndromes) also potentially contribute to carcinogenesis. UV exposure appears to promote the induction of skin cancer by two mechanisms. The first involves direct mutagenesis of epidermal DNA, which promotes the induction of neoplasia. The second is associated with immune suppression, which allows the developing tumor to escape immune surveillance and grow progressively (Katiyar and Mukhtar, 2001).

It is known that UV exposure results in photochemical modification of the genetic material (DNA), but most of this damage is accurately and efficiently repaired by the cell. However, if the amount of damage is too great, some of the alterations to the DNA may remain as permanent mutations. DNA absorbs UVB light, and the absorbed energy can break bonds in the DNA. Most of the DNA breakages are repaired by proteins present in the cell's nucleus, but unrepaired genetic damage of the DNA can lead to skin cancers. As already mentioned previously, solar UVR induces a variety of photoproducts in DNA, including cyclobutane-type pyrimidine dimers, pyrimidine-pyrimidone (6-4) photoproducts, thymine glycols, cytosine damage, purine damage, DNA strand breaks and DNA-protein cross-links. It has been proposed that if unrepaired damage occurs to regulatory genes (e.g., tumor suppressor genes), this may be involved in the process of carcinogenesis. In this context, mutations to and activation of genes may be important. Other responses likely to result from UV exposure of cells include increased cellular proliferation, which could have a tumor-promoting effect on genetically altered cells, as well as changes in components of the immune system present in the skin (International programme on chemical safety, Environmental Health Criteria 160).

Solar radiation was tested for carcinogenicity in a series of exceptional studies in mice and rats. Large numbers of animals were studied, and well characterized benign and malignant skin tumors developed in most of the surviving animals. Although the reports are deficient in quantitative details, the results provide convincing evidence that sunlight is carcinogenic for the skin of animals (IARC, 2010).

"It seems that in rapidly dividing epithelium, such as the epidermis, nuclear damage triggered by some xenobiotics may not be so important because of the constant introduction of new healthy cells, whereas a DNA mutation has a much higher probability to become fixed to a transformed phenotype in tissues (e.g., liver) with slow cell turnover" (Fuch et al., 2001).This may explain at least in part why the absolute number of clinically well-recognizedhuman skin carcinogens is so small. According to estimation of Douglas et al. (2010), physiologic UV doses create mutations at a frequency of $\sim 10^{-4}$/gene per cell division. The specific mutations needed to activate an oncogene would be rarer. The probability of mutating five genes needed for cancer formation, such as an oncogene and both alleles of two particular tumor suppressor genes, is at best 10^{-20}. With 10^6 proliferating keratinocytes per cm^2 in human skin, and $\sim 1\ cm^2$ exposed, less than one person in 10^{10} would develop a tumor. However, clonal expansion increases by 1,000-fold the number of targets for the next mutation and increases the probability of tumor formation. It is widely believed that cancer development inhumans and laboratory animals is caused by sequential mutations and clonal outgrowthof somatic cells.

Increasing evidence has implicated a role for free radicals and oxidativestress in all three stages of the carcinogenic process. Radicals may be involved in theinitiation step, either in the oxidative activation of a procarcinogen to its carcinogenicform or in the binding of the carcinogenic species to DNA or both (Guyton and Kensler, 1993; Trush and Kensler, 1991; Pryor, 1997), thus making oxidative stress an important cofactor for carcinogen activation.Promotion always involves radicals, at least to some extent (Cerutti, 1985; Troll and Wiesner, 1985; Marks and Fu¨rstenberger, 1985;Kensler and Taffe, 1986; Crawford et al., 1988; Sun, 1990; Cheng et al., 1992; Agarwal and Mukhtar, 1993; Feig et al., 1994; Kensler et al., 1995; Slaga, 1998), while their role in progression is controversial (Pryor, 1997). For further information on redox modulation and oxidative stress in dermatology, see review by Fuchs et al. (2001).

A 1% decrease in the ozone layer will cause an estimated 2% increase in UVB irradiation; it is estimated that this will lead to a 4% increase in basal carcinomas and 6% increase in squamous-cell carcinomas (Graedel et al., 1993). Ninety percent of the skin carcinomas are attributed to UVB exposure (Wayne, 1991), and the chemical mechanism by which it causes skin cancer has been identified (Tevini, 1993). The cumulative dose of sunlight required to cause basal cell carcinoma (BCC) or squamous-cell carcinoma (SCC) in adults is fairly large, approximately 10,000 and 70,000 hours of exposure, respectively (Brash et al., 2010). There appears to be a correlation between brief, high-intensity exposures to UV and eventual appearance (as long as 10 to 20 years) of melanoma (Sparling. B. www.nas.nasa.gov). Different patterns of sun exposure appear to lead to different types of skin cancer among susceptible individuals.

Cumulative lifetime sun exposure is strongly associated with SCC incidence. BCC and actinic keratoses AK instead seem to depend on reaching a certain threshold of UV exposure, often attained in youth, such that individuals develop BCC at a relatively early age, and the incidence does not increase with further exposure (Brash et al., 2010). Intermittent sun exposure seems to be the most important risk factor for melanoma. Individuals whose first sun bed exposure occurred as a young adult, or who had long durations or high frequencies of tanning bed exposure, already have a 70% higher risk for melanoma (Gallagher et al., 2005).The intensive UV exposure early in life influences cancer formation since children are particularly sensitive to sunlight. Due to more years that are provided for mutant cells created in youth,they acquire the additional genetic mistakes/mutations required for cancer formation. Besides, cells divide faster in children, and DNA molecule is most vulnerable when being divided.

Facts about skin cancer (source: http://www.ehealthmd.com/library/skincancer):

- About 1.3 million Americans are diagnosed with skin cancer each year.
- There are three kinds of skin cancer. The rarest, melanoma, is the most serious.
- Almost half of all Americans will have some type of skin cancer at least once by the time they reach age 65.
- Most cases of skin cancer occur in people aged 50 and over.
- Childhood sun exposure may decide an individual's risk of skin cancer.
- People with certain skin types have the highest risk of skin cancer.
- Some individuals may inherit a defective gene that increases the risk of malignant melanoma.
- The risk of skin cancer may be rising because of damage to Earth's protective ozone layer.
- A routine skin self-examination is important in early detection of skin cancer.
- The cure rate for skin cancer would be almost 100 percent if all were detected early and treated.

Malignant Melanoma of the Skin and UV Radiation

Melanoma is a malignant tumor of melanocytes. Melanoma is one of the less common types of skin cancer but causes the majority (75%) of skin cancer related deaths ("Early Detection and Treatment of Skin Cancer," 2000). One in seven invasive melanomas is lethal. Approximately 130,000 malignant melanomas occur globally each year, substantially contributing to mortality rates in fair-skinned populations. An estimated 66,000 deaths occur annually from melanoma and other skin cancers (WHO, 2010).

It is estimated that 1 out of 70 Americans will experience a malignant melanoma in their lifetime.

Information from a case-control study of all patients with cutaneous malignant melanoma first diagnosed in Scotland in 1987, has been used to derive a personal risk-factor chart. Four strongest risk factors were identified to predict the relative risk of cutaneous melanoma: total number of benign pigmented naevi above 2 mm diameter; freckling tendency; number of clinically atypical naevi (over 5 mm diameter and having an irregular edge, irregular pigmentation, or inflammation); and a history of severe sunburn at any time in life (MacKie et al., 1989).

Descriptive studies in whites in North America, Australia and several other countries show a positive association between incidence of and mortality from melanoma and residence at lower latitudes. Studies of migrants suggest that the risk of melanoma is related to solar radiant exposure at the place of residence in early life. The body site distribution of melanoma shows lower rates per unit area on sites usually unexposed to the sun than on usually or regularly exposed sites. When expressed as lesions per unit area, melanomas are 10- to 20-fold more frequent on the face and male ears than on intermittently exposed sites such as the lower legs in women, shoulders, back, or neck (Green et al., 1993). In men, the incidence of invasive melanoma on the ears, a chronically sun-exposed site, was extraordinarily high, with annual rates of over 200 per 10(5) units of surface area in the Queensland population. Next highest rates of over 100 melanomas per 10(5) units were found on the face, neck, shoulders and back in men and on the face and shoulders in women. Comparison with site-specific incidence rates in the same population 7½ years previously showed that incidence of invasive disease had significantly increased for all these sites, though the largest relative increase in this period occurred on the forearm in both men and women (Green et al., 1993).Green et al. (1993) reported that "in contrast to predictions based on apparent frequency of sun exposure at subsites on the upper limbs, the relative concentration of melanomas on the shoulder suggests that wearing sleeveless garments outdoors in the sun should be avoided whenever possible. Also, the similar densities of leg and forearm melanomas seem inconsistent with the relative degree of exposure of each and further suggest that women's adoption of ankle-length skirts or trousers, in preference to knee-length skirts, would be a worthwhile modern control measure." Increases in melanomas have been greatest in intermittently sun-exposed sites such as the trunk and limbs, with little change in melanomas' frequency in head and neck, most probably due to increased recreational sun exposure (Brash et al., 2010). Assessment of intermittent exposure is complex; nonetheless, most studies show positive associations with measure of intermittent exposure, such as particular sun-intensive activities, outdoor recreation or vacations. Increased sun radiation due to decreased ozone layer might have significant role in skin cancer incidence. On the other hand, increased incidence of melanoma could be attributed also to the fact thatpeople live longer, have more wealth and more leisure time for recreational activities and vacations under the sun. A large number of case-control studies are pertinent to the relationship between melanoma and exposure to the sun. Results are generally consistent with positive associations with residence in sunny environments throughout life, in early life and even for short periods in early adult life. Positive associations are generally seen between measurements of cumulative sun damage expressed biologically as microtopographical changes or history of keratoses or nonmelanocytic skin cancer (IARC, 2010).

The evidence relating lifetime cumulative exposure to melanoma risk comes from two sources: migrant studies and studies of lifetime exposure, controlling for intermittent and occupational exposure. Data from Australia and Italy show that individuals who migrate from areas of low exposure to ultraviolet (UV) radiation, such as the United Kingdom, to areas of high exposure, such as Australia or Israel, before they reach an ageof tenyears have a lifetime risk of developing melanoma that is similar to that of people in the new country (Iscovich and Howe, 1998; McMichael and Giles, 1988; Khlat et al., 1992). Alternatively, according to National Cancer Institute, adolescents or older individuals who migrate from areas of low solar exposure to areas of high solar exposure have a risk that is more similar to that of people from their area of origin than to that of people in the new area. These data have often been cited as indicating that childhood sun exposure is more important than adult sun exposure in melanoma development.

However, the data could also be interpreted as suggesting that the length of high-level exposure is more critical than the age at exposure. Thus, people who migrate early in life to a high-insolation region have a longer potential period for intense exposure compared than do those who migrate later in life. Data from Connecticut have shown that cumulative lifetime exposure to ultraviolet-B (UVB) radiation does not differ between melanoma cases and controls; rather, intermittent sun exposure is the more important risk factor (Lea et al., 2007). The risks related to intermittent sun exposure are even greater if this pattern is experienced both early in life and later in life. These data can also be interpreted as suggesting that sun exposure patterns are rather consistent and stable throughout one's lifetime, i.e., that individuals who receive a great deal of intermittent sun exposure during early life are also likely to receive a great deal of intermittent sun exposure during later life.

Nonetheless, an intermittent pattern of sun exposure over many years appears to significantly increase melanoma risk (National Cancer Institute). It could be summarized that both chronic sun damage and intermittent sun exposure are important risk factors for skin cancer formation. The action spectrum for the induction of melanoma by UVR is unknown. Although UVB is considered by some (Sober, 1987; Koh et al., 1990) to be the waveband primarily responsible, the possibility that the action spectrum lies within the UVA, visible or even infrared parts of the solar spectrum cannot, as yet, be discounted (Loggie and Eddy, 1988), although UVA is 20-fold more frequent in sunlight spectrum but requires 1,000-fold greater doses for the induction of cell damage.

Comparisons of skin cancer data from Norway and Australia/New Zealand indicate that squamous cell carcinoma and basal cell carcinoma are mainly related to annual solar UVB influences, while UVA influences play a larger role for cutaneous malignant melanoma (Moan et al., 2008). Moan et al. (1999) proposed a hypothesis for melanoma induction: "UV radiation absorbed by melanin in melanocytes generates products that may activate the carcinogenic process. Products formed by UV absorption in the upper layers of the epidermis cannot diffuse down as far as to the melanocytes. Thus, melanin in the upper layer of the skin may be protective, while that in melanocytes may be photocarcinogenic."

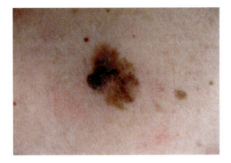

Figure 27. Example of a malignant melanoma (Author of the picture: assistant professor Mateja Dolenc—Voljč, MD).

A: Asymmetry

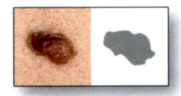

B: Borders

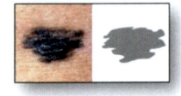

C: Color

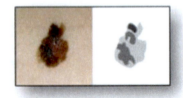

D: Diameter

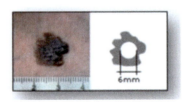

The best defense against melanoma as a whole is to encourage sun-protective behaviors, regular skin examinations and patient skin self-awareness.

A melanoma is often not recognizable to the naked eye, and at first looks hardly any different from a mole or a birthmark. The A-B-C-D-E rule can be useful in making an early diagnosis. If a mole is asymmetrical (A), has no distinct border (B), if its color changes (C), if it is larger than 5mm in diameter (D), if it has evolution (E), such as changes in color, shape, size, elevation, skin surface, and symptoms such as itching or bleeding of a lesion—all are hallmark signs of malignancy (http://www.euromelanoma.org/uk/melanoma).

Non-Melanoma Skin Cancer (NMSC)

Between twoand threemillion non-melanoma skin cancers, e.g., basal cell carcinomas and squamous cell carcinomas, are diagnosed each year but are rarely fatal and can be surgically removed. Fewer than one in 10,000 basal cell carcinoma (BCC) will metastasize. This number increases to 1 in 40 for SCC. BCC is the most common malignancy in people of European descent, with an associated lifetime risk of 30% (Miller and Weinstock, 1994). Non-melanoma skin cancer occurs mostly in light-skinned people and then predominantly on skin areas most exposed to sunlight, such as the face. The results of descriptive epidemiological studies suggest that exposure to sunlight increases the risk ofnonmelanocytic skin cancer. These tumors occur predominantly on the skin of the face and neck, which ismost commonly exposed to sunlight, although the distribution of basal-cell carcinomas is not as closely relatedto the distribution of exposure to the sun as is that of squamous-cell carcinomas. There is a strong inverserelationship between latitude and incidence of or mortality from skin cancer and, conversely, a positiverelationship between incidence or mortality and measured or estimated ambient UVR (IARC, 2010). Migrants to Australia from the British Isles have lower incidence of and mortality from nonmelanocytic skin cancer than the Australian-born population. People who work primarily outdoors have higher mortality from these cancers, and there is some evidence that outdoor workers have higher incidence. In several cross-sectional studies, positive associations have been seen between measures of solar skin damage and the prevalence of basal- and squamous-cell carcinomas. Measures of actual exposure to the sun have been less strongly associated with these cancers, possibly because of errors in measurement andinadequate control for potential confounding variables. In a study of U.S. fishermen, estimates of individual annual and cumulative exposure to UVB were positively associated with the occurrence of squamous-cell carcinoma but not with the occurrence of basal-cell carcinoma (IARC, 2010). The so called UV "signature" mutations are often found in mutated p53 genes, a key tumor suppressor gene in human squamous cell and basal cell carcinomas (Brash, 1997).

Epidemiological studies show that more than 90% of epidermal squamous cell carcinomas and more than 50% of basal cell carcinomas display UV-induced mutations that inactivate p53 (Brash et al., 1996). The p53 gene is mutated in about 50% of all human cancers. The P53 protein is a transcription factor that controls genes involved in the cell cycle control, apoptosis, and DNA repair (Latonen, 2005). In attempting to replicate past cyclobutane pyrimidine dimer lesions, the cell often makes the same mistake of misincorporating two consecutive bases, resulting in mutations characteristic for UV damage

(Brash, 1997). This is the key link between UV exposure and skin cancer and directly implicates*Intermittent exposure hypothesis.*

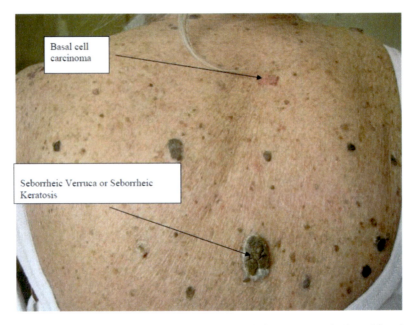

Figure 28. Example of basal cell carcinoma and multiple Seborrheic Verrucae. (Author of the picture: assistant professor Mateja Dolenc—Voljč, MD).

Intermittent Exposure Hypothesis

Although the evidence from epidemiological studies indicates an association between melanoma and sunlight exposure, it does not appear that cumulative sun exposure explains the relationship, as it does for non-melanoma skin cancer (NMSC). Instead, an intermittent exposure hypothesis proposes that infrequent intense exposure of unacclimatized skin to sunlight is related to increasing melanoma incidence and is more important than chronic sun exposure. This hypothesis is supported by the observation that most studies have shown that an increased risk of melanoma is associated with a past history of severe sunburn in childhood and adolescence (Armstrong, 1988; MacKie and Aitchison, 1982). This could be attributed also to the effect of hormesis (see also the chapter dedicated to the effect of hormesis), which explains action resulting from a response of an organism to low intensity of a stress (e.g., UVR exposure). Stress response then activates increased protection mechanisms and DNA repair systems.

According to World Health Organization- International Agency for Research on Cancer, in the Monographs on the evaluation of carcinogenic risks to humans' solar and ultraviolet, radiation is classified:

"Solar radiation is *carcinogenic to humans (Group 1).* There is *sufficient evidence*in humans for the carcinogenicity of solar radiation. Solar radiation causes cutaneous malignant melanoma and nonmelanocytic skin cancer. There is *sufficient evidence* for the carcinogenicity of solar radiation in experimental animals. There is *sufficient evidence* for the carcinogenicity of broad-spectrum ultraviolet radiation in experimental animals. There is *sufficient evidence* for the carcinogenicity of ultraviolet A radiation in experimental animals. There is *sufficient evidence* for the carcinogenicity of ultraviolet B radiation in experimental animals. There is *sufficient evidence* for the carcinogenicity of ultraviolet C radiation in experimental animals. Ultraviolet A radiation is *probably carcinogenic to humans (Group 2A)*. Ultraviolet B radiation is *probably carcinogenic to humans (Group 2A)*. Ultraviolet C radiation is *probably carcinogenic to humans (Group 2A)*."

Although DNA damage due to ROS is not a rare event since it is estimated that human cell sustains an average of 10^5 oxidative hits per day due to cellular oxidative metabolism (Fraga et al., 1991), DNA is functionally very stable, so that the incidence of cancer is much lower than one would expect, taking into account the high frequency of oxidative hits. Nevertheless, avoidance of excessive cumulative and sporadic sun exposure is important in reducing the risk of skin cancer and skin aging. Additionally, antioxidants might act by enhancing the DNA enzyme repair systems through a post-transcriptional gene regulation of transcription factors (Xanthoudakis et al., 1992; Hirota et al., 1997; Schenk et al., 1994). The repair capacity of human skin cells, therefore, directly relates to the probability of initiation of the carcinogenesis process and eventually tumor formation. Cellular antioxidant defense mechanisms are, therefore, crucial for the prevention or removal of the damage caused by the oxidizing component of UV radiation.

The most important strategy to reduce the risk of sun UV radiation damage is to avoid the sun exposure and to engage in the use of sunscreens. The next step is the use of exogenous antioxidants orally or by topical application and interventions in preventing oxidative stress and in enhanced DNA repair (for more information see section on antioxidants and alternative methods to decrease oxidative stress). Yarosh (2010) claims that properly conceived efforts to alleviate skin aging have the benefit of reducing rates of skin cancer since people are more motivated by improving their physical appearance than lowering their perceived risk of disease. Thus, the most successful anticancer efforts will arrive as treatments for skin aging.

UVR and Immune System

UVR also has impact on immune system (e.g., UV radiation damages and depletes antigen presenting Langerhans cells in the skin; erythemal doses of UV radiation induce systemic immune suppression by the release of cytokines, soluble mediators, and altered function of antigen presenting cells to induce antigen-specific regulatory T cells. Cytokines and soluble factors from UV-damaged keratinocytes enter the circulation and exert systemic suppressive effects on the immune response) (Strickland, 2009). UV-induced immune suppression is caused by both passive (damage to antigen presenting cells and subsequent inability to activate effector T cells) and active (induction of antigen-specific regulatory T cells) mechanisms (Strickland, 2009). Many of the influences of UVR on the immune system are suppressive. UV-induced immunosuppression and ROS generation by phagocytic cells could have influence on skin damage formation and accumulation, on cancer and aging process. Photoimmunology is the study of the effects of light on the immune system. Immunodermatology studies skin as an organ of immunity in health and disease. The skin is the largest organ of the body. It is also an immune organ. Besides the interdigitating network of antigen-presenting Langerhans cells and macrophages and lymphocytes that enter the dermis through lymph vessels, epidermal skin cells themselves can influence the immune response by their production of cytokines such as IL-10, TNF-alpha, and many others (Schwarz et al., 1994). Photomedicine is an interdisciplinary branch of medicine that involves the study and application of light with respect to health and disease.

A growing body of evidence suggests that environmental levels of UV radiation may suppress cell-mediated immunity and thereby enhance the risk of infectious diseases and limit the efficacy of vaccinations. UV-induced immune suppression is also an essential event in skin cancer formation (Kripke, 1984). Sun exposure, specifically the UVB component, causes immunosuppression. UVB exposure can suppress the resistance of a mouse's immune system against UVB-induced tumors (Fishern and Kripke, 1977; Daynes et al., 1977). Skin tumors induced in mice by UV radiation were highly antigenic and would be rejected when transplanted into genetically identical mice that had not been exposed to UV. These same tumors would grow when transplanted into immunosuppressed mice, showing that the immune system could readily recognize and reject UV-induced skin cancers. What was surprising, however, was that when these same tumors were transplanted into mice that were treated with a subcarcinogenic dose of UV radiation, transplanted UV-induced tumors would grow while skin tumors induced by chemical carcinogens would still be rejected. These results indicated that UV radiation not only caused skin tumors but prevented their rejection by the immune system (Strickland, 2009).

Furthermore, the induction of hypersensitivity to contact allergens may be suppressed by prior exposure of the skin to UVB radiation, both in mice and in humans (Kripke, 1984; Toews et al., 1980).

According to Jenkins et al. (2009), immunosuppression is due to spare the skin from an overly destructive immune system reactions (Jenkins et al., 2009). With aging, there is a reduction in epidermal Langerhans cells, the skin's immune antigen-presenting effector cells (Yaar and Gilchrest, 2003). There is also decreased production of the epidermal cytokine interleukin -1a and as a result decreased production of downstream cytokines including IL-6, granulocyte-macrophage colony stimulating factor and IL-8, among others (Elias and Ghadially, 2002).

Exposure to suberythemal doses of UV have been shown to exacerbate a variety of infections in rodent models. According to WHO, "UV radiation affects infections both at the site of exposure and at distant sites. Epidermal cells like Langerhans cells and melanocytes and keratinocytes secrete cytokinesafter UV exposure. Cytokines such as IL-1 and TNF-α then induce a cascade of other cytokines that can activate collagen degrading enzymes, suppress the immune system, dilate blood vessels, and attract inflammatory cells (Heck et al., 2004). In this way, cells with DNA damage have profound effect on cells in the skin and elsewhere that may not have been exposed to UV. Recent work indicates that systemic infections without skin involvement may be affected. Enhanced susceptibility appears to result from T-helper cell activity. The mechanisms associated with this suppression appear to be the same as those identified with suppression to contact and delayed type hypersensitivity responses. Suppression of these immune responses appears to be mediated by release of soluble mediators from UVB-exposed skin, which alters the antigen presentation by Langerhans and other cells so that they fail to activate TH 1 cells. The resulting immune suppression is antigen specific, can occur regardless of whether or not antigen is applied at the site of exposure, and is relatively long lasting. UV exposure also prevents the development of protection immunity to a variety of infections in mice and rats" (WHO, Ultraviolet radiation, Environmental Health Criteria: 160).

A number of studies additionally suggest that UV exposure at environmental levels suppress immune responses in both rodents and man. In rodents, this immune suppression results in enhanced susceptibility to certain infectious diseases with skin involvement and some systemic infections. Mechanisms associated with UV-induced immunosuppression and host defense mechanismsthatprovide for protection against infectious agents are similar in rodents and man. It is, therefore, reasonable to assume that exposure to UV may enhance the risk of infection and decrease the effectiveness of vaccines in humans (WHO, Ultraviolet radiation, Environmental Health Criteria: 160). Relatively few investigations have been reported of the effects of UVR on immunity in humans, but changes do occur. The primary evidence cited for immune surveillance in preventing UV-induced skin cancer is the 10- to 20-fold increase in actinic keratoses (AK) and squamous cell carcinoma (SCC) on previously sun-exposed skin in transplant patients receiving chronic immune suppression to prevent organ rejection (Brash et al., 2010). There is also evidence that contact allergy is suppressed by exposure to UVB and possibly to UVA radiation. The number of Langerhans' cells in the epidermis is decreased by exposure to UVR and sunlight, and the morphological loss of these cells is associated with changes in antigen-presenting cell function in the direction of suppression; this change may be due not only to simple loss of function but also to active migration of other antigen-presenting cells into the skin. A reduction in natural killer cell activity also occurs, which can be produced by UVA radiation. These changes are short-lived, and their functional significance is unknown. It was suggested that there may be a genetic susceptibility to UV-induced suppression, because skin cancer patients are more easily UV suppressed than cancer-free controls (Streilein, 1991).

Pigmentation of the skin may not protect against some UVR-induced alterations of immune function. Several immune responses are suppressed by UVR in mice and other rodents. Suppression of contact hypersensitivity has received most attention, and this response may be impaired locally, at the site of exposure to radiation, or systemically, at a distant, unexposed site. "The two forms of suppression have different dose dependencies—systemic suppression requiring much higher doses—and their mechanisms appear to differ, but the efferent limb of each involves generation of hapten-specific T-suppressor cells that block induction but not elicitation of contact hypersensitivity. Systemic suppression of delayed hypersensitivity to injected antigens can also be produced by exposure to UVB radiation, and several observations suggest that the mechanism of this suppression differs from that of systemic suppression of contact hypersensitivity. Alterations in immune function induced by exposure to UVR play a central role in photocarcinogenesis in mice. UVR-induced T-suppressor cells block a normal immunosurveillance system that prevents the growth of highly antigenic UVR-induced tumors. It is not known whether this mechanism operates in humans" (IARC, 2010).

Apart from the photodermatoses, where the skin lesions are caused by sunlight, there are diseases that are aggravated by sun exposure, e.g., lupus erythematosus, an autoimmune disease (Cripps and Rankin, 1973). There are, however, also skin diseases where sunlight improves the condition of the skin. Psoriasis, for example, is a widespread noninfectious skin disease; exposures to UVB radiation form an effective medical treatment (Van Weelden et al., 1988).

UV causes depletion of cellular antioxidants and antioxidant enzymes (SOD, catalase), initiates DNA damage leading to the formation of thymidine dimers, activates the neuroendocrine system leading to immunosuppression and release of neuroendocrine mediators, and causes increased synthesis and release of pro-inflammatory mediators from a variety of skin cells. The pro-inflammatory mediators increase the permeability of capillaries leading to infiltration and activation of neutrophils and other phagocytic cells into the skin. The net result of all these effects is inflammation and free radical generation (both reactive oxygen and nitrogen species) (Pillai, 2005).

Sunburn

Sunburn, or erythema, is an acute injury following excessive exposure to solar UVR. Sunburns are an acute inflammation reaction of the skin and tissue just beneath it that follows excessive exposure of the skin to UVR. The affected area becomes red, hot, tender, and swollen, and in severe cases, blisters may form. Low-dose or short exposure to UV irradiation is tolerated bythe skin without noticeable or clinically relevant changes.Only after a certain threshold is reached does delayed and prolongedvasodilatation develop, allowing passage of lymphocytes andmacrophages into the tissue and induction of an inflammatoryresponse that is clinically visible as erythema. In epidemiology studies, sunburn is usually defined as burn with pain and/or blistering that lasts for twoor more days. Cumulative sun exposure is the additive amount of sun exposure that one receives over a lifetime. A frequentlyused measure of UV irradiation–induced erythema is determinationof the minimal erythema dose (MED). One MED is the minimal amountof energy required to induce a uniform, clearly demarcated redness16 to 24 h after exposure to UV irradiation. Even a single minimum erythema dose (1 MED) can damage the dermal matrix. Cumulative sun exposure may reflect the additive effects of intermittent sun exposure, or chronic sun exposure, or both. The redness of the skin that results is due to an increased blood content of the skin by dilatation of the superficial blood vessels in the dermis, mainly the subpapillary venules (Diffey, 1991).Skin color is an important factor in determining the ease with which the skin will sunburn. Whereas fair-skinned people require only about 15 to 30 min of midday summer sunshine to induce an erythemal reaction, people with moderately pigmented skin may require one to two h exposure, and those with darkly pigmented skin (i.e. negroes) will not normally sunburn. Other phenotype characteristics that may influence the susceptibility to sunburn are hair color, eye color and freckles (Azizi et al, 1988,;Andreassi et al, 1987). Based on a personal history of response to 45 to 60 min of exposure to midday summer sun in early June (Fitzpatrick, 1975), individuals can be grouped into six sun-reactive skin types (Table 6).

Types 1 and 2 are at high risk of skin cancer, particularly when exposed to intense sunlight.

There are anatomical differences in erythemal sensitivity (Diffey, 1991). The face, neck and trunk are two to four times more sensitive than the limbs (Olson et al., 1966). Vertical surfaces of an upright person receive about one-half of the ambient UVR, whereas horizontal surfaces, such as the epaulet region of the shoulder, receive up to 75%.

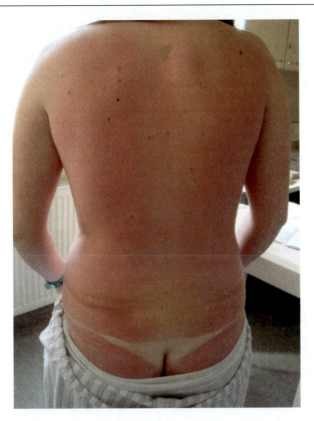

Figure 29. Picture of the sunburn of a girl using a sun bed (author of the picture: assist. Tanja Planinšek Ručigaj, MD).

In addition to erythema and tanning, thickening (hyperplasia) of the epidermis is a significant component of a mild sunburn reaction (Diffey, 1991). A single moderate exposure to UVB can result in up to a three-fold thickening of the stratum corneum within one to three weeks, and multiple exposures every one to two days for up to seven weeks will thicken the stratum corneum by about three- to five-fold (Miescher, 1930). Skin thickness returns to normal about one to two months after ceasing irradiation.

Table 6. Fitzpatrick's skin types. The following six skin phenotypes were defined on the basis of response to sun exposure at the beginning of summer (Fitzpatrick, 1988)

1.	Type I: Extremely fair skin, always burns, never tans.
2.	Type II: Fair skin, always burns, sometimes tans.
3.	Type III: Medium skin, sometimes burns, always tans.
4.	Type IV: Olive skin, rarely burns, always tans.
5.	Type V: Moderately pigmented brown skin, never burns, always tans.
6.	Type VI: Markedly pigmented black skin, never burns, always tans.

Thickening of the skin, especially of the stratum corneum, after sun exposure can lead to a significant increase in protection against UVR by a factor of five or even higher. In Caucasians, skin thickening is probably more important than tanning in providing endogenous photoprotection, although in darkly pigmented races, skin pigmentation is the most important means of protection against solar UVR.

More on solar ultraviolet radiation effects on biological systems can be read in excellent review byDiffey (1991).

Tanning

Less intense or shorterduration exposure to UVR results in an increase in skin pigmentation that provides some protection against further UVR-induced damage. The increased skin pigmentation occurs in two phases, immediate pigment darkening and delayed tanning. Intermediate pigment darkening occurs during exposure to UVR and results from oxidation and redistribution of existing melanin. This reaction may fade rapidly or persist for several days. Delayed tanning results from increased synthesis of epidermal melanin and requires 24 to 72 hours to become visible.

Melanocytes are specialized dendritic cells interspersed among basal keratinocytes and serve the primary function of producing melanin in intracellular organelles melanosomes that are then distributed to surrounding keratinocytes (Hakozaki et al., 2010).

Following solar UVR exposure, there is an increase in the number of functioning melanocytes, and activity of the enzyme tyrosinase is enhanced (Fitzpatrick et al., 1983). This leads to the formation of new melanin and hence an increase in the number of melanin granules throughout the epidermis. Melanins are the major UV-absorbing chromophores in skin, exhibiting an extremely broad spectrum of absorption over the UVB, UVA and visible ranges. Melanins are complex polymeric proteins that are produced by melanocytes and transferred to keratinocytes. It should be stressed that melanin cannot offer 100% protection to our skin against harmful effects of solar radiation.

Gilchrest et al. (1999) explained how ultraviolet irradiation stimulates melanogenesis in the skin. A direct effect of UV photons on DNA results in upregulation of the gene for tyrosinase, the rate-limiting enzyme in melanin synthesis, as well as an increase in cell-surface expression of receptors for at least one of the several known keratinocyte-derived melanogenic factors, MSH. Direct effects of UV on melanocyte membranes, releasing DAG and arachidonic acid, may also play a role in the tanning response. Diacylglycerol may activate PKC-beta, which, in turn, phosphorylates and activates tyrosinase protein; the pathways by which products of other inflammatory mediator cascades may act on melanogenesis are unknown. The tanning response also relies heavily on UV-stimulated increased production and release of numerous keratinocyte-derived factors including bFGF, NGF, endothelin-1 and the POMC-derived peptides MSH, ACTH, beta-LPH and beta-endorphin (Gilchrest et al., 1999). Ultraviolet-induced melanogenesis may be one part of a eukaryotic SOS response to damaging ultraviolet irradiation that has evolved over time to provide a protective tan in skin at risk of further injury from sun exposure (Gilchrest et al., 1999).

The distribution and size of melanin particles also plays an important role in protecting epidermal cells. Melanin particles have a distribution within the stratum corneum and epidermal cells depending upon skin type. In dark skin types (5 and 6), theseparticles are positioned within cells to provide optimum optical protection for the cell nuclei and in adequate size in the stratumcorneum (Kolliaset al., 1991).

According to Euro melanoma (http://www.euromelanoma.org/uk/home) "fake tan (auto bronzing) is by far safer than a suntan. A fake tan produces a natural looking tan through a chemical reaction in the skin. It, therefore, gives the desired cosmetic result in someone who is very keen to have a tan, without him or her having to sunbathe. Application of fake tan needs to be carried out every one to two weeks in order to maintain the tan since the top layers of the skin are constantly being renewed. However, the actual tanning produces by 'fake tan' is not at all protective against UV-radiation and consumers should be aware of this important factor."

Development of Different Human Skin Colors

The earliest members of the hominid lineage probably had a mostly unpigmented or lightly pigmented integument covered with dark black hair, similar to that of the modern chimpanzee. The evolution of a naked, darkly pigmented integument occurred early in the evolution of the genus Homo. A dark epidermis protected sweat glands from UV-induced injury, thus insuring the integrity of somatic thermoregulation (Jablonski and Chaplin, 2000). There are many hypotheses for skin darkening (reviewed by Juzeniene et al., 2009): shielding of sweat glands and blood vessels in the skin, protection against skin cancer and overproduction of vitamin D, camouflage, adaptation to different ambient temperatures, defense against microorganisms, protection against folate photodestruction. The primary selective pressure within the tropics was to protect folate by maintaining dark pigmentation. Photolysis of folate and its main serum form of 5-methylhydrofolate is caused by UVR and by reactive oxygen species generated by UVA. Competition for folate between the needs for cell division, DNA repair, and melanogenesis is severe under stressful, high-UVR conditions and is exacerbated by dietary insufficiency (Jablonski and Chaplin, 2000). Hypotheses for skin lightening are: sexual selection, adaptation to cold climates, enhancement of vitamin D photoproduction, and changing food habits leading to lower intake of vitamin D.

As hominids migrated outside of the tropics, varying degrees of depigmentation evolved in order to permit UVB-induced synthesis of previtamin D(3). The lighter color of female skin may be required to permit synthesis of the relatively higher amounts of vitamin D(3) necessary during pregnancy and lactation (Jablonski and Chaplin, 2000).

Solarium or SunBeds

Besides natural sunlight, there is an increasing influence of the use of artificial UV radiation. Sunbeds are broadly used for cosmetic tanning purposes. The expression "sun bed" includes tanning equipment consisting of a UV-emitting lamp or a number of such lamps incorporated in a bed, canopy or panel, or any combination thereof. There are four distinct types of lamps in use, each with different UV-emission characteristics. Those are UVA, low-pressure fluorescent tubes; UVA, filtered high-intensity discharge lamps; UVB, low-pressure fluorescent tubes; UVB, filtered high-intensity discharge lamps (International programme on chemical safety, Environmental Health Criteria 160).The emission characteristics and the health risks associated with the use of each type of lamp are different. The last two lamp types are associated with high levels of UVB and are now little used. They have been almost universally replaced by the predominantly UVA emitting lamp types.

According to Melanoma Awareness Newsletter (http://www.melanomaawareness.org/spring2008.pdf), on an average day in the UnitedStates, more than onemillionpeople tan in tanning salons.Nearly 70 percent of tanningsalon clients are girls andwomen, primarily aged 16 to 29years.Nearly 30 million people tanindoors in the United Statesannually. Of these, 2.3 millionare teens.

The "RAYS: Your Grade" survey (http://www.aad.org/RaysYourGrade/) polled adults in 32 U.S. metropolitan regions spanning 29 states and tested their knowledge, attitudes and behaviors toward tanning and sun protection. Nearly three-quarters (73%) of adults feel that people look more attractive with a tan. Nearly half (47%) of adults incorrectly believe that sun exposure is healthy. More than one-third (37%) of adults incorrectly believe their skin type means they don't have to worry about sun exposure. Four out of five (80%) adults are concerned about skin cancer and feel it is important to protect themselves. Half (50%) of adults have been sunburned at least once in the past year. About one-quarter (23%) of adults never examine their own skin for changes to moles and other skin blemishes. More than half (52%) of adults know that getting a base tan is not a healthy way to protect skin from sun damage. A large majority (71%) of adults do not apply sunscreen on an average day.

(Skin) Age Spots and Hyperpigmentation

Hyperpigmentation is caused by increased melanin deposition in the epidermis or dermis. There are three main types of skin hyperpigmentation. Melasma (also known as "Chloasma faciei") is a general term describing darkening of the skin, mostly on the face. Melasma is a common, acquired hypermelanosis that primarily affects sun-exposed areas in women. The symptoms of melasma are dark, irregular patches commonly found on the upper cheek, nose, lips, upper lip, and forehead. Chloasma is typically used to describe skin discolorations caused by hormones, such as pregnancy, birth control pills or estrogen replacement therapy. Frequently, melasma and chloasma are used interchangeably. Solar (Actinic) lentigenes is the technical term for darkened spots on the skin caused by the sun. Lentigenes describes a darkened area of skin that is quite common in adults with a long history of unprotected sun exposure. Photomelanosis is caused by increased pigmentation due to sun exposure. The pigmentation occurs on exposed skin, commonly on the face, neck and the back. The pigmentation may be patchy or as diffused darkening of the exposed skin.

Age spots are also called liver spots, lentigo simplex and senile lentigines. They are flat, gray, brown or black spots that occur on more than 90% fair-skinned people after age 50. Age spots range from frecklesize to a few inches in diameter. They are most common on skin areas most exposed to the sun. The more sun damage or sun skin was exposed, the more likely age spots will emerge. Age spots do show up more as a person gets olderdue to a longer time of sun exposure.

Adult melanocytes are able to stop to proliferate, and terminally differentiated melanocytes are still metabolically active but post-mitotic. The altered differentiated functions of senescent melanocyte are not well known. Alterations of melanosomes, melanin-synthesizing enzyme in mitogen-activated protein kinase (MAPK), and in cell-cycle progression have been reported. All these altered functions may have a real impact in tissue (Medrano, 1998). The knowledge of the mechanisms of human skin color is of prime importance to develop skin care products, increasing the skin radiance and fighting spot formation (Roquet and Bonte, 2002). Disturbed keratinocytes-melanocytes interactions during melanosome transfer and skin melanosome distribution patterns could be related to spot formation. Melanocytes located in the basal layer of epidermis produce melanin-loaded melanosomes, which are distributed to neighboring keratinocytes. UV radiation leads to an accumulation of melanosomes in melanocytes and treatment with melanocyte-stimulating hormone MSH induces exocytosis of melanosomes. UV and MSH increase the phagocytose of melanosomes by keratinocytes (Virador et al., 2002). Keratinocytes and fibroblasts, whose paracrine effects on melanocytes (rather than melanocytes itself), play an important role in the epidermal pigmentation (Okazaki, 2010 and references cited there). Human keratinocytes and fibroblasts express or secrete several melanogenic cytokines. It has been reported that also overexpression of these melanogenic cytokines is responsible for the age-related pigmentary cutaneous disorders (Kadono et al., 2001; Hattori et al., 2004).

Several proven targets for pigmentation control are known, but recent genomic and proteomic understanding of melanogenesis, the melanocyte, melanocyte-keratinocyte interactions and melanocyte-fibroblast interaction has revealed potentially hundreds of proteins and other effectors involved in the pigmentation process (Hakozaki et al., 2010). The regulation of melanin production is very complex and involves more than 80 genes (Hearing, 1999; Schallreuter, 2007).

The formation of skin spots on photoexposed areas is thus a very complex problem but may be viewed as a double problem. The direct and indirect processes stimulated by UV irradiation (endothelin-1, thymin dimers, NO) increase the melanin production (Manaka et al., 2001; Tajima et al., 1998; Craven et al., 1998). Their local aggregation can also generate new reactive oxygen species (Nofsinger et al., 2002). A disturbance of cell-cell signaling (cadherin E, P, etc.) can cause melanin to be transferred to basal keratinocytes instead to suprabasal cells, resulting in pigment accumulation (Andersen, 1997). Accumulation of pigment in such cells could also be due to local defect of keratinization and to oxidation products, like lipofuscin. Changes due to UV irradiation and aging could make these cells, pigment-loaded by error, less easy to eliminate. Furthermore, melanocytes getting the information that their protective pigment distribution pattern is abnormal will continue to oversynthesize pigment, leading to more, uncontrolled accumulation.

Freckles, age spots, spider veins on the face, rough and leathery skin, fine wrinkles that disappear when stretched, loose skin, a blotchy complexion, actinic keratoses (thick wart-like, rough, reddish patches of skin), and skin cancer can all be traced to sun exposure. Primary prevention of UVR exposure and sun protection is the most important step for reducing age-spot formation. Comprehensive sun protection includes:

- Avoiding deliberate tanning, including use of indoor tanning devices.
- Staying out of the sun between 10:00 a.m. and 4:00 p.m., when the sun's rays are the strongest.

- Wearing protective clothing, such as a wide-brimmed hat and long sleeves, when outdoors during the day.
- Applying sunscreen year round. Sunscreen should be broad spectrum (offers UVA and UVB protection) and have a Sun Protection Factor (SPF) of 30 or higher. Sunscreen should be applied 20 minutes before going outdoors to all skin that will be exposed. It should be reapplied after sweating or being in water.

More radical measures (once spots are formed) include chemical peels or microdermabrasion. Increasingly, laser treatments are seen as the best way of dealing with extensive or deep sun spots.

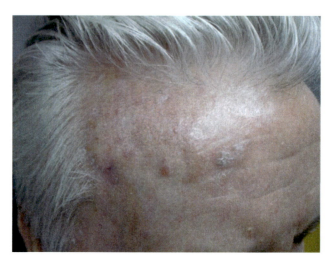

Figure 30. Picture of initial actinic keratoses (Keratoses actinicae frontis) (author of the picture: Ana Benedicic, MD, MSc).

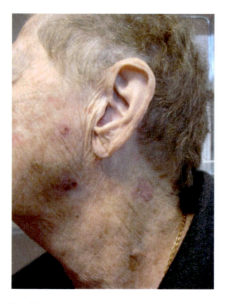

Figure 31. Picture of a progressed actinic keratoses (author of the picture: Ana Benedicic, MD, MSc).

Photosensitization

Photoexcitation is the mechanism of electron excitation by photon absorption, when the energy of the photon is too low to cause photoionization. In chemistry, photoisomerization is molecular behavior in which structural change between isomers is caused by photoexcitation. Photosensitization is a process of transferring the energy of absorbed light. After absorption, the energy is transferred to the (chosen) reactants. Photosensitization is also a clinical condition in which skin (areas exposed to light and lacking significant protective hair, wool, or pigmentation) is hyperreactive to sunlight due to the presence of photodynamic agents. Molecules of photosensitizing agents present in the skin are energized by light. When the molecules return to the less-energized state, the released energy is transferred to receptor molecules that quickly initiate chemical reactions in various skin components. Tissue injury is thought to result from the production of reactive oxygen intermediates or from alterations in cell membrane permeability.

Deleterious biological effects are mainly due to the UVB portion of the sun's spectrum, but it was shown that also wavelengths in the UVA range can produce similar biological effects by specific mechanisms (Applegate et al., 1995; Fuchs et al., 1989; Moysan et al., 1993; Moysan et al., 1995). These mechanisms involve endogenous chromophores such as quinones, steroids, flavins, free porphyrins, and heme-containing enzymes, which act as photosensitizers when induced by UVA irradiation. Most adverse effects of UVA in the skin are assumed to be the result of oxidative damage mediated through UVA absorption by cellular chromophores such as urocanic acid (Menon and Morrison, 2002), riboflavin (Sato et al., 1995; Kipp and Young, 1999), and melanin precursors that act as photosensitizers (Kvam and Tyrell, 1997; Schraffetter-Kochanek et al., 1997). Reactive oxygen species, including singlet oxygen, superoxide radical anion, hydroxyl radical, and hydrogen peroxide, are produced during these photosensitization reactions in such a manner that the pro-antioxidant balance can be disturbed (Shindo et al., 1994). The resulting photooxidative stressdue to these harmful ROS is considered to play a major role in causing modifications of DNA, lipids, proteins, and carbohydrates in human skin (Applegate et al., 1999; Moysan et al., 1995; Punnonen et al., 1991; Treina et al., 1996).

Photosensitization can be difficult to differentiate clinically from actual sunburn (*The Merck Manual*). Clinical signs are easily recognized in cases of marked photosensitivity but are similar to the primary actinic effects of sunburn in early or mild cases. Treatment involves mostly palliative measures. While photosensitivity continues, sun exposure should be avoided; one should stay in shadow or in darkness. There is a long list of drugs that can cause photosensitization reactions. Antineoplastics, antimicrobials, diuretics, retinoids, hypoglycemic agents, and even antihistamines are capable of triggering photosensitivity reactions in certain individuals. Photosensitizers are found in some cosmetics or as ingested photosensitizing drugs that reach the skin, including some phenothiazines (used as tranquilizers), as well as fluoroquinolone and tetracycline antibiotics (Halliwell and Gutteridge, 2007). Photosenzitizers can be found also in plants. Celery, parsnips and parsley contain psoralenes. Psoralene is a naturally occurring furocoumarin, extracted from Psoralea corylifolia and other plants. After photoactivation with UV radiation, it appears to bind DNA through single- and double-stranded cross-linking. St. John's Wort (*Hypericum hirsutum*) produces hypericin, which is also a photosensitizer.

Beneficial Effects of UV

Until now, just harmful effects of UVR on different cellular molecules of the skin were discussed. However, small amounts of UV are beneficial for people and essential in the production of vitamin D. UV radiation is also used to treat several diseases, including rickets, psoriasis, atopic dermatitis and jaundice. This takes place under medical supervision, and the benefits of treatment versus the risks of UV-radiation exposure are a matter of clinical judgment.

According to Diffey (1991), the only thoroughly established beneficial effect of solar ultraviolet radiation on the skin is the synthesis of vitamin D3. Solar radiation in the UVB waveband photochemically converts 7-dehydrocholesterol in the epidermis to previtamin D3. This previtamin immediately isomerizes to vitamin D3 in a reaction controlled by skin temperature and which takes two to three days to reach completion. Previtamin D3 is photolabile, and excessive exposure to sunlight causes its photolysis to biologically inert photoproducts, lumisterol and tachysterol. In fact, production of previtamin D3 is limited to no more than 5% to 15% of the total 7-dehydrocholesterol content in the skin, no matter how long a person is exposed to sunlight. Once vitamin D3 is made in the skin, it enters the blood for transport to the liver to be metabolized to 25-hydroxyvitamin D (Webb and Holick, 1988). If vitamin D3 does not enter the circulation before sun exposure the following day, it can be rapidly degraded in the skin by sunlight to suprasterol 1, suprasterol 2 and 5,6-transvitamin D3—products which are believed to be biologically inert (Webb et al., 1989). Thus sunlight, through its photochemical activity, is able to regulate the production of both previtamin D3 and vitamin D3 in the skin.

Only short exposures to sunlight are required to synthesize vitamin D3 in the skin; from spring until autumn, 15 min exposure to the hands, arms and face between 9 am and 4 pm is adequate to provide our vitamin D3 requirement (Diffey, 1991). There is still the ongoing debate between the adequate sun exposure to create sufficient vitamin D and the risk arising from skin cancer from moderate increased sun exposure (Holick, 2004; Grant and Holick, 2005). It has been roughly estimated that a sufficiency of vitamin D synthesis in skin can be provided by exposure of 40% of the body to 25% of the UVB minimal erythemal dose (Grant and Holick, 2005). An untanned person with fair skin may receive mild sunburn in as little as 25 minutes at noon (depending on the time of year and the latitude) but would have to lie in the sun for at least two hours to receive the same dose after 3 pm (International programme on chemical safety, Environmental Health Criteria 160).

Alternative to sun exposure vitamin D production is the intake of synthetic vitamin D with supplements. But on the other hand, supplements of vitamin D can cause side effects from excess vitamin D, while sun-exposure cannot lead to excessive vitamin D amounts. However, it can lead to excessive skin damage formation.

Conclusion

The ultraviolet spectrum of the solar light is the most damaging exogenous source for our skin. Photoaging affects the sun-exposed areas and is characterized clinically by fine and coarse wrinkling, roughness, dryness, laxity, teleangiectasia, loss of tensile strength and pigmentary changes. There is also an increase in development of benign and malignant neoplasms on photoaged skin (Sjerobabski, Masnec and Poduje, 2008).

UVR penetrates our skin, reaches the cells and is absorbed by DNA, leading to the formation of photoproducts that inactivate the functions of DNA. UVA radiation acts mostly indirectly through the generation of ROS, producing high amounts of singled oxygen, which can further initiate lipid peroxidation, oxidation of proteins or generation of DNA strand breaks (Scharffetter-Kochanek et al., 2000). UVB action is mostly by direct interaction with DNA via the inductionof DNA damage. Both UVA and UVB can induce MMP. The epidermis and dermis are both affected by UVB, but the dermis is also affected to a significant extent by UVA. It has long been thought that the majority of human photo-lesions are due to UVB rays; now it is believed that UVA plays a substantial role in photoaging.

But DNA is not the only biomolecule damaged by UVR. Free radicals and oxidants produced by UVR oxidize also lipids and proteins in the cell. The skin then springs into action with an inflammatory response, characterized by erythema (sunburn), the release of proteases and cytokines. Infectious agents that may try to take advantage of this compromised situation are sought out and destroyed. Then, a temporary period of immune suppression follows. During that time, repair systems are activated that excise DNA lesions and replace the damaged DNA, and non-functional proteins are turned-over by proteases. Hormesis effect activates the synthesis of melanin and antioxidant protection, and damaged lipids are cleaved and replaced. Irreparable cells are removed by apoptosis (Yarosh, 2003). However, these repair mechanisms are not 100% effective. The damaged components are not always completely repaired. The problem arises in the cases of intensive acute sun exposure or in the cases of chronic sun exposure over longer decades, which manifests as skin photoaging.To what extent each mechanism—mtDNA mutagenesis, protein oxidation, downregulation of collagen synthesis and increased expression of matrix metalloproteinases—contributes to premature skin aging is still not answered.

As photoaging via sunlight or artificial UV-exposure is the major impacting factor for skin appearance, new defense strategies have been suggested, including the appropriate UVA+UVB sunscreen choice in addition to an antioxidant-rich diet, the inductionof photoprotective melanogenesis by means of thymidine-dinucleotide (pTpT) formulations, the use of phytoestrogens and metal chelating agents to inhibit the collagenase activation, the avoidance of refined hyperglycemic carbohydrates so as to slow down the glycation/oxidation of proteins, the use of DPTT, aminoguanidine and carnosine formulations to inhibit the collagen cross-linking as well as retinoic acid to stimulate the DNA repair mechanisms and collagen synthesis (Ionescu, 2005).

UV protection includes not only reduction of sun exposure but also use of sun protective filters, UV protective clothes, DNA repair enzymes, and antioxidant supplementation. More on the antioxidant action on the skin can be read in the further chapter.

Chapter 7

Skin, Free Radicals and Antioxidants

Oxidative phosphorylation in the mitochondria is an important energy-producing process for eukaryotic cells, but this process can also result in producing potentially cell-damaging side products, e.g., free radicals and other ROS. Oxygen is the final proton acceptor in this cascade of electron/proton transfer and results in harmless water. The electron transfer, however, is not completely efficient, and oxygen is not totally reduced to water. It is estimated that approximately 1% to 3% oxygen is reduced to superoxide instead to water. Low amounts of these ROS are important for cellular-signaling pathways. At least two classical signaling pathways, the mitogen-activated protein kinases (MAPK) and signaling leading to activation of NF-κB, are activated by oxidants. Oxidants can modulate cell-signaling events by modifying cell-surface receptors, phosphatases and protein phosphorylation, etc. Excessive ROS, however, can induce oxidative stress, leading to cell damage that can culminate in cell death. Therefore, the cell has developed an antioxidant network to scavenge excessively produced ROS. In general, the balance between the production and scavenging of ROS leads to homeostasis (Wittgen and van Kempen, 2007). But it seems that there isalways a bit more free radicals produced leading to constant oxidative stress and cell damage thataccumulates with time.

Antioxidants attenuate the damaging effects of ROS and can impair and/or reverse many of the events that contribute to epidermal toxicity and disease. However, increased or prolonged free radical action can overwhelm ROS defense mechanisms, contributing to the development of cutaneous diseases, disorders and skin aging. Although the skin possesses extremely efficient antioxidant activities, during aging, ROS levels rise and antioxidant activities decline. Oxidants and antioxidants play an important role in maintaining a balance between free radicals produced by metabolism or derived from environmental sources. Cellular antioxidants may change their redox state, be targeted for destruction, regulate oxidative process involved in signal transduction, and affect gene expression and pathways of cell proliferation and death. Free radicals can be generated also from the environmental exposures. It is well documented that solar UV exposure to mammalian skin induces a number of pathological conditions, such as sunburn cell formation, hyperplastic response, and DNA damage that contributes to the development of several disease states, including immunotoxicity and skin aging. In addition, UV exposure to the skin results in the generation of reactive oxygen species (ROS), such as singlet oxygen, peroxy radicals, superoxide anion, and hydroxyl radicals, which damage cellular DNA and non-DNA cellular targets (Peak et al., 1988; Beehler et al., 1992; Berton et al., 1997; Li et al., 1996) and accelerate the skin-aging process. UV-induced generation of ROS in the skin develops oxidative stress, when their formation exceeds the antioxidant defense ability of the target cell (Katiyar and Mukhtar,2001). More on this subject was written in the previous chapter. Intracellular and extracellular oxidative stress initiated by reactive oxygen species (ROS) advance skin aging, which is characterized by wrinkles and atypical pigmentation (Masaki, 2010). Skin is a major target of oxidative stress due to reactive oxygen species (ROS) that originate in the environment and in the skin itself. ROS are generated during normal metabolism, are an integral part of normal cellular function, and are usually of little harm if intracellular mechanisms that reduce their damaging effects work properly (Kevin, 2002). Most important,mechanisms include antioxidative enzymatic and non-enzymatic defenses as well as repair processes. But the problem arises with age, when endogenous antioxidative mechanisms and repair processes do not work anymore in the effective way.

Chapter 7.1.

General Overview of Antioxidative Protection

Defenses against ROS

A biological antioxidant has been defined as any substance that, when present at low concentrations compared to those of an oxidizable substrate, significantly delays or prevents oxidation of that substrate (Halliwell and Gutterigde, 1999).

Antioxidant functions are associated with lowering oxidative stress, DNA damage, malignant transformation, and other parameters of cell damage in vitro as well as epidemiologically with lowered incidence of certain types of cancer and degenerative diseases, such as ischemic heart disease and cataract. They are of importance in the process of aging. Reactive oxygen species occur in tissues and cells and can damage DNA, proteins, carbohydrates, and lipids. The main cellular components susceptible to damage by free radicals are lipids (peroxidation of unsaturated fatty acids in membranes), proteins (denaturation), carbohydrates and nucleic acids. These potentially deleterious reactions are controlled in part by antioxidants that eliminate pro-oxidants and scavenge free radicals.

Since some free-radical production in cells is inevitable and can be very damaging, a defense system against the deleterious actions of free radicals has evolved (Cheeseman and Slater, 1993). These are known as antioxidant defenses, and the two main categories are those whose role is to prevent the generation of ROS and those that intercept any radicals that are generated (Cheeseman and Slater, 1993).

The defense system exists in aqueous and membrane compartments of cells and can be enzymatic and non-enzymatic. A second category of natural antioxidants are repair processes, which remove the damaged biomolecules before they accumulate to cause altered cell metabolism or viability (Cheeseman and Slater, 1993). Oxidatively damaged nucleic acids are repaired by specific enzymes, oxidized proteins are removed by proteolytic systems, and oxidized lipids are repaired by phospholipases, peroxidases and acyl transferases (Cheeseman and Slater, 1993).

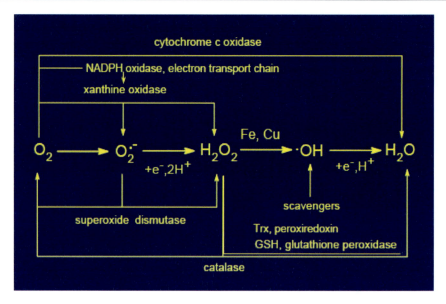

Figure 32. Mechanisms of formation and detoxification of reactive oxygen species (figure from Rafael Radi: Formation and Properties of Reactive Oxygen and Nitrogen Species, Techniques in Free Radical Biology, FEBS Practical Course, Debrecen, Hungary, 2010).

Primary Endogenous Antioxidant Defenses

Superoxide Dismutase (SOD)

From bacteria to humans, a primary cellular defense against oxygen toxicity involves one or more forms of the enzyme superoxide dismutase (SOD). Since SOD is present in all aerobic organisms and most (if not all) cellular compartments that generate activated oxygen, it has been assumed that SOD plays a central role in the defense against oxidative stress (Beyer and Fridovich, 1991; Bowler et al., 1991). SODs are a group of metalloenzymes that catalyze the conversion of superoxide anion to hydrogen peroxide and dioxygen (Hohmann and Mager, 1997). In the reaction catalyzed by SOD, two molecules of superoxide form hydrogen peroxide and molecular oxygen, and are thereby a source of cellular hydrogen peroxide. A dismutation reaction means that free radical reactants produce non-radical products. The reaction catalyzed by SOD is extremely efficient, limited only by diffusion.

$$2O_2^{\cdot -} + 2H^+ \rightarrow H_2O_2 + O_2$$

In eukaryotic cells, $O_2^{\cdot -}$ can be metabolized to H_2O_2 by two metal-containing SOD isoenzymes, an 80-kDa tetrameric Mn-SOD present in mitochondria, and the cytosolic 32-kDa dimeric Cu/Zn-SOD. Exposure of yeast cells to hyperoxia or paraquat has been shown to induce the synthesis of the mRNA and protein for both SODs. Each subunit binds to a single Cu and Zn atom, which are absolutely necessary for catalysis. Superoxide is ushered into the catalytic site via a positively charged electrostatic channel, thereby rendering this a highly efficient enzyme with a catalytic rate constant of 10^9 $M^{-1}s^{-1}$. In mitochondria, superoxide is formed in relatively high concentrations due to the leakage of electrons from respiratory chain. Although MnSOD is localized in mitochondria, it is encoded by a nuclear gene and the protein is imported into mitochondrial matrix via a 27-amino acid amino-terminal mitochondrial targeting sequence.

Catalase

Hydrogen peroxide formed by SOD, through a number of enzymatic activities and by the non-enzymatic reaction of the hydroperoxyl radical, is scavenged by catalases, ubiquitous hem proteins that catalyze the dismutation of hydrogen peroxide into water and molecular oxygen (Santoro and Thiele, 1997).

$$2 H_2O_2 \rightarrow O_2 + 2H_2O$$

The enzyme is found in all aerobic eukaryotes and is important for the removal of hydrogen peroxide, generated in peroxisomes by oxidases during β-oxidation of fatty acids and purine catabolism. One antioxidative role of catalases is to lower the risk of hydroxyl radical formation from H_2O_2 via Fenton reaction catalyzed by Cr or Fe ions.

Glutathione Peroxidase (GPx)

All glutathione peroxidases may catalyze the reduction of H_2O_2 using glutathione (GSH) as a substrate. They can also reduce other peroxides (e.g., lipid peroxides in cell membranes) to alcohols.

$$ROOH + 2\ GSH \rightarrow ROH + GSSG + H_2O$$

The catalytic mechanism proposed for the reduction of hydroperoxides by GPx involves oxidation of the active site selenolate (Se^-) to selenic acid (SeOH). Upon addition of one molecule of GSH, the selenic acid is transformed to a selenylsulfide adduct with glutathione (Se-SG), which can be regenerated to the active selenolate and glutathione disulfide (GSSG) by addition of a second molecule of GSH (Santoro and Thiele, 1997). GPx has a higher affinity for H_2O_2 than catalase. GPx is responsible for detoxification of low H_2O_2 amounts, while in higher H_2O_2 amounts, catalase takes the leading part in cellular detoxification (Halliwell and Gutteridge, 1999).

Glutathione-Related Systems

Beside enzymatic defenses involving catalase, superoxide dismutase and glutathione peroxidase, cells also possesses a non-enzymatic defense system for the protection of cellular constituents against free radicals and reactive oxygen species (ROS) and for maintaining the cellular redox state. Glutathione (GSH) is a tripeptide γ-L-glutamyl-L-cystin glycine. It is one of the major antioxidant molecules of the cell and is thought to play a vital role in buffering the cell against ROS. Glutathione (GSH) is the most abundant intracellular thiol-based antioxidant, prevalent in millimolar concentrations in all living aerobic cells, including bacteria (Chesney et al., 1996).It functions mainly as a sulfhydryl buffer, but GSH also detoxifies compounds either via conjugation reactions catalyzed by glutathione S-transferases or directly, as in the case with peroxide in the GPx-catalyzed reaction (Santoro and Thiele, 1997) or with Cr(VI) (Jamnik and Raspor, 2003). GSH can function as an antioxidant in many ways. It can react chemically with a singlet oxygen, superoxide and hydroxyl radical (McKersie, 1996), and, therefore, function directly as a free radical scavenger. GSH may stabilize membrane structure by removing acyl peroxides formed by lipid peroxidation reactions (Price et al., 1990). GSH is the reducing agent that recycles ascorbic acid from its oxidized to reduced form by the enzyme dehydroascorbate reductase (Halliwell and Gutteridge, 1999). Glutathione is one of the most important compounds for maintaining cellular integrity due to its reducing property (its standard oxidation-reduction potential $E°`= - 0.23V$) and wide involvement in cellular metabolism. This molecule acts as a radical scavenger, with the redox-active sulfhydryl group reacting with oxidants to produce oxidized glutathione (GSSG). The ratios of reduced-to-oxidized glutathione (GSH/GSSG) in normal cells are high (> 10/1), so there must be a mechanism for reducing GSSG back to GSH. This is achieved by glutathione reductase enzymes, which catalyze the following reaction:

$$GSSG + NADPH + H^+ \rightarrow 2GSH + NADP^+$$

The NADPH required is provided by several enzyme systems, but the best known is the oxidative phase of pentose phosphate pathway (Halliwell and Gutteridge, 1999). GSSG is reduced by glutathione reductase at the expense of NADPH. NADPH is regenerated by glucose-6-phosphate dehydrogenase. Biosynthesis of glutathione is catalyzed by two enzymes, Gsh1 (γ-glutamylcysteine synthetase) and Gsh2 (glutathione synthetase) (Izawa et al., 1995).

Both glutathione reductase and glucose-6-phosphate dehydrogenase are involved in the glutathione recycling system (Izawa et al., 1995).

Generation of ROS and the activity of antioxidant defenses appear more or less balanced *in vivo*. In fact, the balance may be slightly tipped in favor of ROS so that there is continuous low-level oxidative damage in the human body. This creates a need for a second category of natural antioxidant defense repair processes, which remove damaged biomolecules before they can accumulate and cause altered cell metabolism.

Secondary Antioxidant Defenses

Although extremely important, the antioxidant enzymes and compounds are not completely effective in preventing oxidative damage, and, consequently, cellular macromolecules become oxidatively damaged. To deal "with the damage that does still occur, a series of damage removal/repair enzymes, for proteins, lipids and DNA, is synthesized. Many of these essential maintenance repair systems become deficient in senescent cells, thus a high amount of biological "garbage" is accumulated (e.g., intralysosomal accumulation of lipofuscin) (Terman and Brunk, 2006; Brunk et al., 1992). Age-related oxidative changes are most prominent in non-proliferating cells, such as neurons and cardiac myocites, because there is a lack of "dilution effect" of damaged structures through cell division (Terman, 2001). The DNA repair ability correlates with species-specific lifespan, being necessary but not sufficient for longevity (Cortopassi and Wang,, 1996). There is an age-related decline in proteasome peptidase activities and proteasome content in different tissues (e.g., rat liver, human epidermis), which leads to accumulation of oxidatively modified proteins (Grune et al., 1997). Proteasomes are part of the protein-removal system for most eukaryotic cells. They contain proteases, which degrade damaged or unnecessary proteins from the cell. Proteasome activity declines with age in the human epidermis (Bulteau et al., 2000). Proteasome activities and function are decreased upon replicative senescence, whereas proteasome activation confers enhanced survival against oxidative stress, lifespan extension and maintenance of the young morphology longer in human primary fibroblasts (Chondrogianni et al., 2010). Also, keratinocytes that undergo replicative senescence are known to have a reduction in proteasome levels (Petropoulos, 2000). Authors suggest that that proteasome is downregulated during replicative senescence as well as in aged cells in vivo, possibly resulting in the accumulation of modified proteins. The total amount of oxidatively modified proteins for an 80-year-old human is estimated to be up to 50% (Stadtman, 1992). Besides, elevated levels of oxidized lipids, DNA and glycoxidation macromolecules are found in aged organisms (Beckman and Ames, 1996; Shringarpure and Davies, 2002; Sell et al., 1996). Torres and Perez (2008) have shown that proteasome inhibition is a mediator of oxidative stress and ROS production by affecting mitochondrial function. Authors propose that a progressive decrease in proteasome function during aging can promote mitochondrial damage and ROS accumulation. It is likely that changes in proteasome dynamics could generate a prooxidative condition at the immediate extracellular microenvironment that could cause tissue injury during aging, in vivo (Torres and Perez, 2008).

Numerous studies have reported age-related increases in somatic mutation and other forms of DNA damage, suggesting that an important determinant of the rate of aging at the cell and molecular level is the (in)capacity for DNA repair (Promislow, 1994; Burkle et al., 2002). A key player in the immediate cellular response to ROS-induced DNA damage is the enzyme poly(ADP-ribose) polymerase-1 (PARP-1), which recognizes DNA lesions and flags them for repair. Grube and Burkle (1992) discovered a strong positive correlation of PARP activity with the species lifespan; cells from long-lived species having higher levels of PARP activity than cells from short-lived species.

ROS-generating compounds induce base oxidation, generate strand breaks, and increase the frequency of intrachromosomal recombination (Frankenberg et al., 1993; Brennan et al., 1994; reviewed in Costa and Moradas-Ferreira, 2001). Oxidized bases have to be removed and replaced by a system of secondary antioxidant defenses.

The most active DNA-repair enzymes, excision-repair enzymes, all operate on the basis of damage or mutilation occurring to only one of the two strands of the DNA double-helix such that the undamaged strand can be used as a template to repair the damaged strand. The damaged area of the injured strand is cut-away (excised) by a nuclease (or glycosylase) enzyme, and a new strand (or a single nucleotide) is constructed.In the nucleus, a base excision repair system acts synergistically with the nucleotide excision repair, mediated by Rad1p (Swanson et al., 1999; reviewed in Costa and Moradas-Ferreira, 2001).

The excision repair of oxidized bases involves two DNA glycosylases, Ogg1p and Ntg2p, which remove the damaged bases (7,8-dihydro-8-oxoguanine, 2,6-diamino-4-hydroxy-5-nmethylformamidopyrimidine, thymine glycol, and 5-hydroxycytosine) (Karahalil et al., 1999; Alseth et al., 1999; You et al., 1999 cit. Costa and Moradas-Ferreira, 2001).

Lipid peroxides or damaged lipids can be metabolized by peroxidases or lipases, and oxidized proteins can either be accumulated or hydrolyzed by more or less specific proteases (Lushchak, 2001).

Overall, antioxidant defense seems to be in approximate balance with the generation of oxygen-derived species *in vivo*. There appears to be no great reserve of antioxidant defenses in mammals, but as previously mentioned, some oxygen-derived species perform useful metabolite roles (Stocker and Frei, 1991). The production of H_2O_2 by activated phagocytes is the classic example of the deliberate metabolic generation of ROS for useful purposes (Halliwell and Cross, 1994).

Generation of $O_2^{-\cdot}$, HOCl and H_2O_2 by phagocytes is known to play an important part in killing various bacterial and fungal strains. $O_2^{-\cdot}$ is also produced by several cell types other than phagocytes, including lymphocytes, fibroblasts and vascular endothelial cells (Babior and Woodman, 1990). Such $O_2^{-\cdot}$ might be involved in intercellular signaling and could have important biological functions, although more research is needed (Stocker and Frei, 1991). H_2O_2 is used by the enzyme thyroid peroxidase to help make thyroid hormones.

Exogenous Antioxidant Defenses: Compounds Derived from the Diet

Although all the protective mechanisms against the oxidative stress mentioned, normal metabolism is associated with unavoidable mild oxidative stress resulting in biomolecular damage that cannot be totally repaired or removed by cellular degradative systems, including lysosomes, proteasomes, and cytosolic and mitochondrial proteases. Consequently, irreversibly damaged and functionally defective structures (biological "garbage") accumulate within long-lived post-mitotic cells, such as cardiac myocytes and neurons, leading to progressive loss of adaptability and increased probability of death and characterizing a process of aging, or senescence (Terman and Brunk, 2006). In this respect, the intake of exogenous antioxidants from fruit and vegetables could play an important role in mediating oxidative stress and its cellular damage. Natural antioxidants like vitamin C and E, carotenoids and polyphenols (e.g., flavonoids) are generally considered to be beneficial components of fruits and vegetables. The antioxidative properties of these compounds are often considered responsible for the protective effects of these food components against cardiovascular diseases, certain forms of cancers, photosensitivity diseases and aging (Rietjens et al., 2001). However, many of the reported health claims are based on observational epidemiological studies in which specific diets were associated with reduced risks for specific forms of cancer and cardiovascular diseases and with the reduction of stress.

Identification of the actual ingredient in a specific diet responsible for the beneficial health effect remains an important bottleneck for translating observational epidemiology to the development of functional food ingredients. For antioxidant-type functional food ingredients, toxic pro-oxidant actions at higher doses may be important (Rietjens et al., 2001). It is estimated that ¾ of sun exposure is non-intentional. Our skin is exposed to majority of UV radiation when we are outdoors working, walking, etc. and not when we are intentionally exposed to the sun on the beach. At this time, we also do not use sun-creams with UVA/UVB protection.

Table 7. ROS-induced amount of cell damage and lifespan

	Short-lived species	Long-lived species
ROS formation	↑	↓
ROS protection	↓	↑
Oxidative damage repair	↓	↑
Probability of damage (redundancy, buffering, etc.)	↑	↓

The only protectionforour skin is its endogenous protection (melanine and enzymatic antioxidants) and antioxidants we consumed with the food (vitamin A, C, E, etc). Therefore, this chapter is dedicated to the endogenous and exogenous skin protection with antioxidants.

Skin Antioxidants

Cellular redox homeostasis is carefully maintained by an elaborate endogenous antioxidant defense system, which includes endogenous antioxidant enzymes, proteins, and low-molecular-weight scavengers. Some of them aresuperoxide dismutase (SOD), catalase, glutathione peroxidase (GPx), glutathione (GSH) and others (uric acid, coenzyme Q, lipoic acid). Generation of ROS and the activity of antioxidant defense appear more or less balanced *in vivo*. In fact, as already mentioned, the balance may be slightly tipped in favor of the ROS so that there is continuous low-level oxidative damage in the human body. This creates a need for a second category of endogenous antioxidant defense system, which removes or repairs damaged biomolecules before they can accumulate and before their presence results in altered cell metabolism.

The alternative could be increased intake of exogenous antioxidants from fruit and vegetables.Antioxidants like vitamin C and E, carotenoids, and polyphenols (e.g., flavonoids) are, at present, generally considered to be the main exogenous antioxidants.Clinical studies have found that eating a diet rich in fruits, vegetables, whole grains, legumes and omega-3 fatty acids can help skin retain its healthy glow and look youthful.Antioxidants can be classified into water-soluble and lipophilic antioxidants, into enzymatic and non-enzymatic antioxidants and according to their function into:

- Free radical scavengers (e.g., vitamin C)
- Scavengers of non-radical oxidants (e.g., catalase)
- Compounds that inhibit generation of oxidants (e.g., metal chelators)
- Compounds that induce the production of antioxidants (e.g., isothiocyanates)

Skin Antioxidants

The skin is equipped with a network of protective antioxidants. They include enzymatic antioxidants such as glutathione peroxidase, superoxide dismutase and catalase, and nonenzymatic low-molecular-weight antioxidants such as vitamin E isoforms, vitamin C, glutathione (GSH), uric acid, and ubiquinol (Shindo et al., 1993).

Various other components present in skin are potent antioxidants including ascorbate, uric acid, carotenoids and sulphydrils. Water-soluble antioxidants in plasma include glucose, pyruvate, uric acid, ascorbic acid, bilirubin and glutathione. Lipid soluble antioxidants include alpha-tocopherol, ubiquinol-10, lycopene, ß-carotene, lutein, zeaxanthin and alpha-carotene. In general, the outer part of the skin, the epidermis, contains higher concentrations of antioxidants than the dermis (Shindo et al., 1994).

In the lipophilic phase, α-tocopherol is the most prominent antioxidant, while vitamin C and GSH have the highest abundance in the cytosol. On molar basis, hydrophilic non-enzymatic antioxidants including L-ascorbic acid, GSH and uric acid appear to be the predominant antioxidants in human skin (Thiele et al., 2006). Their overall dermal and epidermal concentration are more than 10- to 100-fold greater than those found for vitamin E or ubiquinol.

Aging- and photoaging-dependent changes of enzymic and nonenzymic antioxidants in the epidermis and dermis of human skin in vivo was analyzed by Rhie at al. (2001). The study showedthat the activities of superoxide dismutase and glutathione peroxidase are not changed during skin-aging processes in human skin in vivo.

Interestingly, the activity of catalase was significantly increased in the epidermis of photoaged (163%) and naturally aged (118%) skin (n = 9), but it was significantly lower in the dermis of photoaged (67% of the young skin level) and naturally aged (55%) skin compared with young (n = 7) skin.

The activity of glutathione reductase was significantly higher (121%) in naturally aged epidermis. The concentration of alpha-tocopherol was significantly lower in the epidermis of photoaged (56% of young skin level) and aged (61%) skin, but this was not found to be the case in the dermis. Ascorbic acid levels were lower in both epidermis (69% and 61%) and dermis (63% and 70%) of photoaged and naturally aged skin, respectively.

The antioxidant capacity of the human epidermis is far greater than that of dermis. This was demonstrated in the study by Shindo et al. (1994) where enzymic and non-enzymic antioxidants in human epidermis and dermis from six healthy volunteers undergoing surgical procedures was measured.

The concentration of every antioxidant (referenced to skin wet weight) was higher in the epidermis than in the dermis. Among the enzymic antioxidants, the activities of superoxide dismutase, glutathione peroxidase, and glutathione reductase were higher in the epidermis compared to the dermis by 126.61 and 215%, respectively. Catalase activity in particular was much higher (720%) in the epidermis. Glucose-6-phosphate dehydrogenase and isocitrate dehydrogenase, which provide reduced nicotinamide adenine dinucleotide phosphate (NADPH), also showed higher activity in the epidermis than the dermis by 111% and 313%, respectively.

Among the lipophilic antioxidants, the concentration of alpha-tocopherol was higher in the epidermis than the dermis by 90%. The concentration of ubiquinol 10 was especially higher in the epidermis, by 900%.

Among the hydrophilic antioxidants, concentrations of ascorbic acid and uric acid were also higher in the epidermis than in the dermis by 425 and 488%, respectively. Reduced glutathione and total glutathione were higher in the epidermis than in the dermis by 513 and 471%.

A similar study was done by Shindo et al. (1993) where enzymic and non-enzymic antioxidants in epidermis and dermis of hairless mice were compared. Catalase, glutathione peroxidase, and glutathione reductase were higher in epidermis than dermis by 49%, 86%, and 74%, respectively. Superoxide dismutase did not follow this pattern.

Lipophilic antioxidants (alpha-tocopherol, ubiquinol 9, and ubiquinone 9) and hydrophilic antioxidants (ascorbic acid, dehydroascorbic acid, and glutathione) were 24% to 95% higher in epidermis than in dermis. In contrast, oxidized glutathione was 60% lower in epidermis than in dermis.

The stratum corneum (SC) was found to contain both hydrophilic and lipophilic antioxidants. Vitamins C and E (both $\alpha\gamma$ and α-tocopherol) as well as GSH and uric acid were found to be present in the SC (Weber et al.,1999; Thiele et al., 1998).

Surprisingly, they were not distributed evenly, but in gradient fashion, with low concentrations on the outer layers and increasing concentrations toward the deeper layers of the SC. This phenomenon may be explained by the fact that O2 partial pressure is higher in the upper SC, which already causes a mild oxidative stress resulting in the partial depletion of antioxidants.

Moreover, the further up corneocytes are located, the longer they have been a part of the SC and the longer they have been exposed to the ambient environmental oxidative stress (Weber et al., 1999; Weber and Packer, 2001).

Besides oxygen, UVexposure could also decrease the amount of antioxidants present in the upper layer of SC. Similarly, the highest expression of human 8-oxoguanine-DNA glycosylase 1 (hOGG1), which repairs 8-oxo-7,8-dihydro-2'-deoxyguanosine (8-oxo-dG), was in the superficial epidermal layer (stratum granulosum) as revealed by the study of Javer et al. (2008). Study of the hOGG1 mRNA expression also showed the highest level in the upper region of the epidermis. This was not regulated by UV irradiation but by the differentiation state of keratinocytes as calcium-induced differentiation increased hOGG1 gene expression. UVA-induced 8-oxo-dG was repaired more rapidly in the upper layer of human skin compared to the lower layers.

Results of the study conducted by Javer et al. (2008) indicate that weaker expression of the nuclear form of hOGG1 enzyme in the basal cells of the epidermis may lead to a lack of DNA repair in these cells and, therefore, accumulation of UVA-induced oxidative DNA mutations.

Keratinocytes and skin fibroblasts contain milimolar levels of GSH, α-tocopherol, ascorbate, and DNA repair enzymes. In general, keratinocytes are more resistant than most animal cells to killing by H2O2, organic peroxides or peroxynitrite.

In mice, levels of catalase, GPx, glutathione reductase, α-tocopherol, ubiquinol, ascorbate and GSH (but not SOD) are higher in epidermis than in dermis (Shindo et al., 1993). Thioredoxin and thioredoxin reductase in skin have also been suggested to contribute to antioxidant defense.

Dietary antioxidants play a major role in maintaining the homeostasis of the oxidative balance. Vitamin C (ascorbic acid), vitamin E (tocopherol), beta-carotene and other micronutrients such as carotenoids, polyphenols and selenium have been evaluated as antioxidant constituents in the human diet.

It is important to obtain many different water and lipid soluble antioxidants by intake of different kinds of fruit and vegetables since all antioxidants work in synergy, e.g., glutathione is an important substrate for enzymatic antioxidant functions and is capable of nonenzymatic radical scavenging. All antioxidants can act also in a pro-oxidative form.

For example, at low glutathione concentrations, UVB-induced mtDNA deletions have been prevented, but at high levels of glutathione, when it acts as an electron donor, the pro-oxidative properties reveal and the mtDNA deletions return (Ji et al., 2006). Thiols associated with membrane proteins may also be important to the antioxidant systems. Tocopherols and tocotrienols (vitamin E) and ascorbic acid (vitamin C) as well as the carotenoids react with free radicals, notably peroxyl radicals, and with singlet molecular oxygen (1O2), this being the basis of their function as antioxidants. RRR-alpha-tocopherol is the major peroxyl radical scavenger in biological lipid phases such as membranes or low-density lipoproteins (LDL). L-Ascorbate is present in aqueous compartments (e.g., cytosol, plasma, and other body fluids) and can reduce the tocopheroxyl radical; it also has a number of metabolically important cofactor functions in enzyme reactions, notably hydroxylations.

Upon oxidation, these micronutrients need to be regenerated in the biological setting, hence the need for further coupling to nonradical reducing systems such as glutathione/glutathione disulfide, dihydrolipoate/lipoate, or NADPH/NADP+ and NADH/NAD+. Carotenoids, notably beta-carotene and lycopene, as well as oxycarotenoids (e.g., zeaxanthin and lutein), exert antioxidant functions in lipid phases by free-radical or 1O2 quenching (Sies et al., 1992).

Skin Antioxidants Protect Against UVR

UVR exposure affects the skin antioxidants. Ascorbate, GSH, SOD, catalase and ubiquinol are depleted in UV-B exposed skin, both dermis and epidermis. Levels of electron paramagnetic resonance (EPR)-detectable ascorbyl radical rise on UV exposure of skin.

Studies of cultured skin cells and murine skin in vivo have indicated that UVR-induced damage involves the generation of reactive oxygen species and depletion of endogenous antioxidant systems (McArdle, et al., 2002).

For example, in the study by Shindo et al. (1993),enzymatic and non-enzymiatic antioxidants in epidermis and dermis and their responses to ultraviolet light of hairless mice were compared. Mice were irradiated with solar light to examine the response of cutaneous layers to UV irradiation.

After irradiation, epidermal and dermal catalase and superoxide dismutase activities were greatly decreased. alpha-Tocopherol, ubiquinol 9, ubiquinone 9, ascorbic acid, dehydroascorbic acid, and reduced glutathione decreased in both epidermis and dermis by 26% to 93%. Oxidized glutathione showed a slight, non-significant increase. Because the reduction in total ascorbate and catalase was much more severe in epidermis than dermis, authors concluded that UV light is more damaging to the antioxidant defenses in the epidermis than in the dermis. Many other studies confirmed that acute exposure of human skin to UVR in vivo leads to oxidation of cellular biomolecules that could be prevented by prior antioxidant treatment. The identification of free radical reactions as promoters of the aging process implies that interventions aimed at limiting or inhibiting them should be able to reduce the rate of formation of aging changes with a consequent reduction of the aging rate and disease pathogenesis. There have been many studies performed where different antioxidants or combinations of antioxidants and different phytochemicals were tested in order to find evidence against ROS-induced damage. Some of them are presented in the next paragraphs.

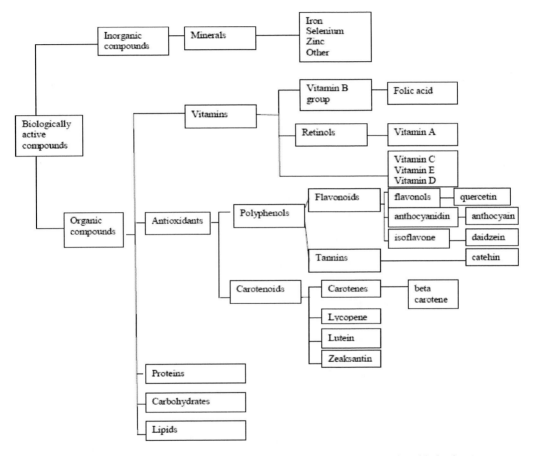

Figure 33. Classification (after Juvan et al., 2005) of biologically-active compounds; with the focus on antioxidants and phytochemicals.

Vitamin C

Natural antioxidants are generally considered to be beneficial fruit and vegetable components. Vitamin C is present in almost all foods of plant origin. It is an essential micronutrient in man, due to the absence of L-gulonolactone oxidase. Any insufficient intake of fresh fruits or vegetables leads to vitamin-C deficiency and to scurvy. Vitamin C has several important roles, and there are many enzymesutilizing ascorbate as a cofactor. The term *vitamin C* refers to both ascorbic acid (AA) and dehydroascorbic acid (DHA), since both exhibit anti-scorbutic activity. Ascorbic acid, the functional and primary *in vivo* form of the vitamin, is the enolic form of an α-ketolactone (2,3-didehydro-L-threo-hexano-1,4-lactone). The two enolic hydrogen atoms give the compound its acidic character and provide electrons for its function as a reductant and an antioxidant. Its one-electron oxidation product, the ascorbyl radical, readily dismutates to ascorbate and DHA, the two-electron oxidation products. Both the ascorbyl radical and DHA are readily reduced back to ascorbic acid *in vivo*. Because of its ability to donate electrons, ascorbic acid is an effective antioxidant. The vitamin readily scavenges reactive oxygen species (ROS) and reactive nitrogen species (RNS) (e.g., hydroxyl, superoxide, singlet oxygen, and peroxynitrite, nitroxide radicals, respectively) as well as peroxyl and hypochlorite (Frei et al., 1989; Halliwell and Whiteman, 1997). The one- and two-electron oxidation products of ascorbate are relatively non-toxic and easily regenerated by the ubiquitous reductants glutathione and NADH or NADPH. Both the one- and the two-electron oxidation products of the vitamin are readily regenerated *invivo* — chemically and enzymatically—by reduced glutathione, nicotinamide adenine dinucleotide (NADH), and nicotinamide adenine dinucleotide phosphate (NADPH) -dependent reductases (May et al., 1998; Park and Levine, 1996). In addition to scavenging reactive oxygen species and reactive nitrogen species, vitamin C can regenerate other small molecule antioxidants, such as α-tocopherol, glutathione (GSH), urate, and β-carotene, from their respective radical species (Halliwell, 1996). Many cells possess enzymes that can convert dehydroascorbate or ascorbate radical back to ascorbate at the expense of GSH or NADH. Glutathione dependent dehydroascorbate reductase enzymes have been identified in plants and in several mammalian tissues. Evidence that GSH and ascorbate interact *in vivo* is provided by studies on animals treated with the inhibitors of GSH synthesis (Halliwell and Gutteridge, 1999). Severe glutathione depletion in newborn rats is lethal, but death can be prevented by high doses of ascorbate (but not DHA). For more information on vitamin C anti- and pro-oxidative properties, see the review article "Metal Ions Mediated Pro-Oxidative Reactions with Vitamin C: Possible Implications for Treatment of Different Malignancies," Ionescu and Poljsak, *Int. J. Canc. Prev*, 2010. Some important information about vitamin C and its chemical structures as well as risk assessment can be found in Final report of the safety assessment of L-Ascorbic Acid, Calcium Ascorbate, Magnesium Ascorbate, Magnesium Ascorbyl Phosphate, Sodium Ascorbate, and Sodium Ascorbyl Phosphate as used in cosmetics (Elmore, 2005). Different forms of vitamin C e.g., L-Ascorbic Acid, Calcium Ascorbate, Magnesium Ascorbate, Magnesium Ascorbyl Phosphate, Sodium Ascorbate, and Sodium Ascorbyl Phosphate, function in cosmetic formulations primarily as antioxidants. Ascorbic Acid is used as an antioxidant and pH adjuster in a large variety of cosmetic formulations (Elmore, 2005). Calcium Ascorbate and Magnesium Ascorbate are described as antioxidants and skin-conditioning agents—miscellaneous for use in cosmetics—but are not currently used. Sodium Ascorbyl Phosphate functions as an antioxidant in cosmetic products and is used at concentrations ranging from 0.01% to 3%. Magnesium Ascorbyl Phosphate functions as an antioxidant in cosmetics and was reported being used at concentrations from 0.001% to 3%. Sodium Ascorbate also functions as an antioxidant in cosmetics at concentrations from 0.0003% to 0.3%. Related ingredients (Ascorbyl Palmitate, Ascorbyl Dipalmitate, Ascorbyl Stearate, Erythorbic Acid, and Sodium Erythorbate) have been previously reviewed by the Cosmetic Ingredient Review (CIR) Expert Panel and found "to be safe for use as cosmetic ingredients in the present practices of good use." Ascorbic Acid is a generally recognized as safe (GRAS) substance for use as a chemical preservative in foods and as a nutrient and/or dietary supplement. Calcium Ascorbate and Sodium Ascorbate are listed as GRAS substances for use as chemical preservatives. Because of the concern that certain metal ions may combine with antioxidant ingredients in a product to produce pro-oxidant activity, formulators should be cautioned to be certain that these ingredients are acting as antioxidants in cosmetic formulations. The bioavailability of vitamin C is dosedependent. Saturation of transport occurs with dosages of 200 to 400 mg/day. Vitamin C is not proteinbound and is eliminated with an elimination half-life ($t_{(1/2)}$) of tenhours. In Western populations, plasma vitamin C concentrations range from 54 to 91 micro mol/L. According to Diplock et al. (1998), with regard to the safety of administration of supplementary vitamins, vitamin C is safe at levels of supplementation up to 600 mg/d, and higher levels, up to 2000 mg/d, are without risk.

Vitamin C and Skin Studies

Oral vitamin C supplements (500 mg/day) were taken by 12 volunteers for eightweeks, resulting in significant rises in plasma and skin vitamin C content (McArdle et al., 2002). Supplementation had no effect on the UVR-induced erythemal response. The skin malonaldehyde content was reduced by vitamin C supplementation, but surprisingly, reductions in the skin content of total glutathione and protein thiols were also seen. Authors speculate that this apparently paradoxical effect could be due to regulation of total reductant capacity by skin cells, such that vitamin C may have been replacing other reductants in these cells. Ascorbic Acid was a photoprotectant in clinical human UV studies at doses well above the minimal erythema dose (MED). An opaque cream containing 5% Ascorbic Acid did not induce dermal sensitization in 103 human subjects. A product containing 10% Ascorbic Acid was non-irritant in a four-day minicumulative patch assay on human skin, and a facial treatment containing 10% Ascorbic Acid was not a contact sensitizer in a maximization assay on 26 humans (McArdle, 2002). Ascorbic Acid was a photoprotectant when applied to mice and pig skin before exposure to ultraviolet (UV) radiation. The inhibition of UV-induced suppression of contact hypersensitivity was also noted. Magnesium Ascorbyl Phosphate administration immediately after exposure in hairless mice significantly delayed skin tumor formation and hyperplasia induced by chronic exposure to UV radiation. The conclusions from the Dietary nutrient intakes and skin-aging appearance among middle-aged American women study(2007) were: "Higher intakes of vitamin C and linoleic acid and lower intakes of fats and carbohydrates are associated with better skin-aging appearance. Promoting healthy dietary behaviors may have additional benefit for skin appearance in addition to other health outcomes in the population." In another study, topical vitamin C 5% cream applied for sixmonths led to clinical improvement in the appearance of photoaged skin with regard to firmness, smoothness, and dryness compared to vehicle (Humbert et al., 2003). Additionally, it was reported that topical vitamin C stimulates the collagen-producing activity of the dermis (Nusgens, et al., 2002). Many other studies have found that vitamin C can increase collagen production, protect against damage from UVA and UVB rays, correct pigmentation problems, and improve inflammatory skin conditions.

Vitamin E

Tocopherols are a series of organic compounds consisting of various methylated phenols. The most important is α-tocopherol (vitamin E), which is a potent, lipid-soluble, chain-breaking antioxidant. Structural analyses have revealed that molecules having vitamin E antioxidant activity include four tocopherols (α, β, γ, δ) and four tocotrienols (α, β, γ, δ). Vitamin E is a membrane-bound antioxidant and free radical scavenger that appears to offer protection against injuries caused by O_2, O_3, and NO_2, and nitrosamine formation. This is done by the vitamin E giving up one of its electrons to the electron-deficient free radical, making it more stable. While Vitamin E performs its antioxidant functions, it also protects the other antioxidants from being oxidized. As demonstrated in vitro, when ascorbic acid or coenzyme Q10 are present, the tocopheroxyl radical is rapidly reduced and the active form of vitamin E is regenerated. α-tocopherol is known to efficiently scavenge lipid peroxyl and alkoxyl radicals by intercepting lipid chain propagation. The skin is equipped with an elaborate system of antioxidant substances and enzymes that includes a network of redox active antioxidants.

Among these, vitamin E has also been identified as the predominant antioxidant both in murine and human skin and shows a characteristic gradient with lower levels towards the outer stratum corneum layers. While hydrophilic antioxidants are less abundant in the hydrophobic SC environment than in the nucleated epidermal layers, vitamin E appears to be the predominant antioxidant in human SC (Theiel et al., 2006). Skin exposure to UV and ozone alone and in combination resulted in a significant potentiation of the UV-induced vitamin E depletion (Packer and Valacchi, 2002), which means that vitamin E is efficiently quenching ROS during O3 and UVR skin exposure. Depletion of SC vitamin E is one of the earliest oxidative stress markers in human skin exposed to UVR and other environmental stress (Thiele, 2001).

In a study by Werninghaus and coworkers (1994), a relatively small group of 12 healthy volunteers received 295 mg (400 IU) α-tocopherol acetate or a placebo daily for six months, along with their regular diets. Mean MEDs were similar in both groups before supplementation but increased in some subjects and decreased in others after supplementation. Plasma concentrations of α-tocopherol increased during the study, but no parallel increase was detected in the skin. This finding was explained by the fact that the skin samples were taken 24 h after exposure and thus α-tocopherol may have been depleted from the skin.

Moreover, the study spanned several months, and because individual MEDs were shown to be higher in summer than in winter (Bykov, 1999), seasonal changes may have obscured any effects. In contrast with the findings of La Ruche and Cesarini (1991), no change in the number of sunburn cells was found in the subjects who received the supplement. Besides its antioxidative properties, vitamin E was shown to modulate arachidonic acid metabolism (Traber and Packer, 1995).

The interaction of vitamin E with the eicosanoid system may result in an anti-inflammatory effect and thereby complement the photoprotective effects of other antioxidants in the skin (Boelsma et al., 2001).

One study showed that the number of sunburn to cells was decreased by treatment with the antioxidant tocopherol and may result from both direct protection from free radicals and indirect protection by means of increased epidermal thickness. (Ritter et al, 1997).

Additionally, Packer et al. (2001) showed that vitamin E has skin barrier-stabilizing properties.

Safety Assessment of Tocopherols

Safety and risk assessment of tocopherol and its compounds were published in *Int J. Toxicol* by Zondlo Fiume in 2002. Brief abstract: "tocopherol and its several ester and ether derivatives all function as antioxidants in cosmetic formulations; they also have other functions, such as skin conditioning. Tocopherol may be isolated from vegetable oils or synthesized using isophytol and methylhydroquinone. Tocopheryl Acetate, Tocopherol, and Tocopheryl Linoleate are used in 2,673 formulations, generally at concentrations of up to 36%, 5%, and 2%, respectively, although Tocopheryl Acetate is 100% of vitamin E oil (Zondlo and Fiume, 2002). Tocopherol, Tocopheryl Acetate, Tocopheryl Linoleate, and Tocopheryl Succinate were all absorbed in human skin.

"In rat skin, Tocopheryl Acetate is hydrolyzed to Tocopherol. Tocopherol is a natural component of cell membranes thought to protect against oxidative damage. Tocopherol, Tocopheryl Acetate, and Tocopheryl Succinate each were reported to protect against ultraviolet radiation-induced skin damage. These ingredients are generally not toxic in animal feeding studies, although very high doses (≥ 2 g/kg/day) have hemorrhagic activity. These ingredients are generally not irritating or sensitizing to skin or irritating to eyes, although a Tocopheryl Acetate did produce sensitization in one animal test, and Tocophersolan was a slight eye irritant in an animal test" (Zondlo Fiume, 2002).

Tocopherol has been shown to reduce the photocarcinogenic effect of ultraviolet radiation in mice. Similar studies with Tocopheryl Acetate and Tocopheryl Succinate, however, demonstrated some enhancement of photocarcinogenesis, although the effect was not dose related.

Observational epidemiological studies provide the basis for relating the intake of vitamin E-rich food to decreased incidence of risk of mortality due to cardiovascular diseases (Stephens et al., 1996). However, the results from large-scale intervention studies are inconclusive, reporting adverse, as well as beneficial, or no effects at all of daily supplementation with α-tocopherol (Virtamo, 1999; Stocker, 1999).

Human intervention studies in which smoking male volunteers were exposed during five to eight years to daily supplementation with vitamin E did not reveal any effect on the overall mortality of male smokers but did show increased mortality resulting from hemorrhagic stroke (The alpha-tocopherol, beta-carotene cancer prevention study group 1994, Halliwell and Gutteridge, 1999). The inconsistency in the effects of vitamin E may be related to the complex function and chemical behavior of vitamin E, being able to have antioxidant, neutral or pro-oxidative effect.

The pathway depicted implies that increased levels of α-tocopherol result, upon subsequent oxidative stress, in increased levels of α-tocopherol radicals. These α-tocopherol radicals can initiate processes of, e.g., lipid peroxidation by themselves (Rietjens et al., 2001). When antioxidant networks are balanced, this pro-oxidant action of vitamin E is inhibited by co-antioxidants, which can reduce the radical back to vitamin E.

Increasing the levels of only α-tocopherol may, especially under conditions of increased oxidative stress, result in increased levels of α-tocopherol radicalsthatcan no longer be efficiently detoxified by co-antioxidants. This provides the possibility for pro-oxidant toxicity of the α-tocopherol radical (Rietjens, 2001). This biochemical rationale explains why foods containing comparatively small levels of vitamin E but also co-antioxidants provide greater health benefits than vitamin E supplements (Rietjens, 2001).

Table 8. Outcomes of some epidemiological studies where selected antioxidant supplements were tested on humans (Bjelakovic et al., 2004)

Study	Subjects	Vitamin	Results
Bjelakovic et al.	Meta-analize	A, C, E, selenium	Gastrointestinal cancer- no effect
Hennekens et al, Omenn et al. Miller et al.	Randomised and placebo-controlled trial	Beta caroten	↑ mortality due to all reasons ↑ mortality - cardiovascular ↑ mortality - cancer
Hennekens et al, Omenn et al. Miller et al.	Randomised and placebo-controlled trial	Vitamin E	No effect
US Nurses health study Health professionals follow-up study		Vitamin E	Every day, high intake for long period ↓ cardiovascular disease

Intake and Bioavailability of Vitamin E

Vitamin E has a very low human toxicity and an intake of 1000 mg/d is without risk; 3200 mg/d has been shown to be without any consistent risk. Serum alpha- and gamma-tocopherol range from 21 micro mol/L (North America) to 27 micro mol/L (Europe) and from 3.1 micro mol/L to 1.5 micro mol/L, respectively. alpha-Tocopherol is the most abundant tocopherol in human tissue. The bioavailability of all-rac-alpha-tocopherol is estimated to be 50% of R,R,R-alpha-tocopherol. The hepatic alpha-tocopherol transfer of protein (alpha-TTP) together with the tocopherol-associated proteins (TAP) is responsible for the endogenous accumulation of natural alpha-tocopherol. Elimination of alpha-tocopherol takes several days with a t((1/2)) of 81 and 73 hours for R,R,R-alpha-tocopherol and all-rac-alpha-tocopherol, respectively. The t((1/2)) of tocotrienols is short, ranging from 3.8 to 4.4 hours for gamma- and alpha-tocotrienol, respectively. Gamma-Tocopherol is degraded to 2, 7, 8-trimethyl-2-(beta-carboxyl)-6-hyrdoxychroman by the liver prior to renal elimination (Schwedhelm et al., 2003).

Vitamin A (Retinol and Carotenes)

Retinoids constitute a group of natural and synthetic compounds characterized by vitamin A-like biological activity. Retinol is among the most usable forms of vitamin A, which also include retinal (aldehyde form), retinoic acid (acid form) and retinyl esters (ester forms). These chemical compounds are collectively known as retinoids, and all possess the biological activity of all-*trans* retinol as a common feature in their structure. Vitamin A and other natural retinoids play a critical role in embryogenesis, reproduction, vision, immunity and epithelial cell differentiation. Retinoids are obtained from the diet, absorbed by the intestine, stored in the liver as retinyl esters (Res), and transported in the circulation to target cells as ell-trans-retinol (ROL). Retinoids are used in medicine, primarily due to the way they regulate epithelial cell growth. Retinoids are important signaling molecules in vertebrates and act to alter the transcriptional activation or repression of numerous genes (Mangelsdorf et al., 1994; Roos et al., 1998).

Retinol is an active form of vitamin A. It is found in animal liver, whole milk, and some fortified foods. Retinol is ingested in a precursor form; animal sources (liver and eggs) contain retinyl esters, whereas plants (carrots, spinach) contain pro-vitamin A carotenoids. Hydrolysis of retinyl esters results in retinol, while pro-vitamin A carotenoids can be cleaved to produce retinal. Vitamin A is a vitamin that is needed by the retina of the eye in the form of a specific metabolite, the light-absorbing molecule retinal. This molecule is absolutely necessary for both scotopic and color vision. Vitamin A (retinol and retinyl esters) is present also in the epidermis as free and esterified retinol (Rocquet and Bonte, 2002). Acute exposure to UVA completely depletes the epidermis of vitamin A and causes lipid peroxidation. In contrast, exposure to UVB results only in the loss of vitamin A (Sorg et al., 2002).

Vitamin A can be found in two principal forms in foods:

- Retinol, the form of vitamin A absorbed when eating animal food sources, is a yellow, fat-soluble substance. Since the pure alcohol form is unstable, the vitamin is found in tissues in a form of retinyl ester. It is also commercially produced and administered as esters, such as retinyl acetate or palmitate. In foods of animal origin, the major form of vitamin A is an ester, primarily retinyl palmitate, which is converted to the retinol in the small intestine. The retinol form functions as storage form of the vitamin and can be converted to and from its visually active aldehyde form, retinal (Wikipedia).
- Carotenoids are dark-colored dyes found in plant foods that can turn into a form of vitamin A. One such carotenoid is beta-carotene. Beta-carotene is an antioxidant. Of all the carotenoids, ß-carotene has been the focusof most attention because it makes the most important quantitativecontribution to human nutrition. The carotenes alpha-carotene, beta-carotene, gamma-carotene; and the xanthophyll beta-cryptoxanthin (all of which contain beta-ionone rings), but no other carotenoids, function as vitamin A in herbivore and omnivore animals, which possess the enzyme required to convert these compounds to retinal. In general, carnivores are poor converters of ionine-containing carotenoids, and pure carnivores such as cats and ferrets lack beta-carotene 15,15'-monooxygenase and cannot convert any carotenoids to retinal (resulting in *none* of the carotenoids being forms of vitamin A for these species).

As some carotenoids can be converted into vitamin A, attempts have been made to determine how much of them in the diet is equivalent to a particular amount of retinol, so that comparisons can be made of the benefit of different foods. The situation can be confusing because the accepted equivalences have changed. For many years, a system of equivalencies in which an international unit (IU) was equal to 0.3 µg of retinol, 0.6 µg of β-carotene, or 1.2 µg of other provitamin-A carotenoids was used (USDA, 2008). Later, a unit called retinol equivalent (RE) was introduced—1 RE corresponded to 1 µg retinol, 2 µg β-carotene dissolved in oil (it is only partly dissolved in most supplement pills, due to very poor solubility in any medium), 6 µg β-carotene in normal food (because it is not absorbed as well as when in oils), and 12 µg of either α-carotene, γ-carotene, or β-cryptoxanthin in food (these molecules only provide 50% of the retinol as β-carotene, due to only half the molecule's being convertible to usable vitamin).

Research has shown that the absorption of provitamin-A carotenoids is only half as much as previously thought, so in 2001 the U.S. Institute of Medicine recommended a new unit, the retinol activity equivalent (RAE)—1 µg RAE corresponds to 1 µg retinol, 2 µg of β-carotene in oil, 12 µg of "dietary" beta-carotene, or 24 µg of the three other dietary provitamin-A carotenoids (Institute of Medicine, 2001).

Blood serum carotenoids in Western populations range from 0.28 to 0.52 micro mol/L for beta-carotene, from 0.2 to 0.28 for lutein, and from 0.29 to 0.60 for lycopene. All-trans-carotenoids have a better bioavailability than the 9-cis-forms. Elimination of carotenoids takes several days with a t((1/2)) of five to seven and two to three days for beta-carotene and lycopene, respectively. The bioconversion of beta-carotene to retinal is dose-dependent, and ranges between 27% and 2% for a 6 and 126mg dose, respectively (Schwedhelm et al., 2003). Several oxidized metabolites of carotenoids are known.

Vitamin A and Skin Studies

1. Carotenoids

Carotenoids are antioxidants and act as accessory pigments and are involved in dissipation of an excess light energy through the xanthophyll cycle, quenching excited triplet state molecules and singlet oxygen as their way of providing photoprotection (Demmig-Adams and Adams, 2002). The antioxidant activity of carotenoids and biochemical properties influencing signaling pathways have been discussed as basic mechanisms of prevention (Stahl and Sies, 2005). Beta-carotene is a major constituent of commercially available products administered for systemic photoprotection. β-carotene supplements are frequently used as so-called oral sun protectants, but studies proving a protective effect of oral treatment with β-carotene against skin responses to sun exposure are scarce and conflicting results have been reported (Stahl et al., 2006). Studies on the systemic use of beta-carotene provide evidence that 15 to 30 mg/d over a period of about 10 to 12 wk produces a protective effect against UV-induced erythema. Similar effects have been attributed to mixtures of carotenoids or after long-term intake of dietary products rich in carotenoids. Supplementation with carotenoids contributes to basal protection of the skin but is not sufficient to obtain complete protection against severe UV irradiation (Stahl and Krutmann, 2006). Studies showed that the efficacy of β-carotenein systemic photoprotection depends on the duration of treatment and on the dose (Stahl, 2000). For successful intervention, treatment with carotenoids is needed for a period of at least ten weeks (Sies and Stahl, 2004).

Although the photoprotective effects of beta-carotene are thought to originate from its antioxidant properties, some studies documented pro-oxidant effects of beta-carotene. Objective of the study by (Cho et al. 2010) was to determine the effects of twodifferent doses of dietary beta-carotene on wrinkles and elasticity, procollagen gene expression and ultraviolet (UV)-induced DNA damage in human skin. Results showed that beta-carotene improved facial wrinkles and elasticity significantly only in the low-dose group. The minimal erythema dose decreased significantly only in the high-dose group. Type I procollagen mRNA levels were significantly increased to 4.4 +/- 1.6 times the baseline level only in the low-dose group, and procollagen immunostaining increased accordingly. UV-induced thymine dimer staining was reduced in the low-dose group but tended to increase in the high-dose group. In the low-dose group, 8-hydroxy-2'-deoxyguanosine staining was significantly reduced. From this study, it can be concluded that 30 mg/day of beta-carotene supplementation is demonstrated to prevent and repairphotoaging (Cho et al., 2010).

Another study investigated the effects of oral vitamin E and beta-carotene supplementation on ultraviolet radiation-induced oxidative stress in human skin (McArdle et al., 2004). Results revealed that vitamin E or beta-carotene supplementation had no effect on skin sensitivity to UVR. Although vitamin E supplements significantly reduced the skin malondialdehyde concentration, neither supplement affected other measures of UVR-induced oxidative stress in human skin, which suggested no photoprotection of supplementation.

A study by Stahl et al. (2000) was performed where carotenoids' and tocopherols' antioxidant effect was investigated againstscavenging reactive oxygen species generated during photooxidative stress. It was investigated whether antioxidant oral supplementation may protect the skin from ultraviolet light-induced erythema. The antioxidants used in this study provided protection against erythema in humans and may be useful for diminishing sensitivity to ultraviolet light.

The study conducted by Varani et al. (2000) concluded that vitamin A antagonizes decreased cell growth and elevated collagen-degrading matrix metalloproteinases and stimulates collagen accumulation in naturally aged human skin (Varani et al., 2000). Their findings indicate that naturally aged, sun-protected skin and photoaged skin share important molecular features including connective tissue damage, elevated matrix metalloproteinase levels, and reduced collagen production. In addition, vitamin A treatment reduced matrix metalloproteinase expression and stimulated collagen synthesis in naturally aged, sun-protected skin, as it does in photoaged skin.

An increase in the yellow component of the skin was also shownin 12 subjects whose habitual diet was supplemented with 50mg of a natural carotenoid mix daily for six weeks (Heinrich et al., 1998). Parallelwith this increase in theyellow component of the skin, thedegree of redness in the skin after exposure to constant UVirradiation decreased as supplementation progressed. Moreover,on the basis of alterations in skin color, carotenoid concentrationsin the skin increased.

Heinrich et al. (2003) additionally compared the erythema-protective effect of beta-carotene (24 mg/d from an algal source) to that of 24 mg/d of a carotenoid mix consisting of the three main dietary carotenoids, beta-carotene, lutein and lycopene (8 mg/d each). In a placebo-controlled, parallel study design, volunteers with skin type II (n = 12 in each group) received beta-carotene, the carotenoid mix or placebo for 12 weeks. Serum beta-carotene concentration increased three- to fourfold in the beta-carotene group, whereas in the mixed carotenoid group, the serum concentration of each of the three carotenoids increased one- to threefold. No changes occurred in the control group. The intensity of erythema 24 h after irradiation was diminished in both groups that received carotenoids and was significantly lower than baseline after 12 wk of supplementation. Long-term supplementation for 12 weeks with 24 mg/d of a carotenoid mix supplying similar amounts of beta-carotene, lutein and lycopene ameliorates UV-induced erythema in humans. According to the authors, the effect is comparable to daily treatment with 24 mg of beta-carotene alone.

In another study, the supplement, providing 30 mg of a natural carotenoidmix (29.4 mg ß-carotene, 0.36 mg α-carotene, 0.084mg cryptoxanthin, 0.072 mg zeaxanthin, and 0.054 mg lutein)daily was provided to 22 subjects for eightweeks in a trial by Leeet al. (2000). The concentration of carotenoids was enhanced at30-mg increments every eightweeks to a final dose of 90 mg/d. After 24 weeks of supplementation, serum beta-carotene levels were increased from 0.22 microg/ml to 1.72 microg/ml. Similarly, alpha-carotene serum levels increased from 0.07 microg/ml to 0.36 microg/ml. Supplementationwith 60 and 90 mg carotenoids/d resulted in a dose-dependentincrease in MEDs. Moreover, serum ß-carotene concentrationsincreased after each subsequent supplementation; however, concentrationsin the skin were not present. The authors also showed thatthe twohighest concentrations of the carotenoid mix inhibitedserum lipid peroxidation. It was concluded that the dose ofsunlight required to produce a minimal perceptible erythemaincreased with increasing doses of carotenoids and that supplementation with natural carotenoids may partially protect human skin from UVA- and UVB-induced erythema, although the magnitude of the protective effect is modest.

Skin contains carotenoids at levels that correlate with blood levels. β-carotene and lycopene are rapidly degraded in skin exposed to sunlight. Ribaya-Mercadoet al. (1995) showed that lycopene was present in the skin in concentrationssimilar to those of ß-carotene and that exposure ofthe skin to UV light decreased skin lycopene concentrationsmore so than skin ß-carotene concentrations.

In contrast, intake of a much lower dosage of ß-carotene(30 mg/d) for tenweeks increased the yellow component of the skinat all body skin sites, as measured by chromametry, althoughthis color change was not visible (Gollnick et al., 1996). After the ten-wk supplementationperiod, supplementation continued in conjunction with exposureto natural sunlight for 13 d, i.e., approximately equivalent toa two-week vacation in the sun. During this period, the developmentof erythema in subjects who had taken ß-carotene wasmuch less pronounced than in the placebo group. During sun exposure,serum ß-carotene concentrations decreased to subphysiologicconcentrations in the placebo group. Such low concentrationsare possibly associated with an increased cancer risk. In thesupplemented group, however, concentrations did not fall belowreference values during sun exposure. Gollnick et al. (1996) concludedthat presupplementation with moderate dosages of ß-carotene(30 mg/d) before and during sunlight exposure provides protectionagainst sunburn, possibly because of the increased absorptioncapacity of the skin or because ß-carotene concentrationsin the skin do not decrease to below concentrations consideredto be critical. The study also showed that the combination ofsystemic and topical photoprotection by sunscreens offers asynergistic effect.

In a study by Wolf et al. (1988), 23 healthy volunteers received150 mg of an oral carotenoid preparation containing 60 mg ß-caroteneand 90 mg canthaxantin daily for fourwk. No differences in MEDswere shown in a comparison of values before and after carotenoidsupplementation. Concentrations in serum increased during treatment,but concentrations in the skin were not reported. Additionally,no effects of ß-carotene were detected when UV irradiation–inducedunscheduled DNA synthesis was investigated, suggesting thatcarotenoids were not protective against DNA lesions repairableby excision repair. The authors concluded that (1) carotenoids do not reduce UVB-, UVA-, or psoralen ultraviolet A (PUVA)-induced erythema in human skin; that (2) reactive oxygen species may not be involved in PUVA-erythema production or, alternatively, carotenoids may not quench these radicals sufficiently in vivo; and that (3) carotenoid protection against UVB-induced carcinogenesis does not operate by reducing the number of mutagenic lesions in DNA.

An extensive study was performed a few years later by Garmynet al. (1995). In this study, 16 healthy women underwent dietaryrestriction for threewk to reduce plasma baseline ß-caroteneto low-normal concentrations. Five days after ingestion of asingle dose of 120 mg ß-carotene, there was no significantchange in the intensity of erythema after a constant dose ofUV radiation. Moreover, an intake of 90 mg ß-carotene/dfor 23 d in conjunction with the habitual diet did not changethe intensity of erythema. Although ß-carotene concentrationsincreased in both plasma and skin under both conditions, therewere no effects of supplementation on biological features, e.g.,the number of sunburn cells and clinical appearances (intensityof erythema after acute exposure to sunlight).

Carotenoids have been shown to inhibit UV-induced epidermal damage and tumor formation in mouse models (Mathews-Roth & Krinsky, 1987).

The use of sunscreens on the skin can prevent sunburn, but whether long-term use can prevent skin cancer is not known. Also, there is evidence that oral beta-carotene supplementation lowers skin-cancer rates in animals, but there is limited evidence of its effect in human beings (Green et al., 1999). In a community-based randomized trial performed by Green et al. (1999) with a two-by-two factorial design, individuals were assigned to four treatment groups: daily application of a sun protection factor 15-plus sunscreen to the head, neck, arms, and hands, and beta-carotene supplementation (30 mg per day); sunscreen plus placebo tablets; beta-carotene only; or placebo only. Participants were 1,621 residents of Nambour in southeast Queensland, Australia. The endpoints after 4.5 years of follow-up were the incidence of basal-cell and squamous-cell carcinomas both in terms of people treated for newly diagnosed disease and in terms of the numbers of tumors that occurred. The 1,383 participants underwent full skin examination, and 250 of them developed 758 new skin cancers during the follow-up period. There were no significant differences in the incidence of first new skin cancers between groups randomly assigned daily sunscreen and no daily sunscreen. Similarly, there was no significant difference between the beta-carotene and placebo groups in incidence of either cancer. In terms of the number of tumors, there was no effect on incidence of basal-cell carcinoma by sunscreen use or by beta-carotene, but the incidence of squamous-cell carcinoma was significantly lower in the sunscreen group than in the no daily sunscreen group (1,115 vs. 1,832 per 100,000). The authors concluded that there was no harmful effect of daily use of sunscreen in this medium-term study. Cutaneous squamous-cell carcinoma, but not basal-cell carcinoma, seems to be amenable to prevention through the routine use of sunscreen by adults for 4.5 years. There was no beneficial or harmful effect on the rates of either type of skin cancer, as a result of beta-carotene supplementation (Green et al., 1999).

A randomized, placebo-controlled clinical trial on the efficacy of oral β-carotene (50 mg/day over fiveyears) in prevention of skin cancer in patients with recent nonmelanoma skin cancer showed no significant effect of β-carotene on either number or time of occurrence of new nonmelanoma skin cancer (Greenberg et al., 1990). In a separate trial among healthy men, 12 years of supplementation with β-carotene (50 mg on alternate days) produced no reduction of the incidence of malignant neoplasms, including nonmelanoma skin cancer (Hennekenset al., 1996). It must be pointed out that these intervention trials were conducted with patients whose skin cancer was primarily UVinduced, and it remains to be seen whether antioxidants are clinically effective in prevention of cutaneous chemocarcinogenesis (Fuch et al., 2001).

Irradiation of the skin in the infra-red (IR) range of the spectra, applied at physiological doses, can also produce free radicals. The magnitude of destruction of antioxidants, such as carotenoids, can serve as a marker of the extent of the stress factor, characterized by the quantity of produced free radicals. In a recent study, measurements on the degradation of cutaneous carotenoids following IR skin irradiation of 12 healthy volunteers (skin type II), was performed by Darvin et al. (2011). The amount of destroyed carotenoids after IR irradiation was higher in the case of pretreatment with beta-carotene than for the untreated skin, indicating that the superficial part of antioxidants is most important for protecting against external stressors. Additionally, topically applied carotenoids as a single antioxidant component are less stable than the carotenoids in the skin incorporated by nutrition and accumulated in a mixture with different antioxidant substances.

A number of experimental studies indicate protective effects of beta-carotene against acute and chronic manifestations of skin photodamage. However, most clinical studies have failed to convincingly demonstrate its beneficial effects so far. Nevertheless, intake of oral β-carotene supplements before sun exposure has been recommended on a population-wide basis. Studies on skin cells in culture have revealed that beta-carotene acts not only as an antioxidant but also has unexpected pro-oxidant properties (Biesalski and Obermueller-Jevic, 2001). For this reason, further studies with focus on in vivo β-carotene-induced pro-oxidative properties and its relevance on human health are needed.

2. Retinoids and Skin Studies

In cosmetics, vitamin A derivatives are used as anti-aging chemicals. Vitamin A is absorbed through the skin and increases the rate of skin turnover and gives an increase in collagen, giving a more youthful appearance (Kafi et al., 2007). Topical retinoids remain the mainstay for treating photoaging given their proven efficacy in both clinical and histological outcomes. The application of retinoids might not only clinically and biochemically repair photoaged skin, but their use might also prevent photoaging (Serri and Iorizzo, 2008). Evidence from a randomized clinical trial showed that, in spite of the many surgical procedures effective in ameliorating the clinical appearance of photoaged skin, the most effective medical therapy with proven benefits in photoaged skin are topical retinoids, in particular tretinoin, isotretinoin, and tazarotene. Tretinoin is the acid form of vitamin A and is also known as all-*trans* retinoic acid or ATRA. It is available as a cream or gel (brand names Aberela, Airol, Renova, Atralin, Retin-A, Avita, or Stieva-A). Available topical retinoids include prescription tretinoin (Retin-A®), adapalene (Differen®), and tazarotene (Tazorac®) and over-the-counter Retinol® and Retinol-A®. These drugs are derivatives of vitamin A, which might have anti-aging properties (Helfrich et al., 2008). In addition to retinoids, many other cosmeceutical agents are now available. The gold standard among cosmeceuticals for the treatment of photodamaged skin is the topical retinoids, such as tretinoin. Topical pretreatment with tretinoin inhibits the induction and activity of MMPs in UVB-irradiated skin through prevention of AP-1 activation. Topical tretinoin was first observed to ameliorate the clinical signs of photoaging by Cordero (1983) and Kligman et al. (1986). In a pilot study, Kligman et al. (1986) found that all-trans-RA cream (tretinoun, Retin-A), which is used for the treatment of acne vulgaris, could partially reverse structural skin damage associated with photoaging. In the late 1980s, the first double-blinded, randomized, vehicle-controlled clinical trials investigating the use of tretinoin for photoaged skin were performed. In these studies, investigators found that surface roughness, dyspigmentation, and fine wrinkles demonstrated the most improvement with topical tretinoin therapy (0.1% tretinoin cream) in the first four to ten months of therapy (Weiss et al., 1988). Numerous subsequent clinical studies have confirmed these initial observations using 0.05% tretinoin for three to six months (Leyden et al., 1989; Lever et al., 1990; Weinstein et al.,1991; Olsen et al., 1992).

A study was done to compare the effects of dietary administration of a vitamin A drug (13-cis-retinoic acid) to the natural form of vitamin A (retinyl palmitate). Female mice were administered a chemical carcinogen to evaluate the incidence and severity on mouse skin tumor promotion. The results showed that retinyl palmitate inhibited the number and weight of tumors, whereas 13-cis-retinoic acid resulted in a decrease in weight but not in number of tumors promoted (Gensler et al., 1987).

In another study, tumors were chemically induced in a group of Swiss mice over a 23-week period. The topical application of 13-cis-retinoic acid was compared to natural vitamin A (retinyl palmitate). This study showed that both retinyl palmitate and 13-cis-retinoic acid inhibited the development of skin papillomas and also had a marked effect on skin cancers (Abdel-Galil et al., 1984). Vitamin A may be one of the better-documented vitamins to protect against several types of human cancers. One of its mechanisms is to induce healthy differentiation and apoptosis of aged cells. The value of vitamin A in protecting the skin is to help facilitate cell renewal and possibly prevent skin cancers.

Griffiths et al. (1993) investigated whether collagen synthesis was reduced in photodamaged human skin and, if so, whether it could be restored by treatment with topical tretinoin. The study found that treatment of photodamaged skin with tretinoin produced an 80 percent increase in collagen I formation. The formation of collagen I was significantly decreased in photodamaged human skin, and this process was partly restored by treatment with tretinoin.

In large-scale, double-blind, placebo-controlled, six-month trials, 0.05% tretinoin emollient cream (Renova, Retinova) reduced fine wrinkles and skin roughness, and it produced histological changes such as epidermal thickening, increased granular layer thickness, stratum corneum compaction, and decreased melanin content. The study conducted by Gilchrest(1997) concluded topical tretinoin is safe and effective in the treatment of photodamage.

The clinical and histologic effects of an emollient cream formulation of topical tretinoin at concentrations of 0.05% and 0.01% were examined in 251 subjects with mild to moderate photodamaged facial skin in a randomized, double-blind, vehicle-controlled, multicenter study conducted by Weinstein et al. (1991). Seventy-nine percent of the subjects who received 0.05% tretinoin for 24 weeks showed overall improvement in photodamaged skin compared with improvement in 48% of the vehicle-treated control subjects. Significant reductions were found in fine wrinkling, mottled hyperpigmentation, roughness, and laxity after 0.05% tretinoin therapy when compared with controls.

In a double-blind, placebo-controlled study conducted by Voorhees (1990), 0.1% topical tretinoin reduced the effects of photoaging maximally after tenmonths, with no further improvements if treatment was continued until 22 months.

The utility of topical tretinoin in combination with sun protection has now been formally established as a useful approach to the treatment of sun-damaged skin (Leyden, 1998).

Retinoid-mediated improvement of photoaging is associated with increased collagen I formation (Griffiths et al., 1993), reorganization of packed collagen fibers (Yamamotoet al., 1995), and increased number of type VII anchoring fibrils (Chen et al., 1997).However, up to 92% of subjects used tretinoin in various clinical studies have reported "retinoid dermatitis," i.e., erythema and scaling at the site of application (Weiss et al., 1988; Rittie et al., 2006).Irritation can be minimized by reducing dose and frequency of treatments.

The study conducted by Varani et al. (1998), using human skin in organ culture and epidermal keratinocytes and fibroblasts in monolayer culture, show that retinoic acid stimulates growth of both keratinocytes and fibroblasts and stimulates extracellular matrix production by the fibroblasts. Adult skin from sun-exposed and sun-protected sites responds equally well to retinoic acid, whereas neonatal skin is much less responsive under the same conditions.

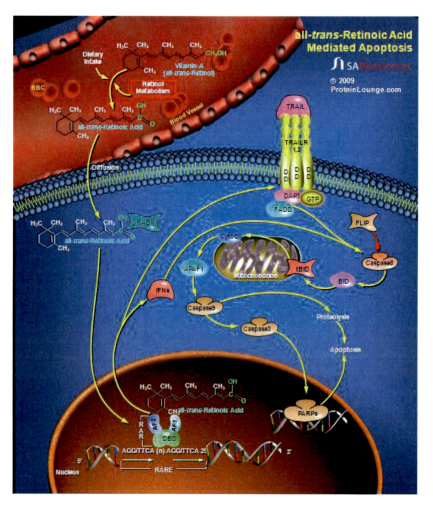

Figure 34. Retinoic acid, a lipophilic molecule and a metabolite of vitamin-A (all-trans-retinol), affects gene transcription and modulates a wide variety of biological processes like cell proliferation, Differentiation, including apoptosis. retinoic acid-mediated gene transcription depends on the rate of transport of retinoic acid to target cells and the timing of exposure of retinoic acid to RARs (retinoic acid receptors) in the target tissues. (source: SABiosciences, a QIAGEN company. http://www.sabiosciences.com/).

Authors conclude (i) that retinoids may be able to repair intrinsically aged skin as well as photoaged skin, and (ii) that retinoids modulate human skin cell function in a manner that is age-related and not simply a response to photodamage. Most of the research concerning cosmeceutical retinoid ingredients is based upon the effects of retinoic acid on the skin. Clinical trials concerning retinol and retinaldehyde are scant and lacking in statistical evaluation for significance (Levin and Momin, 2010).

Lycopene

Tomato and tomato products are recognized to confer a wide range of health benefits. Lycopene is the pigment principally responsible for the characteristic deep-red color of ripe tomato fruits and tomato products. Epidemiological studies have provided evidencethat high consumption of tomatoes effectively lowers the risk of reactive oxygen species (ROS)-mediated diseases such as cardiovascular disease and cancer by improving the antioxidant capacity. Lycopene is a non-provitamin A carotenoid present in human blood and tissues. Lycopene is present in the human blood (approximately 0.5 micromol/liter plasma), and the tissue levels vary from 1 nmol/g wet wt in adipose tissue to up to 20 nmol/g wet wt in adrenals and testes. The composition and structure of the food also have an impact on the bioavailability of lycopene and may affect the release of lycopene from the tomato tissue matrix. Lycopene bioavailability in processed tomato products is higher than in unprocessed fresh tomatoes. Food processing may improve lycopene bioavailability by breaking down cell walls, which weakens the bonding forces between lycopene and tissue matrix, thus making lycopene more accessible and enhancing the cis-isomerization. This makes its presence in the diet of considerable interest (Shi and Le Maguer, 2000). The major dietary sources of lycopene for the human are tomatoes and tomato products. There are several biochemical mechanisms potentially underlying the protective effects of lycopene. These include antioxidant activity such as the quenching of singlet oxygen and the scavenging of peroxyl radicals, induction of cell-cell communication, and growth control. Lycopene was reported to be a more stable and potent singlet oxygen quenching agent compared to other carotenoids (Bhuvaneswari and Nagini, 2005). Although it has no provitamin A activity, lycopene does exhibit a physical quenching rate constant with singlet oxygen almost twice as high as that of beta-carotene. In vitro and in vivo studies support this assumption (Sies and Stahl, 1998).

Stahl (Stahl et al., 1998) reported that carotenoid mixtures protect oxidative damage in the synergistic way. Antioxidant activity of carotenoids in multilamellar liposomes assayed by inhibition of formation of thiobarbituric acid-reactive substances was in the ranking: lycopene> alpha-tocopherol> alpha-carotene> beta-cryptoxanthin > zeaxanthin = beta-carotene> lutein. Mixtures of carotenoids were more effective than the single compounds. This synergistic effect was most pronounced when lycopene or lutein was present.

Additionally, Stahl et al. (2001) designed the study to investigate whether intervention with a natural dietary source rich in lycopene protects against UV-induced erythema in humans. Tomato paste (40 g), providing approximately 16 mg/d of lycopene, was ingested with 10 g of olive oil over a period of tenwk by ninevolunteers. Controls (n = 10) received olive oil only. At wk ten, dorsal erythema formation was 40% lower in the group that consumed tomato paste compared with controls. The data demonstrate that it is feasible to achieve protection against UV light-induced erythema by ingestion of a commonly consumed dietary source of lycopene.

The photoprotective effect of beta-carotene supplementation alone was compared with that of a carotenoid mixture consisting of beta-carotene, lutein and lycopene. After a standard dose of UV irradiation, the intensity of erythema was diminished to a similar extent in both groups (Albanes et al., 1996). In the study of Aust et al. (2005), the photoprotective effects of synthetic lycopene in comparison with a tomato extract (Lyc-o-Mato) and a drink containing solubilized Lyc-o-Mato (Lyc-o-Guard-Drink) was investigated. With these different sources, the volunteers ingested similar amounts of lycopene (about 10 mg/day). After 12 weeks of supplementation, significant increases in lycopene serum levels and total skin carotenoids were observed in all groups. All groups demonstrated a reduction in erythema formation following UV irradiation, but the protective effect was more pronounced with the tomato extract in both capsule and drink formats (Aust et al., 2005).

Additionally, lycopene was reported to enhance UVA-induced oxidative stress in C3H cells, and authors of the study suggest that under UVA irradiation, lycopene may produce also oxidative products that are responsible for the pro-oxidant effects (Yeh et al., 2004).

Synergistic Effect between Antioxidants

As it was shown in previous studies, the combination of different antioxidants applied simultaneously can provide a synergistic effect. Antioxidants are most effective when used in combination. Vitamin C regenerates vitamin E, and selenium and niacin are required to keep glutathione in its active form. Ascorbate can regenerate α-tocoferol from its phenoxyl radical in many model systems (Guo and Packer, 2000); namely, the tocopherol radical (TO$^\cdot$) formed can be repaired subsequently through the one-electron oxidation of ascorbic acid (AscH$^-$), thereby regenerating α-tocoferol and producing ascorbate radical (Asc$^{\cdot-}$):

$$AscH^- + TO^\cdot \rightarrow Asc^{\cdot-} + TOH$$

Asc$^{\cdot-}$ can be removed by dismutation, yielding AscH$^-$ and dehydroascorbate (DHA). Both Asc$^{\cdot-}$ and DHA can be reduced by the enzyme system, which uses NADH or NADPH as sources of reducing equivalents(Halliwell and Gutterigde, 1999). In addition, it is well known that DHA can be enzymatically or non-enzymatically reduced to ascorbate with GSH, an important endogenous thiol antioxidant. Mendiratta et al. (1998) reported that ascorbate regeneration from DHA in human erythrocytes is largely GSH dependent.

It has been demonstrated that vitamin C can regenerate α-tocopherol from its chromanoxyl radical (Packer et al., 1979), and the vitamin C radical may be recycled by GSH non-enzymatically under slightly acidic conditions (Stocker et al.,1986) that are present in the stratum corneum (Ohman and Vahlquist, 1994). In another study, much higher doses of 2 g α-tocopherol/d, 3g ascorbate/d, a combination of both vitamins, or a placebowere administered to 40 healthy volunteers for 50 d (Fuchs and Kern, 1998). Bioavailabilitywas established by the increased concentrations of α-tocopheroland ascorbate in buccal mucosal keratinocytes after supplementation.MEDs increased markedly after intake of the combination of α-tocopheroland ascorbate. Obviously, because MEDs also increased slightlyin subjects who received either vitamin alone or placebo, seasonalinfluences may have interfered with the measurements.

Nevertheless,the interaction between vitamins E and C likely explained theirmore pronounced photoprotective effect compared with that ofeither vitamin alone (Boelsma et al., 2001). Although this study convincingly showedthat vitamin supplementation effectively protects the skin againstsunburn, the doses of vitamins used were much higher than amountsgenerally ingested from habitual diets (Boelsma et al., 2001).

The protective effect of a combination of vitamins E and C wasalso shown in the study by Eberlein-König et al. (1998). In their study,subjects received lower dosages of 671 mg vitamin E/d and 2g vitamin C/d for a relatively short time, eightd. Despite theselower dosages, mean MEDs increased compared with baseline ineight of ten subjects receiving the supplement.

Another study examined the photoprotective potential of the dietary antioxidants vitamin C, vitamin E, lycopene, beta-carotene, and the rosemary polyphenol, carnosic acid, was tested in human dermal fibroblasts exposed to ultraviolet-A (UVA) light (Offord et al., 2002). Researchers concluded that vitamin C, vitamin E, and carnosic acid showed photoprotective potential. Lycopene and beta-carotene did not protect on their own but in the presence of vitamin E. Their stability in culture was improved, and the rise in MMP-1 mRNA expression was suppressed, suggesting a requirement for antioxidant protection of the carotenoids against formation of oxidative derivatives that can influence the cellular and molecular responses.

The beneficial effects of a combination of ß-caroteneand other antioxidants were investigated by Postaire et al. (1997).In their study, tensubjects received a supplement providing 13mg ß-carotene, 2 mg lycopene, 5 mg tocopherol, and30 mg ascorbic acid daily for eightwk. The aim of the study was to demonstrate that modification of the cellular redox-equilibrium occurs as a consequence of antioxidant nutrients intake (carotenoids, vitamin E and vitamin C) and that these nutrients play a role in the pigmentation of the skin without any UV exposure. Significant increase of melanin concentrations in skin was found after four, five, six, and eight weeks of dietary antioxidant intake.

Synergistic effect between antioxidants was confirmed also in the study from Cesarini et al. (2003). Authors investigated, in 25 healthy individuals, the capacity of an antioxidant complex (AOC)—vitamins (lycopene, beta-carotene, alpha-tocopherol), selenium—to reduce UV-induced damages. Study concludes that after the oral intake of an antioxidant complex, many parameters of the epidermal defense against UV-induced damages were significantly improved. The oral intake of AOC could provide a safe, daylong and efficient complement to photo-protective measures provided by topical and physical agents and may contribute to reducing the DNA damages leading to skin aging and skin cancers.

A clinical, randomized, double-blind, parallel group, placebo-controlled study was conducted by Greul et al. (2002), in healthy young female volunteers (skin type II) investigating the preventive, photoprotective effect of supplementation with Seresis, an antioxidative combination containing both lipid and water-soluble compounds: carotenoids (beta-carotene and lycopene), vitamins C and E, selenium and proanthocyanidins. Supplementation with Seresis decreased the UV-induced expression of MMP-1 and 9, which might be important in photoprotective processes. By the combination of antioxidants, such as in the formulation of Seresis, a selective protection of the skin against irradiation can be achieved.

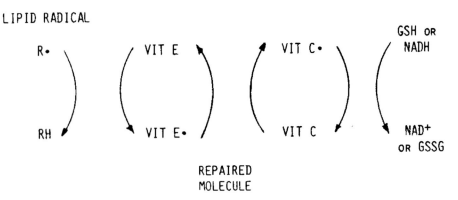

Scheme 2. Synergistic action of vitamin E and C and glutathione (Figure adopted from Halliwell and Gutteridge, 1999).

It was also reported that the combination of carotenoids and CoQ10 in topical skin care products may provide enhanced protection from inflammation and premature aging caused by sun exposure (Fuller et al., 2006).

Werninghaus et al. (1994) reported that vitamin E given orally at 400IU/day for a period of six months affords no significant increase in UV protection. Similarly, in a study with 12 volunteers, vitamin C given at 500 mg/day over eight weeks had no effect on the UV-induced erythemal response (McArdle et al., 2002), indicating again the importance of antioxidants to be supplemented together to obtain the synergistic effect.

Vitamin D

Ultraviolet (UV) radiation has both beneficial and harmful effects on the human body. Its most important beneficial effect may be vitamin D production in the skin, also known as vitamin D photosynthesis. This is of particular interest for the elderly, who often show vitamin D-deficiency. Vitamin D is essential for normal growth, calcium absorption, and skeletal development. Vitamin D is naturally present in few foods; most comes from the photo-conversion of 7-dehydrocholesterol in skin. The limiting factor in this conversion is the availability of ultraviolet light less than 310 nm (Neer, 1975). The two major forms are vitamin D_2 or ergocalciferol, and vitamin D_3 or cholecalciferol. These are known collectively as calciferol. Vitamin D is carried in the bloodstream to the liver, where it is converted into the prohormone calcidiol. Circulating calcidiol may then be converted into calcitriol, the biologically active form of vitamin D, either in the kidneys or by monocyte-macrophages in the immune system. Vitamin D insufficiency can result in thin, brittle, or misshapen bones, while sufficiency prevents rickets in children and osteomalacia in adults, and, together with calcium, helps to protect older adults from osteoporosis. Intentional UV exposure has been recommended by different institutions in order to increase vitamin D levels. Nevertheless, UV radiation directly causes DNA damage and is verifiably responsible for carcinogenesis, potentially resulting in lethal skin cancers. Because UV radiation is neither a reliable nor a safe method of achieving healthy vitamin D levels, intentional UV radiation is not recommended to increase vitamin D levels. Diffey (2010) showed that current advice about modest sun exposure during the summer months does little in the way of boosting overall

25(OH)D levels, while sufficient sun exposure that could achieve a worthwhile benefit would compromise skin health. On the contrary, the study performed by Rhodes et al. (2010) revealed that recommended summer sunlight exposure levels can produce sufficient (> or =20 ng ml(-1)) but not the proposed optimal (> or =32 ng ml(-1)) 25(OH)D levels at UK latitudes. Assuming midday UVB levels, sufficient but suboptimal vitamin D status is attained after a summer's short (13 minutes) sunlight exposures to 35% skin surface area (Rhodes et al., 2010).

In order to prevent skin cancer, UV protection is to be conducted as commonly recommended, by minimizing sun exposure, and especially sunburn, with appropriate sun protective behaviors, e.g., usage of sunscreen and clothing (hat, sunglasses, long sleeves, and pants). Infants must be protected with extra care (Barysch et al.,2010). Even in the summer months, the amount is suboptimal in some population groups in the northern latitudes (i.e., above the 35th parallel) (Viethl et al., 2001). More debate is required regarding optimal vitamin D bioavailability, either from moderate sun exposure (risk of photoaging and skin cancer) or from fortified foods and supplements.

The B Vitamins

The B vitamins are eight water-soluble vitamins that play important roles in cell metabolism and in regulation of the oxidative stress. The B vitamins were once thought to be a single vitamin, referred to as vitamin B. In general, supplements containing all eight are referred to as a vitamin B complex. Riboflavin (vitamin B2), niacin (vitamin B3) and pyridoxine (vitamin B6) are required for optimal skin health. Riboflavin is an important coenzyme in the conversion of carbohydrates, fats and proteins into energy and typically takes the form of flavin adenine dinucleotide (FAD) or flavin mononucleotide (FMN). It plays a crucial role in preventing cellular oxidative damage through its involvement in the recycling of glutathione. Deficiency causes skin disorders like seborrheic dermatitis (Lakshmi, 1998) and other disorders e.g., ariboflavinosis. Symptoms may include cheilosis (cracks in the lips), high sensitivity to sunlight, angular cheilitis, glossitis (inflammation of the tongue), seborrheic dermatitis or pseudo-syphilis (particularly affecting the scrotum or labia majora and the mouth), etc. Also, niacin (NAD and NADP) is required for energy production and inhibits the oxidation of cellular components and regulates oxidative stress. Besides, it is required for steroid hormones, essential for skin function (Jenkins et al., 2009). Nicotinamide, the amide form of vitamin B3, is an inexpensive agent thatis used for a variety of dermatological applications with little or no toxicity even at high doses. Nicotinamide has photoprotective effects against carcinogenesis and immune suppression in mice and is photoimmunoprotective in humans when used as a lotion or orally (Damian, 2010). Nicotinamide normalizes subsets of apoptosis, immune function and energy metabolism-related genes that are downregulated by UV exposure; nicotinamide prevents also UV-induced cellular ATP loss and protected against UV-induced glycolytic blockade (Park et al., 2010). UV irradiation depletes keratinocytes of cellular energy, and nicotinamide, which is a precursor of nicotinamide adenine dinucleotide, may act at least in part by providing energy repletion to irradiated cells (Damian, 2010). Also, Sivapirabu et al. (2009) reported that topical nicotinamide modulates cellular energy metabolism and provides broad-spectrum protection against ultraviolet radiation-induced immunosuppression in humans. Nicotinamide, which protected against both UVB and UVA, is thus a promising agent for skin cancer prevention. Oral nicotinamide, at doses of either 1,500 or 500 mg daily, significantly reduced UV immunosuppression with no immune effects in unirradiated skin as reported in the study of Yiasemides et al. (2009). Oral nicotinamide is safe and inexpensive and looks promising as a chemopreventive supplement for reducing the immunosuppressive effects of sunlight. Deficiency of vitamin B3, along with a deficiency of tryptophan causes pellagra. Symptoms include aggression, dermatitis, insomnia, weakness, mental confusion, and diarrhea. In advanced cases, pellagra may lead to dementia and death. Also, pyridoxine is involved in cellular energy production and amino acid metabolism. It is important for the healthy function of tissue that needs to regenerate quickly. Deficiency may lead to microcytic anemia (because pyridoxyl phosphate is the co-factor for heme synthesis), depression, dermatitis, high blood pressure (hypertension), water retention, and elevated levels of homocysteine. Deficiency also adversely affects the maturation of newly formed collagen. Also, Vitamin B_9 (folic acid and folate inclusive) is essential to numerous bodily functions. Both synthetic folic acid and the most biologically abundant extracellular reduced folate, 5-methyltetrahydrofolate, are degraded under conditions of ultraviolet radiation (UVR) exposure. Skin is a proliferative tissue with increased folate nutrient demands due to a dependence upon continuous epidermal cell proliferation and differentiation to maintain homeostasis. Regions of skin are also chronically exposed to UVR, which penetrates to the actively dividing basal layer of the epidermis, increasing the folate nutrient demands in order to replace folate species degraded by UVR exposure and to supply the folate cofactors required for repair of photodamaged DNA. Localized folate deficiencies of skin are a likely consequence of UVR exposure (Williams and Jacobson, 2010). Williams and Jacobson (2010) additionally reported that folate deficiency creates a permissive environment for genomic instability, which is an early event in the process of skin carcinogenesis. The effects of folate restriction, even in severely depleted, growth-arrested keratinocytes, were reversible by repletion with folic acid. B vitamins are found in all whole, unprocessed foods. Processed carbohydrates, such as sugar and white flour, tend to have lower B vitamin content than their unprocessed counterparts. B vitamins are particularly concentrated in meat and meat products such as liver, turkey, and tuna (Stipanuk, 2006). Other good sources for B vitamins are whole grains, potatoes, bananas, lentils, chili peppers, tempeh (traditional soy product), beans, nutritional yeast and brewer's yeast.

Coenzyme Q

Coenzyme Q_{10} (also known as ubiquinone, ubidecarenone, coenzyme Q) (CoQ10) is a 1,4-benzoquinone, where Q refers to the quinone chemical group, and 10 refers to the number of isoprenyl chemical subunits. This oil-soluble substance is present in most eukaryotic cells, primarily in the mitochondria. Coenzyme Q10 is a naturally occurring antioxidant and a prominent component of mitochondrial electron transport chain. The processes of aging and photoaging are associated with an increase in cellular oxidation. This may be in part due to a decline in the levels of the endogenous cellular antioxidants, among them also coenzyme Q10 declines significantly with age and UV stress (Podda et al., 1998).Coenzyme Q10 is a biosynthesized quinone with 10 isoprene side chains in humans. Antioxidant action is a property of the reduced form of coenzyme Q10, ubiquinol (CoQ10H2) and the ubisemiquinone radical (CoQ10H·) (Siemieniuk and Skrzydlewska, 2005). Its essential role is as an electron carrier in the mitochondrial respiratory chain. Coenzyme Q is recognized as an obligatory cofactor for the function of uncoupling proteins (for further reading, see also paragraph on uncoupling) and a modulator of the transition pore. Furthermore, recent data reveal that CoQ10 affects expression of genes involved in human cell signaling, metabolism, and transport, and some of the effects of exogenously administered CoQ10 may be due to this property. Coenzyme Q is the only lipid soluble antioxidant synthesized endogenously. In its reduced form, CoQH2, ubiquinol, inhibits protein and DNA oxidation, but it is the effect on lipid peroxidation that has been most deeply studied. Ubiquinol inhibits the peroxidation of cell membrane lipids and also that of lipoprotein lipids present in the circulation (Littarru and Tiano, 2007). Moreover, coenzyme Q10 is one of the most important lipophilic antioxidants, preventing the generation of free radicals as well as oxidative modifications of proteins, lipids, and DNA, and it can also regenerate the other powerful lipophilic antioxidant, alpha-tocopherol (see also section on synergistic effect and regeneration of antioxidants). Thus, coenzyme Q10 may prevent both initiation and the propagation of lipid peroxidation in contrast to α-tocopherol, which exerts its antioxidant activity through chain-breaking mechanisms, thus acting only by inhibiting propagation (Ernster and Orsmark-Andree, 1993).

CoQ and the Skin Studies

Coenzyme Q10 (CoQ10), which has both energizing and antioxidative effects, is also reported to have anti-aging action. Levels of Coenzyme Q10 (CoQ10), are reduced in skin cells from aging donors, and according to Blatt et al. (2005), topical supplementation can ameliorate processes involved in skin aging.

The study of Prahl et al. (2008) shows significant age-dependent differences in mitochondrial function of keratinocytes isolated from skin biopsies of young and old donors. From the data, researchers postulate that energy metabolism shifts to a predominantly non-mitochondrial pathway and is, therefore, functionally anaerobic with advancing age. CoQ10 positively influences the age-affected cellular metabolism and enables to combat signs of aging starting at the cellular level. As a consequence, topical application of CoQ10 is beneficial for human skin as it rapidly improves mitochondrial function in skin in vivo.

The study of Hoppe et al. (1999) has investigated whether topical application of CoQ10 has the beneficial effect of preventing photoaging. Authors were able to demonstrate that CoQ10 penetrated into the viable layers of the epidermis and reduced the level of oxidation measured by weak photon emission. Furthermore, a reduction in wrinkle depth following CoQ10 application was also shown. CoQ10 was determined to be effective against UVA-mediated oxidative stress in human keratinocytes in terms of thiol depletion, activation of specific phosphotyrosine kinases and prevention of oxidative DNA damage. CoQ10 was also able to significantly suppress the expression of collagenase in human dermal fibroblasts following UVA irradiation. It was recently reported that Coenzyme Q10 protects against oxidative stress-induced cell death and enhances the synthesis of basement membrane components in dermal and epidermal cells (Muta-Takada et al., 2009).Coenzyme Q10 (CoQ10) was reported to reduce ROS production and DNA damage triggered by UVA irradiation in human keratinocytes in vitro. Further, CoQ10 was shown to reduce UVA-induced MMPs in cultured human dermal fibroblasts (Inui et al., 2008). Besides, in the clinical trial study, it was found that the use of 1% CoQ10 cream for five months reduced wrinkle score grade observed by a dermatologist (Inui et al., 2008). It seems that the biochemistry ofCoQ10 may inhibit the production of IL-6, which stimulates fibroblasts in dermis by paracrine manner to upregulate MMPs production, and contribute to protecting dermal fiber components from degradation, leading to rejuvenation of wrinkled skin (Inui et al., 2008).There was observed also the influence of CoQ10 on endogenous antioxidant defense. It was reported that CoQ10 strongly inhibits oxidative stress in the skin induced by UVB via increasing SOD2 and GPx (Kim et al., 2007).It was reported that it is considered that CoQ10 appears to have also a cutaneous healing effect in vivo (Choi et al., 2009).

Also, idebenone, a synthetic analog of Coenzyme Q 10, has potent antioxidant activity; it reduces skin roughness, increases skin hydration, reduces fine lines, and was associated with an improvement in overall global assessment of photoaged skin (McDaniel, et al.,2005).

Glutathione

Glutathione (GSH) is another powerful endogenous antioxidant. Glutathione is synthesized from glutamate, cysteine, and glycine and occurs in milimolar concentration in cells but only in trace amounts in plasma. GSH may be involved in a number of antioxidant reactions that are relevant to UV-mediated oxidative stress including detoxification of hydrogen peroxide (as a cofactor of GSH peroxidase), detoxification of free radicals, reduction of protein disulphides, and competition with protein thiols for oxidizing species.

In cell culture models using human skin cells, it has been clearly shown that glutathione depletion leads to a large sensitization to UVA (334 nm, 365 nm) and near-visible (405 nm) wavelengths as well as to radiation in the UVB (302 nm, 313 nm) (Tyrrell and Pidoux, 1986,1988). There is a direct correlation between the levels of sensitization and cellular glutathione content. Additional evidence that glutathione is a photoprotective agent in skin cells is derived from experiments thathave demonstrated that glutathione levels in both dermis and epidermis are depleted by UVA treatment (Connor and Wheeler, 1987).

Carnosine

Antioxidants cannot completely protect proteins. Nature's second line of defense is to repair or remove damaged proteins. This is where carnosine (beta-alanyl-L-histidine) demonstrates its most profound anti-aging effect. Carnosine is found exclusively in animal tissues. Carnosine has the potential to suppress many of the biochemical changes (e.g., protein oxidation, glycation, AGE formation, and cross-linking) that accompany aging and associated pathologies. Studies show that carnosine is effective against cross-linking and the formation of advanced glycation end products (AGE) (Aldini et al., 2010).

Due to carnosine's antiglycating activity, reactivity toward deleterious carbonyls, zinc- and copper-chelating activity and low toxicity, carnosine and related structures could be effective against age-related protein carbonyl stress. Carnosine's ability to react with deleterious aldehydes such as malondialdehyde, methylglyoxal, hydroxynonenal, and acetaldehyde may also contribute to its protective functions. It is suggested that carnivorous diets could be beneficial because of their carnosine content, as the dipeptide has been shown to suppress some diabetic complications in mice. It is also suggested that carnosine's therapeutic potential should be explored with respect to neurodegeneration (Hipkiss et al., 2006). Other, and much more speculative, possible functions of carnosine considered include transglutaminase inhibition, stimulation of proteolysis mediated via effects on proteasome activity or induction of protease and stress-protein gene expression, upregulation of corticosteroid synthesis, stimulation of protein repair, and effects on ADP-ribose metabolism associated with sirtuin and poly-ADP-ribose polymerase (PARP) activities (Hipkiss et al., 2009).

L-carnosine has been reported to delay the replicative senescence and extend the lifespan of cultured human diploid fibroblasts. Shao et al. (2004) studied the effect of carnosine on the telomeric DNA of cultured human fetal lung fibroblast cells. Cells continuously grown in 20 mM carnosine exhibited a slower telomere shortening rate and extended lifespan in population doublings. When kept in a long-term nonproliferating state, they accumulated much less damages in the telomeric DNA when cultured in the presence of carnosine (Shao etal., 2004).

Glycated proteins produce 50-fold more free radicals than nonglycated proteins and carnosine may be the most effective anti-glycating agent known (see also the chapter on glycation and AGEs). However, mechanisms of its anti-aging potentials are not fully established, and further studies are needed.

Selenium

Selenium is an another important trace element needed in a complex antioxidant network of the human body. Selenium (Se) is an essential element for animals and humans that is obtained from dietary sources including cereals, grains and vegetables. The Se content of plants varies considerably according to its concentration in soil. Plants convert Se mainly into Se-methionine (Se-Met) and incorporate it into protein in place of methionine (Met). Selenocystine (Se-Cys), methyl-Se-Cys and gamma-glutamyl-Se-methyl-Cys are not significantly incorporated into plant protein and are at relatively low levels irrespective of soil Se content. Higher animals are unable to synthesize Se-Met, and only Se-Cys was detected in rats supplemented with Se as selenite (Tapiero et al., 2003).

Selenite (SeL) or selenomethionine (SeM) are the most common selenium (Se) compounds taken as dietary antioxidants to reduce oxidative stress. Because the public may frequently supplement Se compounds at high doses, the possible pro-oxidant effect of Se becomes a concern (see also the chapter "Should we take antioxidant supplements?"). In the in vitro system, the chemical form of Se is an important factor in eliciting cellular responses. Although the cytotoxic mechanisms of selenite and other redoxing Se compounds are still unclear, it has been suggested that they derive from their ability to catalyze the oxidation of thiols and to produce superoxide simultaneously. "Selenite-induced cytotoxicity and apoptosis in human carcinoma cells can be inhibited with copper (CuSO(4)) as an antioxidant. High doses of selenite result in induction of 8-hydroxydeoxyguanosine (8-OHdG) in mouse skin cell DNA and in primary human keratinocytes. It may cause DNA fragmentation and decreased DNA synthesis, cell growth inhibition, DNA synthesis, blockade of the cell cycle at the S/G(2)-M phase and cell death by necrosis. In contrast, in cells treated with methylselenocyanate or Se methylselenocysteine, the cell cycle progression was blocked at the G(1) phase and cell death was predominantly induced by apoptosis" (Tapiero et al., 2003).

As already mentioned, Se can increase oxidative stress and oxidative damage of DNA. What happens when Se reacts with other antioxidants present in the cell? Se compounds and other dietary antioxidants, such as vitamin (Vit) C or Vit E, are often supplemented and taken together with Se compounds. However, the cellular effects of these interactions of Se with antioxidants are still unknown. The study by Shen et al. (2001) was designed to investigate the interactive effects of SeL or SeM plus Vit C, trolox (a water-soluble Vit E), or copper sulfate (CuSO(4)) on cell viability and induction of 8-OHdG adduct formation in DNA of primary human keratinocytes NHK (Shen et al., 2001). "Coincubation of Vit C or CuSO(4) with SeL appeared to protect NHK against SeL-induced cytotoxicity. However, synergistic effects were observed between SeL and trolox resulting in enhanced cytotoxicity. On the other hand, SeM + Vit C, SeM + trolox, and SeM + CuSO(4) did not affect cell viability. In the absence of Se supplementation, Vit C, trolox, or CuSO(4) alone did not induce 8-OHdG adduct formation, regardless of dose. When NHK cells were coincubated with SeL and Vit C or CuSO(4), they protected NHK from SeL-induced DNA damage with a reduction in 8-OHdG generation. In contrast, treatment of SeL + trolox elevated generation of 8-OHDG: Furthermore, treatments of SeM plus trolox or CuSO(4) elevated 8-OHdG adduct formation. In terms of apoptosis measured as internucleosomal DNA fragmentation, copper protected NHK against SeL-induced apoptosis in cultured NHK." The data from the study from Shen et al. (2001) suggest that the use of CuSO(4) may play a protective role in SeL-induced cytotoxicity, DNA oxidative damage, and apoptosis and that there may be potentially deleterious interactions among common high-dose antioxidant supplements taken by the public (Shen et al., 2001). The results of this study indicate the need fortesting not only a single substance but all possible interactions between different substances relevant for interactions in our cells. On the other hand, accumulating evidence indicates that Se compounds possess anticancer properties. Se is specifically incorporated into proteins in the form of selenocysteine and non-specifically incorporated as selenomethionine in place of methionine. The effects of Se compounds on cells are strictly compositional and concentrationdependent. At supranutritional dietary levels, Se can prevent the development of many types of cancer. At higher concentrations, Se compounds can be either cytotoxic or possibly carcinogenic. The cytotoxicity of Se is suggested to be associated with oxidative stress (Letavayová et al., 2006). In the case of selenium, the ingestion of the therapeutic dose is beneficial, but on the other hand, lack of selenium or its overdose can have harmful effects on the health.

Zinc

Zinc (Zn) is another metal thatis important for cell's antioxidative defense. Zinc possesses antioxidant properties, which protect against premature aging of the skin and muscles of the body, although studies differ as to its effectiveness (Milbury and Richer, 2008). Zinc is also involved in the healing process after an injury. Many of the elderly are deficient in Zinc, and this may impair wound healing. Zinc effects on the resistance of cultured cells towards oxidative stress in vitro were examined by Richard et al. (1993). An intracellular oxidative stress was performed with UVB or UVA radiation. Results showed that

Zn-treated fibroblasts were more resistant than cells grown in normal medium (Richard et al., 1993). Additionally, Zn can positively influence the effects of oxidative stress on cultured human retinal pigment epithelial (RPE) cells (Tate et al., 1999). Good sources of zinc include beef, lamb, pork, crabmeat, turkey, chicken, lobster, clams and salmon, milk, cheese, yeast, peanuts, beans, and wholegrain cereals, brown rice, whole wheat bread, potato and yogurt. Of all these vegetarian zinc foods, pumpkin seeds offer one of the most concentrated non-meat food sources of zinc.

Polyphenol Compounds

Interest in polyphenols has recently increased due to a broad spectrum of medical, pharmacological and therapeutic efficacies, including free radical scavenging, metal-chelating and antioxidant ability, anti-inflammatory, cardioprotective and anticarcinogenic properties (Rice-Evans, 2001). Phenolic compounds or polyphenols constitute one of the most numerous and widely distributed groups of substances in the plant kingdom, with more than 8,000 phenolic structures currently known. Polyphenols are products of the secondary metabolism of plants (Glauce Socorro de Barros Viana et al., 2010). Flavonoids represent the most common and widely distributed group of plant phenolics. Structural variations within the aromatic rings subdivide the flavonoids into several families: flavonols, flavones, flavanols, isoflavones, and antocyanidins, among others. These flavonoids often occur as glycosides, the glycosiylation rendering the molecule more water-soluble and less reactive toward free radicals.

Polyphenols are partly responsible for the sensory and nutritional qualities, as well as astringency and bitterness of plant food. Vegetables in the outer part of the plant contain primarily flavonoid glycosides, while berries have high anthocyanin content. Apples and citrus fruits are rich in phenolic acids and flavonoids. Nuts are rich in tannins, and oil seeds primarily contain phenolic acids. Catechins and proanthocyanidins accumulate principally in the lignified portion of grape clusters, especially in the seeds. Olive oil contains both phenolic acids and hydrolysable tannins (Kovac et al., 1992). Coffee beans are rich in chlorogenic acid, while cocoa beans contain epicatchin, tannins and anthocyanins. The poliphenols in wine include phenolic acids, anthocyanins, tannins, and other flavonoids.

Phenolic compounds act as antioxidants, with mechanisms involving both free radical scavenging and metal chelation (de Barros Viana et al., 2010). In vitro antioxidant potential of phenolic compounds was even more effective than vitamin E and C, on a molar basis (Rice-Evans et al., 1997). Besides antioxidant potential, flavonoids possess also anti-thrombotic, anti-cancer, anti-viral, anti-microbic and anti-inflammatory effects (Gerritsen et al., 1995; Muldoon and Kritchevsky, 1996). Additionally, cells respond to polyphenols through direct interactions with receptors or enzymes involved in signal transduction that may result in modification of the redox status of the cell and may trigger a series of redox-dependent reactions (Halliwell et al., 2005; Moskaug et al., 2005; Forman et al., 2002).

Bioflavonoids

Flavonoids are water-soluble polyphenolic molecules containing 15 carbon atoms. Flavonoids belong to the polyphenol family. Over 4,000 flavonoids have been identified, many of which occur in fruits, vegetables and beverages (tea, coffee, beer, wine and fruit drinks). The flavonoids consist of sixmajor subgroups: chalcone, flavone, flavonol, flavanone, anthocyanins and isoflavonoids. Flavonoids may be further divided into subclasses: anthocyanidins, flavan-3-ols, flavanones, flavonols, flavones, isoflavones.

Flavonoids are compounds found in fruits, vegetables, and certain beverages that have diverse beneficial biochemical and antioxidant effects.Together with carotenes, flavanoids are also responsible for the coloring of fruits, vegetables and herbs. Foods that contain high amounts of flavonoids include blueberries, red beans, cranberries, and blackberries. Many other foods, including red and yellow fruits and vegetables and some nuts, also contain flavonoids. Flavonoids are becoming very popular because they have many health-promoting effects. The contribution of flavonoids to the total antioxidant activity of components in food can be very high because daily intake can vary between 50 to 500 mg. Many bioflavonoids prevent the cellular damage caused by free radicals. The capacity of flavonoids to act as antioxidants depends upon their molecular structure. The position of hydroxyl groups and other features in the chemical structure of flavonoids are important for their antioxidant and free radical-scavenging activities. Flavonols such as quercetin glycosides and rutin are predominantly absorbed as aglycones, bound to plasma proteins and subsequently conjugated to glucuronide, sulfate, and methyl moieties. The $t((1/2))$ ranges from 12 to 19 hours. The bioavailability of catechins is low, and they are eliminated with a $t((1/2))$ of two to four hours. Catechins are degraded to several gamma-valerolactone derivatives, and phase II conjugates have also been identified (Schwedhelm et al., 2003).

Red Wine Flavonoids and Resveratrol

Red wine contains high levels of flavonoids, mainly quercetin and rutin. The high intake of red wine (and flavonoids) by the French might explain why they suffer less from coronary heart disease than other Europeans, although their consumption of cholesterol-rich foods is higher (French paradox).

It has long been known that moderate drinking is associated with a lower risk of heart disease, most likely because it increases "good cholesterol" (high-density lipoprotein) and reduces platelet clumping and associated clot formations. A Dutch study found that men who consumed approximately 20 grams of alcohol a day (wine, beer and other types of spirits) added 2.5 years to their life expectancies at the age of 50 compared to men who did not drink at all (Giltay et al., 2007). And more significantly, they found that men who only consumed wine added five years to their life expectancies. Lead researcher Marinette Streppel of the University of Wageningen in the Netherlands and colleagues, in the *Journal of Epidemiology and Community Health* where the study was published, suggest that the cardio-protective effect of wine could be due to a protective effect of polyphenol compounds in red wine, although other explanations cannot be ruled out (Streppel et al., 2009). Resveratrol, a molecule found in various plants including grapes, red wine, berries and peanuts, is reported to slow aging in simple eukaryotes and has been suggested as a potential caloric-restriction mimetic. Resveratrol has also been reported to act as a sirtuin activator, and this property has been proposed to account for its anti-aging effects. Novel compounds related to resveratrol or sirtinol are being tested that are able to modulate sirtuin activity (Pallas et al., 2008). Sirtuins regulate many fundamental biological processes in response to a variety of environmental and nutritional stimuli. The protein implicated in the protective process of CR and life-extension is the silent information regulator 2 (SIR2, SIRT1 in mammals), an enzyme that belongs to the nicotinamide adenine dinucleotide $(NAD)^+$ -dependent protein deacetylases. SIRs regulate gene silencing, DNA repair, rDNA recombination and aging, apart from regulating programmed cell death. In this context, increasing SIRT1 has been found to protect cells against amyloid-beta-induced ROS production, DNA damage, etc. Resveratrol that utilizes SIRT1 pathway modulators could thus be used in treating aging-related disorders. Besides resveratrol, red wine contains very complex mixture of polyphenols, alcohol and other chemicals, such as procyanidine, that could also have significant effects on longevity (Corder et al., 2006). Additionally, sirtuin activity is regulated by NAD biosynthetic pathways, and nicotinamide phosphoribosyltransferase (NAMPT) plays a critical role in the regulation of mammalian sirtuin activity. Recent studies have provided a proof of concept for the idea that nicotinamide mononucleotide (NMN), the NAMPT reaction product, can be used as a nutriceutical to activate SIRT1 activity (Imai, 2010).

Application of resveratrol to the skin of hairless mice effectively prevented the UVB-induced increase in skin thickness and the development of the skin edema (Afaq and Mukhtar, 2002). Immunohistochemical studies have revealed that this inhibitory effect is associated with a reduction of UVB-induced H2O2 formation.

Isoflavones from soy products (genistein, daidzein, glycitein), are another class of flavonoids that function as antioxidants and in addition possess phytoestrogenic properties that can be effective for menopausal symptoms and to promote bone density in post-menopausal women. Soy bioflavonoids have been implicated in collagen/elastin synthesis promoters, too.

Green Tea

Tea flavonoids have many health benefits. Tea flavonoids reduce the oxidation of low-density lipoprotein and lower the blood levels of cholesterol and triglycerides.

Because of a characteristic aroma and health benefits, green tea is consumed worldwide as a popular beverage. Green tea flavonoids are potent antioxidant compounds in vitro. The major flavonoids in green tea are kaempferol and catechins (catechin, epicatechin, epicatechin gallate (ECG), and epigallocatechin gallate (EGCG)).

The epicatechin derivatives present in green tea possess antioxidant, anti-inflammatory and anti-carcinogenic properties. The major and most highly chemopreventive constituent in green tea responsible for the biochemical or pharmacological effects is (-)-epigallocatechin-3-gallate (EGCG) (Katiyar, 2003).

The in vitro and in vivo animal and human studies suggest that green tea polyphenols are photoprotective in nature and can be used as pharmacological agents for the prevention of solar UVB light-induced skin disorders including photoaging, melanoma and nonmelanoma skin cancers after more clinical trials in humans. Green tea polyphenols were shownto reduce UV light-induced oxidative stress and immunosuppression(Katiyar et al., 2000). The polyphenolic compounds from green teawere tested against chemical carcinogenesis and photocarcinogenesisin murine skin. These green tea polyphenols were found to affordprotection against chemical carcinogenesis as well as photocarcinogenesisin mouse skin. According to the study of Katiyar (2003), topical treatment or oral consumption of green tea polyphenols (GTP) inhibit chemical carcinogen- or UV radiation-induced skin carcinogenesis in different laboratory animal models. Topical treatment of GTP and (-)-epigallocatechin-3-gallate (EGCG) or oral consumption of GTP resulted in prevention of UVB-induced inflammatory responses, immunosuppression and oxidative stress, which are the biomarkers of several skin-disease states (Katiyar et al., 1999). Topical application of GTP and EGCG prior to exposure of UVB protects against UVB-induced local as well as systemic immune suppression in laboratory animals, which was associated with the inhibition of UVB-induced infiltration of inflammatory leukocytes. Katiyar demonstrated that treatment of EGCG to human skin resulted in the inhibition of UVB-induced erythema, oxidative stress and infiltration of inflammatory leukocytes. His research team also showed that treatment of GTP to human skin prevents UVB-induced cyclobutane pyrimidine dimers formation, which is considered to be mediators of UVB-induced immune suppression and skin cancer induction. According to a recent study of Katiyar et al.,(2010), drinking GTPs prevents UV-induced immunosuppression, and inhibiting UV-induced immunosuppression may underlie the chemopreventive activity of GTPs against photocarcinogenesis (Katiyar et al., 2010). Additionally, oral administration of green tea or caffeine in amounts equivalent to three or five cups of coffee per day to UVB-exposed mice increased levels of p53, slowed cell cycling, and increased apoptotic sun burn cells in the epidermis (Lu., et al., 2008). This represents a new photoprotection strategy thatselectively targets DNA-damaged cells for apoptosis while leaving normal cells unaffected (Yarosh, 2010).

Green tea polyphenols have received attention as protective agents against UV-induced skin damage. Analysis of published studiesdemonstrates that green tea polyphenols have anti-inflammatoryand anticarcinogenic as well as anti-aging properties. These effects appear to correlatewith antioxidant properties of green tea polyphenols, which could be used as new photoprotection agents. But the general problem considering flavonoids are their metabolites, which may have lower antioxidant capacity than their parent compounds found in foods, and they are present in human plasma and tissues only at low concentrations. Nevertheless, flavonoids exert also non-antioxidant physiological effects (e.g., cell signaling pathways), and these effects potentially exert health benefits in humans.

Other Flavonoids and the Skin Studies

Silymarin, a naturally occurring polyphenolic flavonoid antioxidant, was shown to exhibit preventive and anticancer effects against skin cancer. For example, silymarin strongly prevents both photocarcinogenesis and skin tumor promotion in mice, in part, by scavenging free radicals and reactive oxygen species and strengthening the antioxidant system (Singh and Agarwal, 2002). Skin cancer chemopreventive effects of a silymarin were also reported in the study by Ahmad et al. (1998). Skin cancer chemopreventive effects werereported to be mediated via impairment of receptor tyrosine kinase signaling and perturbation in cell cycle progression.

Additionally, chemoprevention of skin cancer by the flavonoid fraction of *Saraca asoka* (Family—*Caesalpiniaceae*—widely used in the Ayurvedic (traditional Indian) system of medicine especially due to its wound healing property) was reported (Cibin et al., 2010).

The protective effect of three flavonoids quercetin, hesperetin and naringenin were also evaluated. Study by Bonina et al. (1996)revealed that topically applied flavonoids could be excellent candidates for successful employment as protective agents in certain skin diseases caused, initiated or exacerbated by sunlight irradiation.In the study of Chondrogianni et al.(2010), authors have identified quercetin (QUER) and its derivative, namely quercetin caprylate (QU-CAP), as a proteasome activator with antioxidant properties that consequently influence cellular lifespan, survival and viability of HFL-1 primary human fibroblasts. The potential protective effects of the flavanol catechin, the flavonol quercetin, the flavones, luteolin and rutin, and the isoflavones, genistein and daidzein, against the photooxidative stress induced by ultraviolet A radiation (UVA) and by phototoxic reactions resulting from the interaction of UVA with drugs and chemicals, has been assessed with cultured human skin fibroblasts (Filipe et al., 2005). Genistein has been shown to possess antioxidant and anticarcinogenic effect on skin (Wei et al., 1995). Contrasting effects of flavonoids were also observed. The flavanol, the flavonol and the flavones may protect against lipid peroxidation and cell death-induced UVA. On the other hand, an amplification of the photodamage may be observed with isoflavones. A concentration-dependence study demonstrated that among the protective flavonoids, quercetin is the most efficient. It was reported that epicatechin and its methylated metabolite attenuate UVA-induced oxidative damage to human skin fibroblasts. The study by Basu-Modak et al. (2003) provided clear evidence that this dietary flavanol has the potential to protect human skin against the deleterious effects of sunlight.

Cocoa

Cocoa, the major ingredient of dark chocolate, is an excellent source of catechins, which are polyphenols of the flavanol group, and which are believed to protect against conditions with increased oxidative stress. Cocoa contains relatively high amounts of epicatechin and has been found to have nearly twice the antioxidant content of red wine and up to three times that of green tea in vitro (Lee et al., 2003).In a study published in a 2006 issue of the *Journal of Nutrition,* researchers found that cocoa containing high levels of two dietary flavonols (epicatchin and catechin) protected skin from sun damage, improved circulation to skin cells, affected hydration, and made the skin look and feel smoother. In a crossover design study, ten healthy women ingested a cocoa drink (100 ml) with high (329 mg) or low (27 mg) content of flavanols. The major flavanol monomer in both drinks was epicatechin, 61 mg in the high-flavanol, and 6.6 mg in the low-flavanol product per 100 ml. Subsequent to the intake of high-flavanol cocoa, dermal blood flow was significantly increased by 1.7-fold at t = 2 h and oxygen saturation was elevated 1.8-fold. No statistically significant changes were found upon intake of low-flavanol cocoa. Maximum plasma levels of total epicatechin were observed one h after ingestion of the high-flavanol cocoa drink, 11.6 ± 7.4 nmol/l at baseline, and 62.9 ± 35.8 nmol/l at 1 h. No change of total epicatechin was found in the low-flavanol group (Neukam et al., 2007).

In the study of Heinrich et al. (2006), two groups of women consumed either a high-flavanol (326 mg/d) or low-flavanol (27 mg/d) cocoa powder dissolved in 100 mL water for

12 wk. Epicatechin (61 mg/d) and catechin (20 mg/d) were the major flavanol monomers in the high-flavanol drink, whereas the low-flavanol drink contained 6.6 mg epicatechin and 1.6 mg catechin as the daily dose. Photoprotection and indicators of skin condition were assayed before and during the intervention. Following exposure of selected skin areas to 1.25 x minimal erythemal dose (MED) of radiation from a solar simulator, UV-induced erythema was significantly decreased in the high-flavanol group, by 15 and 25%, after sixand 12 wk of treatment, respectively, whereas no change occurred in the low-flavanol group. Evaluation of the skin surface showed a significant decrease of skin roughness and scaling in the high-flavanol cocoa group compared with those at wk 12. Dietary flavanols from cocoa contribute to endogenous photoprotection, improve dermal blood circulation, and affect cosmetically relevant skin surface and hydration variables.

Additionally, Lee et al. (2006) reported that Cocoa polyphenols inhibit phorbol ester-induced superoxide anion formation in cultured HL-60 cells and expression of cyclooxygenase-2 and activation of NF-kappaB and MAPKs in mouse skin in vivo.

Heinrich et al. (2006) demonstrated that long-term ingestion of high-flavanol cocoa provides photoprotection against UV-induced erythema and improves skin condition in women. Daily ingestion of cocoa polyphenols improved also skin-barrier function.

French Maritime Pine Bark Extract - Pycnogenol

Pycnogenol is a standardized extract of the bark of the French maritime pine, Pinus pinaster Ait., that has multiple biological effects, including antioxidant, anti-inflammatory and anticarcinogenic properties. "Loaded with bioflavonoids and other biologically active phytonutrients, or plant nutrients, Pycnogenol is backed by clinical research and a long history of use.

"Between 65% and 75% of Pycnogenol are procyanidins comprising of catechin and epicatechin subunits with varying chain lengths. Other constituents are polyphenolic monomers, phenolic or cinnamic acids and their glycosides. Owing to the basic chemical structure of its components, the most obvious feature of pycnogenol is its strong antioxidant activity.

"In fact, phenolic acids, polyphenols, and in particular flavonoids, are composed of one (or more) aromatic rings bearing one or more hydroxyl groups and are, therefore, potentially able to quench free radicals by forming resonance-stabilized phenoxyl radicals" (D'Andrea, 2010).

The procyanidin-rich French maritime pine bark extract Pycnogenol (PBE) has been investigated for its effect in protecting human skin against solar UV-simulated light-induced erythema. Data from the study conducted by Saliou et al. (2001) indicate that oral supplementation of PBE reduces erythema in the skin. Inhibition of NF-kappaB-dependent gene expression by PBE possibly contributes to the observed increase in MED.

Tixier research group (1984) shows evidence by in vivo and in vitro studies that binding of pycnogenols to elastin affects its rate of degradation by elastases as occurs in inflammatory processes (Tixier et al., 1984).

The study of Sime and Reeve (2004) indicates that topical Pycnogenol offered significant and dose-dependent protection from solar-simulated UV radiation-induced acute inflammation, immunosuppression and carcinogenesis, when applied to the skin after daily irradiation. Additionally, Pycnogenol appears to have potential in providing photoprotection for humans in a complementary role with sunscreens, having demonstrable activity when applied to the skin after, rather than before, UV exposure (Simeand Reeve, 2004).

Cho et al. (2007) reported that oral administration of the antioxidant mixture of vitamin C, vitamin E, pycnogenol and evening primrose oil significantly inhibited wrinkle formation caused by chronic UVB irradiation through significant inhibition of UVB-induced MMP activity accompanied by enhancement of collagen synthesis on hairless mouse skin.

Red Ginseng

The study of Cho et al. (2009) reports that a red ginseng extract-containing Torilus fructus and Corni fructus mixture improves facial wrinkles, a clinical sign of photoaging, and this improvement is associated with biochemical and histological evidence of increased collagen synthesis in the dermis.Red ginseng contains many bioactive constituents, including various ginsenosides that are believed to have antioxidant, immunostimulatory, and anti-aging activities. Controlled human study has explored its effects on photoaged skin (Cho et al., 2009). This study determined whether long-term intake of a red ginseng extract-containing Torilus fructus and Corni fructus mixture reduces facial wrinkles and increases collagen synthesis in human skin. Facial wrinkles, elasticity, epidermal water content, erythema, and pigmentation were measured objectively. Facial wrinkles were significantly improved, type I procollagen gene and protein expression was increased, MMP-9 gene induction was prevented, and fibrillin-1 fiber length was elongated only in the treatment group. No changes were seen in the facial elasticity, epidermal water content, facial erythema and pigmentation, and epidermal thickness in either group.

Conclusion

A wide variety of polyphenols or other phytochemicals have been reported to possess substantial skin photoprotective effects, such as green tea polyphenols, grape seed proanthocyanidins, resveratrol, silymarin, genistein, and others on UV-induced skin inflammation, oxidative stress and DNA damage, etc. On the other hand, large intakes of beta-carotene must be viewed with caution because they have been shown to confer detriment to a population at high risk of lung cancer when administered after many years of high-risk (smoking) behavior. Until further work clarifies the situation in heavy smokers with respect to taking supplements, larger doses should be avoided by such individuals. There is little reliable information about the human toxicology of flavonoids and related non-nutrient antioxidant constituents of the diet (See also paragraph "Should we take supplements?"). Consumer demand for healthy food products provides an opportunity to develop antioxidant-rich food as new functional foods, as well as food-grade and pharmaceutical-grade and bioactive antioxidants as new nutraceutical products. Many of the discussed compounds showed photoprotective effect. When considering the fact that inadvertent sun exposure (when no topical protection is used) represents two-thirds of the total erythemal dose accumulated per year (Godar et al., 2001), it is important to consider also dietary intake of different natural antioxidants from vegetables and fruit as the preventive approach.

Fatty Acids

Although fatty acids are not declared as antioxidants, their impact on the skin (their anti-inflammatory effect, lipid oxidation effect, UV-induced damage prevention effect, etc.) is discussed in this paragraph.

Fats are indispensable to life not only as an energy source but also for their structural role in the skin, retina, nervous system, lipoproteins, and biological membranes. They are also precursors of important hormones and constitute the vehicle for the absorption of liposoluble vitamins. Nutritionists recommend a balanced lipid intake corresponding to a total amount of fats equal to 25% to 30% of total calories with a ratio in monounsaturated and polyunsaturated fatty acids (Viola and Viola, 2009).

Lipid compounds include monoglycerides, diglycerides, triglycerides, phosphatides, cerebrosides, sterols, terpenes, fatty alcohols, and fatty acids. Fatty acids are carboxylic acids with a long hydrocarbon chain, usually straight, as the fourth substituent group on the carboxyl (–COOH) group that makes the molecule an acid. Saturated fatty acids are those in which every carbon atom carries its full "quota" of hydrogen atoms, and, therefore, there are only single bonds between adjacent carbon atoms. Unsaturated fatty acids have one or more carbon-carbon double bonds in the molecule. Chemically, these double bonds can take up hydrogen, which is the process of hydrogenation, forming saturated fatty acids. Fatty acids with two or more double bonds are polyunsaturated fatty acids, often abbreviated to pufa. In general, fats from animal sources are high in saturated and relatively low in unsaturated fatty acids; vegetable and fish oils are generally higher in unsaturated and lower in saturated fatty acids. Essential fatty acids are fatty acids that humans and other animals must ingest for good health because the body requires them but cannot make them from other food components. There are only two EFAs: alpha-linolenic acid, an omega-3 fatty acid, and linoleic acid, an omega-6 fatty acid (Whitney Ellie and Rolfes, 2008; Burr et al.,1930).

Aging causes a progressive decline in our ability to internally synthesize the essential fatty acids (EFAs) required by the skin to maintain a youthful, moist appearance. The most important oils to supplement are the omega-3s that can make the skin smoother, softer, and more radiant-looking. Common food sources of n-3 polyunsaturatedfatty acids (PUFAs) are cold liver oil, fish oil,and marine animals with a high amount of fat, such as mackerel,salmon, and menhaden. When skin is properly nourished, it shows less of the effects of aging. The oral ingestion of fish, flax, or perilla oil provides abundant quantities of the omega-3 fatty acids that are beneficial to the health and appearance of the skin. Low-fat diets have been studied as an approach to prevent skin cancer. Animal studies have revealed that high-fat diets shorten the time between UV exposure and tumor formation and increase the number of tumors per animal (Brash et al., 2010). Following initial studies indicating that fish oils could reduce UV-induced erythema in hairless mice (Orengo et al., 1989), further studies have shown that high doses of dietary n-3 polyunsaturated fatty acids can reduce the sunburn in humans. In a study by Orengo et al (1992), ten subjects enriched theirdiets daily with fish oil containing 2.8 g EPA and 1.2 g docosahexaenoicacid (DHA; 22:6n-3) and tenother subjects received a placebo. After four wk, a small but statistically significant increase in the MED was seen in the fish-oil group, which corresponded to a sun-protection factor slightly >1. Fish-oil supplementation did not change prostaglandin E_2 (PGE_2) concentrations significantly. This study showed that at a relatively low dose (2.8 g EPA and 1.2 g DHA) of fish oil and within a short period of time, consumption of n-3 PUFAs was photoprotective.

Many different studies were performed in order to investigate the effect of fatty acids on health. In the study of Rhodes et al. (1994) (cit. Boelsma et al., 2001), authors have examined the effect of dietary fish oil rich in omega-3 fatty acids upon susceptibility to UVB-induced erythema and epidermal lipid peroxidation. Fifteen volunteers took 10 g fish oil, containing 18% eicosapentaenoic acid and 12% docosahexaenoic acid, daily for three or six months. Dietary supplementation resulted in an increase in the MED after six months; ten weeks after fish-oil supplementation ended, the MED decreased again. However, parallel to an increase in total n-3 fatty acids in the epidermis, lipid peroxidation products increased in irradiated skin. Although fish-oil consumption reduced UV irradiation–induced erythema, the susceptibility of the skin to lipid peroxidation increased because of the unstable nature of n-3 fatty acids. Thus, omega-3 fatty acids may act as an oxidizable buffer, protecting more vital structures from free radical damage. The photoprotective effect of fish oil has also been examined in light-sensitive patients with polymorphic light eruption (PLE). Thirteen patients with polymorphic light eruption received dietary supplements of fish oil rich in omega-3 polyunsaturated fatty acids for three months. After fish oil supplementation, patients showed reduction in both basal and UVB-dependent prostaglandin E2 levels and some improvement in the clinical threshold for PLE provocation (Rhodes et al., 1995). In the study by Rhodes et al. (1995), dietary supplementation of 16 individuals with a similar amount of fish oil (10 g/d) resulted in an increase in the MED after only three months. Because prostaglandins mediate the vasodilatation, authors examined the effect of fish oil on ultraviolet (UV) B-induced prostaglandin metabolism. PGE_2 concentrations in skin fluid decreased after fish-oil consumption both in non-irradiated and irradiated skin. The authors suggested that the reduced responsiveness to UV irradiation-induced erythema after long-term supplementation with fish oil may have been due, at least in part, to the inhibition of PGE_2 concentrations in the skin. The photoprotection against UVA-provocation of a papular response suggests a clinical application for fish oil in polymorphic light eruption. In following study by Rhodes et al. (Rhodes et al., cit. Boelsma et al., 2001), the protective role of dietary EPA supplementation against the acute effects of a single dose of UVB irradiation was investigated. Twenty-eight subjects received 4 g 98% EPA or 98% oleic acid daily for three mo. In the EPA-supplemented group, UVB irradiation-induced erythema and p53 induction decreased, whereas no significant changes were found in the oleic acid group. These changes in sunburn sensitivity and p53 expression indicate the ability for high levels of dietary EPA to protect against UV-induced genotoxicity.

Boelsma et al. (2001) reported that the important health effect of oral n-3 PUFA intakes from fish oil may be ascribed to their anti-inflammatory effects. One potential mechanism was proposed by Lands (1992) regarding n-3 polyunsaturates competition with n-6 polyunsaturates for metabolism by cyclooxygenase and lipooxygenase, resulting in the production of less inflammatory prostaglandins and leukotriens. Moreover, n-3 PUFAs are unstable and may preferably be damaged by free radicals, thereby protecting other structures from attack by free radicals. Nevertheless, to protect against excessive formation of free radicals and lipid peroxidation, appropriate amounts of antioxidants (e.g., vitamin E, CoQ as well as water soluble antioxidants to regenerate them) should also be consumed (Boelsma et al., 2001). The precise mode of action by which n-3 polyunsaturates can reduce UV-induced erythema is still unclear (Jenkins et al., 2009). Besides, the omega-3 fatty acids EPA and DHA in available nutritional supplements appear to stabilize mitochondrial membranes (Demaison et al., 1994; Oudart H, et al., 1997; Pehowich, 1999)and thus influence intrinsic skin aging.

Recently, Kim et al. (2010) observed that the amounts of free fatty acids (FFA) and triglycerides (TG) in the epidermis of photoaged or acutely UV-irradiated human skin were significantly decreased. The expressions of genes related to lipid synthesis, including acetyl-CoA carboxylase (ACC), fatty acid synthase (FAS), stearoyl-CoA desaturase (SCD), sterol regulatory element binding proteins (SREBPs), and peroxisome proliferator-activated receptors (PPARgamma) were also markedly decreased.

The population-based case-control study (Green et al., 1993) contrasted nutrient intakes of 41 women with cutaneous malignant melanoma to those of 297 women sampled from the same community (Brisbane, Australia). Diet was assessed by a comprehensive foodfrequency questionnaire. According to Green et al. (1993), the strong inverse relation observed between high intakes of polyunsaturated fatty acids and melanoma ($P < 0.01$) adds sufficient weight to prior findings for this persisting causal hypothesis to be abandoned.

Cosgrove et al. (2007) reported that higher intakes of vitamin C and linoleic acid and lower intakes of fats and carbohydrates are associated with better skin-aging appearance. Higher linoleic acid intakes were associated with a lower likelihood of senile dryness and skin atrophy. A 17-g increase in fat and a 50-g increase in carbohydrate intakes increased the likelihood of a wrinkled appearance and skin atrophy among middle-aged American women.

Fatty acids play very important role on mitochondrial membrane and thus on free radical release. Available comparative evidence supporting the mitochondrial free radical theory of aging consistently indicates that two basic molecular traits are associated with the rate of aging and thus with the maximum lifespan: the presence of low rates of mitochondrial oxygen radical production and low degrees of fatty acid unsaturation of cellular membranes in post-mitotic tissues of long-lived homeothermic vertebrates in relation to those of short-lived ones (Pamplonaet al., 2002). Lipids play varied and critical roles in metabolism, with function dramatically modulated by the individual fatty acid moities in complex lipid entities. In particular, the fatty acid composition of membrane lipids greatly influences membrane function (Hulbert et al., 2005).Saturated and monounsaturated fatty acids are very resistant to peroxidative damage, while the more polyunsaturated a fatty acid, the more susceptible it is to peroxidation. Furthermore, the products of lipid peroxidation can oxidatively damage other important molecules. Membrane fatty acid composition is correlated with the maximum lifespans of mammals and birds. Exceptionally long-living mammal species and birds have a more peroxidation-resistant membrane composition compared to shorter-living similar-sized mammals (Hulbert 2008).

The recent discovery that the fatty acid composition of tissue phospholipids varies in a systematic manner among species has led to the proposal that membrane fatty acid composition is an important determinant of the metabolic rate characteristic for each species. Additionally, it was noted that in the rat membrane fatty acid composition is a regulated parameter being more influenced by the balance between n-3 and n-6 polyunsaturates in the diet than it is by general diet content of saturated, monounsaturated and total polyunsaturated fats (Hulbert 2007).

The ω-3 and ω-6 polyunsaturated fatty acids (PUFAs) are separate essential dietary fatty acids that play a key role in many physiologic processes in higher animals. The content of these PUFAs is relatively well described for many individual food components. But the relative proportions of ω-3 and ω-6 PUFAs vary greatly across meals (Turner et al., 2010).

The importance of membrane fatty acid unsaturation can be demonstrated on honey bees. In the honey bee (Apis mellifera), depending on what they are fed, female eggs become either workers or queens. Although queens and workers share a common genome, the maximum lifespan of queens is an order-of-magnitude longer than workers. The mechanistic basis of this longevity difference is unknown. The explanation was provided by Haddadet al. (2007). "The cell membranes of both young and old honey bee queens are highly monounsaturated with very low content of polyunsaturates. Newly emerged workers have a similar membrane fatty acid composition to queens but within the first week of hive life, they increase the polyunsaturate content and decrease the monounsaturate content of their membranes, probably as a result of pollen consumption. This means their membranes likely become more susceptible to lipid peroxidation in this first week of hive life. The results support the suggestion that membrane composition might be an important factor in the determination of maximum lifespan."

Mechanisms that prevent or decrease the generation of endogenous damage during the evolution of long-lived animals seem to be more important than trying to intercept those damaging agents or repairing the damage already inflicted (Pamplonaet al., 2002). Prevention of free radical formation is thus more efficient than its neutralization once free radicals have been formed.

Creatine

Also, creatine does not offer direct antioxidant protection but rather its protective skin effect is from increasing cell energy reserves. Cellular energy level, however, might have an impact on endogenous antioxidant defense and cellular damage repair systems. As already explained in previous chapters, cutaneous aging is characterized by a decline in cellular energy metabolism, which is mainly caused by detrimental changes in mitochondrial function. Skin cells try to compensate any loss of mitochondrial energetic capacity by extra-mitochondrial pathways such as glycolysis or the creatine kinase (CK) system. Stress-induced decline in mitochondrial energy supply in human epidermal cells correlated with a decrease in mitochondrial CK activity (Lenz et al., 2005). Creatine acts like an energy store thatis able to provide additional energy in situations of fast energy demand. After cellular uptake, creatine (Cr) is phosphorylated to phosphocreatine (PCr) by the creatine kinase (CK) reaction using ATP. Creatine is metabolized to creatinine, which is cleared via renal excretion, and daily turnover of creatine to creatinine for a 70-kg male has been estimated to be round 2 g (Blatt et al., 2010). Creatine is synthesized in human cells, but from the age of 30, a reduction of the cellular concentration in the skin was observed in the study of Ponticos et al. (1998). Previous evidence suggested that AMPK activates fatty acid oxidation, which provides a source of ATP, following continued muscle contraction. The novel regulation of AMPK described in the study of Ponticos et al. (1998) provides a mechanism by which energy supply can meet energy demand following the utilization of the immediate energy reserve provided by the creatine kinase-phosphocreatine system. While glycolysis pathway could stimulate the oxidative stress situation, creatine kinase system could even reduce the electron "jam" in the respiratory chain by providing a sink for free ATP-coupled energy by building-up phosphocreatine (PCr) stores for phosphorylation (Blatt et al., 2010).

Lenz et al. (2005) reported that human skin cells that are energetically recharged with the naturally occurring energy precursor, creatine, are markedly protected against a variety of cellular stress conditions, like oxidative and UV damage in vitro and in vivo. Additionally, Berneburg et al. (2005) reported that supplementation of normal human fibroblasts with creatine during repeated UVA exposure showed a mitigation of mtDNA mutations as well as the normalization in oxygen consumption and MMp-1 production. (Berneburg et al., 2005).

Maes et al. (2004) treated cells with creatine, which is known to restore the pool of phosphocreatine in the mitochondria. Creatine treatment significantly increased cell survival after UV exposure, stimulated the repair of UVB-induced DNA damage in keratinocytes and caused a significant reduction in the number of sunburn cells in a UVB-exposed reconstituted skin model. Maes and his research group (2004) claims that treatment with creatine seems to provide the necessary boost to the cellular metabolism, which leads to an induction of a significant amount of protection and repair to human skin cells. Once inside the cell, creatine can be stored at high milimolar concentrations (e.g., 40 mM for muscle cell).

All of the results indicate that restoration of the energy pool in mitochondria increased cellular self-defense mechanism (induction of protective and repair mechanisms). Data show the important role played by the mitochondrial energy metabolism on the (skin) aging process and indicate a possible therapy with creatine that can be used to counteract this negative effect.

According to the estimate of the World Health Organization, nearly 80% of the population of the developing countries (over two billion people) rely on traditional medicines, mostly plant derived drugs or phytopharmaceuticals for their primary health care needs. The proliferation of products can cause confusion among consumers, who often ask their dermatologists for advice as to which anti-aging products they should choose. Ideally, the anti-aging claims of cosmeceutical formulations and their components should be demonstrated in controlled clinical trials (Bruce, 2008), but there is a lack of such studies due to their high costs. Besides, FDA does not demand such studies to be performed prior of the foodsupplements being launched in the marked. Since cosmeceutical products are claiming to therapeutically affect the structure and function of the skin, it is rational and necessary to hold them to specified scientific standards that substantiate efficacy claims (Levin and Momin, 2010). Ideally, a cosmeceutical should be clinically tested for efficacy to ensure a proven skin benefit and also to substantiate marketing claims. Governmental limitations of efficacy claims restrict cosmeceutical development because products can only be assessed in terms of their ability to improve skin appearance but not function. Improving function would remove the cosmeceutical from the cosmetic category and place it in the drug category (Draelos, 2009). In order to provide appropriate recommendations to their patients/users, medical doctors, pharmacists and nutritionists must become familiar with the available data on currently marketed products and gain experience with anti-aging regimens. Some studies (usually performed on skin cells in vitro or on animal models) suggest that oral uptake of selected micronutrients and phytochemicals can provide photoprotection of human skin. Nevertheless, photoprotection can only be achieved if an optimal pharmacological dose range is reached in the human skin due to well-known pro-oxidative reactions of antioxidants, e.g., in the case of excessive carotenoid concentrations. However, very few over-the-counter cosmetic "anti-aging" products have been subjected to a rigorous double-blind, vehicle-controlled trial of efficacy, where the therapeutic dose would be established. Nevertheless, research is continuously demonstrating that various phytopharmaceuticals offer significant protection against different diseases and skin aging. Compelling evidence has led to the conclusion that diet is a key environmental factor and a strong tool for the control of skin-aging process. Genetic methods and anti-aging drugs offer much hope for the longer-term aging delay. But what can be done now? In the previous chapters, it was demonstrated that skin aging is mainly caused by oxidative stress, which is induced by exogenous or endogenous sources. Evidence is accumulating that dietary changes and special nutrients may help to reduce oxidative stress, free radical formation and thereby slow down the aging process. Foods rich in antioxidants and other phytochemicals, such as fruits, vegetables, wine and green tea, help protect against oxidative damage and free radical attack of all body cells including the skin. The primary treatment of photoaging is photoprotection, but secondary treatment could be achieved with the use of antioxidants and some novel compounds such as polyphenols. Exogenous antioxidants like vitamin C, E, and many others cannot be synthesized by the human body and must be taken up by the diet. They have been shown to prevent exogenous free radical formation (e.g., UVA and UVB). They could also possess beneficial effects in endogenous ROS prevention. Antioxidants can regulate the transfer of electrons or quench free radicals escaping from electron transport chain. Since the effectiveness of endogenous antioxidant system is diminished during aging, the exogenous supplementation of antioxidants might be a protective strategy against age-associated skin oxidative damage. Several associations between diet, nutrients in serum and skin conditions were observed (e.g., serum vitamin A, skin sebum content and surface pH and between the dietary intake of total fat, saturated fat, monounsaturated fat, and skin hydration), indicating that different nutrients are absorbed and transported into skin cells, and changes in baseline nutritional status may affect skin condition (Boelsma et al., 2003). Many in vitro studies showed promising effects of nutritionalfactors on the skin. The laboratory studies conducted in animal models suggest that many plant compounds have the ability to protect the skin from the adverse effects of UV radiation, including the risk of skin cancers. It is suggested that antioxidants may favorably supplement sunscreen protection and may be useful for skin diseases associated with solar UV radiation-induced inflammation, oxidative stress and DNA damage. At this point, it should be stressed that extrapolation of in vitrodata to the in vivo situation is often difficult. Moreover,in vivo studies of the effects of nutrients on human skin havemainly focused on indirect measures of skin function after supplementation. Many more placebo-controlled human studies are required to support food and supplement product claims regarding skin-beneficial effects. It seems that skin's antioxidative defense is also influenced by nutritive factors. Besides vitamin A, C and E, η-3 fatty acids certain non-vitamin plant-derived ingredients might have beneficial effect on skin aging, skin sun protection or skin cancer. Among them, polyphenols and isoflavones have great potential. Besides the compounds mentioned in our review, many recent studiesshowed potentially interesting effects of some naturally occurring,less well-investigated compounds that may improve skin conditions. This area of research is constantly emerging, and new antioxidants are reported. Nevertheless, endogenous skin protection with the use of selected antioxidants or plant extracts contributes to the protection of sensitive dermal target sites beyond those reached with sunscreens and especially because of lifelong exposure to sunlight, which mainly occurs under everyday circumstances, when no topical protection is applied. According to Stahl et al. (2006), endogenous photoprotection is complementary to topical photoprotection, and these two forms of prevention clearly should be considered mutually exclusive.

To effectively combat age- and sun-related skin changes, a multifaceted approach is required. Any treatment for mature skin must address the many causes of skin changes, that is, collagen production, lipid balance and epidermal texture. Several currently available compounds have scientificallyestablished beneficial effects on skin and are anticipated to be even more effective in combination with other compounds, which might result in a synergistic effect between them.

Endogenous Skin Antioxidants

As already discussed, skin has a network of protective antioxidants. They include endogenous enzymatic antioxidants such as glutathione peroxidase, superoxide dismutase and catalase, and nonenzymatic low-molecular-weight antioxidants such as vitamin E isoforms, vitamin C, glutathione (GSH), uric acid, and ubiquinol (Shindo et al., 1993). All the major antioxidant enzymes are present in skin, but their roles in protecting cells against oxidative damage generated by UV radiation have not been elucidated. In response to the attack of reactive oxygen species, the skin has developed a complex antioxidant defense system including, among others, the manganese-superoxide dismutase (MnSOD). Manganese superoxide dismutase (MnSOD) is the mitochondrial enzyme that disposes of superoxide generated by respiratory chain activity. Of all electrons passing down the mitochondrial respiratory chain, it is estimated that 1% to 2% are diverted to form superoxide (although recent studies claim that this amount is even less); thus production of hydrogen peroxide occurs at a constant rate due to MnSOD activity. MnSOD dismutates the superoxide anion ($O_2^{\cdot-}$) derived from the reduction of molecular oxygen to hydrogen peroxide (H_2O_2), which is detoxified by glutathione peroxidase to water and molecular oxygen. The study of Poswig et al. (1999) revealed that adaptive antioxidant response of manganese-superoxide dismutase following repetitive UVA irradiation can be induced. The authors provide evidence for the increasing induction of MnSOD upon repetitive UVA irradiation that may contribute to the effective adaptive UVA response of the skin during light hardening in phototherapy. The study of Fuchs et al. (1989) on mouse skin showed that acute UV exposures lead also to changes in glutathione reductase and catalase activity in mouse skin but insignificant changes in superoxide dismutase and glutathione peroxidase (Fuchset al., 1989). The study of Sander et al. (2002) confirmed that chronic and acute photodamage is mediated by depleted antioxidant enzyme expression and increased oxidative protein modifications. Biopsies from patients with histologically confirmed solar elastosis, from non-ultraviolet-exposed sites of age-matched controls, and from young subjects were analyzed. The antioxidant enzymes catalase, copper-zinc superoxide dismutase, and manganese superoxide dismutase and protein carbonyls were investigated. Whereas overall expression of antioxidant enzymes was very high in the epidermis, low baseline levels were found in the dermis. In photoaged skin, a significant depletion of antioxidant enzyme expression was observed within the stratum corneum and in the epidermis. Importantly, an accumulation of oxidatively modified proteins was found specifically within the upper dermis of photoaged skin. Upon acute ultraviolet exposure of healthy subjects, depleted catalase expression and increased protein oxidation were detected. Exposures of keratinocytes and fibroblasts to ultraviolet B, ultraviolet A, and H2O2 led to dose-dependent protein oxidation and thus confirmed in vivo results.

Not all skin cells are exposed to the same level of oxidative stress. It was found that keratinocytes respire as much oxygen as fibroblasts, even though maximal activities of the respiratory chain complexes are two- to fivefold lower, whereas expression of respiratory chain proteins are similar. Superoxide anion levels are much higher in keratinocytes, and keratinocytes display much higher lipid peroxidation level and a lower reduced glutathione/oxidized glutathione ratio (Blatt et al., 2010).

It can be concluded that oxidative stress is a problem of skin cells, and endogenous as well as exogenous antioxidants could play an important role in decreasing it.

Part III. The Act: Measures to Decrease Oxidative Stress

Chapter 7.2.

Antioxidant Prevention of Damage Induced by Extrinsic Factors (Environmental Pollutants)

Skin is a highly metabolic tissuethatpossesses the largest surface area in the body and serves as the protective layer for internal organs. Skin is also a major candidate and target of oxidative stress. Most environmental pollutants are also strong oxidants and thus have impact on skin's oxidative stress.

Environmental pollutants enter human body through ingestion, inhalation or dermal absorption. Most environmental oxidants originate from the air due to the incomplete burning of petroleum fuel in cars or from fossil fuel from electrical (thermal) power-plants. Another big environmental oxidant is ozone and tobacco smoke—due to the incomplete burning of tobacco leaf (Ames and Gold, 1998).

Reducing one's exposure to environmental pollutants would be the best approach, but since this is not always possible, the use of antioxidants as "neutralizers" of certain environmental oxidants could reduce the damage of environmental exposure to oxidants. Some of the pollutants with strong oxidizing abilities are later on discussed as well as potential ability of antioxidants to reduce their damaging effects.

Part of this chapter was adopted from *Encyclopedia of Environmental Health*, 2011, Poljsak et al. (2011). (Impact of environmental pollutants on oxidation-reductionprocesses in the cell environment. In Dr Jerome Nriagu (ed).*Encyclopedia of Environmental Health. Elsevier*).

Ozone

The toxic action of O_3 is attributed in part to free radical formation. Mild O_3 exposure contributes to the effect of hormesis by its adaptation by increasing endogenous antioxidant protection (increasing the levels of SOD, catalase and GPx). Constituents of the respiratory tract fluids, which contain O_3 scavengers ascorbate, GSH and urate, absorb and neutralize O_3.

Also α-tocopherol could contribute to protection against O_3 in a way of preventing lipid peroxidation induced by O_3 reactions with polyunsaturated fatty acids (PUFAs).

Antioxidant protection of tocopheryl acetate, ascorbic acid and carotenoids has been reported in model animals exposed to O_3. Increased intake of vitamin E, vitamin C and beta-carotene can reduce the magnitude of lung function decrements in subjects exposed to high O_3 doses both occupationally and recreationally.

Nitrogen Oxides

Tocopherols, ascorbic acid, glutathione and uric acid can scavenge $NO_2^{\cdot}$. Several studies reported the protective effect of ascorbate, tocopherol, melatonin, epigallocatechin gallate and catechin administration as a protective effect prior to $NO_2^{\cdot}$ exposure.

Cigarette Smoke

The antioxidants in the respiratory tract lining fluids do offer some protection against cigarette smoke toxicity. Additionally, observational studies have shown an inverse association between fruit and vegetable intake and lung cancer. Blood plasma exposed to cigarette smoke-borne free radicals is depleted in a number of antioxidants, including ascorbate, α-tocopherol, β–carotene and several other carotenoids. Ascorbate and urate quench $NO_2^{\cdot}$ and RO_2.

Decreases in vitamin C and α-tocopherol, and increased lipid peroxidation could contribute to accelerated atherosclerosis in smokers. Due to faster antioxidant depletion among smokers, the recommended daily intake of ascorbate for smokers is set at a higher level.

On the other hand, some studies point out that high dietary level of vitamin C, α-tocopherol and especially β–carotene might accelerate the development of preneolastic lesions or stimulate cancer among smokers. The results of the randomized primary prevention trials have not supported the view that prolonged high doses of antioxidant supplementation would decrease the risk of lung cancer. Thus, the best defense against cigarette smoking is not doing it.

Particulate Matter (PM)

The mechanism by which particles cause oxidative damage remain unresolved although the bioavailability of metal complexes associated with PM surfaces may be important. Studies have suggested that the formation of superoxide and hydroxyl radicals by bioavailable metals could be responsible for oxidative damage induced by PM *in vitro* and *in vivo*.

Air-borne particle exposure influences also extrinsic skin aging. In the recent study of Vierkötter et al. (2010), the impact of air pollution on skin aging was analyzed. The impact of air pollution on skin aging was significantly correlated to extrinsic skin-aging signs, in particular to pigment spots and less pronounced to wrinkles. An increase in soot and particles from traffic was associated with 20% more pigment spots on forehead and cheeks. These results indicate that particle pollution might influence skin aging as well.

Copper

Both a deficiency in dietary copper and copperoverload might stimulate oxidative stress in cells. A number of nutrients have been shown to interact with Cu and alter its cellular effects. Vitamin E is generally protective against Cu-induced oxidative damage. While most *in vitro* or cell culture studies show that ascorbic acid aggravates Cu-induced oxidative damage, results obtained from available animal studies suggest that the compound is protective. High intakes of ascorbic acid and zinc may provide protection against Cu toxicity by preventing excess Cu uptake. Zinc also removes Cu from its binding site, where it may cause free radical formation. β-carotene, α-lipoic acid and polyphenols have also been shown to attenuate Cu-induced oxidative damage. Further studies are needed to better understand the cellular effects of this essential, but potentially toxic, trace mineral.

Chromium

The affect of ascorbic acid and Trolox (water-soluble analogue of α-tocopherol) on Cr(VI)-induced toxicity was investigated. Antioxidants could influence Cr(VI) to Cr(III) reduction velocity. Fast decomposition of highly permeable H_2O_2, O_2^- and Cr(V) leads to milder DNA damage given that Cr(III) is scarcely able to penetrate the nuclear membrane. Thus, antioxidant pretreatment could influence both types of Cr(VI)-induced cellular damage: (i) a direct pathway of cellular damage mediated by reactive chromium intermediates, and (ii) an oxidative pathway mediated by ROS.

Iron

Iron can stimulate free radical production as a catalyst of Fenton reaction. Most problematic is free iron in a cell. Superoxide has been labeled an endogenous toxin and has been shown to promote iron release from ferritin. Iron release from ferritin is capable of initiating lipid peroxidation and catalyzes the Haber-Weiss reaction, leading to the damage of cell biomolecules. Fortunately, cells have many enzymes capable of removing ROS (e.g., superoxide dismutase, catalase, glutathione peroxidase, etc.). Additionally, precise mechanisms of uptake, distribution and storage of iron have evolved. Ferritin and ceruloplasmin are effective means of preventing oxidative damage catalyzed by free iron.

Ionizing Radiation

Ionizing radiation consists of highlyenergetic particles or waves that can detach (ionize) at least one electron from an atom or molecule. Ionizing radiation occurs in the environment in many forms, originating from both natural (natural background radiation comes from four primary sources: cosmic radiation, solar radiation, external terrestrial sources, and radon) (1) and human-contrived sources. Radon gas could be the second largest cause of lung cancer in America, after smoking.The damaging effects of ionizing radiation on cells due to OH· and other reactive radicals attack induced by ionizing radiation can sometimes be prevented or decreased by reactions with certain antioxidants, like GSH, ascorbic acid, melatonin, α-Phenyl-*N-t*-butylnitrone and others. There are still inconclusive results of studies investigating whether patients undergoing radiotherapy should take additional antioxidant supplements.

UV Radiation

UVradiation to skin might cause a large degree of destruction of enzymatic and non-enzymatic antioxidants immediately after irradiation. Ultraviolet radiation is the most common environmental factor in the pathogenesis of skin cancer.For more information, see chapter on skin photoaging. Many studies suggest that exogenous supplementation of antioxidants prevents UVR-induced photooxidative damage (see also previous chapter on exogenous antioxidants). In recent years, there has been much interest in the use of oral and topical antioxidants as photoprotective agents (vitamin C, vitamin E, carotenoids, such as beta-carotene, green tea extracts and others).

Alcohol

Many observations have shown thatethanol-induced cell injury may be linked, at least partly,to an oxidative stress resulting from increased free radicalproduction and/or decreased antioxidant defense. Pharmacological antioxidants could have beneficial effects in reducing the incidence of ethanol-induced changes in cellular lipids, proteins and nucleic acids. The antioxidants considered could act by reducing free radical production (e.g., chelators of redox-active iron derivatives), trapping free radicals themselves, interrupting the peroxidation process or reinforcing the natural antioxidant defense. The best way to reduce alcohol-induced oxidative stress is to drink alcohol in moderate amounts. Women drinking 20 g or more (two or more drinks) daily had 2.5 (odds ratio) times the risk of melanoma as nondrinkers (95% confidence interval, 0.87 to 7.4) (Green et al., 1993).

Chlorine as Water Disinfectant

Chlorine (Cl_2) as strong oxidizing agent, when added to drinking water (HOCl), could increase oxidative stress in human cells, e.g., by decreasing endogenous antioxidants, oxidizing cholesterol molecules and killing beneficial intestine microorganisms. HOCl can oxidize thiols, ascorbate, NAD(P)H, and lead to chlorination of DNA bases and tyrosine residues in proteins. Chlorination of water decreases its natural antioxidative potential by ten- or even more fold. The users of such water ingest more oxidants and should thus consume more fruit and vegetables to compensate the balance between oxidants and antioxidants. Because of the immense benefits in reduction of infectious diseases, and the simplicity and low cost of water treatment using chlorine, chlorination is still the most appropriate choice as a method of ensuring safe drinking water for most water systems.

Conclusion

There is a growing body of evidence, epidemiological, clinical and experimental, that the involvement of antioxidants can prevent or decrease the damage caused by certain environmental pollutants connected to ROS generation in the cell. Protection against ROS-mediated environmental pollutants can generally take place on two levels: (i) physiochemical protection to lower the dose of exposure, which usually cannot be done by individuals living in polluted areas, unless they move out or (ii) by physiological protection to increase the organism's antioxidative defense. Since we have little influence on increasing the levels of endogenous antioxidants, it would be reasonable to increase the amount of exogenous antioxidants in order to strengthen the organism's defensive properties against environmental oxidative stress.

Part III/2. Decreasing Oxidative Stress Caused by Endogenous (Intrinsic) Factors—the Use of Antioxidants

Chapter 7.3.

Can Antioxidants as Dietary Supplements Offer Appropriate Protection against ROS-Induced Damage?

Due to less-specific data on skin aging, the use of food supplements on more general sense regarding their effects on aging process is discussed in this chapter.

To protect against damage by ROS, all biological systems have evolved complex antioxidant systems composed of low molecular-weight compounds (such as glutathione and vitamin A, C, E) and enzymes, such as catalase, superoxide dismutase and glutathione peroxidase.Uncoupling agents and heat shock proteins could also be considered as antioxidants due to their roles in reducing oxidative stress.

Most studies are in agreement that during aging, increased age-related oxidative damage of cellular DNA, proteins and lipids can cause redox imbalance, resulting in the disruption of cellular regulatory processes.

It, therefore, seems reasonable to expect that reducing the oxidatively damaged cellular component by antioxidants can remedy a situation in which age-related damage and life-shortening pathogenesis interact synergistically (Yu, 1999).

Surveys show that more than half of the U.S. adult population uses food supplements. In 1996, alone, consumers spent more than $6.5 billion on dietary supplements. Today, consumers pay much attention totheir health and prevention of diseases; consumers want a greater opportunity to determine whether supplements may help them and ask questions about dietary supplements: Do dietary supplements offer health benefits or potential health hazards? Can their claims be trusted? Are they safe? Does the Food and Drug Administration approve them?

Under the Dietary Supplement Health and Education Act of 1994 (DSHEA), the dietary supplement manufacturer is responsible for ensuring that a dietary supplement is safe before it is marketed. FDA is responsible for taking action against any unsafe dietary supplement product after it reaches the market. Generally, manufacturers do not need to register their products with FDA nor get FDA approval before producing or selling dietary supplements (http://www.fda.gov/Food/DietarySupplements/default.htm).

By law (DSHEA), the manufacturer is responsible for ensuring that its dietary supplement products are safe before they are marketed. Unlike drug products that must be proven safe and effective for their intended use before marketing, there are no provisions in the law for FDA to "approve" dietary supplements for safety or effectiveness before they reach the consumer. Also, unlike drug products, manufacturers and distributors of dietary supplements are not currently required by law to record, investigate or forward to FDA any reports they receive of injuries or illnesses that may be related to the use of their products. On the other hand, the law essentially gives dietary supplement manufacturers freedom to market more products as dietary supplements and provide information about their products' benefits—for example, in product labeling. FDA or other similar institutions do not authorize or test dietary supplements since they are not intended to diagnose, cure, mitigate, treat, or prevent diseases. The manufacturer just has to prove that new ingredient can reasonably be expected to be safe. Safe means that the new ingredient does not present a significant or unreasonable risk of illness or injury under conditions of use recommended in the product's labeling. Once a dietary supplement is marketed, FDA has the responsibility for showing that a dietary supplement is unsafe before it can take action to restrict the product's use. Contrary, before entering on the market, drugs must undergo clinical studies to determine their effectiveness, safety, possible interactions with other substances, and appropriate dosages, and FDA must review these data and authorize the drugs' use before they are marketed.

A dietary supplement, also known as a foodor nutritional supplement, is a preparation intended to provide nutrients such as vitamins, minerals, fiber, fatty acids or amino acids that are either missing or not consumed in sufficient quantity in one's diet. The idea that antioxidant supplements, such as Vitamin C, Vitamin E, lipoic acid and N-acetylcysteine, might extend human life stems from the free radical theory of aging.

Evidence is presented in the following paragraph to show that synthetic antioxidant supplements cannot offer appropriate or total protection against oxidative stress and damage and that the use of antioxidants to prevent disease is controversial (Meyers, 1996). Since dietary sources contain a wider range of carotenoids and vitamin E tocopherols and tocotrienols from whole foods, *ex post facto* epidemiological studies can draw conclusions that differ from those based on artificial experiments using isolated compounds. For example, it was reported that in a high-risk group like smokers, high doses of beta-carotene increased the rate of lung cancer (Ruano-Ravina et al., 2006). In less high-risk groups, the use of vitamin E appears to reduce the risk of heart disease (Pryor, 2000). Also, in other diseases such as Alzheimer's, the evidence concerning vitamin E supplementation is mixed (Boothby and Doering, 2005; Kontush and Schekatolin, 2004).

Natural antioxidants like vitamin C and E, carotenoids and polyphenols (e.g., flavonoids) are generally regarded as beneficial components of fruits and vegetables. The antioxidative properties of these compounds are often claimed to be responsible for the protective effects of these food components against cardiovascular diseases, certain forms of cancers, and photosensitivity diseases (Rietjens et al., 2001). However, many of the reported health claims have been derived from observational epidemiological studies in which specific diets were associated with reduced risks of specific forms of cancer, cardiovascular diseases, and the reduction of stress. The controversy in beneficial vs. harmful synthetic antioxidant properties may also reflect a misinterpretation of epidemiology. Fruits, grains and vegetables contain multiple components that might exert protective effects against disease. It could be any, or any combination of, those factors that is a true protective agent. For example, high plasma ascorbate levels or high ascorbate intake could simply be a marker of a good diet rather than a true protective factor (Rietjens et al., 2001). Identification of the actual ingredient in a specific diet responsible for the beneficial health effect remains an important bottleneck for translating observational epidemiology to the development of functional food ingredients. For antioxidant-type functional food ingredients, toxic pro-oxidant actions at higher doses may be important(Rietjens et al., 2001). In this chapter, the current state of knowledge regarding antioxidants as dietary supplements and their roles in decreasing the oxidative stress aresummarized.

Antioxidants and Clinical Trials

Endogenous Antioxidants

Several studies have been conducted regarding endogenous defenses. It was observed that maximum lifespan correlates negatively with antioxidantenzyme levels and free-radical production and positively with the rate of DNA repair.Female mammals express more Mn−SOD and glutathione peroxidase antioxidant enzymes than males. This has been hypothesized as the reason why females live longer than males.The maximum lifespan of transgenic mice has been extended by about 20% through overexpression of humancatalase targeted to mitochondria (Schriner et al., 2005).

In contrast, a recent study showed that overexpression of both catalase and superoxide dismutase had no effect on lifespan in mice (Perez et al., 2009). Overexpression of the enzyme that synthesizes glutathione in long-lived transgenicDrosophila (fruit flies) extended maximum lifespan by nearly 50% (Orr et al.,2005). In some model organisms, such as yeast and *Drosophila*, there is evidence that reducing oxidative damage does, as predicted by the free radical theory, extend lifespan.

In mice, interventions that enhance oxidative damage generally shorten lifespan. However, in roundworms (*Caenorhabditis elegans*), blocking the production of the naturally occurring antioxidant superoxide dismutase has recently been shown to increase lifespan(Jeremy et al., 2009).

Although this could be explained by less H_2O_2 formation, since H_2O_2 is far more dangerous as superoxide in producing oxidative damage with the ability of crossing mitochondrial and cellular membranes. Mutant strains of the roundworm *Caenorhabditis elegans* that are more susceptible to free radicals have shortened lifespan and vice versa (Larsen, 1993; Ishii, 2000). Short-term induction of oxidative stress due to caloric restriction increases lifespan in *Caenorhabditis elegans*by promoting stress defense, specifically by inducing the enzyme catalase that reduces the amount of H_2O_2. Michael Ristow and co-workers showed that nutritive antioxidants completely abolish this extension of lifespan by inhibiting a process called mitohormesis.

Adding more SOD and catalase enzymes in genetic experiments has extended the lifespan of model organisms, indicating that catalytic antioxidants have the ability to extend lifespan.

However, according to Villeponeau (2003), genetic approaches currently have severe limitations in humans, and, considering the fact that the catalytic enzymes themselves would be degraded in the digestive tract, the rationale solution would be to search for SOD and catalase mimetics (formore information, see also paragraph on mimetics).

Intake of Exogenous Antioxidants

Use of multivitamins/minerals (MVMs) has grown rapidly over the past several decades, and dietary supplements are now used by more than half of the adult population in the United States. In general, MVMs are used by individuals who practice healthier lifestyles, thus making observational studies of the overall relationship between MVM use and general health outcomes difficult to interpret. Despite the widespread use of MVMs, insufficient knowledge about the actual amount of total nutrients that Americans consume from diet and supplements still exists. This is at least in part due to the fortification of foods with these nutrients, which adds to the effects of MVMs or single-vitamin or single-mineral supplements (National Institutes of Health, 2006).According to National Institutes of Health (2006), "most of the studies examined on antioxidant use do not provide strong evidence for beneficial health-related effects of supplements taken singly, in pairs, or in combinations of three or more. Within some studies or subgroups of the study populations, there is encouraging evidence of health benefits, such as increased bone mineral density and decreased fractures in postmenopausal women who use calcium and vitamin D supplements. However, several other studies also provide disturbing evidence of risk, such as increased lung cancer risk with beta-carotene use among smokers. The current level of public assurance of the safety and quality of MVMs is inadequate, given the fact that manufacturers of these products are not required to report adverse events and the FDA has no regulatory authority to require labeling changes or to help inform the public of these issues and concerns. It is important that the FDA's purview over these products is authorized and implemented" (National Institutes of Health, 2006). On the other hand, most epidemiological studies support a relationship between the consumption of diets rich in antioxidants and the health of the consumer. Based on the analysis of the available epidemiological data, a daily intake of at least 400 g of fruits and vegetables (or five to ten portions) has been recommended by the World Health Organization.

Micronutrient deficiency may explain, in good part, why the quarter of the population that eats the fewest fruits and vegetables (five portions a day is advised) has about double the cancer rate for most types of cancer when compared to the quarter with the highest intake. For example, 80% of American children and adolescents and 68% of adults do not eat five portions a day (Ames, 2001).People who eat fruits and vegetables, which happen to be good sources of antioxidants, have a lower risk of heart disease and some neurological diseases (Stanner et al., 2007), and there is evidence that some types of vegetables, and fruits in general, protect against a number of cancers (World Cancer Research Fund, 2007). These observations suggested the possibility that antioxidants help to prevent these conditions. However, this hypothesis has now been tested in many clinical trials and does not seem to be true, since antioxidant supplements have no clear effect on the risk of chronic diseases such as cancer and heart disease (Stanner et al., 2004; Shenkin, 2006).Many clinical trials in which individuals received one or more synthetic antioxidants failed to obtain beneficial results. Results of clinical trials on exogenous antioxidants intake are thus conflicting and contradictory. This indicates that other substances in fruits and vegetables (possibly flavonoids), or a complex mix of substances, may contribute to the better cardiovascular health and decreased cancer incidence observed in individuals who consume more of these foods (Cherubini et al., 2005; Lotito and Frei, 2006). There is also the problem regarding the dosing of synthetic antioxidants. Larger amounts of antioxidants are suggested to be consumed in order to effectively fight oxidative stress by some scientists and pharmacologic companies. We should not exceed the RDA values of vitamins, although again there are claims that RDA levels are too low. For example, there are observed differences for the different routes of administration. The oral route can be neutralized or affected during transit to the bowel, where variable amounts are "sequestrated" by the liver, so that the "bioavailability" of the original supplement for other tissues/organs is reduced (e.g., the case of reduced glutathione). Another approach should consider the administration of metabolic precursors of the antioxidant. For instance, the reduced glutathione is rapidly oxidized in the plasma and cannot be administered using the intravenous route; in this case, the clinician can consider the possibility of administering some cysteine-enriched peptides capable of reconstituting the glutathione into the cells. In dealing with antioxidant supplementation, one must be aware of several other uncertainties (Rose, 1996; Palozza, 1998; Rumsey and Levine, 1998) associated with the use of dietary supplements before assessing the full impact of intervention: (1) gut absorption of dietary antioxidants, (2) maintenance of antioxidant plasma levels, (3) membrane transport, (4) regulation of intracellular antioxidant balance, (5) compensatory actions among the various antioxidants, and (6) antioxidants converting to pro-oxidants (e.g., ascorbate and carotenoids) under certain physiological conditions (Yu et al., 1998). It is a difficult task to develop compounds that can get through the intestinal tract and into the bloodstream and still be able to enter through the cell membranes with the chemical properties necessary to react with DNA (or protect it) and perform their desired function. Due to our current lack of understanding concerning the overall regulation of an integrated antioxidant status, these uncertainties are great challenges to investigators engaged in anti-aging research (Yu, 1999). As already mentioned, the results of epidemiological studies in which people were treated with synthetic antioxidants are inconclusive and contradictory, providing findings that prove either a beneficial effect, no effect, or a harmful effect of the synthetic antioxidant supplements. None of the major clinical studies using mortality or morbidity as an end point has found positive effects of supplementation with antioxidants such as vitamin C, vitamin E or β-carotene. The intake of only one antioxidant could alter the complex system of endogenous antioxidative defense of cells or alter the necrosis or apoptosis pathways. We have to realize that the use of synthetic vitamin supplements is not an alternative to regular consumption of fruits and vegetables. It is probable that many antioxidants are still undiscovered. Furthermore, the combination of antioxidants in fruits and vegetables causes their reciprocal regeneration and intensifies their defense against free radicals. However, deficiency of vitamins B-12, folic acid, B-6, C or E, iron or zinc appears to mimic radiation in damaging DNA by causing single- and double-strand breaks, oxidative lesions or both. Evidence is accumulating that a multivitamin/mineral supplement could improve the health of specific populations such as the poor, the young, the obese and the elderly. This is confirmed by the experiment on transgenic knockout mice with SOD II genes, which revealed that exogenous antioxidants can offer some protection. SOD II knockout mice die about ten days after birth (Chan et al., 1995). This death is primarily due to oxidative stress damage resulting from the failure to dismutate the superoxide radical. Repletion of the scavenging by exogenous catalytic "salen" (salicylic aldehyde and ethylenediamine) antioxidants extended the life of the SOD II knockout animals to about 30 days (Melov et al., 2001). Complete rescue of the exogenous antioxidants does not occur because they cannot penetrate the blood-brain barrier, and the mice suffered from a spongiform encephalopathy. Thus, it is important where in the cell a specific antioxidant quenches the free radicals, since different cells of the human body present large differences regarding proliferative activity, apoptotic rate, ROS production and DNA repair capability.Besides, Tolamsoff et al. (1980)

found that the ratio of SOD-specific activity to specific metabolic rate increased with increasing maximum lifespan potential for all species that they examined. These data show an important correlation between lifespan and energy metabolism and between oxidative stress and antioxidative defense systems (Ishii and Hartman, 2003). Harman (1968) and Comfort (1971) reported that increases in average life expectancy of some groups of mice receiving one of a number of different free radical reaction inhibitors were associated with lower body weights. This effect may result from the adverse effects on mitochondrial function: antioxidants decrease ATP formation (Jamnik, 2007; Pardini, 1970; Horum, 1978) through partial uncoupling of mitochondrial respiration, and under these circumstances superoxide radical and hydrogen peroxide formation is also decreased since the oxidation of respiratory components is greater (Bandy and Davidson, 1990). In contrast to the results obtained with mice, both the average and maximum lifespan of *Drosophila* (Horrum et al., 1978; Miquel and Johnson, 1975) and nematodes (Epstein and Gershon, 1972) are increased by antioxidants. These effects, at least in *Drosophila*, are associated with decreased respiration (Miquel et al., 1982) and thus decreased ATP formation. Increases in the maximum lifespan of nematodes are attributed to their capacity to live during reduced rates of ATP production. CR in yeast also decreased mitochondrial ROS generation, although it raised mitochondrial respiration rates (Barros et al., 2004). Furthermore, CR in yeast decreased NADH levels due to lower glucose metabolism and/or increased levels of the Pcn1 enzyme that hydrolyses nicotinamide to nicotinic acid, which can then be used to make more NAD+. In 2002, a team led by Professor Bruce Ames at UC Berkeley discovered that feeding aged rats a combination of acetyl-L-carnitine and alpha-lipoic acid (both substances are already approved for human use and sold in health food stores) produced a rejuvenating effect (Lui et al., 2002). Feeding old rats the normal mitochondrial metabolites acetyl carnitine and lipoic acid for a few weeks restores mitochondrial function, lowers oxidants to the level of a young rat, and increases ambulatory activity (Ames, 1989). Acetyl-L-carnitine is a high-energy mitochondrial substrate and appears to reverse many age-associated deficits in cellular function, in part by increasing cellular ATP production (Shigenaga et al., 1994). Thus, these two metabolites can be considered necessary for health in old age and are, therefore, conditional micronutrients. However, some recent studies showed that antioxidant therapy has no effect and can even increase mortality (*The Alpha-Tocopherol, Beta-Carotene Cancer Prevention Study Group, 1994;Omenn et al., 1996;Bjelakovic et al., 2004;Miller et al., 2005; Heart Protection Study Collaborative Group, 2002;Age-Related Eye Disease Study Research Group, 2001*).

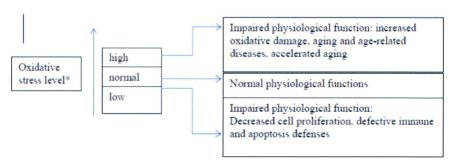

Figure 35. Oxidative stress level should be optimal. Increased oxidative stress is harmful, as well as increased "antioxidative stress". *Figure adapted from Cutler and Mattson. Measuring oxidative stress and interpreting its relevance in humans. In: Oxidative stress and Aging (Eds: Cutler RG and Rodriguez, H.). World Scientific, 2003.

There are several possible explanations for the potential negativeeffect of antioxidant supplements. Reactive oxygen species inmoderate concentrations are essential mediators of defense against unwanted cells. Thus, if administrationof antioxidant supplements decreases free radicals, it may interferewith essential defensive mechanisms for ridding the organismof damaged cells, including those that are precancerous andcancerous (Salganik, 2001). Thus, antioxidant supplements may actually causesome harm (Vivekananthan et al., 2003; Bjelakovic et al., 2004a; Bjelakovic et al., 2004b; Miller et al., 2005; Bjelakovic et al., 2007; Caraballoso et al., 2003). Our diets typically contain safelevels of vitamins, but high-level antioxidant supplements couldpotentially upset an important physiologic balance (Vivekananthan et al., 2003; Bjelakovic et al., 2004a; Bjelakovic et al., 2004b; Miller et al., 2005; Bjelakovic et al., 2007; Caraballoso et al., 2003). A systematic review and meta-analysis done by Bjelakovic et al. (2007) concludes that long-term treatment with beta-carotene, vitamin A, andvitamin E may increase mortality. There are still many gaps in our knowledge ofthe mechanisms of bioavailability, biotransformation, and actionof antioxidant supplements. Proponents of the theory claim that this phenomenon can be explained by hormesis: addition of antioxidants can lead to a decrease of the normal biological response to free radicals and to a more sensitive environment for oxidation. On the other hand, antioxidants might indeed trigger mild oxidative stress due to their pro-oxidative properties (e.g., ascorbic acid) (Poljsak et al., 2008).

Selman et al. (2006) suggested different possible explanations regarding the general inability of antioxidants in supplementation studies to consistently deliver the promise of increased lifespan in animal modelsor reduced disease risk in humans and as to why it could have a varied causality (see McCall and Frei, 1999).

(i) Perhaps *in vivo* some antioxidants may act more as a pro-oxidants than an antioxidant (Childs et al., 2001; Rehman et al., 1998), possibly necessitating increased activation of the defense system to maintain the status quo.
(ii) Alternatively, vitamin C and other antioxidants may successfully scavenge ROS (Carr and Frei, 1999), but this may not be translated into damage reduction and lifespan enhancement. Vitamin C may negatively affect the endogenous scavenging and repair systems, either directly (Nemoto et al., 1997; Podmore et al., 1998), or indirectly via systems that sense reduced radical production.

Diets high in fruits and vegetables, which are high in antioxidants, promote health and reduce the effects of aging. However, antioxidant vitamin supplementation has no detectable effect on the aging process, so the effects of fruits and vegetables may be unrelated to their antioxidant contents (*Thomas, 2004;Ward, 1998*). One reason for this might be the fact that consuming antioxidant molecules such as polyphenols and vitamin E will produce changes in other parts of the metabolism, and these other non-antioxidant effects may be the real reason for their importance in human nutrition (Azzi, 2007;Aggarwal and Shishodia, 2006) and their positive effect on aging and chronical degenerative diseases prevention.

Each part of a cell is protected by a different antioxidant nutrient, and this explains why only a comprehensive intake of nutrients can protect us. For example, some nutrients defend against free radical attack in the blood surrounding the cell, others defend the outside of the cell membrane, others defend inside the cell, and still other nutrients protect the cell mitochondria—the energy factories of human cells. There seems to be an effect between exogenous antioxidants that tends to depress endogenous antioxidant levels. Changing the level of one antioxidant causes a compensatory change in others, while the overall antioxidant capacity remains unaffected. Dosing cells with exogenous antioxidants might decrease the rate of synthesis or uptake of endogenous antioxidants, so that the total "cell antioxidant potential" remains unaltered. Thus, the key to the future success of dietary antioxidant supplementation should be the suppression of oxidative damage without disruption of the well-integrated antioxidant defense network. Recent evidence emerging from dietary restriction studies shows such possibilities, as in upregulating the antioxidant defense system in the most appropriate manner without causing a redox imbalance. The selective enhancement of the defense system could be a major strategy for a successful intervention by antioxidant administration (Yu, 1999).

Additionally, for overall life expectancy, it has even been suggested that moderate levels of oxidative stress may increase lifespan in the worm *Caenorhabditis elegans* by inducing a protective response to increased levels of reactive oxygen species (Schulz et al., 2007). However, the suggestion that increased life expectancy results from increased oxidative stress conflicts with results seen in the yeast*Saccharomyces cerevisiae* (Barros et al. 2004), and the situation in mammals is even less clear (Sohal et al., 2002; Sohal, 2002; Rattan, 2006). Nevertheless, antioxidant supplements do not appear to increase life expectancy in humans (Green, 2008).

It could be postulatedthat antioxidants would be therapeutically effective in an agedmammal exposed to a stressor that generates exaggerated oxidativeinjury as revealed by the study of Zhang et al. (2004), which made an effort to determine whethera therapeutic intervention that reduces the degree of oxidativedamage can protect old animals from heat-stress-induced liverinjury. Due to the ubiquitous distribution of antioxidants in the body, there is a necessity to have a formula with a wide and complete spectrum of actions. Unfortunately, a unique formula capable of fitting the above criteria is not available. In fact, it is well known that vitamin E is a powerful antioxidant, but its activity is reduced when the partial oxygen pressure is reduced, a situation in which ß-carotenes are most effective. On the other hand, vitamin C is particularly capable of recycling oxidized vitamin E but, as opposed to vitamin E, it is not liposoluble and, therefore, cannot reach fatty tissues, although diffusion of the coenzyme Q10 is not problematic. Therefore, since a unique antioxidant is only partially effective, it is indispensable that the clinician considers a cocktail of antioxidants, e.g., a formula containing multiple antioxidants with a wide range of activity (e.g., synergistic effect between vitamin E, ß-carotenes, vitamin C and coenzyme Q10). See also the paragraph on the synergistic effect between antioxidants.

Pro-Oxidant Activities of Antioxidants and Their Impact on Cancer

Antioxidants that are reducing agents can also act as pro-oxidants, since they are capable of reacting with molecular oxygen (e.g., ascorbic acid), and generate superoxide radicals under aerobic conditions. These will dismutate to H_2O_2 that can enter cells and react with superoxide or reduced metal ions to form highly damaging hydroxyl radicals (Anderson and Phillips, 1999). The presence of redox cycling metal ions with antioxidants might result in a synergistic effect, resulting in increased free radical formation or the so-called pro-oxidant effect. See also chapter "The role of macro and micro nutrients."

Increasing cellular viability with antioxidants prior to toxic compound-induced toxicity (e.g., Cr(VI), UVradiation, ionizing radiation) might not always be beneficial. Carcinogen-induced growth arrest and apoptosis are at the molecular decision point between carcinogen toxicity and carcinogen carcinogenesis (Carlisle, 2000). When normal growing cells come in contact with carcinogens, they may respond by undergoing growth arrest, apoptosis and necrosis. A population of genetically damaged cells may also emerge, which exhibits either intrinsic or induced resistance to apoptosis (Carlisle 2000). Such cells may be predisposed to neoplasia as a result of their altered growth/death ratio, disrupted cell cycle control, or genomic instability. This, however, raises the question of whether decreasing carcinogen toxicity with antioxidants might actually increase the incidence of cancer by allowing the inappropriate survival of genetically damaged cells. This hypothesis was confirmed by human intervention studies in which smoking male volunteers were exposed for five to eight years to daily supplementation with vitamin E and beta-carotene. The overall mortality of male smokers increased in those taking supplements of beta-carotene, and was most probably due to its effect on cell proliferation (*The Alpha-Tocopherol, Beta-Carotene Cancer Prevention Study Group*, 1994; Halliwell and Gutteridge, 1999). Randomized trials have demonstrated the anti-neoplastic and neoplastic effects of antioxidants, with neoplastic effects associated with patients at higher risk owing to smoking and alcohol consumption or patients undergoing chemo- or radiation therapy. This hypothesis was recently confirmed also by the study of Schafer et al. (2009), which revealed an unanticipated mechanism for cell survival in altered matrix environments by antioxidant restoration of ATP generation. Antioxidant activity may promote the survival of pre-initiated tumor cells in unnatural matrix environments and thus enhance malignancy. The main problem of antioxidant supplements is that most free-radical scavengers act in oxidation-reduction reactions that are reversible, and some, such as ascorbate, can act both as antioxidants and pro-oxidants, depending on the conditions (Podmore, 1998). More studies are warranted in which the effects of antioxidant supplementation on more than one biomarker of oxidative damage are determined. The discrepancies between different studies may be also due to the differential ability of the various macromolecules, i.e., DNA, lipids, and proteins, to bind metal ions and the redox activity of the bound metal ions (Halliwell and Gutteridge, 1986). Whether an antioxidant functions as an antioxidant or pro-oxidant is determined by at least threefactors: 1) the redox potential of the cellular environment; 2) the presence/absence of transition metals; and 3) the local concentrations of that antioxidant (Ionescu, 1998; Gonzales et al., 2005; Ionescu 2006). Antioxidants may thus have dichotomous activities with respect to tumorigenesis, namely, suppressing tumorigenesis by preventing oxidative damage to DNA (Gao, 2007; Narayanan, 2006) and promoting tumorigenesis by allowing survival of cells that are metabolically impaired (e.g., in altered matrix environments). In support of this, expression of SOD2, a mitochondrial protein that reduces oxidative stress caused by a respiratory chain leak, is increased in more advanced and higher-grade mammary tumors (Ivshina et al., 2006; Sorlie et al., 2001). Furthermore, a recent study has revealed that enhanced pentose phosphate pathway (PPP) flux and increased antioxidant capacity correlates with metastasis of breast cancer cells to the brain (Chen et al., 2007). These controversial and sometimes contradictory outcomes fromexperiments involving the manipulation of antioxidants by eitherpharmacological or genetic approaches add further support tothe notion that aging is a complicated and multifaceted phenomenonthat cannot be explained by a single theory. For this reason, it is important to recognize that physiological observables have multiple molecular causes, and studying them in isolation leads to inconsistent patterns of apparent causality when it is the simultaneous combination of multiple factors that is responsible. This explains, for instance, the decidedly mixed effects of antioxidants that have been observed (Kell, 2010). As already pointed out by Kregel and Zhang (2006), extrapolating findingsfrom flies, worms and rodents to humans, while useful as apotential means of optimizing human health and longevity, shouldbe approached with caution. Given our complex genetic andphysiological make-up, it is important to directly assess therole of oxidative stress in human aging processes.

Conclusion

The results of epidemiologic studies where people were treated with synthetic antioxidants are inconclusive and contradictory: from the proven beneficial effect, proven no difference, to the proven harmful effect of synthetic antioxidant supplements. None of the major clinical studies using mortality or morbidity as an end point has found positive effects of supplementation with antioxidants such as vitamin C, vitamin E or β-carotene. The intake of only one antioxidant could alter the complex system of endogenous antioxidative defense of cells or could alter the necrosis or apoptosis pathways. It is wrong to search the "redox magic bullet"among different compounds with increased redox potential. Better approach is to focus on detailed understanding of the complex redox system of our cells and to investigate the synergistic effects of different antioxidants on total oxidative stress. We have to realize that the use of synthetic vitamin supplements is not an alternative to regular consumption of fruit and vegetables. It is probable that many antioxidants are still undiscovered; furthermore, the combination of antioxidants in fruit and vegetables causes their reciprocal regeneration and consecutively intensifies their defense from free radicals. However, deficiency of vitamins B-12, folic acid, B-6, C or E, or iron or zinc appears to mimic radiation in damaging DNA by causing single- and double-strand breaks, oxidative lesions or both (Ames, 2001). Evidence is accumulating that a multivitamin/mineral supplement could improve the health of specific populations, e.g., the poor, the young, the obese, the elderly and people exposed to increased ROS from the environment.

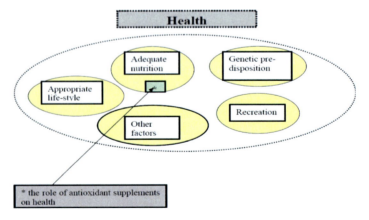

Figure 36. Health is a state of complete physical, mental, and social well-being. It is a complex equilibrium of many variables (e.g., nutrition, lifestyle, genetics, etc). The figure shows the minor role of antioxidants on health as total.

The current lack of sufficient data does not permit the systematic recommendation of antioxidants. Nevertheless, antioxidant-rich diets with fruit and vegetables should be recommended (Bonnefoy, 2002).

Should Supplements of Antioxidants Be Taken?

The impoverishment of the soil (resulting from the abnormal exploitation of the soil itself, acid rain, increasing desertification, pollution, etc.), the often-uncontrolled use of pesticides, the processes of refinement of vegetables, and the processes of transformation, storage and even cooking of foods, can affect the antioxidant content of fruits and vegetables. Therefore, as a precaution, many nutritionists today suggest the indiscriminate use of antioxidants. Inadequate dietary intakes of vitamins and minerals are widespread, most likely due to excessive consumption of energy-rich, micronutrient-poor, refined food (Ames, 2006). However, the use of antioxidant supplements should be limited only to document cases of oxidative stress (see section concerning how to measure oxidative stress). Importantly, before starting any supplementation, an attempt should be made to measure the oxidative stress and to identify and remove the possible cause for the increased production of free radicals and thus increased oxidative stress. In addition, methods today allow us to estimate the level of oxidative stress of an individual (see chapter concerning how to detect and measure oxidative stress). As in the case of a medical doctor who does not prescribe pills for lowering high blood pressure before measuring blood pressure level, it, therefore, should be reasonable to first test oxidative stress status before starting therapy with antioxidant supplements.

The nutritional status and needs of elderly people are associated with age-related biological and often socioeconomic changes. Decreased food intake, a sedentary lifestyle, and reduced energy expenditure in older adults altogether become critical risk factors for malnutrition, especially protein and micronutrients. Surveys indicate that the elderly are particularly at risk for marginal deficiency of vitamins and trace elements. Changes in bodily functions, together with the malnutrition associated with advancing age, increase the risk of developing a number of age-related diseases. Chronic conditions pose difficulties for the elderly in carrying out the activities of daily living and may increase the requirements for certain nutrients due to changes in absorptive and metabolic capacity (Meydani, 2001). Free radicals and oxidative stress have been recognized as important factors in the biology of aging and of many age-associated degenerative diseases. In this regard, modulation of oxidative stress by caloric restriction, as demonstrated in animal models, is suggested as one mechanism to slow the aging process and the decline of body functions. Therefore, dietary components with antioxidant activity have received particular attention because of their potential role in modulating oxidative stress associated with aging and chronic conditions (Meydani, 2001).

There are some exceptions where supplements of vitamins might be beneficial: for example, fish oils have proved to be useful source of long chain ω-3 fatty acids for those who do not like oil-rich fish, and supplements are recommended for vulnerable groups, for example, folic acid for women of child-bearing age, iron supplements for women with heavy menstrual losses, vitamin D for young children, pregnant women and older (housebound) people, and calcium for those at high risk of osteoporosis. Additionally, folic acid, vitamin B6 and vitamin B12 have been shown to reduce homocysteine levels in the blood and appear to lower cardiovascular risk (Bunout et al., 2000). Also, magnesium may be useful in treating high blood pressure (Touyz and Milne, 1999), cardiovascular diseases (Rubenowitz et al., 2000), Alzheimer's (Glick, 1990) and osteoporosis (Toba et al., 2000). Omega-3 fatty acids appear to reduce the risk of cardiovascular disease (Von Schacky, 2010) and cancer (Bougnoux et al., 2006). Garlic extracts fight viral and bacterial infections and prevent chronic inflammation (Cellini et al., 1996). Functional foods, for example those with added fiber or probiotics, may also be of benefit.

Some critics of the oxidative theory claim that the failure of antioxidant interventions to stop or reverse the aging process and to quell the current pandemic of age-related diseases (e.g., cardiovascular disease) brings the oxidative hypothesis into question (Howes, 2006). Nevertheless, since aging is a complex dysregulation of many redox systems, single - antioxidant administration should not necessarily be expected to influence the aging process. Complex multiple-antioxidant interventions or complete dietary changes might be more successful in this aspect (Gilca et al., 2007).

The thesis that pro-oxidant effect of a specific antioxidant depends on its unbalance with other antioxidants, minerals and other nutrients, among them many still unknown, opens many questions regarding the best way to minimize the oxidative damage through food intake. Enough fruits and vegetables seem to be just the first step to this goal. Experiments on pigs show that supplementation of diet with different types of fruits and vegetables (apples, strawberries and tomatoes) have different effects on lowering the level of oxidative stress; so docs their combination (Pajk Žontar et al; 2006). Which combination of fruits and vegetables arebest for humans? A controlled intervention should take into account the subject's blood redox potential and its total antioxidant activity. According to well-known biologists' thesis, no animal species is optimally adapted to environment (Dawkins, 1999), especially in changeable environment. Despite the new finding on speeding up of genetic changes in humans (Hawkes, 2007), human genes have not changed much during the last 10,000 years, but all produced food has due to normal selection that agriculture does (Watson, Berry 2007). Moreover, today's fruits and vegetables are depleted of some essential micronutrients because of the intensified type of production (Poljšak, 2006) or because of post-harvest processes—transport, storage, etc. (Tijskens, 2004).

Finally, the present evidence is insufficient to recommend either for or against the use of antioxidant supplementsto prevent chronic diseases. Advances in research and improved communication and collaboration among scientists, health care providers, patients, the pharmaceutical and supplement industries, and the public are required.

What is the content of nutrients of specific fruits and vegetables we eat? How to measure with non-invasive methods the specific needs of vitamin C and other nutrients of each individual? The path of food supplements seems to be at the present time even more uncertain. However, there is a general trend towards the increased intake of processed food and food supplements. In most countries of the world, the consumption of fruits and vegetables is below the minimal level of 400 g per day advised by WHO and FAO (FAO/WHO, 2004). Even in countries that in the past had high consumption of fruits and vegetables, their consumption has been lowering (López-Torres, Barja, 2008). The addition of different food supplements to one's diet seems to be, besides consumption of fruits and vegetables, for different reasons, and especially in different clinical conditions, a need as well. But more research is needed to find solutions that are closer to optimal human diet and will have "the best effect in reducing oxidative stress of an organism. The fact that clinical trials or laboratory tests where model organisms were pretreated with supplements of antioxidants did not show increased maximum lifespan could be explained with the fact that mitochondrial DNA, a major site of oxidative damage and the leading reason for the aging process, is not protected by exogenous antioxidants. Additionally, endogenous antioxidant defense is regulated to provide a net protection that is difficult to change significantly by the addition or deletion of a single antioxidant. Nevertheless, exogenous antioxidant intake (preferably from fruits and vegetables) has a positive effect on nuclear DNA, as it was observed in epidemiological studies where consumption of fruit and vegetables was associated with decreased incidence of most chronic degenerative diseases. This could be also because antioxidants may elicit effects on gene expression via redox sensitive transcription factors. The transcription factors AP-1 and NF-κB appear to be crucial in modulating the oxidant/antioxidant response (Griffiths and Rayment, 2003). Thus, activity of DNA repair could be modulated by the redox status of the cell, which, in turn, is affected by antioxidants (Xanthoudakis et al., 1992; Hirota et al., 1997; Schenk et al., 1994). This could be explained with decreased incidence of cancer and heart diseases among people who consume significant amounts of fruits and vegetables, rich in antioxidants. Cutler (2003) described "The oxidative stress compensation model" which explains why dietary supplements of antioxidants have minimum effect on longevity. Cutler explains that most humans are able to maintain their set points of oxidative stress and so no matter how much additional antioxidant supplements they consumed in their diets, further decrease in oxidative stress does not occur. However, antioxidant supplements do appear to be affective in lowering an individual's oxidative stress if his/her initial oxidative stress is above normal or above his/her set point of regulation (Cutler, 2003). This hypothesis was confirmed with the already-mentioned study on mice given dietary supplements of vitamin E. Mice on a vitamin E-deficient diet have usually high tissue levels of SOD, but when placed on vitamin E-supplement diet, they had lower levels of SOD. Besides compensational/adaptation model, this experiment indicates also the fact that exogenous antioxidant intake can significantly affect the activity of endogenous antioxidative protection. Thus, antioxidant supplements would only be of help to an organism if they were needed to correct a high level of oxidative stress that could not be controlled by endogenous antioxidants. All of this points to the need of determination of individual's oxidative stress before supplement therapy starts. But how can oxidative stress of an individual be established? We try to answer this question in the following paragraph.

Part III/3 Decreasing the Formation of Endogenous Oxidative Stress— Preventing the Formation of Free Radicals

Chapter 7.4.

Methodology for the Detection of Oxidative State in Biological Systems

Free radicals and reactive oxygen species are involved in toxic mechanisms of action of certain air pollutants, metals, ionizing and non-ionizing radiation, alcohols, and pesticides being in contact with the skin or ingested with the food and water. The most efficient preventive step to avoid the exogenous free radical exposure would be to avoid as much as possible exposure of the skin to certain environmental pollutants. But since this is not always possible, protection could be obtained by adequate antioxidant balance. But what is appropriate antioxidant status? Can it be measured? Increasing interest in the role of free radicals in the pathogenesis of disease has led to an increased need for techniques to measure free radicals and their reactions *in vivo* and, most importantly, in the clinical situation. A vast array of analytical techniques has been developed to measure the various end-products of ROS reactions with cellular components, although not all are applicable to clinical situations where the only samples normally available are blood, urine and expired breath. Besides, it is not possible for a reactive free radical produced in an tissue and having a lifetime measured in microseconds to diffuse into the blood such that it can be detected at a distant site. The researcher is thus strictly limited to the determination of secondary products in a body fluid distant from the locus of production of the original damage (Holley and Cheeseman, 1993).

Free radicals have a very short half-life, which makes them very hard to measure in the laboratory. Multiple methods of measurement are available today, each with its own benefits and limits (for further reading, see review article by Poljsak and Jamnik, 2010). The problem of ascertaining the true importance of free radicals (and other reactive oxygen species—ROS) in biological systems has been that these evanescent species are difficult to measure *in vivo*. In order to establish the mechanism of toxicity as ROS mediated, direct and indirect methods are used. Direct methods relate to ROS measurement of superoxide, H_2O_2 and $OH^.$. These species are very reactive and their quantitation can be difficult. The only technique that can detect free radicals directly is the spectroscopic technique of electron spin resonance (ESR), sometimes called electron paramagnetic resonance (EPR). Therefore, indirect methods are used. Indirect methods usually measure changes in endogenous antioxidant enzyme activity (catalase, SOD, GPx, NADPH) and non-enzymatic defense such as measurement of glutathione. Indirect methods, also called fingerprinting methods, measure the products of damage by ROS on cellular components. Indirect methods measure changes in endogenous antioxidant defense systems and the damage on cellular components caused by ROS.

Measurement of Total Antioxidant Status

Patients who are deficient in antioxidants show evidence of increased oxidative damage *in vivo*, and epidemiological studies have shown that low antioxidant status is linked to the development of diseases. These observations have stimulated interest in the possibility that measurement of antioxidant status may have a role in the clinical arena (Lunec and Griffiths, 2000). Protection at the cellular level is mainly guaranteed by enzymes such as superoxide dismutase (SOD), catalase and glutathione peroxidase, whereas in plasma non-enzymatic antioxidants are playing the major role. Radical-scavenging antioxidants are consumed during the reactions with ROS, and antioxidant status could be used indirectly to assess free radical activity. One approach is to measure individual antioxidants (e.g., ascorbate, α-tocopherol, urate) in blood, plasma or tissue homogenates. All of the individual molecules that are currently recognized as antioxidants should be measured (Lunec and Griffiths, 2000). However, this approach will present several problems: 1) it will be time consuming, expensive and technically demanding, 2) it might fail to yield information about the synergistic effects between individual antioxidants, and 3) it might not account for the influence of not yet discovered antioxidant substances. The other approach is to measure total antioxidant capacity or activity by subjecting the samples to controlled oxidative stress conditions and measuring either the rate of oxidation or how long it takes for oxidation to occur. The most commonly used method for determining the antioxidant capacity of a food product is a measurement technique called Oxygen Radical Absorbance Capacity (ORAC). Even though there are a number of analytical techniques and indicators available to determine antioxidative potential, such as electron spin resonance (ESR), chemimodification, TEAC (Trolox Equivalent Antioxidant Capacity), FRAP (Ferric Reducing Ability of Plasma), oxidation reduction potential (ORP) and photosensitization, all of the methods have inherent limitations and specific practicalities. Serafini (2008) classified Total Antioxidant Capacity (TAC) assays into two groups on the basis of the chemical reaction involved:

- single-electron-transfer mechanism
- hydrogen atom-transfer mechanism

Assays involving the single-electron-transfer mechanism include:

(1) Ferric reducing ability of plasma (FRAP)
(2) Trolox equivalent antioxidant capacity (TEAC)

Assays involving the hydrogen-atom-transfer mechanism include:

(1) Total radical-trapping antioxidant parameter (TRAP)
(2) Fluorescence lipid-oxidation (Fluo-Lip)
(3) Oxygen radical antioxidant capacity (ORAC)

According to the International Observatory of Oxidative Stress, Free Radicals and Antioxidant Systems, most specific tests for oxidative stress evaluation are based on the general principle that the imbalance between the production and the elimination of free radicals becomes evident in the body due to an increased concentration/activity of a number of compounds resulting from the oxidant attack (e.g., hydroperoxides levels, glutathione peroxidase activity), and/or a decreased concentration/activity of one or more components of the antioxidant system (vitamins, minerals, enzymes) in the tissues and/or extracellular fluids.

On the basis of the above concepts, the presently available laboratory tests evaluate either the oxidant component (free-radical production) or the antioxidant component (antioxidant activity) of the oxidative stress. In determining the most adequate test, it is proper that the assessment of oxidative stress be "global," i.e., able to evaluate both the pro-oxidant and antioxidant components. Therefore, one should select at least two different assays: the first to measure the level of free-radical production and the second to measure the antioxidant capacity or potential.

In order to provide a reliable assessment of oxidative stress, it is preferable to perform the tests on blood because the by-products from cell oxidation accumulate primarily in this extracellular fluid, and it represents the location of the first antioxidant barrier.

The d-ROMs test, developed by the Italian chemist Mauro Carratelli, uses an accurate measurement of the oxidant status to provide the clinician with information that otherwise would not be obtainable by any of the available biochemical tests and indicates the general wellness status of the body, a status that largely depends on the rhythm of biological oxidations. Therefore, the values of the d-ROMS test are a faithful "mirror" of either endogenous (cell respiration) or reactive (inflammation) oxidative processes, and hence they provide reliable information on the rate of the physiological process of aging in a determined instance. As far as we know, the d-ROMs test is the only reliable test now available on the market to evaluate the oxidant status in clinical practice.

The Assessment of Antioxidant Status: The BAP Test

The blood plasma of living organisms contains several compounds that are collectively capable of opposing the oxidant potential of oxidant reactive chemical species. Any compound, either "endogenous" (albumin, transferrin, ceruloplasmin, bilirubin, uric acid, reduced glutathione, etc.) or "exogenous" (tocopherols, carotens, ubiquinol, ascorbate, methionine, flavonoids, polyphenols, etc.), is also able to block the potential damage of free radicals if it is able to give electrons. The reactivity of a free radical is indeed the result of a lack of electrons. Each of the above-listed antioxidants has its own antioxidant power or capacity, i.e., it is able to oppose free radicals with an effectiveness that is dependent on the reduction-oxidation potential, the "oxidant" action of free radicals. Such a power is due to the property of the components of the barrier to give "reducing equivalents" (e.g., electrons or hydrogen atoms) to the oxidant species, thus avoiding their elimination by such reactive species from essential biochemical components and hence prevention of the triggering of dangerous chain reactions. From a methodological point of view, starting with the concept that the simplest oxidation existing in the natural world is the change of iron from a ferrous to ferric form as in the generation of the rust, one can consider as antioxidant a solution, such as blood plasma, which is able to bring back iron from its ferric to ferrous form. It is on this basis that Mauro Carratelli developed the BAP test. The BAP test is used to measure the biological antioxidant potential and is a photometric test that can be performed in a laboratory. It allows for the substantial measuring of the blood concentration of antioxidants as agents able to reduce iron from its ferric (Fe^{3+}) to ferrous form (Fe^{2+}). At the moment, there are no data available on antioxidants detected and quantified by the BAP test for comparison with data derived from other tests measuring the ability of serum/plasma to reduce transition metals (e.g., FRAP and CuRAP assays). The BAP test provides a global measurement of many antioxidants, including uric acid, ascorbic acid, proteins, a-tocopherol, bilirubin, and so on. In other words, as with other tests for the measurement of antioxidant status (e.g., Total Antioxidant Status by Randox, ORAC), the BAP test has not been designed to provide any information about the concentration of a single antioxidant because this information alone is of very limited clinical value. The BAP test was shown to correlate positively and significantly with the FRAP assay; it integrates well with the results of the d-ROMs test, and it can be considered as its "complementary" test.

Progress in understanding the effects of treatment on oxidative damage in human diseases will be greatly facilitated when biomarkers of oxidative damage are routinely included in clinical trials of therapeutic agents. The need for simple, accurate and non-invasive techniques that have rapid throughput is the hallmark of the clinical biochemistry/pathology laboratory.

Who Should Be Tested?

According to the International Observatory of Oxidative Stress, Free Radicals and Antioxidant Systems, it is clear that all healthy people should undergo the d-ROMs test because all individuals are potentially exposed to the risk of producing exaggerated amounts of free radicals. The primary aim of tests is to identify and prevent oxidative stress and its unwanted consequences (early aging, diseases). The tests should be even more systematically performed on all clinically asymptomatic subjects who are exposed for a number of reasons to factors capable of increasing the production of free radicals (e.g., radiations, pollutants, smoke) and/or reducing the clearance of reactive species (e.g., unbalanced diet). In these cases also, the aim of tests is to identify and prevent oxidative stress and its unwanted consequences (early aging, diseases). Moreover, a test to identify the level of oxidative stress should be carried out on all patients with oxidative stress-related diseases (over one hundred) such as Alzheimer's disease, Parkinson's disease, stroke, infarction, Crohn's diseases, rheumatoid arthritis, AIDS, some cancers, accelerated skin aging, etc. In all of these cases, the aims of the tests are to monitor oxidative stress and prevent its consequences, to monitor the efficacy of a specific therapy on the current disease, and importantly, to monitor the efficacy of a specific therapy, in combination with an eventual antioxidant integration to combat the oxidative stress associated with the current disease. On this subject, it must be stressed that many of the above-mentioned diseases have a chronic course, and oxidative stress tends to raise the impact of an additional health risk factor. Therefore, it must be controlled in order to optimize the results of the therapy.

Other Methods Important in the Aging Process

Determination of Glycated Hemoglobin
(*Hemoglobin A1c, Hba$_{1c}$, A1C,* or *Hb$_{1c}$*)

Glycated hemoglobin (glycosylated hemoglobin, *hemoglobin A1c, HbA$_{1c}$, A1C,* or *Hb$_{1c}$*; sometimes also HbA1c) is a form of hemoglobin used primarily to identify the average plasma glucose concentration over prolonged periods of time. It is formed in a non-enzymatic pathway by hemoglobin's normal exposure to high plasma levels of glucose. A buildup of glycated hemoglobin within the red cell, therefore, reflects the average level of glucose to which the cell has been exposed during its life cycle. Measuring glycated hemoglobin assesses the effectiveness of therapy by monitoring long-term serum glucose regulation. The HbA$_{1c}$ level is proportional to average blood glucose concentration over the previous four weeks to three months.

It can be found out how the body handles carbohydrates by performing the glycated hemoglobin test (a.k.a. HbA1c test). HbA1c test shows how much of your hemoglobin has reacted with glucose and is a good measure of the overall level of glycation and cross-linking in the body. HbA1c also correlates with your average blood sugar level over the threemonths preceding the test. The normal HbA1c range for healthy individuals is 4% to 5.9%. Some experts believe that the values in the lower half of the range are optimal for health and longevity.

Better carbodyrate metabolism can be improved by more exercise, weight reduction, a diet based on low-glycemic foods, blood-sugar lowering supplements and so forth. See also the section concerning glycosylation. There is some way to go until validated precise methods are available for measuring biomarkers of oxidative damage in human subjects in vivo under minimally invasive conditions. With respect to oxidative damage in DNA, HPLC and GC-mass spectrophotometry methods have both merits and limitations. Lipid oxidation products in plasma are best measured as isoprostanes or as lipid hydroperoxides using specific HPLC techniques. Development of isoprostane measurement will advance specificity and precision. The measurement of oxidative damage to proteins has some potential, but such methods have not been effectively exploited (Diplock et al.,1998).

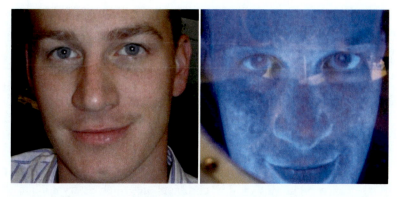

Figure 37. Derma View Skin Analyzer machine points to problem areas of sun-damaged skin. The DermaView utilizes ultraviolet or black light and prints the picture of the face.

Derma View

The DermaView skin analyzer uses harmless black light to locate damage to an individual's skin that cannot necessarily be sees with the naked eye.

Telomere Testing

Age-adjusted telomere length is a method to assess biological age using structural analysis of chromosomal change in the telomere. Telomere Score can be calculated. The calculation is based on the patient's telomere length on white blood cells (T-lymphocytes). This is the average compared to telomere length on lymphocytes from a sample of the American population in the same age range. The higher the telomere score, the "younger" the cells. Serial evaluation of telomere length is an indicator of how rapidly one ages relative to a normal population (www.spectracell.com).

Markers of Skin Aging: Antioxidants and UV-Induced ROS in Skin Equivalent Models

In order to examine the impact and role of UV-induced free radicals in the skin, it is essential to detect and visualize them in a real time. However, due to extremely short-lived nature of free radicals, this is very difficult. Several techniques were developed for assessing skin damages in human skin equivalent models (Date and Hakozaki 2010). Several evaluation methods such as chemiluminescence probe, photon emission detection, and fluorescence detection have been developed. With the use of a combination of a human skin equivalent model and 8-OHdG immunohistochemistry, Toyokuni et al. (2006) examined the effect of pre-treatment of several antioxidants. UVB-induced DNA modification in a skin equivalent model was evaluated by utilizing produced 8-OHdG level as a biomarker. The formation of 8-OHdG was effectively suppressed by the pre-treatment of antioxidative compounds ascorbate, β-carotene and Cu, Zn-superoxide dismutase. Date et al. (2006) used electron spin resonance technique to detect ROS in a human skin equivalent model. Authors tested the application of the antioxidants known to scavenge specific ROS such as mannitol (OH˙) scavenger, SOD (O2˙-) scavenger, ascorbate (O2˙-, OH˙ and 1O2 scavenger), β-carotene (1O2 quencher). The results showed diminishing of the ESR signal of DMPO-OH (to detect O2˙- and OH˙) by mannitol, SOD, as well as suppression of the ESR signal of TMPD-1O2) to detect 1O2 by β-carotene. Chemiluminescent technique to detect or visualize ROS in a human skin-equivalent modelwas also used by Date et al. (2006). Authors tested antioxidative compounds ascorbate, β-carotene, SOD and yeast ferment filtrate. All tested antioxidants greatly reduced UVB-induced chemiluminescent intensities immediately after the measurement. The fluorescence of tryptophan and collagen cross-links in the dermal matrix may serve as in vivo markers of skin aging, photoaging, and as a way of assessing exposure to UVA radiation (Tian et al., 2001). The fluorescence properties of skin chromophores such as tryptophan and collagen cross-links might be useful markers of aging and photoaging.

As the fluorescence of pepsin-digestible collagen cross-links was found to increase with aging and decrease with photoaging, authors investigated the characteristics of this dependence. Several groups of hairless mice were followed over a period of 18 months to document changes in skin fluorescence with aging. Other groups of animals were exposed to either broad-band or narrow-band ultraviolet A radiation to determine the effects of ultraviolet A exposure on the fluorescence of the dermal collagen cross-links and to determine an action spectrum for the induced changes. Authors found that the intensity of pepsin-digestible collagen cross-links in vivo increases linearly with age and that the fluorescence of epidermal tryptophan decreases linearly with age.

Authors also found that the fluorescence of pepsin-digestible collagen cross-links decreases immediately following exposure to ultraviolet A, whereas epidermal tryptophan fluorescence increases. Both changes were dosedependent, but the increase in tryptophan fluorescence occurred exclusively in young animals (two to six mo old). Authors foundout that the ultraviolet-induced fluorescence decrease of pepsin-digestible collagen cross-links is wavelength-specific. The results seem to indicate that in vivo fluorescence of epidermal tryptophan moieties and collagen cross-links in the dermal matrix may serve as markers for skin aging, photoaging and for immediate assessment of exposure to ultraviolet A radiation.

Cyclic Voltammetry

Cyclic voltammetry is proposed as a new method for evaluating the antioxidant capacity of skin based on the reducing properties of lowmolecularweight antioxidants. Ruffien-Cizsak et al. (2006) reported that their experiments using cyclic voltammetry were performed simply by recording the anodic current at 0.9 V/SCE of a platinum microelectrode placed directly on the epidermis surface without any gel or water.

This method ensured a direct, rapid (less than one min), reliable (accuracy 12%) and non-invasive measurement of the global antioxidant capacity of the stratum corneum with a high spatiotemporal resolution (Ruffien-Ciszak et al., 2005).

The cyclic voltammetry was also used to investigate a potential test method to monitor changes through possible degradation of a collagen/glycosaminoglycan tissue-engineering scaffold in vitro (Ismail et al., 2007). Cyclic voltammetry and linear sweep voltammetry were additionally used in order to evaluate the global antioxidant properties of dermocosmetic creams (Guitton et al., 2005).

Skin releases low molecular weight antioxidants (LMWA) from its epidermal layers. Cyclic voltammetry measurements have shown that rat skin releases three major groups of reducing antioxidants at peak potentials of 476 and 889 and 1,044 mV, while human skin releases two major groups at peak potentials of 779 and 1,068 mV.

In rats, the overall concentrations of the LMWA secreted decreased significantly with age. The major components of the LMWA composing the first anodic wave in rats were identified as uric acid and ascorbic acid. Uric acid and other as yet uncharacterized LMWA, but not ascorbic acid, were released in human skin (Cohen et al., 2004).

Important aspects of skin aging that can be addressed include also skin hydration, barrier, matrix, pigmentation and skin antioxidant capacity (Osburne et al., 2009). Other markers of oxidative stress and damage thatcould be used on skin cells for direct and indirect estimation of skin aging and /or damage:

Marker of oxidative stress or Type of Damage

the ratio of reduced glutathione (GSH) versus its oxidized form (GSSG); free radical formation through the colorimeter thiobarbituric acid method and more specific by spin trapping agents and electron spin resonance measurements of the stable adducts formed;
DNA/RNA Damage
8-hydroxyguanosine (8-OHG)
8-hydroxydeoxyguanosine (8-OHdG)
Abasic (AP) sites
Double-strand DNA breaks
Comet Assay (general DNA damage)
Lipid Peroxidation
4-Hydroxynonenal (4-HNE)
Malondialdehyde (MDA)
8-iso-Prostaglandin F2alpha (8-isoprostane)
Oxidative Protein Damage
Protein Carbonyl Content (PCC)
3-Nitrotyrosine
Advanced Glycation End Products (AGE)
Advanced Oxidation Protein Products (AOPP)
Reactive Oxygen Species
Universal ROS
Hydrogen Peroxide
Antioxidants
Catalase
Superoxide Dismutase
Oxygen Radical Antioxidant Capacity (ORAC)
Hydroxyl Radical Antioxidant Capacity (HORAC)

Chapter 8

Alternative Methods to Decrease Oxidative Stress and Retard the Aging Process

The best evidence that certain compounds or methods decreases oxidative stress and have influence on longevity would be obtained by human trials or epidemiological studies. However, case-control or cohort studies that would investigate human longevity would be performed for 50 or more years to obtain some results. Showing causality requires manipulating an experimental system, but this usually cannot be bone so easily with humans. Until now, many epidemiological studies suggest that substances or behavior may have beneficial effects on longevity or diseases associated with aging. But these studies usually show only correlative and not causative effects between the application of particular substance and longevity (Rockenfeller and Madeo, 2010). On the other hand, just epidemiological studies cannot give a real explanation for the effects on longevity. Explanations of some methods to decrease oxidative stress are just hypothetical since they are based just on biochemical explanations or on tests done on animals, which cannot be directly extrapolated on humans. For this reason, many different approaches and studies as well as the mechanisms of the processes regarding methods and strategies that might decrease oxidative stress in this paragraph will be presented. In the following sections, we discussdifferent processes related to decreasing the oxidative stress of an organism or methods thatwould keep the respiratory chain in skin cells working, in order to avoid electron "jam" and consequently increased free radical production.

The reduction of oxidative stress could be achieved in three levels: by lowering exposure to environmental pollutants (described in detail in chapter entitled "Antioxidant prevention of damage induced by extrinsic factors"), by increasing levels of antioxidants (described in chapter entitled "Exogenous antioxidants: compounds derived from the diet"), or by lowering the generation of oxidative stress by stabilizing mitochondrial energy production and efficiency (discussed in this chapter). Or as Villeponteau (2003) would explain, "stabilizing mitochondria structure and energy efficiency is an obvious target for decreasing oxidative free radicals. This is analogous to making a more fuel-efficient and cleaner-burning gasoline engine that generates far less oxidative pollutants." Decreased oxidative stress of the body could have beneficial influence also on skin cells.

Table 9. Oxidative stress is regulated by ROS formation, antioxidative protection and prevention of ROS generation *

Oxidative stress : Balance between ROS formation and antioxidative protection					
Prevention of ROS generation	ROS generation		ROS damage	Protective system	Protective system
	Endogenous sources	Exogenous (from the environment) sources			
Food that decreases ROS and inflammation	Increased respiration (metabolism)	Ozone, NOx, SOx, PM, tobacco smoke	Air pollution	Damage to DNA	Ascorbic acid, tocopherols, carotens, polyphenolics, other vitamins, vitamin cofactors and minerals, other organic antioxidants	Antioxidants
Caloric restriction					
Avoiding environmental pollution			Damage to membranes		
Regular and moderate exercise	Increased mitochondrial leakage	Cupper, Iron, Chromium, Nickel…	Metals	Damage to proteins	Chelating agents	Metal chelator
Appropriate sleeping habits	inflammation	Ionizing, nonionizing	Radiation	Mutations, cytotoxicity, accelerated aging, impaired immune system, other	DNA repair, elimination of damaged Proteins	Repair system
		Alcohol, pesticides, herbicides	Biocides			
Positive thinking and avoidance of emotional stress	Other	Processed food, other	Other			
Others					

*Source: Poljšak et al. (2011).

Since more and more evidence suggests that antioxidant supplements (although highly recommended by the pharmaceutical industry and taken by many individuals) do not offer sufficient protection against oxidative stress, on the accumulation of oxidative damage, or lead to an increased lifespan, some "alternative" methods to decrease oxidative stress are discussed and explained in the next paragraphs. This chapter was adopted from my book *Decreasing Oxidative Stress and Retarding the Aging Process*, Nova SciencePublishers, 2010. The aim of this chapter is to stimulate the scientific discussion and further research into this matter.

Since the methods described apply for all cells of the human body, they could be useful also to prevent aging of the human skin. Probably the same molecular mechanisms underlying the aging of skin and its appendages, including the pigmentary system, underlie age-dependent degenerative changes of the inner organs and entire organism (Trüeb, 2005). However, it should be taken into consideration the fact that research data on skin cells are lacking.

The Induction of Adaptive Responses to Stress Conditions: The Role of Hormesis Effect as an Example of a Beneficial Type of Stress

The term "hormesis" describes beneficial actions resulting from the response of an organism to a low-intensity stressor. The word hormesis is derived from the Greek word *hormaein*, which means "to excite." The adaptive response to a mild stress induces the organism's ability to maximize metabolic efficiency to cope with a new challenging environment. Evidence strongly suggests that most of stresses under sub-lethal levels can be beneficial for the survival of the organism (Laval, 1988;Wiese et al., 1995). Several things happen during cellular adaptive response: transient growth arrest, and the increase in transcription of stress-related genes, antioxidant defense genes and/or repair enzymes. Stressors can also induce a stress response leading to enhanced somatic maintenance (e.g., via molecular chaperones and detoxification enzymes) and resistance to stress. This response can also cause some resistance to aging, suggesting that some overlap exists between the forms of molecular damage that result from some types of stress and those occurring during aging (Gems and Gartridge, 2008). The anti-aging action of caloric restriction stimulated by mild nutritional deprivation is regarded as a good example of this hormetic phenomenon. Studies have reported the anti-aging and life-prolonging effects of a wide variety of so-called stressors, such as pro-oxidants, aldehydes, caloric restriction, irradiation, UVradiation, heat shock and hypergravity. It should be stressed that the basic concept behind the idea of hormesis is to provoke the intrinsic capability of a body rather than to supply exogenous natural or synthetic antioxidants to try to compensate for age-related decline of physiological activities in the overall maintenance mechanisms of life (Goto et al., 2003).

Stress responses involve sensing and activation of signal transduction pathways that adjust the genomic expression program. The induction of both specific and general stress responses increases cellular resistance to subsequent lethal stress. Early responses result in the post-translational activation of pre-existing defenses, as well as activation of signal-transduction pathways that initiate late responses, namely the *de novo* synthesis of stress proteins and antioxidant defenses (Figure 38). Both specific and general stress responses are triggered by oxidative challenges as well as represented by exposure to other mild stress (e.g., oxidative stress, osmotic stress, temperature stress, starvation) (Costa and Moradas-Ferreira, 2001).An oxidative stress response is triggered when cells sense an increase of ROS, which may result also from the exposure of cells to low concentrations of oxidants or the decrease of antioxidant defenses. In order to survive, cells induce the antioxidant defenses and other protective factors, such as stress proteins. Finkel and Holbrook (2000) stated that the best strategy to enhance endogenous antioxidant levels may actually be oxidative stress itself, based on the classical physiological concept of hormesis.

The concept of hormesis has gathered a large body of supportive evidence showing that repetitive mild stress exposure has anti-aging effects (Rattan, 2008; *Gems and Partridge, 2008*).Some of the mild stresses used in experimental studies for the application of hormesis in aging research and interventions are heat shock, irradiation, pro-oxidants, hypergravity and food restriction (*Gems and Partridge, 2008;* Le Bourg and Rattan, 2008). The role of antioxidants in the effect of hormesis is not yet clear. Pretreatment with antioxidants can exert a dual role regarding the hormesis effect. Pretreatment with antioxidants can:

I. produce mild oxidative stress resulting in the auto oxidative (e.g., ascorbic acid) production of O_2^- (Paolini et al., 1999), H_2O_2 and OH^- (Clement et al., 2001). Cells usually tolerate such mild stress, which often results in the induction of the synthesis of antioxidant defense systems (e.g., GSH, GPx, SOD) in an attempt to restore the oxidant/antioxidant balance (Halliwell and Gutteridge, 1999). Additionally, the increased DNA damage (e.g., formation of 8-OHdG) might trigger the induction of the DNA repair system (Cooke et al., 1998). Indeed, exposure to a mild stress induced by the pro-oxidative action of antioxidants could evoke an improved resistance to a severe stress (see chapter on pro-oxidative reactions of antioxidants).

II. Hormesis may also be induced by ROS. Free radicals may induce an endogenous response culminating in an increased defense capacity against exogenous radicals (Tapia, 2006). Recent experimental evidence strongly suggests that this is, indeed, the case, and that such induction of endogenous free-radical production extends the lifespan of the model organism. Most importantly, this induction of lifespan is prevented by antioxidants, providing direct evidence that toxic radicals may mitohormetically exert life-extending and health-promoting effects (Schulz, 2007). Since mitochondrial activity had increased in the aforementioned studies, this effect cannot be explained by an excess of free radicals that might mark mitochondria for destruction by lysosomes, and the free radicals act as a signal within the cell indicating which mitochondria are ready for destruction, as proposed by Nick Lane(2006).The underlying mechanism of the process that prevents cellular damage by reactive oxygen species (ROS) was confirmed also in experiments on yeast in the study of Kelley and Ideker (2009).Whether this concept applies to humans remains to be shown, although recent epidemiological findings support the process of mitohormesis and even suggest that some antioxidant supplements may increase disease prevalence in humans (Bjelakovic et al., 2007) (for detailed explanation of the study from Bjelakovic et al. (2007), see chapter on "Should we take antioxidants?").

Caloric restriction (CR) can also work as a hormesis agent. The hormesis hypothesis of caloric restriction (Anderson et al., 2003; Iwasaki et al., 1988; Mattson et al., 2002) states that the underlying mechanism of dietary restriction is the activation of a defense response that evolved to help organisms to cope with the adverse conditions. Dietary restriction is a mild stressthatprovokes a survival response in the organism, which boosts resistance to stress and counteracts the causes of aging. The theory unites previously disparate observations about ROS defenses, apoptosis, metabolic changes, stress resistance, and hormonal changes and is rapidly becoming accepted as the best explanation for the effects of caloric restriction (Sinclair and Howitz, 2006). The work of Yu and Lee (1991), Koizumi et al. (1987) and Chen and Lovry (1989) strongly suggest that food restriction (energetic stress) enhances the overall antioxidant capacity to maintain the optimal status of intracellular environments through the concerted interactions of cellular components to regulate ROS, and membrane stability against peroxidative stress preserved the cytosolic system (Lee and Yu, 1991). While the (mito)hormesis hypothesis of CR was a purely hypothetical concept until late 2007, the recent work by Michael Ristow's group in a worm *Caenorhabditis elegans* suggests that restriction of glucose metabolism extends lifespan primarily by increasing oxidative stress to stimulate the organism into having an ultimately increased resistance to further oxidative stress (Schulz, 2007). Many of the current theories on dietary restriction can be united in the hormesis hypothesis. Hormesis hypothesis of dietary restriction attempts to unite various theories on the proximate causes of aging. To sum up, caloric restriction provokes a mild stress response, causing enhanced cell defenses and metabolic changes, coordinated by the endocrine system. In a similar way, the "xenohormesis hypothesis" suggests that many of the health benefits of dietary phytochemicals, particularly those of secondary metabolites produced by plants under stress, may work because they activate an evolutionary ancient mechanism that allows animals and fungi to pick up on chemical stress signals from plants (Sinclair and Howitz, 2006). Xenohormesis hypothesis claims that organisms have evolved to respond to stress - signaling molecules produced by other species in their environment. In this way, organisms can prepare in advance for a deteriorating environment and/or loss of food supply (Lamming et al., 2004).

Retardation of aging can be achieved with caloric restriction. However, retardation of aging in mice can also be achieved by intermittent fasting without an overall reduction in caloric intake (Anson et al., 2003). Intermittent fasting greatly increases cellular stress resistance to oxidative stress (Duan and Mattson, 1999; Yu and Mattson, 1999; Duan et al., 2001, 2003a), and people will much easier adopt intermittent fasting. More on CR is written in next chapters. Heat and cold can also work as hormesis agents. The study of Rattan et al. (2004) investigated heat-induced hormesis by challenging cells and organisms with mild stress that often results in anti-aging and life-prolonging effects. Thermal stress induces a heat-shock response involving increased expression of heat-shock proteins (chaperonins). These lead to protection against heat-induced molecular damage, particularly partial denaturation of proteins, by promoting the restoration of protein function via molecular chaperone activity. Heat shock proteins (HSPs) help alleviate stress by protecting cellular proteins from being damaged, allowing newly synthesized proteins to fold into a biologically function state despite the stress and targeting proteins that have been damaged beyond repair for degradation. In a series of experimental studies, it was demonstrated that repeated mild heat stress (RMHS) has anti-aging hormetic effects on growth and various cellular and biochemical characteristics of human skin fibroblasts undergoing aging *in vitro*. More on heat shock and chaperons can be read in the following chapter. Exposure of worms and flies to agents or conditions that cause mild biological stress increases lifespan as well as resistance to other, seemingly unrelated stresses, such as low doses of paraquat, aldehydes, irradiation, heat shock, crowding and hypergravity (Sinclair and Howitz, 2006). If induction of stress resistance increases lifespan and hormesis induces stress resistance, then it is expected that hormesis would result in increased lifespan (Gems and Partridge, 2008).

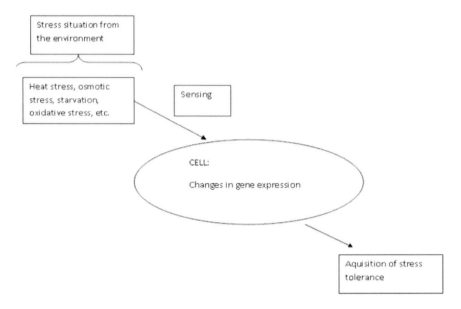

Figure 38. Adaptive responses to stress conditions. Temporary adaptation to oxidative stress in cells was found where cell cultures were exposed to lower levels of oxidant (pre-treatment) before being exposed to lethal doses of the same oxidant.

It can be concluded that stress responses involve sensing and activation of signal transduction pathways that adjust the genomic expression program. The induction of both specific and general stress responses increases cellular resistance to subsequent lethal stress (Costa and Moradas-Ferreira, 2001).

But how can hormesis affect aging process? Healthy aging may be achieved by hormesis through mild and periodic, but not severe or chronic, physical and mental challenges, and by the use of nutritional hormesis incorporating mild stress-inducing molecules (Rattan, 2008). Consideration should be given to strategies that boost host-defense mechanisms that are known to be activated in response to oxidative stress. So far, the best mechanism for boosting such responses seems to be stress itself (Finkel and Holbrook, 2000). As already mentioned, during elevated temperatures, heat shock proteins are formed. Conditions in sauna could also trigger heat shock response and induce HSPs. HSPs would thus not only protect the existing proteins from thermal damage, but they would also tag for disposal all proteins altered by pre-existing unrepaired insults. Sauna therapy may act to increase the amount of the heat shock protein Hsp90, which is induced by even modest heating of mammalian tissues. Sauna therapy has been already used to treat a number of different diseases or to increase health. Also vigorous exercise may induce moderate heat stress; increasing body temperature due to the increased metabolism and heat production of the skeletal muscle tissue might induce HSPs. Endurance training adaptation causes increased efficiency in ATP synthesis at the expense of potential increase in oxidative stress that is likely to be compensated by enhanced activities of antioxidant enzymes (Hollander et al., 1999) and proteasome (Radak et al., 1998). See also paragraph "Exercise and ROS" in this chapter.

Also UVR can induce hormetic effects. When skin is exposed to more UVB radiation than it is accustomed to, it has the ability to adapt. The epidermal layers become thicker, and melanin pigment is formed and dispersed throughout the epidermis. The adaptation of the skin to UVB radiation is effected mainly by hyperplasia, a thickening of the most superficial layer of the skin, the epidermis. In a series of repeated exposures, as given in UVB phototherapy, adaptation typically proceeds by steps of about 20% (Van der Leun, and van Weelden, 1986). This means that with the next exposure, the UV dose required for eliciting an observable reddening of the skin, the "minimal erythema dose" (MED), is increased by about 20%. A calculation shows that about 15 of such exposures are necessary to adapt the skin from its winter condition to the increased UVB irradiance in summer. These reactions limit the effects of subsequent exposures to UVB radiation (Van der Leun et al., 1993).According to van der Leun et al. (1993), the outcome of increased UVB skin exposure is not always an increase of the grossly observable effect. Some effects of UVB radiation on health will indeed increase, some will not be influenced appreciably and some will even decrease in the case of increased UVB irradiance.

Statistics in several countries showed indoor workers to have a higher risk of melanoma than outdoor workers, in contrast to the experience with non-melanoma skin cancer (van der Leun et al., 1993). Does it mean that cutaneous melanomas had nothing to do with sunlight?The fact that outdoor workers have a lower risk than indoor workers is most probably ascribed to adaptation due to the regular exposures. Indoor workers are exposed very little during their work. When they go on a weekend or holiday trip, they may suddenly receive a high dose of UV radiation to which the skin is not adapted (van der Leun et al., 1993).

The study of Kewada et al. (2010) revealed that hairless mice get fewer wrinkles if they spend time in an oxygen chamber after exposure to UVB. Researchers exposed mice to UVB from a fluorescent lamp three times a week for five weeks. After each session, half the mice spent two hours in a hyperbaric chamber on 90 percent oxygen, which increased the amount of oxygen dissolved in their blood. After the trial, the mice on oxygen had fewer wrinkles and less thickening of the epidermis than those who had gone untreated. A number of transcription factors—proteins that bind to specific sections of DNA—play a role in skin damage, including one which responds to low oxygen levels. The team suggests that when skin is exposed to high-pressure oxygen, it interferes with these pathways, decreasing skin damage. This study confirmed the hormesis hypothesis applied on skin where oxygen (although harmful source of free radicals) triggers protective mechanisms of skin defense.

Low oxidative stress induced by pro-oxidative form of vitamin C and hydrogen peroxide could be used as hermetic mechanism. "Indeed, the cellular lifespan of cultivated human skin epidermis keratinocytes NHEK-F was shown to be extended up to 150% of population doubling levels (PDLs) by repetitive addition with two auto-oxidation-resistant derivatives of ascorbic acid (Asc), Asc-2-O-phosphate (Asc2P), and Asc-2-O-alpha-glucoside (Asc2G), respectively, but not to be extended with Asc itself. In contrast, hydrogen peroxide (H(2)O(2)) as dilute as 20 microM, which was non-cytotoxic to the keratinocytes, or at 60 microM being marginally cytotoxic achieved the cellular longevity, unexpectedly, up to 160 and 120% of PDLs, respectively, being regarded as a hormesis-like stimulatory effect"

(Yokoo et al., 2004). "The PDL-dependent shortening of telomeric DNA of 11.5 kb finally down to 9.12 to 8.10 kb upon Hayflick's limit was observed in common for each additive-given cells, but was decelerated in the following order: 20 microM H(2)O(2) > Asc2P = Asc2G > 60 microM H(2)O(2) > Asc = no additive, being in accord with the order of cell longevity. Intracellular reactive oxygen species (ROS) was diminished by Asc2P, Asc2G or 20 microM H(2)O(2), but not significantly by Asc or 60 microM H(2)O(2) as estimated by fluorometry using the redox indicator dye CDCFH. Yokoo et al. suggest that longevity of the keratinocytes is believed to be achieved by slowdown of age-dependent shortening of telomeric DNA rather than by telomerase; telomeres may suffer from less DNA lesions due to the continuous and thorough repression of intracellular ROS, which was realized either by pro-vitamin C such as Asc2P or Asc2G that exerted an antioxidant ability more persistent than Asc itself or by 20 microM H(2)O(2), which diminished intracellular ROS assumedly through a hormesis-like effect" (Yokoo et al., 2004).

Heat-Shock Proteins (Hsps)

The phenomenon of hormesis is represented by mild stress-induced stimulation of maintenance and repair pathways, resulting in beneficial effects for cells and organisms. The term "heat shock" is a residue from their initial discovery in *Drosophila* as a protein family induced in response to hyperthermia (Ashburner and Bonner, 1978).

Virtually all cells—from prokaryotes to highly differentiated mammalian tissues—respond to a sudden increase in temperature with increased production of a limited set of proteins, called heat shock proteins or stress proteins (hsp). All cells, including the prokaryotic microorganisms and the highly differentiated eukaryotic cells in human tissues, contain a small set of normally silent genes that are rapidly activated by a heat shock that raises the temperature only 5% to 10% above that of the normal physiologic range for that organism. Concomitantly, many active genes are turned off. Other stress factors such as alcohol, heavy metals, oxidants (e.g., UV light) and agents leading to protein denaturation are equally able to induce a similar response. Induction of hsp is followed by a transient state of increased resistance to further stress. Many hsp function as "molecular chaperones" by binding to partially folded or misfolded proteins thus preventing their irreversible denaturation during stress exposure (Trautinger et al., 1996). Hsp provide a protective function to cells, allowing them to recover from an inducing stress and survive subsequent stress that could otherwise be lethal. The high observation of the stress response and of genes involved suggests that this adaptive response is critical for the survival of both prokaryotic and eukaryotic organisms subjected to hostile environmental conditions.

The 70 kilodalton heat shock proteins (Hsp70s) are a family of ubiquitously expressed heat shock proteins. Proteins with similar structure exist in virtually all living organisms. The Hsp70s are an important part of the cell's machinery for protein folding and help to protect cells from stress (Tavaria et al., 1996; Morano 2007). Various stressors, including UV light, induce heat shock proteins (HSPs) and the induction, particularly that of HSP70, provides cellular resistance to such stressors. The anti-inflammatory activity of HSP70, such as its inhibition of nuclear factor kappa B (NF-kappaB), was recently revealed (Matsuda et al., 2010).

If oxidized proteins cannot be repaired, they are degraded. Within the cell, the proteasome is responsible for the degradation of oxidized proteins. Damaged proteins in the epidermis can be degraded by the proteasome system, provided that aggregation has not gone too far. Proteasome activity seems to decline with age, perhaps contributing to the photoaging phenomenon (Halliwell and Gutteridge, 2007).

In *C. elegans*, brief thermal stress sufficient to induce thermotolerance also causes small but statistically significant increases in lifespan (Lithgow et al., 1995). Significantly, the dose-response relationships for thermotolerance and longevity are very similar (Cypser and Johnson, 2002); furthermore, in *C. elegans* populations subjected to mild heat stress, expression levels of the small heat-shock protein gene hsp-16 in individual worms are predictive of both thermotolerance and lifespan (Wu et al., 2006). These beneficial effects of a repeated stress challenge include the maintenance of stress protein profile, reduction in the accumulation of oxidatively and glycoxidatively damaged proteins, stimulation of proteasomal activities for the degradation of abnormal proteins, improved cellular resistance to other stresses, and enhanced levels of cellular antioxidant ability. These results further support the view that increased stress resistance causes increased lifespan. Over-expression of certain HSPs in the mitochondria can significantly extend the longevity of normal-lived animals (Aikagi et al., 2003; Kurapati et al., 2000; Morrow et al., 2004).

Hormesis, Hsps and the skin

The expression of heat shock proteins (Hsp) is induced in all cells by exposure to heat and other environmental stress, and Hsp can protect cells from damage through further exposure. Hsp are highly conserved, and it is likely that they are essential for survival in a potentially harmful environment. In human epidermis, Hsp are associated with differentiation, photoprotection, and skin disease (Jonak et al., 2009). The high evolutionary conservation of this reaction suggests its importance for the survival of cells and tissues under hostile environment conditions. Ultraviolet radiation (UV) exerts many potentially harmful effects on prokaryotic and eukaryotic cells, and Hsp may help the cell to cope with UV-induced damage.

Since the balance of antioxidant molecules in cells and tissue is altered following UVR, it may be this effect along with increased levels of lipid oxidation that acts as a signal for activation of other cellular processes. These include general signs of oxidative stress such as the alteration of heat shock proteins, heme oxygenase, ferritin, and other proteins that may help the cell to combat free radical presence (Laurent-Applegate and Schwarzkopf 2001).

Based on a series of experimental studies, the team of Rattan et al. (2004) has reported that repeated mild heat stress (RMHS) has anti-aging hormetic effects on growth and various cellular and biochemical characteristics of human skin fibroblasts and keratinocytes undergoing aging in vitro.

The effects of repetitive mild heat shock (e.g., 30 min, 41 degrees C or 41 degrees C heat shock for oneh twice a week) on growth and various cellular and biochemical characteristics of human skin fibroblasts undergoing aging in vitro were analyzed. Human skin cells maintained several characteristics of young cells until late in life. Whereas the growth rates, population doubling rates, and cumulative population doubling levels achieved in vitro remained unaffected, age-related changes in cellular morphology, cell size, cytoskeletal organization, autofluorescence and neutral beta-galactosidase activity were significantly slowed down by repeated mild heat shock. Hormetic effects of repeated mild heat stress include the maintenance of the stress protein profile, reduction in the accumulation of oxidatively and glycoxidatively damaged proteins, stimulation of the activities of the proteasome and its 11S activator, improvement in cellular resistance to ethanol, hydrogen peroxide, and ultraviolet rays, and increased antioxidative activity of the cells (Rattan, 2004).Additionally, RMHS given to human cells increased the basal levels of various chaperones, reduced the accumulation of damaged proteins, stimulated proteasomal activities, enhanced the levels of various antioxidant enzymes, enhanced the activity and amounts of sodium-potassium pump, and increased the phosphorylation-mediated activities of various stress kinases (Rattan, 2009).

Results from Rattan show that the slower accumulation of damaged proteins in fibroblasts exposed to repeated mild heat shock (RMHS) results partly from the increased ability of these cells to cope with oxidative stressand to synthesize HSP responsible for protein capping and refolding. The basal concentration of reduced glutathione was higher and that of oxidized glutathione was lower in RMHS cells. Whereas the basal level of heat shock protein HSP27 decreased in both RMHS and control cells during serial passaging, the increase of the basal level of HSP70 with increasing passage level was significantly higher in RMHS cells (Verbeke et al., 2001). Additionally, Fonager et al. (2002) investigated if RMHS treatment affected the basal levels of four major stress proteins Hsp27, 70, 90 and Hsc70. The basal levels of Hsp27, Hsc70, and Hsp70 increased significantly in late passage senescent cells, which is indicative of an adaptive response to cumulative intracellular stress during aging. RMHS increased the levels of these Hsp even in early passage young cells and were maintained high throughout their replicative lifespan. Again, these alterations were accompanied by an improved functional and survival ability of the cells in terms of increased proteasomal activities, increased ability to decompose $H(2)O(2)$, reduced accumulation of lipofuscin and enhanced resistance to ethanol, $H(2)O(2)$ and UVA radiation (Foneger et al., 2002).

Rattan et al. (2009) have recently observed novel hormetic effects of mild heat stress on improving the wound-healing capacity of skin fibroblasts and on enhancing the angiogenic ability of endothelial cells. Rattan et al. (2009) also tested potential hormetins, such as curcumin and rosmarinic acid, in bringing about their beneficial effects in human cells by inducing stress-response pathways involving heat shock proteins and hemeoxygenase HO-1. Results from the Rattan studies indicate that mild stress-induced hormesis can be a useful approach for the modulation, intervention, and prevention of skin aging and age-related impairments.

Hsp have been detected in resting as well as stress-exposed epidermal and dermal cells and experimental evidence points to the fact that these proteins mediate protection from UV-induced cell death in vitro and in vivo. Experimental studies further indicate that UV itself might be able to induce the expression of specific hsp. Thus, hsp might provide an adaptive cellular response to increasing exposure to UV (Trautinger et al., 1996).

In cultured human skin fibroblasts, UVA induces "heat-shock" proteins, including heam oxygenase-1 (Hsp32), co-upregulated with ferritin. Keratinocytes are unusual in expressing Hsp72 constitutively, although levels rise under UV light. By contrast, keratinocytes have higher basal levels of haem oxygenase (HO-2) but little inducible (HO-1) activity. This may be explained by the fact that considerable UV radiation reaches the keratinocytes at the base of the epidermis, whereas higher exposures are needed to reach the dermal fibroblasts (Halliwell and Gutteridge, 1993).

In a human in vivo study, immunohistochemical results have shown a dose- and wavelength-dependentperturbation of SOD and Hsp70 following a single irradiation with artificial UV light sources of skin that is not sun exposed in normal life. The most prominent antioxidant depletion was seen resulting from irradiation with UVA I light. Biologically equivalent doses of UVA I II (with regard to erythema induction) also lead to depletion of SOD and Hsp70, but less than UVA I, whereas solar UV-simulating light only provokeda weak antioxidant depletion (Laurent-Applegate and Schwarzkopf,2001).

Although molecular mechanisms of hormesis are yet to be elucidated, there are indications that relatively small hormetic effects become biologically amplified, resulting in significant improvement of cellular and organic functions and survival. Hormesis, therefore, can be an effective approach for modulating aging, for preventing or delaying the onset of age-related diseases, and for improving the quality of life in old age (Rattan, 2004). A prerequisite for the utilization of the hormesis effect and HSPs is the development of the nontoxic HSP inducers and their evaluation for clinical efficacy and safety.

The idea of hormesis deserves future study in the oxidative stress theory of aging as well as on the skin damage and aging process. There still remains the answer to the following questions: "Are the best antioxidants poisons? Is a little of something bad actually good for us?"

Mild stress-induced hormesis can be an effective way for reducing the accumulation of molecular damage and thus slowing down aging from within. Cell death induced by ultraviolet radiation (UV) can be inhibited by previous heat shock, and UV itself can induce Hsp experimentally. Regulation of Hsp can be pharmacologically modified, and topical and systemic inducers and inhibitors of Hsp expression are under development. Whether phototherapy exerts its clinical efficacy by modulation of Hsp has not been sufficiently studied. The UV-wavelength ranges, intensities and doses that are required to interfere with the heat shock response in the skin still remain to be elucidated (Jonak et al., 2009). Since hsps might provide an adaptive cellular response to increasing UV and enhancing the expression of hsps might turn out as a new way to deal with the immediate and long-term consequences of UV exposure, prerequisite for the utilization of this concept is the development of non-toxic heat shock inducers and their evaluation for clinical efficacy and safety.

Caloric Restriction and Reactive Oxygen Species

The first results of experiments conducted on the impact of caloric restriction (CR) on longer lifespan were published in 1935, by McCay and his collaborators (McCay et al., 1935). Many other researchers have later confirmed these findings with experiments on different prokaryotic organisms (Yu, 1982, 1985; Walford et al., 1986; Bartke et al., 2001; Bodkin et al., 2003; Mattson et al., 2003; Houthoofd et al., 2003; Ishii et al., 2003; Li et al., 2003). Later it was found out that retardation of aging can also be achieved by intermittent fasting without an overall reduction of caloric intake (Gredilla et al., 2001; Anson et al., 2003). "Caloric restriction is the only experimental manipulation that considerably increases both mean and maximum lifespan in a phylogenetically wide variety of animals" (Gredilla and Barja, 2003).

Additionally, many studies have been performed concerning the positive effect of caloric restriction on health (Roe, 1981; Masoro, 1993; Ramsey, 2000, Lane et al., 2000; Mattson, 2000). Although not all types of prokaryotic and eukaryotic organisms have been used in these experiments, it can be asserted with a large degree of certainty that caloric restriction has similar effects on all animals.

It is well established that CR increases both mean and maximum lifespan in laboratory animals (Wendruch and Sohal, 1997). It has been shown during the last two decades that caloric restriction reduces the mitochondrial production of free radicals (as the most important internal source of reactive oxygen species) and enhances the repair defense of organisms (Halliwell and Gutteridge, 2005). Oxidative damage is reduced most probably due to a decreased metabolic rate, although no alterations in mitochondrial oxygen consumption have been found (Gredilla and Barja, 2003). However, Heilbronn et al. (2006) showed that caloric restriction induced a decrease of energy production in humans, although there was no unequivocal effect on markers of oxidative stress. A growing body of evidence supports the hypothesis that CR with no malnutrition and an adequate mineral intake also works by decreasing oxidative stress (Sohal and Weindruch, 1996; Gredilla et al., 2001). A leading hypothesis concerning the mechanism through which CR prevents aging asserts that this process decreases the generation of reactive oxygen species (ROS) and hence the oxidation of cellular components (Herman, 1993, Merry, 2004; Sohal, 2002, Barja, 2002). CR promotes a metabolic shift resulting in more efficient electron transport in the mitochondrial respiratory chain (Weindruch et al., 1996; Sohal, 1996). Faster and more efficient electron transport may lead to a lower production of ROS by mitochondria, one of the major intracellular ROS sources. This occurs because of reduced leakage of electrons from the respiratory chain and/or lower oxygen concentrations in the mitochondrial microenvironment (Korshunov, 1997; Starkov, 1997). One hypothesis regarding the mechanisms whereby CR extends life is that dietary restriction decreases free-radical production in mitochondria as a result of the decreased "burning" of glucose (Sohal and Weindruch, 1996). It was reported that long-term CR led to a 45% decrease in the rate of mitochondrial H_2O_2 generation and 30% decrease in oxidative damage to mtDNA in the rat heart (Gredilla et al., 2001b), and a 28% reduction in the rate of mitochondrial ROS generation and 30% decrease in oxidative damage to mtDNA in rat skeletal muscle (Drew et al., 2003). Furthermore, when rats or mice are maintained on a meal-skipping dietary restriction regimen, the expression of the two major classes of cytoprotective genes are increased in brain cells, namely, growth factors and protein chaperones (Lee et al., 2000c,b; Duan et al., 2001; Duan and Mattson, 1999; Yu and Mattson, 1999). Growth factor protects neurons by inducing the expression of genes that encode proteins that suppress oxidative stress and stabilize calcium homeostasis (Mattson and Lindvall, 1997). Work on the genetics of aging in yeasts, *C. elegans, Drosophila*, and rodents suggests that caloric restriction might act through conserved signaling pathways to control eukaryotic longevity in response to environmental conditions (Kenyon, 2001).

The results of various studies do not support the view that induction of antioxidant enzymes occur in CR animals. Although CR animals produce fewer free radicals, their metabolic rates (oxygen consumption per gram of tissue) arenot reduced. A main causal factor pertaining to the reduction of oxidative stress in animals subjected to continued CR relates to a decrease in mitochondrial free radical generation. Reduced ROS production in isolated functional mitochondria has been reported for the heart, brain and kidney of mice (Sohal et al., 1994).

In rodents, caloric restriction slows aging and extends lifespan. At least four studies have shown that caloric restriction reduces 8-OHdG damage in various organs of rodents. One of these studies (Hamilton et al., 2001) showed that caloric restriction reduced accumulation of 8-OHdG with age in the rat brain, heart and skeletal muscle, and in the mouse brain, heart, kidney and liver. Wolf et al. (2005) showed that dietary restriction reduced accumulation of 8-OHdG with age in the rat brain, heart, skeletal muscle and liver. Reduction of oxidative DNA damage is, therefore, associated with a slower rate of aging and an increased lifespan.

The normal level of caloric intake (without intermittent fasting), therefore, produces too many toxins for an optimal level of health and longevity. The problem is that the ingestion of a normal quantity of calories has a different effect on reproductive function than on longevity. The findings of experiments on caloric reduction corroborate this thesis. Tests performed on different species ranging from unicellular organisms to primates have shown that a reduction of 30% to 50% of caloric intake (whilst retaining the intake of essential nutrients) extends lifespan by about 30% to 50%, while also improving the health of the organism (Gredilla and Barja, 2003). On the other hand, reduction of caloric intake reduces fertility and causes a retardation of sexual maturation (Gredilla and Barja, 2003; Missirlis, 2003).

Therefore, eating enough from the point of view of health and longevity is in evident contradiction with eating enough from a reproductive point of view. In the case of aging as a biological function, the caloric restriction effect may well be an example of the aging function being modulated in order to optimize the organism's lifespan in response to external conditions. Temporary extension of lifespan under famine conditions would be beneficial for group survival because extending lifespan in combination with less-frequent reproduction would prolong the resources required to maintain a given population.

The fact that animals that are severely short of food increase their investment in cellular maintenance functions is at first sight puzzling, particularly since one of the leading physiological explanations of aging, the disposable soma theory (according to disposable soma theory, aging results from and is controlled by the metabolic allocation of the organism's metabolic resources to maintenance and repair—Kirkwood, 1977) suggests that aging occurs because natural selection favors a strategy in which investments in somatic maintenance are limited in order to spare precious resources for growth and reproduction. Thus the fact that food-restricted rodentsupregulate their maintenance seems at first sight counterintuitive. A suggestion to resolve this paradox (suggested by Kirkwood and Mathers, 2009) is that the primary role of the food-restriction response is to shift resources away from reproduction during periods of famine—when the likelihood of reproductive success is small—and to invest as much of the resultant saving as possible into increased somatic maintenance. The potential benefit is that the animal gains an increased chance of survival with a reduced intrinsic rate of senescence, thereby permitting reproductive value to be preserved for when the famine is over (Harrison and Archer, 1989; Holliday, 1989; Phelan and Austad, 1989).

In rodent models, calorie restriction with adequate nutrient intake decreases the risk of developing chronic disease and extends maximum lifespan. It is not yet known whether caloric restriction affects primary aging and extends maximum lifespan in long-lived mammals (Fontana and Klein, 2007). Nonetheless, the data currently available from ongoing studies have shown that many of the metabolic, hormonal, anti-inflammatory, and body-compositional changes that occur in calorie-restricted rodents also occur in calorie-restricted monkeys (Fontana and Klein, 2007). Caloric restriction in adult men and women causes beneficial metabolic, hormonal, and functional changes, but the precise amount of calorie intake or body fat mass associated with optimal health and maximum longevity in humans is not known (Fontana and Klein, 2007). On the other hand, excessive calorie restriction might cause malnutrition and could have adverse clinical effects. In addition, it is possible that even moderate calorie restriction may be harmful in specific patient populations, such as lean persons who have minimal amounts of body fat (Fontana and Klein, 2007). It is not possible to determine a safe threshold of calorie restriction for all persons because of the influence of many different factors, such as initial body composition, daily energy expenditure, and duration of calorie restriction (Fontana and Klein, 2007). The World Health Organization (WHO, 2000), the National Institutes of Health (NIH, 1998), and other bodies (e.g., U.S. Department of Health and Human Services. *Healthy People,* (2010))has proposed that a body mass index (BMI) between 18.5 to 24.9 is normal, because BMI values below or above this range increase the risk for premature mortality. Besides, BMI predicts mortality in different ways; obesity is a risk factor for mortality at age 60, but leanness is a risk factor for mortality at age 80.

Several laboratories have been instrumental in addressing the question of whether dietary restriction effect is due to the total reduction in food intake or the lack of the specific component (Sinclair and Howitz, 2006). Yu and colleagues found that dietary-restricted animals consume about the same total number of calories during their lifespans as *ad libitum* fed animals (36,000 Kcal), leading to speculation that life might be related to the total number of calories consumed per rat per lifetime (Yu et al., 1985). Neither the restriction of minerals nor fat affected lifespan (Iwasaki et al., 1988). A surprising finding has been found that severe restriction of a single amino acid, methionine, is sufficient to extend rat lifespan (Orentreich et al., 1993; Richie et al., 1994). Thus, the important determinant of longevity is not necessarily the restriction of calories, but rather any nutrient deficiency that can invoke a survival response (Braeckman et al., 2001; Lamming et al., 2004; Turturro et al., 2000) as predicted by the hormesis hypothesis of dietary restriction.

It is difficult to determine whether calorie restriction has beneficial effects on longevity in humans because there are no validated biomarkers that can serve as surrogate markers of aging, and because it is impractical to conduct randomized, diet-controlled, long-term survival studies in humans (Johnson, 2006). Nonetheless, data from epidemiologic studies suggest that calorie restriction can have beneficial effects on the factors involved in the pathogenesis of primary and secondary aging and life expectancy in humans (Fontana and Klein, 2007). Food shortages during World War II in some European countries were associated with a sharp decrease in coronary heart disease mortality, which increased again after the war ended (Strom and Jensen, 1951; Hindhede, 1921). In addition, inhabitants of Okinawa island, who ate 30% fewer calories than average Japanese residents, had 35% lower rates of cardiovascular disease and cancer mortality than the average Japanese population and had one of the highest numbers of centenarians in the world (Kagawa, 1978). However, these associations do not prove causality between decreased calorie intake and increased survival (Fontana and Klein, 2007). Despite many similarities in the metabolic adaptation to calorie restriction observed in rodents and humans, it is not known if such restriction affects maximum lifespan in humans. In fact, it has been proposed by some scientists that calorie restriction can only minimally extend maximum lifespan in human and nonhuman primates because of differences in "metabolic stability," "evolutionary entropy," and "dietary reaction norms" between species (Demetrius, 2006; Phelan and Rose, 2006).

Willcox and co-authors in their article (2006) discussed the question "Should we restrict our calories?" First, they presented some scientists who studied the mechanisms of aging and suggested that it is unlikely that the maximum lifespan of humans can be extended by any intervention, including caloric restriction (Hayflick, 2004). It has also been argued that while CR is likely to be almost universal in its beneficial effects on longevity, the benefit to humans is likely to be small, even if humans restrict their caloric intake substantially and over long periods of time (Phelan and Rose, 2005). The latter argument derives from observations of complex differences between species (such as amount of energy allocated to reproduction) and the fact that underlying physiological mechanisms that determine longevity are not necessarily the same between species. Some authors warn that there are potential health concerns, particularly if practiced incorrectly (too severe) or at vulnerable (too young, too old, pregnancy) life stages (Le Bourg, 2005; Dirks and Leeuwenburgh, 2006). On the other hand, Willcox and co-authors (2006), while fully acknowledging that the nature of the life-extending action of CR may differ among species, believe these views to be overly pessimistic and not reflective of the available evidence. Especially cautious approaches to lowering calories (mild CR) among adults while maintaining optimal nutrient intakes would still likely result in significant health benefits. In fact, findings show that even 8% CR has beneficial effects on specific biochemical and inflammatory biomarkers (Dirks and Leeuwenburgh, 2006). Furthermore, Willcox and co-authors (2006) provide the following reasons for a more optimistic view of the potential benefits of the CR lifestyle for human beings: "First, the accumulated evidence of 70 years of CR studies suggests that CR is an extremely ancient and very important survival mechanism that appeared early in the evolution of eukaryotes. Therefore, it appears to be strongly conserved throughout the phylogenetic scale (from yeast to mammals). As such, it would be unusual if it did not work in some positive capacity in humans as well. Second, studies in progress with non-human primates (who share over 95% of our genes and have similar reproductive physiology) on a CR regimen, while not yet conclusive, are showing early results consistent with previous animal data. Third, short-term and longer-term studies of humans under a true CR paradigm have shown dramatic changes in physiology and metabolic shifts similar to other animals." Fourth, research of Willcox team shows that older Okinawans (ages 65 plus) exhibit a CR-like phenotype and ate a low calorie diet over a prolonged period of time (Willcox et al., 2006). The available data support the notion that calorie restriction with adequate nutrient intake in humans causes many of the same metabolic adaptations and reduction of multiple chronic disease risk factors that occur in calorie-restricted animal models, even when restriction is started in midlife. Therefore, even if calorie restriction does not prolong maximum lifespan, it could increase life expectancy and the quality of late life by reducing the burden of chronic disease (Fontana and Klein, 2007). Interestingly, all human cultures advise regular periods of fasting for both religious and nonreligious reasons (Levine, 2008). Thus, fasting may have conferred a selective advantage over non-fasting populations.

In examining calorie restriction with optimal nutrition, it is observed that with less food and an equal nutritional value, there is a higher ratio of nutrients to calories. This may lead to more ideal essential and beneficial nutrient levels in the body. Many nutrients can exist at levels exceeding those needed by the organism, without sideeffects as long as they are in balance and not beyond the body's ability to store and circulate these nutrients. Many nutrients serve as antioxidants and will be at higher levels in the body because there will be lower levels of free radicals due to the lower food intake. As already mentioned, when food availability is low, the cells of the organism are faced with an energetic stress that may induce changes in gene expression that result in adaptive changes in cellular metabolism and an increased ability of the organism to resist stress (Mattson et al., 2003). Many of the effects of calorie restriction are likely mediated by regulating gene expression through (1) upregulation of genes involved in cellular repair and survival, stress resistance, and protection against oxidative damage; (2) downregulation of genes involved in mediating inflammation; and (3) prevention of some changes in gene expression that occur with aging (Dhahbi et al., 2004; Sreekumar et al., 2002; Higami et al., 2004; Park and Prolla, 2005). CR not only upregulate antioxidant defenses and attenuate the formation of ROS but also improve the tissue's ability to remove defective cells by upregulating the incidence of apoptosis. There are some studies thatexamined the role of CR on skin cells.

Thomas (2005) investigated in Fischer 344 rats the effect of CR on age-related histomorphologic features of skin. Rats showed many age-related skin changes, and these were prevented or delayed by the calorie restriction. A recent study in SENCAR mice also confirms that calorie restriction may have beneficial effect on skin aging by inhibiting gene expression in skin tissues relevant to cancer risk (Lu et al. 2007). By reducing the levels of ROS and AGEs formation, CR can have beneficial effect on aging skin.

It is likely that CR could have beneficial effects also on skin aging. Today, there is still lack of data on skin cells and CR. Further studies on validated markers of skin aging should be performed on CR-restricted humans in the future.

The fact that the rate of aging can be significantly slowed by applying an environmental or nutritional intervention such as calorie restriction shows that significant changes in the aging process can be brought about by lifestyle or other nongenetic manipulations. One of them could be CR. However, the question rises whether people are willing to lower the calorie intake in their diets?

Calorie Restriction Mimetics

Since long-term CR is extremely difficult to maintain, the solution could be provided by CR mimetics. Drug companies are currently searching for ways to mimic the lifespan-extending effects of calorie restriction (CR) without having to severely reduce food consumption. Calorie restriction mimetics are agents or strategies that can mimic the beneficial health-promoting and anti-aging effects of CR, the only intervention conclusively shown to slow aging and maintain health and vitality across the phylogenetic spectrum. One such effort is an attempt to find a "mimetic" that would mimic the anti-aging effect of calorie restriction without having to actually radically restrict diet (Chen and Guarente, 2007).

Calorie-restriction mimetics were reviewed by Fontana and Klein (2007). Also, Fontana and Klein believe that even if calorie restriction is shown to increase life expectancy and maximum lifespan in humans, it is unlikely that such restriction will be widely adopted because of the difficulty in maintaining long-term calorie restriction (i.e., low calorie intake) in modern society. Therefore, there has been an increased interest in developing pharmacological agents that act as "calorie-restriction mimetics." Such agents could provide the beneficial metabolic, hormonal, and physiological effects of calorie restriction without having to alter dietary intake or experience any potential adverse consequences of excessive restriction. Several compounds have been proposedas potential calorie-restriction mimetics, such as plant-derived polyphenolic molecules (e.g., resveratrol, quercetin, butein, piceatannol), insulin-action enhancers (e.g., metformin), or pharmacological agents that inhibit glycolysis (e.g., 2-deoxyglucose) (Ingram et al., 2006). FDA approved drug 4-phenylbutyrate, which induces a delayed onset of senescence in *Drosophila* by inhibiting certain histone deacetylases and thereby activating various antioxidants and other genes (Lin et al., 1998). Additionally, resveratrol, which is present in grapes, peanuts, and several other plants, is a potent inducer of the s i r t u i n/S i r 2 family of NAD1-dependent deacetylases. *SIRT1*, one of the seven mammalian sirtuin genes, regulates several biological functions, including cell survival, which has led to the theory that sirtuins mediate some of the effects of calorie restriction in mammals (Guarente and Picard, 2005; Baur et al., 2006). All eukaryotes, including plants, encode sirtuins in their genomes (Frye, 2000; Pandey et al., 2002). Treatment with metformin, a biguanide oral hypoglycemic agent, can decrease the risk of developing diabetes in persons with impaired oral glucose tolerance and of developing cancer in patients with diabetes and causes some of the same changes in gene expression observed in calorie-restricted mice. Dietary supplementation with a glycolytic inhibitor, 2-deoxy-D-glucose (2DG), decreases serum glucose and insulin concentrations, resting heart rate, and blood pressure, and improves the response to neuroendocrine stress in rats (Ingram et al., 2006; Wan et al., 2004). However, there are some claims that 2DG might be harmful. Additionally, antioxidants are commonly used as medications to treat various forms of brain injury. The superoxide dismutase mimetics(Warner et al., 2004) sodium thiopental and propofol are used to treat reperfusion injury and traumatic brain injury (Wilson and Gelb, 2002).It was reported that treatment of nematodes with SOD/catalase mimetics extended lifespan by up to 44% (Melov et al., 2000). Also Deprenyl, a monoamine oxydase B inhibitor, is known to upregulate antioxidant enzymes such as SOD and CAT activities in brain, heart, kidneys, adrenal glands and the speen. Several Chinese herb medicines, including Gingseng and ursolic acid, have been shown to increase activities of SOD and CAT in the liver. Studies clearly demonstrate the importance of free radicals in regulating longevity. However, additional studies are needed to determine whether these and other candidate calorie-restriction mimetics actually affect life expectancy in humans.

Calorie restriction could also influence hormones. Many hormonal signals from peripheral tissues contribute to the regulation of energy homeostasis and food intake. These regulators, which include leptin, insulin and ghrelin, modulate orexigenic (having stimulating effect on appetite) and anorexigenic neuropeptide expression in hypothalamic nuclei. As already discussed, the anti-aging effects of calorie restriction have been explained from an evolutionary viewpoint involving the adaptive response of the neuroendocrine and metabolic response systems to maximize survival during periods of food shortage. In organisms, excess energy is stored in adipose tissues as a triglyceride in preparation for food shortage. Adipose tissue has recently been recognized as an endocrine organ, and leptin, as secreted by adipocytes, seems to be an especially important factor for the adaptive response to fasting and neuroendocrine alterations under calorie restriction. Calorie restriction thus has the potential involvement in decreasing the oxidative stress, in longevity and anti-aging effects of skin, as well.

Exercise and Reactive Oxygen Species

It is well known that moderate and regular exercise enhances health and longevity relative to sedentary lifestyles. Exercising is good for our health because it helps to improve the circulation, which optimizes protection of the organism by providing nutrients, gases and metabolites in the body. Obesity increases the risk of mortality and diabetes, which can be partly ameliorated by exercise and diet. During exercise, oxygen consumption can increase by a factor of more than tenfold. This leads to a large increase in the production of oxidants and results in damage that contributes to muscular fatigue during and after exercise. Nevertheless, evidence will be provided that by performing work and exercise, ROS-induced damage could be reduced.

Mitochondrial uncoupling has been proposed as a mechanism that reduces reactive oxygen species production and could account for the paradox between longevity and activity (Camara et al., 2007). When exercising, the heartbeat and oxygen consumption increases. Elevated consumption of O_2 would lead to elevated production of free radicals. This would be consistent with the proposed link between energy metabolism and aging according to the "rate of living hypothesis." Indeed, a single bout of exercise increases metabolism and oxidative stress during and immediately after exercise (Alessio and Goldfarb, 1988; Ji, 1993). But this is not always so. Any factor that influences the propensity of O_2 to interact with ubisemiquinone (Q-) will likely increase free-radical production. Exercise involves a large flux of energy and a shift in substrate metabolism in mitochondria from state 4 to state 3. This shift causes an increase in superoxide production (Barja, 1999). During aerobic exercise, the rapid consumption of ATP leads to use of the proton gradient to make more ATP, increases electron transport to regenerate the proton gradient, increases oxygen consumption, and increases activity of the Krebs cycle and glycolysis to supply high-energy electrons to drive electron transport. Electron transport is restricted by the chemiosmotic gradient, i.e., electron transport can only go as fast as energy is lost from the gradient. Anything that increases the turnover of energy from the gradient increases the rate of electron transport proportionally. Electron transport is stimulated when the ratio of ATP to ADP is reduced. The rate of binding of ADP to ATP synthetase automatically increases as more ADP is transported into the matrix. Uncoupling agents dissipate the chemical gradient, usually by creating a mechanism by which protons can escape the intermembrane space (or otherwise "short out" the gradient), allowing an increase in electron transport. It is well established that while mitochondrial oxygen consumption is strongly enhanced during the energy transition from state 4 to state 3 during mitochondrial respiration, H_2O_2 production does not increase and is even decreased (Herrero and Barja, 1997b; Venditti et al., 1999). This lack of increase in ROS generation can explain why exercise does not shorten rodent (Holloszy et al., 1985) or human (Lee et al., 1995) longevity. In colder regions of the world, a noticeable change in thyroid hormone levels takes place circa-annually, i.e., levels are higher in winter and lower in summer. Mild exercise could also affect electron transport and reduce ROS formation. When cellular energy demand is low, membrane potential is high, proton leak is high and ROS production is elevated. When cellular energy demand is high (e.g., when exercising) membrane potential is somewhat lower, proton leak is very low and ROS production is much lower (Nicholls, 2002; Arking, 2006).

The benefits of exercise may challenge the time-honored "rate of living" hypothesis (Finch, 2007)—if there is a maximum energy production over the lifespan, then greater expenditures should shorten lifespan. Increased utilization of oxygen in mitochondria would enhance the generation of superoxide and hence hydrogen peroxide. In fact, it has been reported that a bout of treadmill exercise increased protein oxidation as measured by the carbonyl content in rat skeletal muscles (Reznick et al., 1992). While a single bout of exercise of sedentary animals is likely to cause increased detrimental oxidative modification of proteins (Reznick et al., 1992), moderate daily exercise appears to be beneficial by reducing thedamage in rat skeletal muscle (Redak et al., 1998). Organisms challenged by an oxidative stress often decrease their rates of metabolism, which presumably would lead to a corresponding decrease in their rates of free radical generation (Allen and Sohal, 1982; Allen et al., 1984).

However, as already explained, within humans and other mammals, many examples show that energy expenditure and food intake can increase to meet demands but without cost to health and longevity (Speakman, 2005). Exercise is a paradigm for hormesis in this respect (Gems and Partridge, 2008).Due to the effect of hormesis, increased O_2 consumption during sporting activity also increases free radical defense systems. For this reason, a person should practice regular, but moderate physical activity. Intense exercise is known to induce oxidative stress due to an excessive oxygen uptake, higher consumption of ATP and excretion of catecholamines that can result in elevated ROS formation in mitochondria and other enzymatic systems (Packer, 1999). The majority of studies investigating exercise and oxidative stress conclude that endogenous antioxidant defense systems are not able to fully defend against ROS produced during high-intensity exercise associated with isometric exercise, weight lifting, sprinting, bicycling, running, and sports play (Alessio,2006). Although, regular or repeated bouts of exercise are associated with lower resting metabolic rate, higher antioxidant activity, and lower oxidation of LDLs and more protection against oxidation of proteins and DNA (Radák et al., 2000; Vasankari et al., 1997). Additionally, the mechanisms of moderate exercise include improved insulin sensitivity and reductions of oxidative stress and inflammation. Although excessively strenuous exercise can generate harmful levels of free radicals, regular endurance exercise protects against free radicals by increasing muscle levels of (SOD), glutathione peroxidase and reduced glutathione (GSH) (Powers et al., 1999). Exercise can increase genes encoding deacetylase enzymes that silence some potentially harmful genes or decrease genes for insulin and insulin-like growth factor (IGF), macrophage inhibitory factor (MIF), interleukin 6 (IL-6), and C-reactive protein (Fischer et al., 2004; Hammett et al., 2004). Moderate exercise can increase prostaglandin synthesis and increasing protein turnover (Alessio et al., 2000). The release of certain prostaglandins may have protective effects, and protein turnover may facilitate removal of cell fragments and synthesis of new proteins (Alessio 2003). Thus, it is important not to overdo any sporting or physical activity, as this will have the opposite effect withregard to free radical generation. Regular exercise is associated not only with enhanced lifespan in men, but also with good health and function during older age (Yates et al., 2008). Regular exerciseinduces adaptive responses, including attenuation of an increase in ROS production, LIPOX level, NF-κB activation and reduced GSH/GSSG ratio, which appear to be capable of reducing increases of ROS damage in aged groups of rats (Radák, 2004). Exercise also reduces the oxidative load in muscle (Goto et al., 2004; Radak et al., 2002). While single bouts of exercise in sedentary animals can transiently increase the load of oxidized proteins and lipids, regular exercise increases the GSH/GSSG ratio and other antioxidant homeostatic responses (Radak et al., 2001; Radak et al., 2004). Young adult humans who were sedentary but not obese responded to regular aerobic exercise with 15% decrease in oxidized LDL and 28% increase in blood glutathione peroxidase by fourmonths (Elosua et al., 2003). Older coronary patients given three months of aerobic training had 50% lower CRP and twofold higher IL-10 (anti-inflammatory cytokine) (Goldhammer et al., 2005). Prolonged exercise also results in changes in UCP-3 levels (mitochondrial uncoupling protein 3 is a protein that in humans is encoded by the *UCP3* gene), first involving an increase (Jones et al., 2003) and later (in endurance training) a substantial decrease (Hesselink and Schrauwen, 2003). Mitochondrial uncoupling proteins (UCP) are members of the larger family of mitochondrial anion carrier proteins (MACP). UCPs separate oxidative phosphorylation from ATP synthesis with energy dissipated as heat, also referred to as the mitochondrial proton leak (for more information on UPC, see chapter on uncoupling). For this reason, extreme sports could be disadvantageous in accordance with the rate of living/free radical hypothesis and UTS hypothesis (Speakman, 2003). When energy is transferred from food to a working muscle, over 70% of the potential energy is released as heat. Exercise is associated with increased core temperature, and heat is known to disrupt electron transfer in mitochondria. This might result in upregulation of heat shock proteins and have protective effects locally.

The evidence for benefits from antioxidant supplementation in vigorous exercise is mixed. It is still a matter of debate whether exogenous antioxidants should be supplemented in physically active individuals. There is strong evidence that one of the adaptations resulting from exercise is a strengthening of the body's antioxidant defenses, particularly the glutathione system, to regulate the increased oxidative stress(Leeuwenburgh et al., 1994).. It is known that oxygen and chemical oxidants stimulate endogenous antioxidant defenses (Halliwell, 1981). To some extent, this effect may be protective against diseases that are associated with oxidative stress, which would provide a partial explanation for the lower incidence of major diseases and better health of those who undertake regular exercise.In humans, as well as lower mammals, exercise is believed to have many anti-aging benefits. Exercise also most probably influences regulatory gene expressions in many tissues over an organism's lifespan. Studies of Goodrick (1980) suggest that both mean and maximum lifespans may be extended by exercise in rats, and the study of Mlekusch (1996) suggests that the lack of exercise in mice accelerated the senescent process. Since exercise results in acute stress even in conditioned athletes, it is possible that some of its benefits are derived from such a stress-tolerance mechanism. Consideration should be given to strategies for boosting host defense mechanisms that are known to be activated in response to oxidative stress.

Exercising has many other health benefits. As we age, we lose muscle mass, and the muscle we retain is weaker. It was observed that resistance exercise stimulates muscle protein synthesis in both the young and elderly. Moderate exercise is associated with reduced incidence of degenerative diseases of aging and, therefore, it is associated with reduced all-cause mortality (Blair and Wei, 2000), improved metabolic syndrome (Lakka et al., 2003) and cardiorespiratory fitness (Dunn et al., 1999: Gibbons et al., 2000). Being physically active in older age may improve blood flow to the brain and reduce the risk of stroke, dementia and cognitive decline. Being active also enhances mood, self-esteem and well-being. Endurance exercise training increases muscle mitochondrial density and oxidative enzyme activity. Molecular characterization of the expression of about 4,727 genes in the skeletal muscles of endurance athletes and sedentary men showed that the trained man had significantly higher expression of genes involved in molecular chaperones, muscle repair, and oxidative stress pathways, but a lower expression of genes involved in the glyconeogenesis and glycolysis pathways (Yoshioka et al., 2003).

It is widely acknowledged that moderate exercise exerts many health benefits with no contraindications if prescription is tailored to an individual's health status. Ideally, the type of activity should be varied: aerobic activity for the heart, weight-bearing and muscle strength activity for bones, and stretching exercise for increased flexibility. Those who have previously led sedentary lives should start gradually, but even light activity on most days, such as walking, can reap health benefits. The UK Department of Health currently recommends that all adults, including older adults, undertake a minimum 30 minutes of moderate activity, at least five times a week, although benefit is also achieved by taking multiple shorter bouts of physical activity through the day, including lifestyle activities such as climbing stairs or brisk walking, gardening and walking, which are often popular with older people. Regular walking in physically capable older men is not only associated with a lower mortality rate than the one of non-walkers, but the distance walked is inversely related to mortality (Hakim et al., 1998). The Surgeon General's Report on Physical activity and Health (US Department of Health and Human Services. Physical activity and health: a report of the Surgeon General. Atlanta, Georgia: U.S. Department of Health and Human Services, Public Health Service, CDC, National Center for Chronic Disease Prevention and Health Promotion, 1996) recommends participating in regular physical activity four to six days a week (frequency), at 50% to 85% of maximum ability (intensity), for 15 to 60 min per day (time) (Alessio, 2003).To sum up, it is advisable to maintain a high level of activity but do not perform sporting activities to an excessive degree. When 20 men were engaged in vigorous exercise, the rate of oxidative DNA damage products detected in their urine increased by 33% in the study of Poulsen et al. (1996). Additional health concern with strenous exercise is an increased risk of injuries and cardiac dysfunction. Faster aging is predicted in more active tissues and animals because of the greater generation of reactive oxygen species. However, age-related cell loss is greater in less active cell types, such as type II muscle fibers (Amara et al., 2007). Mild uncoupling is a mechanism that protects mitochondrial function and contributes to the paradoxical longevity (e.g., in active muscle fibers). The latest study from Mandic et al. (2009) revealed that modest fitness can extend lifespan, and people who stay even moderately fit as they age may live longer than their sedentary counterparts. It is never too late to start being more active, although the earlier we start, the better. Skin blood flow (SkBF) and endothelial-dependent vasodilatation decline with aging and can be reversed with exercise training. In the recent study, Hodges et al. (2010) tested whether 48 weeks of training could improve SkBF and endothelial function in post-menopausal females. Authors concluded that aerobic exercise produces positive adaptations in the cutaneous vasodilator function to local heating as well as in cutaneous endothelial and endothelial-independent vasodilator mechanisms. Aerobic capacity was also significantly improved. These adaptations were further enhanced with progressive increases in exercise intensity. The aim of the study by Franzoni et al. (2004) was to assess the relationship between age, regular aerobic-endurance training, plasma antioxidant activity and microcirculatory skin blood flow in healthy individuals. Thirty-six male athletes (range: 22 to74 years) and 36 age-sex-matched sedentary controls (range: 20 to 75 years) were studied. The results suggest that regular physical activity is associated with a better microvascular endothelial function in older athletes probably due to increased antioxidant defenses. Keylock et al. (2008) reported that exercise accelerates cutaneous wound healing and decreases wound inflammation in aged mice. Thus, exercise does not have a positive influence only on aging of the organism, but could have a positive effect on skin aging as well.

The Role of Macro- and Micronutrients

Metal Ions that Can Increase ROS in Cells

Many metal ions are necessary for normal cell metabolism, but in higher concentrations, they might represent a health risk. Increased rates of ROS generation have often been suggested as contributors of toxicity during exposure to high levels of metal ions, e.g., iron, copper, lead, cobalt, mercury, nickel, chromium, selenium and arsenic, but not manganese or zinc. These transition metal ions are redox active and can play an important role in ROS production in the cell. Reduced forms of redox-active metal ions participate in the Fenton reaction where a hydroxyl radical is generated from hydrogen peroxide. Addition of a reducing agent, such as ascorbate, leads to a cycle that increases the damage to biological molecules. Furthermore, the Haber-Weiss reaction, which involves the oxidized forms of redox-active metal ions and the superoxide anion, generates the reduced form of the metal ion, which can be coupled to Fenton chemistry to generate a hydroxyl radical.

Fenton reaction:

$$\text{Metal}^{(n+1)} + H_2O_2 \rightarrow \text{Metal}^{(n+1)+} + HO^{\cdot} + H_2O$$

Haber-Weiss reaction

$$\text{Metal}^{(n+1)+} + 2O_2^{\cdot -} \rightarrow \text{Metal}^{(n+1)} + O_2$$

Metals such as iron, copper, chromium, vanadium and cobalt are capable of redox cycling in which a single electron may be accepted or donated by the metal. This action catalyzes reactions that produce reactive radicals and can produce reactive oxygen species. All transition metals, with the exception of copper, contain one electron in their outermost shell and can be considered free radicals. Copper has a full outer shell, but loses and gains electrons, very easily making itself a free radical (Halliwell and Gutteridge, 1985). Iron has the ability to gain and lose electrons (i.e., $Fe^{2+} \leftrightarrow Fe^{3+}$) very easily. This property makes iron and copper two common catalysts of oxidation reactions. Whilst iron (Fe), copper (Cu), chromium (Cr), vanadium (V) and cobalt (Co) undergo redox-cycling reactions, for a second group of metals, mercury (Hg), cadmium (Cd) and nickel (Ni), the primary route for their toxicity is depletion of glutathione and bonding to sulfhydryl groups of proteins. Arsenic (As) is thought to bind directly to critical thiols; however, other mechanisms, involving formation of hydrogen peroxide under physiological conditions, have been proposed. The unifying factor in determining toxicity and carcinogenicity for all these metals is the generation of reactive oxygen and nitrogen species (Valko et al., 2005). Iron is the major component of red blood cells. Iron stores in humans tend to increase with age, partly due to dietary reasons

(Fleming et al., 2002; Beard, 2002). Many metal ions are essential for normal cellular metabolism. However, if they are free (poorly liganded) in the cell and present in higher concentrations, they can stimulate oxidative stress according to Fenton and Haber-Weiss reactions. The transformation of less reactive intermediates into highly reactive forms needs the participation of free metal ions. Oxidative state and bioavailability of redox active metals are the key determinants of their possibility to form ROS. As it was previously explained, the reduced forms of metal ions are involved in Fenton reaction where OH˙ radicals are produced. The oxidative forms participate in Haber-Weiss reaction where reduced forms of metal ions are generated, which can again re-enter Fenton reaction. Thus, it is clear that any increase in the levels of superoxide anion, hydrogen peroxide or redox-active metal ions are likely to lead to the formation of high levels of hydroxyl radical by the chemical mechanisms outlined above. Therefore, the valence state and bioavailability of redox-active metal ions are key determinants in their ability to participate in the generation of reactive oxygen species. Potential anti-aging strategies may involve not only overall reduction of oxidative stress but also the use of iron and other metal chelators hampering Fenton-type chemistry (Terman and Brunk, 2006). Excess copper, chromium and iron have a potentially toxic effect, leading to many pathological conditions that are consistent with oxidative damage to membranes and molecules. Iron is the main catalyst of free radical reactions both *in vitro*(Halliwell and Gutteridge, 1986) and *in vivo* (Sullivan et al., 1987). Hydroxyl radicals are responsible for a large part of the damage done to DNA molecules. However, almost everything reacts so quickly with OH˙ that scavenging of this radical *in vivo* is an unlikely mechanism of action of any antioxidant*in vivo* because huge concentrations of antioxidant would be needed to compete with biological molecules for any OH˙ generated. Iron, copper and H_2O_2 have been thus referred to as the "toxic triad" (Milton, 2004). While there is little that we can do about the production of superoxide and peroxide, we can (by pharmacological or dietary means) try to improve the speciation of iron ions (Kell, 2010). There are two main categories of antioxidant defenses: those who intercept free radicals that are generated and those whose role is to prevent the generation of free radicals. One reason why eukaryotic organisms have compartmentalized DNA in the nucleus, away from the sites of redox cycling that are high in reductants (GSH, NADPH, ascorbic acid), may be to avoid oxidative damage. Indeed, if concentrations of iron or copper are sufficient to saturate the reducing capacity of the cell, these ions may reach the DNA. Some compounds contribute to antioxidant defense by chelating transition metals and preventing them from catalyzing the production of free radicals in the cell. Metal-chelating antioxidants such as transferrin, albumin, and ceruloplasmin avoid radical production by inhibiting the Fenton reaction catalyzed by copper and iron.

Particularly important is the ability to sequester iron, which is the function of iron-binding proteins such as transferrin and ferritin (Imlay, 2003). Many of the polyphenolic compounds (e.g., flavones, isoflavones, stilbenes, flavanones, catechins (flavan-3-ols), chalcones, tannins and anthocyanidins) (Cook et al., 1996; Bravo, 1998; Fang et al., 2002; Fraga et al., 2002; Halvorsen et al., 2002; Havsteen, 2002) so implicated may also act to chelate iron as well (Mandel et al., 2007; Afanas'ev, et al., 1998; More et al., 1994; Moran et al., 1997, Yoshino et al., 1998; for more, see review from Kell, 2010). Besides, magnesium and zinc could prevent the formation of OH˙ in the proximity of DNA by preventing iron and copper ionsfrom binding to DNA because magnesium and zinc cannot be redox-cycling (like iron or copper) and are thus not involved in Fenton-like chemistry (Figure 39). DNAbases are also very susceptible to ROS oxidation caused by the hydroxyl radical formation from the Fenton reaction, and the predominantdetectable oxidation product of DNA bases *in vivo* is 8-hydroxy-2-deoxyguanosine.Oxidation of DNA bases can cause mutations and deletions inboth nuclear and mitochondrial DNA. Mitochondrial DNA is especiallyprone to oxidative damage due to its proximity to a primarysource of ROS and its deficient repair capacity compared withnuclear DNA. Such DNA oxidation and the formation of the 8-OHdG could be prevented if DNA would be saturated with free zinc and magnesium ions. In this way, iron and copper (as catalysts of Fenton reaction) could not form OH$^\cdot$ radical in DNA proximity. Potential anti-aging strategies may involve not only overall reduction of oxidative stress, but also the use of intralysosomal iron chelators to hamper Fenton-type chemistry.

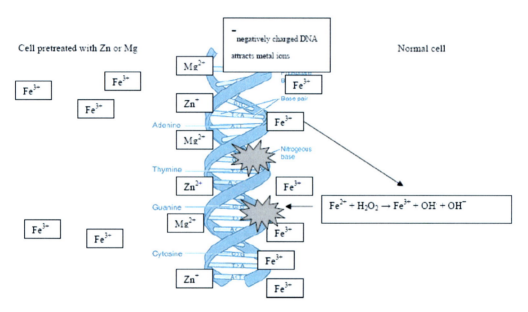

Figure 39. Iron and hydrogen peroxide are capable of oxidizing a wide range of substrates and causing biological damage. Iron (or cupper) -catalyzed free radical formation in DNA proximity can be a source of oxidative DNA damage. Since OH$^\cdot$ cannot be specifically scavenged by antioxidants due to OH's$^\cdot$ extreme reactiveness, it would be better to prevent its formation. One possibility would be by increased intake of magnesium or zinc, which could increase the binding of magnesium or zinc to DNA (negatively charged molecule) and might prevent the binding of iron and copper to DNA and thus decrease the probability of Fenton reaction in the proximity of DNA.

In order to identify compounds that reduce oxidative injury from iron, Lal et al. (2008) evaluated alpha-lipoic acid (LA), a multifunctional antioxidant, in iron-overloaded primary human fibroblasts (IMR-90). Exposure to ferric ammonium citrate (FAC) increased the iron-content of IMR-90 cells and caused a rise in oxidant appearance. The addition of LA improved the cellular redox status and attenuated the iron-mediated rise in oxidants in a dose-dependent manner. Authors conclude that lipoic acid is highly effective in reversing oxidative stress arising from iron overload and that its antioxidant efficacy is further enhanced in combination with acetyl-L-carnitine (ALCAR). ALCAR and LA exhibited superior antioxidant effect at all dose levels.

Selenium and zinc are commonly referred to as antioxidant nutrients, but these chemical elements have no antioxidant action themselves and are instead required for the activity of some antioxidant enzymes, as discussed below.

Selenium was the first of the antioxidant nutrients for which evidence emerged for a role in enhancing DNA repair. Addition of extra selenium (in the form of selenomethionine) induced base excision repair via p53 activation in normal human fibroblasts *in vitro* (Seo et al., 2002). It is possible that higher intakes of zinc in older individuals may help ensure optimal function of both base excision and nucleotide excision repair since several of the proteins involved in these repair systems are zinc finger proteins or zinc-associated proteins (Ho, 2004).

Magnesium plays many roles in the oxidation-reduction steps in mitochondria and is thus an important element in regulating oxidative stress since magnesium deficiency enhances free radical production (Costello andMoser-Veillon, 1992; Kawano et al., 1998). Data indicate on decreased availability of magnesium in the food supply, lower intakes of magnesium by elderly people and widespread supplementation practices.

Antioxidants (both enzymatic and non-enzymatic) provide protection against deleterious metal-mediated free radical attacks. Vitamin E and melatonin can prevent the majority of metal-mediated (iron, copper, cadmium) damage both in vitro systems and in metal-loaded animals. Toxicity studies involving chromium have shown that the protective effect of vitamin E against lipid peroxidation may be associated rather with the level of non-enzymatic antioxidants than the activity of enzymatic antioxidants. However, a very recent epidemiological study has shown that a daily intake of vitamin E of more than 400 IU increases the risk of death and should be avoided. While previous studies have proposed a deleterious pro-oxidant effect of vitamin C (ascorbate) in the presence of iron (or copper), recent results have shown that even in the presence of redox-active iron (or copper) and hydrogen peroxide, ascorbate acts as an antioxidant that prevents lipid peroxidation and does not promote protein oxidation in humans in vitro (Valko et al., 2005).

Another method to decrease iron-induced free radical formation is calorie restriction (CR). Calorie restriction also benefits iron status (Cook et al., 1998) in that it is this improved iron status that, in part, promotes longevity (Reverter-Branchat et al., 2004); for more information on CR, see chapter on calorie restriction.

Mitochondrial Uncoupling

The mitochondria in an eukaryotic cell utilize food to produce energy (in the form of ATP). This process involves storing energy as a proton gradient, also known as the proton motive force, across the mitochondrial inner membrane. This energy is used to synthesize ATP when the protons flow across the membrane (down their concentration gradient) through the ATP synthase enzyme. The flux through the electrontransport chain is relevant to the aging process because it is related to the rate of the production of ROS. Small reductions in metabolic flux through the electron transport chain occur at the cost of increased upstream substrate levels (Mazat et al., 2001). This increased concentration of reduced upstream substrates allows a larger generation of ROS. This idea is supported by the observation that mice with a greater proton leak live longer (Speakman et al., 2004).

It has long been known that respiration and mitochondrial ATP synthesis are coupled. Uncoupling is defined as a condition in which the rate of electron transport can no longer be regulated by an intact chemiosmotic gradient. Uncoupling agents dissipate the chemical gradient, usually by creating a mechanism by which protons can escape the intermembrane space (or otherwise "short out" the gradient), allowing an increase in electron transport.

One postulated mechanism to reduce mitochondrial oxidant production is to increase the rate of metabolic uncoupling (Schulachev, 1996). When oxygen consumption is uncoupled from ATP generation, heat is produced. However, the consumption of oxygen without ATP production would also reduce the level of free molecular oxygen potentially available for superoxide anion formation. The observation that decreased ATP utilization inhibited oxygen consumption and that the respiration rate increased when mitochondria synthesized more ATP led to the concept of respiratory control by ADP phosphorylation. In fact, there is a link between mitochondrial ATP synthesis and cellular ATP demand by a feedback mechanism controlling ATP synthesis induced by mitochondrial respiration. After the seminal proposal made by Peter Mitchell (chemi-osmotic theory), it was demonstrated that the mitochondrial electrochemical proton gradient, generated as electrons pass down the respiratory chain, is the primary source for cellular ATP synthesis.

Since the rate of ROS formation increases when respiratory rates are low, cells also evolved means of accelerating respiration and thus reducing damage caused by free radicals. Once a mechanism to increase respiration was operative, it was subsequently utilized (co-opted in evolutionary terms) to fulfill other physiological roles such as maintenance of body temperature and even the control of energy balance.

Examples of uncoupling agents are the uncoupling proteins (UPCs), a family of transporters belonging to the mitochondrial carrier protein superfamily, which is found in all eukaryotic organisms (Rial and Zardoya, 2009). An uncoupling protein is a mitochondrial inner membrane protein that can dissipate the proton gradient before it can be used to provide the energy for oxidative phosphorylation (Nedergaard et al., 2005).Uncoupling proteins are present in mitochondrial inner membrane and mediate free fatty acid-activated, purine-nucleotide-inhibited H+ re-uptake. UCPs can modulate the tightness of coupling between mitochondrial respiration and ATP synthesis (Jarmuszkiewicz and Woyda-Płoszczyca, 2008). There are at least five types known in mammals: UCP1, also known as thermogenin, UCP2, UCP3, UCP4, and UCP5.

Research data show that the general role of the UPC protein family is protection against oxidative stress, since the acceleration of respiration due to UCP-mediated uncoupling would lead to a reduction in ROS production by the respiratory chain (Krauss and Zhang, 2005). Uncoupling allows heat production while also allowing for the reduction of ROS production because the complexes that generate ROS do so more readily when the proton gradient is high. The function of UCP1 is to generate heat ("thermogenesis"). UCP1 catalyzes the net translocation of protons from the intermembrane space of mitochondria into the matrix but without passing through complex V. Instead, chemiosmotic energy is released as heat. This happens in all cells but is particularly pronounced in the brown fat cells of the body. In most cells, fifty percent of oxidation energy is recovered as ATP in mitochondria through the process of coupling of respiration to ADP phosphorylation. In contrast to mitochondria of most tissues, brown adipocyte mitochondria can escape the obligatorily coupling of respiration and waste almost ninety percent of respiration energy as thermogenesis (Ricquier, 2002). Claims have been made that UCP3 generates little heat, but functions to reduce free radical damage by lowering proton gradient during periods of high metabolic activity. If membrane potential is a key factor that influences free-radical production at complex III (Demin et al., 1998; Brand, 2000), then it would be anticipated that an important factor influencing free-radical production at this site would be the activity of uncoupling proteins on the inner mitochondrial membrane. This is because uncoupling proteins produce another flow of protons across the inner membrane, thereby reducing the membrane potential. UCP2 and UCP3 are induced to uncouple oxidative phosphorylation when confronted with high levels of negatively charged molecules such as superoxide (Echtay et al., 2002). This is also the basis for the "uncoupling to survive" hypothesis (Brand, 2000). Brand et al. (2002) examined levels of protein damage in mitochondria from mice transgenically overexpressing or lacking UCP-3. As predicted from the "uncoupling to survive" hypothesis, mice without UCP-3 had higher levels of oxidative damage relative to the wild-type. However, the UCP-3 overexpressing mice did not have reduced damage relative to the wild-type. Brand et al. (2002) suggested that beyond the basal level of uncoupling, further increases may offer little additional protection. It might be of importance also the balance due to overexpressing UCP.

In addition to the re-entry of protons through ATP synthase, a proton leak represents another mechanism consuming the mitochondrial proton gradient. Mitchell's theory predicted that any proton leak not coupled with ATP synthesis would provoke uncoupling of respiration and thermogenesis (Rousset, 2004). Besides adaptive thermogenesis, uncoupling of respiration allows continuous re-oxidation of coenzymes that are essential for metabolic pathways. In fact, partial uncoupling of respiration prevents an exaggerated increase in the ATP level that would inhibit respiration (Rousset, 2004). Mitochondrial uncoupling has been proposed as a mechanism that reduces reactive oxygen species production and could account for the paradox between longevity and activity (Camara et al., 2007) (also see chapter "Exercise and ROS"). After Ricquier (2002), the ancient function of the UCPs may rather be associated with adaptation to oxygen and control of free radicals than to thermogenesis.

Uncoupling and Heat Production

In endothermic animals, body heat is maintained by signaling the mitochondria to allow protons to run back along the gradient without producing ATP. This can occur since an alternative return route for the protons exists through the uncoupling protein in the inner membrane. As already discussed previously, protein UCP1 (thermogenin) facilitates the return of the protons after they have been actively pumped out of the mitochondria by the electron transport chain. This alternative route for protons uncouples oxidative phosphorylation, and the energy in the proton motive force is instead released as heat.

A mitochondrial uncoupling protein is found in brown adipose tissue. Brown adipose tissue or brown fat is one of the two types of fat or adipose tissue (the other being white adipose tissue) found in mammals. Its primary function is to generate body heat. In contrast to white adipocytes (fat cells), which contain a single lipid droplet, brown adipocytes contain numerous smaller droplets and a much higher number of mitochondria, which contain iron and make it brown (Enerbäck, 2009). As already mentioned, an increase in the activity of uncoupling proteins increases heat production by allowing protons to flow down their gradient without making ATP and may serve as protection against cold, as well as represent a potential means of obesity control.

Mitochondrial metabolism is an important source of heat production. Mechanisms exist for varying the extent to which mitochondria are uncoupled, so as to increase or decrease heat production on a long-term basis. The mechanism of respiratory control can be exploited to increase heat production by dissipating the proton gradient at a faster rate or to slow down heat production by making the electron transport system (ETS) more efficient. One example of that type of regulation is the hormone thyroxine (thyroid hormone). Uncoupling agents dissipate the chemical gradient and allow an increase in electron transport. Thyroxine is also a mildly effective uncoupling agent. In colder regions of the world, a noticeable change in thyroid hormone levels takes place circa-annually, i.e., levels are higher in winter and lower in summer. Rather than utilizing energy from ATP to perform work (like shivering), the goal is to bypass the ATP generation system completely and allow the protons to come back directly into the mitochondrial matrix where they can freely react with oxygen, forming water, and liberating their energy as heat (Speakman, 2003). The first carrier protein known to perform this function was UCP1 (Nicholls and Locke, 1984).

When small animals are exposed to cold, they meet the demands for energy by upregulation of their uncoupling protein levels (Speakman, 2003). Studies on prolonged cold exposure and its effect on oxidative stress are rare. Holloszy and Smith (1986) placed rats in cold water for eight hours each day and found out that there was no decreased longevity in the cold-exposed group, despite the fact that they performed more work and their food intake increased by 40%. Cold exposure is known to have several effects in the free radical scavenging and damage axis (Selman et al., 2000).

Dr. Roy Walford began his career by studying the anti-aging effects of a lowered body temperature. The discoveries of Rikke and Johnson (2004) suggest that the studies of Dr. Walford can now be extended to critically test whether lower body temperature can prolong the lifespan of mammals. Lower temperature decreases the speed/kinetics of certain chemical reactions, including those thatgenerate ROS. Cold-blooded animals needn't expend energy to maintain body temperature and, therefore, generate fewer free-radicals. Also, the rate of chemical reactions more than doubles for each 10°C increase in temperature. Cold-blooded animals may use one-tenth as much energy as warm-blooded animals of the same body weight. The phenomenon of altered lifespan in cold-blooded animals on the basis of temperature was also observed in the fruit fly *Drosophila*. Its mean lifespan is 120 days at 10°C, but only 14 days at 30°C (Halliwell and Gutteridge, 1999). A "Hibernation" hypothesis for the mechanisms underlying the effects of calorie restriction on aging was proposed by Walford and Spindler (1996). Authors demonstrated that in three species of fish, aging could be retarded and lifespan substantially prolonged by lowering body temperature by three to five degrees (Liu and Walford, 1970). A similar study raised crayfish at five different temperatures ranging from 13°C to 33°C. Lipofuscin was measured as a result of free-radical-induced auto-oxidation of cellular structures. The animals raised at the higher temperatures appeared to age more rapidly and had higher lipofuscin levels than did the animals raised at lower temperatures, suggesting proportionality among temperature, rate of living and free-radical production (Sheehy et al., 1995). Exposure of rats to cold temperatures throughout their adult liveswas reported to cause marked reduction in lifespan (Johnson et al., 1963; Kibler et al., 1963; Kibler and Johnson, 1966); however, these studies were also confounded by upper respiratory infections. A more recent study used pathogen-free animals and observed no effects on lifespan (Holloszy and Smith, 1986). Mammals exhibit hypertrophy in response to activity increases, whereas insects and other short-lived poikilotherms do not (Sohal, 1976).

Evidence suggests that mild lowering of body temperature does not result simply in overall metabolic slowdown. Instead, some reactions occur at a slower rate and some at a faster one.

A lower body temperature may actually enhance some enzyme substrate affinities. Indeed, a temperature-sensitive reorganization of the biochemical machinery may be a characteristic for different temperatures (Liu and Walford, 1972). Similarly, it was observed that young, middle-aged, and old mice on the life-extending calorie restriction regime displayed body temperatures 1 to 1.5 degrees lower than unrestricted control mice (Weindruch et al., 1979; Duffy et al., 1987; Jin and Koizumi, 1994; Koizumi et al., 1992). This finding has been found also in calorie-restricted monkeys (Lane et al., 1996). There are many similarities between calorie restriction (CR) and hibernating animals: reduced body temperature, lower blood glucose, increased levels of free radical scavengers, substantial increase in protein synthesis and turnover (Weindruch and Walford, 1988). Many studies of CR in rodents and lower animals indicate that this nutritional manipulation retards aging processes, as evidenced by increased longevity, reduced pathology, and maintenance of physiological function in a more youthful state. The anti-aging effects of CR are believed to relate, at least in part, to changes in energy metabolism. Additionally, a lower temperature was also observed in calorie-restricted monkeys most probably due to metabolic readjustment in order to utilize energy more slowly and efficiently (Halliwell and Gutteridge, 1999). The temporal association between reduced body temperature and energy expenditure suggests that reductions in body temperature relate to the induction of an energy-conservation mechanism during CR. These reductions in body temperature and energy expenditure are consistent with the findings of rodent studies in which the aging rate was retarded by CR, findings that strengthen the possibility that CR may exert beneficial effects in primates analogous to those observed in rodents (Lane et al., 1996).

Temperature manipulation as a way of altering lifespan is much easier in a poikilothermic animal, whose body temperature is not physiologically preset, than in a homeotherm. Altering metabolic rate in homeotherms is a difficult task because their body physiology is designed to yield a body temperature and basal metabolic rate that is relatively independent of the environment (Arking, 2006). In the review of Miller and Austad (2006), evidence is presented for or against the hypothesis that slow growth rates in early life produce delayed aging and extend longevity.

Authors point out that it is worth nothing that the association between small body size and longer lifespan is contrary to the prediction of models that attribute long lifespan to lower metabolic rates. The association of small body size and longer lifespan is supported by two independent sets of data on purebred dogs as well as by the analysis of mixed-breed dogs (Patronek et al., 1997).

Smaller breeds of dogs, with relatively high area/volume ratios, must expend greater energy in maintaining body temperature and are thus expected to have higher-than-average metabolic demands, and indeed a comparison (Speakman et al., 2003) among three breeds found 60 percent higher energy expenditure per kg lean body mass in the small, long-lived breed (Papillion) compared to the larger, short-lived breed (Great Dane). Birds, too, are in general much longer lived than nonflying mammalian species of the same weight, despite metabolic demands, high blood-glucose levels, high body temperature, and high fuel utilization rates typical of flying bird species.

Also, exercise influences the gene expression of UCPs. Uncoupling of oxidation of respiratory substrates and phosphorylation of ADP lowers the efficiency of ATP formation (Goto et al., 2003).

At the same time, it may diminish the formation of ROS by decreasing the mitochondrial membrane potential and thereby stimulating the electron transport and oxygen consumption. This is due to shortening of the half-life of semiquinone, an intemediate of the electron transport system, which can transfer the electron to molecular oxygen, generating superoxide radicals and then hydrogen peroxides (Skulacev, 1998). Many scientists believe that the only regimes proven in numerous experiments to lead to a substantial retardation of aging in vertebrates are: 1) lowering of body temperature in poikilotherms and 2) calorie restriction on a "nutrient-dense" diet (Walford and Spindler, 1996).

Here should be mentioned also the ability of CoQ 10 as the key component of the respiratory chain and creatine, which is a source of a sink for ATP and thus keeps the amount of available ADP for phosphorylation by the mitochondrial respiratory chain high and keeps the mitochondrium in a unrestricted state 3 respiration. For further information, see paragraph on CoQ and creatine.

Nutritional Approaches to Reduce Oxidative Stress

Skin functioning and skin attractiveness are dependent on nutrition.This is evidenced by the development of skin lesions in responseto nutritional deficiencies (Boelsma et al., 2001). Dietary supplementation with thedeficient vitamins, minerals, or essential fatty acids improvesskin conditions in these situations (Roe, 1986). A wide variety of foods have been found that are oxidative stress generators, as well as those that contain compounds to reduce this condition. Some of them are briefly discussed.

Foods that Increase Reactive Oxygen Species Formation

Side-Effects of Processed Food

During heat processing, some nutrients are converted into substances harmful to the organism consuming the food. Some of them are mutagenic or even carcinogenic. Most known classes of cooked toxicants are acrylamides, present in carbohydrates exposed to high temperatures (Jägerstad and Skog, 2005), heterocyclic amines, produced during heat processing of meat and fish (Sugimura et al., 2004; Felton et al., 2004), nitrosamines, present in roasted salted meat (Walker, 1990; Rajar et al., 2006), and polyaromatic hydrocarbons, present in smoked and roasted food (Cross and Sinha, 2006).

The toxicity and lack of nutrients of processed foods might also affect the reproductive process. For example, the lack of vitamin C, folic acid or zinc can damage sperm cells (Ames, 2004). Therefore, cooking is not only a process that increases the quality of food by enhancing its energy value but also one that decreases some other food qualities that might cause a degeneration of the organism.

Some antioxidants such as lycopene and ascorbic acid can be destroyed by long-term storage or prolonged cooking (Xianquan, 2005; Rodriguez-Amaya, 2003). In general, processed foods contain fewer antioxidants than fresh and uncooked foods, since the preparation processes may expose the food to oxygen (Henry and Heppell, 2002). In contrast, cooking can also increase the bioavailability of antioxidants, as in the case of some carotenoids in vegetables (Maiani et al., 2008).

Heat helps to create tasteful flavors that humans have learned to enjoy (Peppa et al., 2003); however, heating has a significant accelerating effect in the generation of glyco- and lipoxidation products.

A high percentage of humans is continually exposed to oxidized oils and fats in the diet, which arise from either shallow or deep-fat frying processes. The most important reaction involved in the oxidative degeneration of lipids is the auto-oxidation of polyunsaturated fatty acids (PUFAs) (Grootveld et al., 2000). For more information, see also chapter on food that increases inflammation.

Alcohol

The National Institute on Alcohol Abuse and Alcoholism has found that "Alcoholism may accelerate normal aging or cause premature aging of the brain." Alcohol consumption could play a dual role in the organism in relation to oxidative stress formation. On the one hand, ethanol is an oxidant that can increase the oxidative stress of the organism, and on the other hand, many observations have been made concerning the beneficial effects of alcohol consumption (e.g., red wine). Alcohol also stimulates the activity of enzymes called cytochrome P450s, which contribute to ROS production. Furthermore, alcohol can alter the levels of certain metal ions in the body, thereby facilitating ROS production. Finally, alcohol reduces the levels of agents that can eliminate ROS (i.e., antioxidants). The resulting state of the cell, known as oxidative stress, can lead to cell injury. Alcoholic beverages are believed to be hormetic in preventing heart disease and stroke(Cook and Calabrese, 2006), although the benefits of light drinking may have been exaggerated (Fillmore et al., 2006). In 2008, a study found that high doses of resveratrol (a constituent of red wine) mimicked some of the benefits of calorie restriction (including reduced effects of aging) in mice (Barger et al., 2008). High doses of resveratrol have been linked to longevity and cancer prevention in other species (Anupam and Bishayee, 2009). For more information on resveratrol, see chapter on red wine and resveratrol.

Avoidance of Excessive Sugar Intake

Sugars such as glucose and fructose can react with certain amino acids such as lysine and arginine and certain DNA bases such as guanine to produce sugar adducts in a process called glycation. These adducts can further rearrange to form reactive species that can then cross-link the structural proteins or DNA to similar biopolymers or other biomolecules such as non-structural proteins. People with diabetes, who have elevated blood sugar, develop senescence-associated disorders much earlier than the general population but can delay such disorders by rigorous control of their blood sugar levels. There is evidence that sugar damage is linked to oxidant damage in a process termed glycoxidation. Hyperglycemia is still considered the principal cause of diabetes complications. Its deleterious effects are attributable, among other things, to the formation of sugar-derived substances—advanced glycation end products (AGEs). AGEs are the result of a chain of chemical reactions after an initial glycation reaction. The intermediate products are known, variously, as Amadori, Schiff base and Maillard products, named after the researchers who first described them.

The modification of collagen by sugar begins with nonenzymatic condensation of sugar aldehyde by means of a free amino group of a protein to yield a Shiff base. This base is then rearranged to yield the more stable Amadori product, which can further react with other such proteins to form the cross-linked AGEs. AGEs are a heterogeneous group of molecules formed from the non-enzymatic reaction of reducing sugars with free amino groups of proteins, lipids and nucleic acids (Peppa, 2003). Damaged proteins and lipids accumulate in lysosomes as lipofuscin. Chemical damage to structural proteins can lead to loss of function; for example, damage to collagen of blood vessel walls can lead to vessel-wall stiffness and thus hypertension, as well as vessel-wall thickening and reactive tissue formation (atherosclerosis), and similar processes in the kidney can lead to renal failure. Damage to enzymes reduces cellular functionality. It is probably no accident that nearly all of the so-called "accelerated aging diseases" are due to defective DNA-repair enzymes (http://en.wikipedia.org/wiki/Senescence). AGEs form at a constant but slow rate in the normal body, starting in early embryonic development, and accumulate with time. Levels of AGEs increase significantly with age in humans and experimental animals (Sell and Monnier, 1995). However, their formation is markedly accelerated in diabetes because of the increased availability of glucose. Elevated blood glucose levels accelerate the rate of production of cross-linked AGEs.

Evidence has accumulated suggesting that the ratio of carbohydrate intake, hyperglycemia and hyperinsulinemia is central to the calorie-induced stimulation of organismal oxidative stress by both enhancement of free radical generation and weakening of antioxidative defenses (Facchini et al., 2000). Additionally, body iron status modifies insulin action and carbohydrate tolerance (Facchini, 1998; Hua et al., 2001; Facchini et al., 2002; Fernandez-real et al., 2002), suggesting that aging can be especially rapid when high carbohydrate intake and iron sufficiency or overloading are coupled in an insulin-resistant phenotype. Insulin is a polypeptide produced by beta cells of the pancreatic islets and is a key metabolic hormone. Insulin promotes storage of glucose and glycogen in liver and of triglycerides in adipose tissue and mediates uptake and utilization of glucose by skeletal muscles. In the absence of adequate insulin action, excessive amounts of glucose accumulate in the circulation, the state called hyperglycemia.There is evidence that hyperglycemia and hyperinsulinemia contribute both interactively to oxidative tissue damage (Brown-Borg and Harman, 2003). Additionally, it is believed that not insulin itself, but the high levels of glucose, which result from a deficiency of insulin action, are responsible for ROS generation.

There is a relationship between a high level of glucose (hyperglycemia) and diabetic complications, but now an even more extensive implication of glucose in other diseases and the aging process has been suggested by many investigators. Human diabetics with altered insulin metabolism appear to suffer accelerated aging and are at a greater risk of developing many of the age-related diseases (Thomas and Inoue, 1998; Tissenbaum and Ruvkun, 1998; Kemnitz et al., 1994; Bodkinet al., 1995). Also, experiments on animals indicatethe importance of insulin-like growth factor receptors in worm C. elegans (Vanfleteren and Braeckman, 1999; Thomas and Inoue, 1998; Tissenbaum and Ruvkun, 1998). Insulin pathway and general metabolism play a role also in long-lived dietary-restricted mammals since insulin and glucose levels fall and altered metabolism is noticed (Kemnitz et al., 1994; Bodkin et al., 1995).The total state of oxidative and peroxidative stress on the healthy body and the accumulation of AGE-related damage are proportional to the dietary intake of exogenous (preformed) AGEs, the consumption of sugars with a propensity towards glycation. Highly reactive sugars (e.g., ribose, threose and glyceraldehyde) or ascorbic acid lead to extensive browning, cross-linking and oxidation. Ascorbic acid (vitamin C) has emerged as powerful glycating agent.(Monnier et al., 2003). A material that undergoes cross-linking usually becomes harder, less elastic and has a tendency to tear or crack. Cross-linking is responsible for hardening of a rubber mat or a garden hose left in the sun. In the aging body, cross-linking contributes to hardening of arteries, wrinkling of the skin and stiffening of joints. On the other hand, protein glycation and advanced glycation was reported to be inhibited by antioxidant components (Vinson and Howard, 1996). For more information, see chapter dedicated to endogenous antioxidants: compounds derived from the diet.

Skin aging and Advanced Glycosylation End Products

Too Much Sugar Causes Wrinkles

As already explained previously, at blame is a natural process known as glycation, in which the sugar in the bloodstream attaches to proteins to form harmful new molecules—advanced glycation end products (AGEs). Glycation (sometimes called non-enzymatic glycosylation) is the result of a sugar molecule, such as fructose or glucose, bonding to a protein or lipid molecule without the controlling action of an enzyme. Enzyme-controlled addition of sugars to protein or lipid molecules is termed glycosylation; glycation is a haphazard process that impairs the functioning of biomolecules, whereas glycosylation occurs at defined sites on the target molecule and is required in order for the molecule to function. Glucose can undergo three types of transformations. It can be biologically transformed through glycolysis, auto-oxidatively modified by redox active metals by the Wolff pathway of the Maillard reaction or transformed, oxidized and degraded via Maillard reaction. In organisms, methylglyoxal is formed as a side-product of several metabolic pathways, the most important source being glycolysis. Methylglyoxal arises from non-enzymatic phosphate elimination from glyceraldehyde phosphate and dihydroxyacetone phosphate, two intermediates of glycolysis. Methylglyoxal is involved in the formation of advanced glycation end products (AGEs); it reacts with free amino groups of lysine and arginine and with thiol groups of cysteine forming AGEs. Methylglyoxal, glyoxal and other auto-oxidized derivatives of sugars induce AGEs that negatively affect essential features of skin cells. It has been reported that AGE formation results in a loss of contractile capacity and cytoskeleton integrity in human skin fibroblasts, which possibly affects tissue cohesion and leads to visible effects of skin aging (Blatt et al., 2010).

The effect of sugars on aging skin is governed by the simple act of covalently cross-linking two collagen fibers, which renders both of them incapable of easy repair. Glucose and fructose link the aminoacids present in the collagen and elastin that support the dermis-producing AGEs. This process is accelerated in all body tissues when sugar is elevated and is further stimulated by ultraviolet light in the skin (Danby 2010).The more sugar one eats, the more AGEs onedevelops. AGEs occur to one's body externally (exogenously), and this is done by heating, mostly cooking sugars with proteins or fats. Baking, broiling and roasting can trigger the production of damaging glycation products, while steaming and boiling helps in preventing the formation in the food we prepare. AGEs formation might also occur within the body, internally (endogenously) through normal course of metabolism and aging. AGEs affect different parts of the body, and the skin is an easy target with its elastin and collagen content.

Wrinkles occur when skin loses its elasticity. The loss of elasticity is caused by extensive formation and accumulation of collagen cross-links. Collagen cross-linking is a result of a chemical process that starts with nonenzymatic attachment of glucose to a collagen molecule. Some of the negative effects of advanced glycation end products include inhibiting the formation and function of skin tightening agents such as collagen fibers and elastin fibers. When enzymes attach glucose to collagen, there is a reason for it and a purpose. Nonezymatic attachment, on the other hand, is random. Collagen cross-linking in this case is uncontrollable and more often than not, unnecessary. Once cross-linking occurs, it is irreversible.

Glycation is an age-related problem in the extracellular proteins, such as collagen and elastin, which are located outside of cells and provide strength and flexibility to tissues. Some of the AGEs form covalent crosslinks with adjacent protein strands. This cross-linking stiffens tissues thatwere formerly flexible or elastic. The process happens gradually, so that cross-links accumulate over the years. Furthermore, AGEs are connected also to increased oxidative stress formation. The end products of advanced glycation that accumulate with aging in long-lived proteins such as those of the extracellular matrix also act as UVA chromophores to become photosensitizers affecting dermal fibroblasts (Wondrak et al., 2002; 2003, 2004). Intracellular AGEs induce oxidative stress, activate NF-κB and hem oxygenase, produce lipid peroxidation products, and cross-link proteins (Kasper and Funk, 2001).

Glucose, in addition to be a substance that can cause damage by randomly reacting with proteins and DNA in the process of glycation or Maillard reaction, is unfortunately also a vital cellular fuel. Most of the energy we get from foods comes from glucose. The level of glucose in the bloodstream is one of the most important physiological parameters because glucose is the primary fuel for the central nervous system. If the blood level of glucose drops below a certain point for a long enough time, a person will lose consciousness, fall into coma and die. High blood glucose seen in diabetes is also harmful. To avoid dangerous swings in glucose level, the body has a sophisticated system for maintaining blood glucose within an appropriate range. Some reserve glucose is always stored in the liver in the form of glycogen (a polymer similar to starch). On top of that, the liver can synthesize glucose from protein if needed. During starvation, the body would gradually break down its muscle protein for the sake of providing the central nervous system with glucose.

Skin cells undergo AGE-related damage. The collagen lattice formed by cross-linked type I collagen is undeformable (unglycated collagen is fully compactible). Cross-linking collagen fibrils also alters the physical and mechanical properties of the extracellular matrixand changes the organization of the intracellular actin cytoskeleton (Howard et al., 1996). Glycated collagen may modify normal cell adhesion (Le Varlet et al., 1999). As adhesion is a fundamental cell function, each alteration can damage cell behavior (apoptosis, etc.) and then change tissue homeostasis. The dermis and elastic fiber network become glycated in people over 35 years of age, and solar irradiation appeared to enhance it (Jeanmaire et al., 2001). The fluorescence of epidermal tryptophan moieties and collagen cross-links in the dermal matrix can also be considered to be good in vivo markers of photoaging (Tian et al., 2001).

In a cross-sectional study involving eightmammalian species, researchers found an overall inverse relationship between skin collagen pentosidine formation rate and longevity

(Sell et al., 1996).Pentosidine, a marker of glycoxidative stress in skin collagen from eight mammalian species as a function of age, was quantified. The rate of increase correlated inversely with maximum lifespan. Dietary restriction, a potent intervention associated with increased lifespan, markedly inhibited glycoxidation rate in the rodent. On the assumption that collagen turnover rate is primarily influenced by the cross-linking due to glycoxidation, these results suggest that there is a progressive age-related deterioration of the process that controls the collagen glycoxidation rate.

It was suggested that markers of skin collagen glycation and glycoxidation rates can predict early deaths in mice. Authors strongly suggest that an age-related deterioration in glucose tolerance is a lifespan-determining process (Sell et al., 2000).

This relationship was confirmed in a follow-up longitudinal study with C57/6 NNia mice. The glycation (furosine) and glycoxidation products of collagen (pentosidine and carboxymethyl-lysine) were determined at 20 months and at death, and a correlation between rate of formation with maximum lifespan was investigated (Sell et al., 2000). Furosine was a strong inverse predictor of lifespan in both ad libitum and calorie-restricted mice, higher levels being associated with early death. Similarly, pentosidine and carboxymethyl-lysine formation rates were inversely related with longevity in ad libitum and calorie-restricted mice, respectively. Glycation and glycoxidation products were also found lower in skin of dietary-restricted animals by Cefalu et al. (1995). These data suggest that glucose tolerance is impaired in aging mice, leading to early death. Alternatively, a process responsible for decreased collagen turnover rate may be responsible for decreased removal rate of damaged cellular organelles from critical lifespan-controlling tissues (for further reading on carbohydrate damage, see review by Monnier et al. (2003)).

The Maillard or browning reaction between sugar and protein contributes to the increased chemical modification and cross-linking of long-lived tissue proteins in diabetes. To evaluate the role of glycation and oxidation in these reactions, authors have studied the effects of oxidative and antioxidative conditions and various types of inhibitors on the reaction of glucose with rat-tail tendon collagen in phosphate buffer at physiological pH and temperature (Fu et al., 1994). Although glycation was unaffected, formation of glycoxidation products and cross-linking of collagen were inhibited by antioxidative conditions. The kinetics of formation of glycoxidation products proceeded with a short lag phase and were independent of the amount of Amadori adduct on the protein, suggesting that auto-oxidative degradation of glucose was a major contributor to glycoxidation and cross-linking reactions. Chelators, sulfhydryl compounds, antioxidants, and aminoguanidine also inhibited formation of glycoxidation products, generation of fluorescence, and cross-linking of collagen without significant effect on the extent of glycation of the protein. Researchers conclude that auto-oxidation of glucose or Amadori compounds on protein plays a major role in the formation of glycoxidation products and cross-linking of collagen by glucose in vitro and that chelators, sulfhydryl compounds, antioxidants, and aminoguanidine act as uncouplers of glycation from subsequent glycoxidation and cross-linking reactions.

Carbonyl stress, with or without oxidative stress, plays an important role in controlling tissue-turnover rate. High glucose levels mediate mitochondrial superoxide and methylglyoxal formation (Nishikawa et al., 2000). Hyperglycaemia increases the production of reactive oxygen species inside cultured bovine aortic endothelial cells. Authors show that this increase in reactive oxygen species is prevented by an inhibitor of electron transport chain complex II, by an uncoupler of oxidative phosphorylation, by uncoupling protein-1 and by manganese superoxide dismutase. Normalizing levels of mitochondrial reactive oxygen species with each of these agents prevents glucose-induced activation of protein kinase C, formation of advanced glycation end products, sorbitol accumulation and NFkappaB activation.

Furthermore, aminoguanidine is an AGE and nitric oxide synthase inhibitor (Onorato et al., 2000), pyridoxamine blocks AGE formation in vivo and normalizes diabetic ketoacidosis, caloric restriction decreases tissue AGE levels, etc.

Monnier et al. (2003) proposed hypothesis that any intervention that would successfully prevent both carbonyl and oxidative stress may be expected to prolong lifespan (and decrease skin aging).

Although short-term studies in healthy animals suggest that feeding a diet high in fructose may increase serum glucose concentrations and increase glycemic stress, the effects of a long-term feeding, i.e., lifespan, are unknown. The study of Lingelbach et al. (2000) was designed to evaluate the long-term effects of dietary carbohydrates on serum and tissue markers of glycemic stress. "Three-month-old male Fischer 344 rats were given free access to or restricted to 60% calorie intake of one of five isocaloric diets that contained as their carbohydrate source either cornstarch, glucose, sucrose, fructose or equimolar amounts of fructose and glucose. Glycated hemoglobin, serum glucose and fructosamine levels were measured as markers of serum glycemic stress. Collagen-associated fluorescence and pentosidine concentrations were measured in skin, aortic, tracheal and tail tendon collagen as markers of advanced glycation end products (AGE). The source of dietary carbohydrate had little effect on markers of glycemic stress and the accumulation of AGE. Restricting the amount of calories consumed resulted in lower serum glucose concentrations, glycated hemoglobin levels and pentosidine concentrations in tail tendon collagen. The data from this study suggest that the rate of collagen glycation is tissue-specific. These results suggest that long-term feeding of specific dietary carbohydrates does not alter serum glucose concentrations or the rate of collagen glycation. Rather, age-related accumulation of AGE is more closely related to calorie intake" (Lingelbach et al., 2000).

Blood fructose, cholesterol, fructosamine and glycated hemoglobin levels, and urine lipid peroxidation products were significantly higher in fructose-fed rats compared with the other sugar-fed and control rats. Acid-soluble collagen and the type-III to type-I ratio were significantly lower, whereas insoluble collagen, the beta-to-alpha ratio and collagen-bound fluorescence at 335/385 nm (excitation/emission) were significantly higher in fructose-fed rats than in the other groups. The data form (Levi and Werman, 1998) suggest that long-term fructose consumption induces adverse effects on aging; further studies are required to clarify the precise role of fructose in the aging process. Another study suggests that fructose diet-induced skin collagen abnormalities are prevented by lipoic acid and taurine (Thirunavukkarasu et al., 2004; Nandhini et al., 2005).

Sugar-induced premature senescence was observed in the skin study on human epidermal keratinocytes. Normal human epidermal keratinocytes (NHEK) show both the Hayflick phenomenon and differentiation in vitro. The aim of the study performed by Berge et al. (2007) was to induce senescence in keratinocytes using two sugars, glucose and glyoxal. "Induction of senescence in early-passage NHEK was characterized by monitoring cell morphology, short-term growth characteristics, cell proliferation, and viability assay. In addition, apoptosis, senescence-associated beta-gal activity, proteasomal activity and glycation, and glycoxidation of total proteins were determined. The results showed that a three-day treatment with 100 mM glucose or 0.1 mM glyoxal induces in early-passage NHEK various cellular and biochemical characteristics comparable to those observed in serially subcultured late passage NHEK. Furthermore, sugar-treated prematurely aged NHEK showed impaired differentiation, as measured by the quantification of involucrin" (Berge et al., 2007).

Additionally, early-passage human skin fibroblasts treated with 1 mM glyoxal for 72 h undergo premature senescence in terms of enlarged cell size, inhibition of cell division, slowing down of cell growth, a decrease in the number of DNA synthesizing cells, and increased resistance to apoptosis (Sejersen and Rattan, 2007).

Therapeutic Interventions

By reducing the chance for sugars to bond with proteins improperly, certain nutrients, supplements and herbs can act as anti-AGEs and thus will provide as aging skin treatments.

AGEs are the subject of ongoing research. Glycation inhibitors include benfotiamine, pyridoxamine, taurine (Nandhini et al., 2005),aminoguanidine (Gugliucci, 2010), and aspirin (Bucala and Cerami, 1992). It is also believed that alpha-lipoic acid can also reduce glycation damage.

Certain dietary measures can be very helpful in reducing the formation of AGEs process. Since glycation is caused mainly due to the rise in sugar levels in the blood stream, it is important to reduce sugar consumption. Dietary changes such as lowering carbohydrate consumption by reducing total carbohydrate intake or consuming carbohydrates with lower glycemic index are often recommended to bring down glucose and insulin levels. It would be suggested to focus more on complex carbohydrates that are high in fiber and nutrients. Several other nutrients like peptides skin care elements (N-acetyl cysteine, glutathione and carnosine), supplements (inositol and alpha lipoic acid), herbs (rosemary, ginger, stinging nettle, turmeric and thyme), and plant phyto-chemicals (grape extract) have been reported to possess anti-glycation effect and could influence AGEs prevention.

Clinical trials with chromium (Cobo and Castiñeira, 1997; Fox and Sabovic, 1998; Guan et al., 2000; Hellerstein, 1998) or α-lipoic acid (Rudich et al., 1999; Konrad et al., 1999; Khamaisi et al., 1999; Jacob et al., 1999) have indicated that these nutritional supplements may be beneficial in modulating insulin levels or glucose levels.

Carnosine (*beta-alanyl-L-histidine*), a dipeptide formed naturally in human tissues, is also believed to inhibit the formation of cross-links between proteinsthathave been glycated or carbonylated (Hipkiss et al., 2001). In animal studies, a nutrient carnosine has been shown to inhibit cross-linking. In particular, carnosine inhibits the protein-protein and DNA-protein cross-linking induced by various aldehydes, including glucose. Whether long-term carnosine supplementation has longevity benefits in humans remains to be determined.

Aspirin may also inhibit the formation of pathological AGE cross-links. For example, chronic users of aspirin have fewer cataracts (Bucala and Cerami, 1992).

Nevertheless, aminoguanidine and aspirin do not seem to break AGEs cross-links thathave already formed. However, other compounds are being studied thatdo. Many of the known cross-link breakers are modified thiazolium salts which include an active site similar in structure to the catalytic ring of thiamine (vitamin B1) (Asif et al., 2000).

The reactivity of the reducing sugars, such as glucose reacting with proteins, nucleic acids or membranes forming adducts, cross-links and then on further reaction with ROS produces AGEs thataccumulate with age resulting in stiffing of tissues such as in skin, the cardiovascular system and in elastic tissues as the urine bladder. Some potential therapeutic and preventive approaches were presented. Mechanisms of their actions are not yet completely established and further human studies are needed.

Avoidance of Chlorinated Water intake

Water intake is very important for appropriate functioning of our organism. It is important to consume enough water during the day and to prevent the dehydration of the organism and internal dehydration of the skin. However, the beneficial role of water ingestion can be minimized by the formation of hypochlorous acid (HOCl) when Cl_2 is added to water for disinfection purposes. HOCl is highly reactive and is capable of oxidizing many biological molecules. Moreover, HOCl reacts with O_2^- to give OH^-, and with H_2O_2 to form singlet O_2. Thus, ingestion of chlorinated water and showering can increase the oxidative stress of an organism (Poljsak, 2011). In areas where water is chlorinated, inhabitants should increase the intake of antioxidants from their diet in order to prevent the oxidative stress of their organism. The average person receives 50% of their chlorine exposure from taking a bath or shower.

Also swimming, especially in strongly chlorinated water, can damage the skin by making it too dry. Chlorine has an extreme drying effect, not only on the hair, but also on the skin. As the skin becomes drier, it also ages more quickly. Additionally, long, hot and too-frequent showers or baths can remove natural oils from the skin. If somebody likes swimming but only has access to chlorinatedpools,lotions specially formulated to create a barrier thatwill prevent skin from absorbing chlorine can be bought. Besides, dermal contact with some organic disinfection by-products such as trihalomethanes in chlorinated drinking water has been established to be an important exposure route (Xu and Weisel, 2005).

Foods that Decrease Oxidative Stress

Nutrition appears to be an important determinant of life expectancy and aging process. This paragraph is written on aging process in general but could be extrapolated on skin cells as well. According to Kirkwood and Mathers (2009), nutrition may have an important effect since, on the one hand, a poor diet will contain factors that are intrinsically damaging either at low levels or when consumed to excess; and on the other, nutrition can have important beneficial effects on the rate of aging, not only because cell-maintenance functions depend on an adequate supply of energybut also because some nutritional ingredients can aid in the protection against damage, e.g., dietary antioxidants.

By increasing our dietary intake of antioxidants, we can help our bodies to defend themselves from oxidative stress. The diet, particularly when including fruits, vegetables, nuts and seeds, provides a rich source of antioxidant substances and vitamins, and other micronutrients with antioxidant characteristics, which are an important exogenous source of compounds that are capable of increasing cellular responses to oxidative stress. Dietary factors that limit damage or that enhance repair would be expected to modify the rate of biological aging.The high incidence of age-related diseases in the increasing population of elderly people has stimulated interest in the search for protective agents that have the ability to prevent premature aging and delaying the onset of degenerative disorders.

Teas

The difference between different teas is how much each one is processed. White teas are the least processed of the commercial teas, followed by green teas, then black. Green tea is harvested when its antioxidant content is at its peak. The leaves are then minimally processed, resulting in tea leaves that are rich in antioxidant polyphenols.

Green tea polyphenols have been extensively studied as cardiovascular disease and cancer chemopreventive agents *in vitro* and in animal studies. The study of Li et al. (2010) suggests that citrus consumption is associated with reduced all-cancer incidence, especially for subjects having simultaneously high green tea consumption. The study of Kuriyama et al. (2006) concluded that green tea consumption is associated with reduced mortality due to all causes and due to cardiovascular disease (CVD) but not with reduced mortality due to cancer. Besides green tea consumption, also coffee, and oolong tea and total caffeine intake was associated with a reduced risk of mortality from CVD (Mineharu et al., 2009). Polyphenols and isothiocyanates present in green tea activate the c-Jun kinase (JNK1) and ERK2 pathways (The JNK/SAPK, c-Jun N-terminal kinases/stress-activated protein kinase, pathway is one of three members of the MAPK (mitogen-activated protein kinase) superfamily, which also includes the ERK and the p38 MAPKinases), inducing an array of detoxification and antioxidant genes that have relationship to the beneficial effects by green tea users (Ouwor and Kong, 2002).

The study of Chan et al. (2009) demonstrated that regular drinkers of tea may enjoy a younger biological age. Telomeres are the endcaps on chromosomes, and telomeric shortening is thought to govern the number of times a cell can divide. Ruth Chan and a team of researchers based in Hong Kong studied 976 Chinese men and 1,030 Chinese women, aged 65+, surveying their dietary habits using a food questionnaire. Overall findings showed that only tea consumption was associated with telomere length. The highest intake of Chinese tea (black or green), at three cups or 750 ml per day, was associated with telomeres that were 4.6 kilobases longer than in people who drank an average of a quarter of a cup per day. The researchers calculated that this average difference in telomere length corresponds to "approximately a difference of five years of life," and stated that "the antioxidative properties of tea and its constituent nutrients may protect telomeres from oxidative damage in the normal aging process."

The study performed by Katiyar et al. (2007) showed that the polyphenols present in green tea (Camellia sinensis) have been shown to have numerous health benefits, including protection from UV carcinogenesis. The oral administration of green tea polyphenols in drinking water or the topical application of epigallocatechin-3-gallate (EGCG) prevents UVB-induced skin tumor development in mice, and this prevention is mediated through: (a) the induction of immunoregulatory cytokine interleukin (IL) 12; (b) IL-12-dependent DNA repair following nucleotide excision repair mechanism; (c) the inhibition of UV-induced immunosuppression through IL-12-dependent DNA repair; (d) the inhibition of angiogenic factors; and (e) the stimulation of cytotoxic T cells in a tumor microenvironment.

Additional study revealed that topical application or oral administration of green tea through drinking water of mice prevents UVB-induced skin tumor development, and this prevention is mediated, at least in part, through rapid repair of DNA. The DNA repair by GTPs is mediated through the induction of interleukin (IL)-12, which has been shown to have DNA-repair ability (Katiyar, 2010). Vayalil et al. (2003) reported that treatment of green tea polyphenols in hydrophilic cream prevents UVB-induced oxidation of lipids and proteins, depletion of antioxidant enzymes and phosphorylation of MAPK proteins in SKH-1 hairless mouse skin. (Vayalil et al., 2003).The tumor-inhibiting property of black tea polyphenol, theaflavin, was reported in the recent study by Sil et al. (2010).In addition to suppressing cell proliferation, promoting apoptosis, and modulating signaling transduction, green tea polyphenols, especially (-)-epigallocatechin-3-gallate, also inhibit cell invasion, angiogenesis, and metastasis (Yang and Wang 2010). Authors report that theaflavin causes an inhibition of the expression and activity of pro-MMP-2 by a process involving multiple regulatory molecules in human melanoma cells, A375.Katiyar et al. (2010) in the recent study additionally report that green tea polyphenols prevent UV-induced immunosuppression by rapid repair of DNA damage and enhancement of nucleotide excision repair genes.

Mediterranean Diet (MD)

The Mediterranean diet includes vegetables, fruits and nuts that are all rich in phenols, flavonoids, isoflavonoids, phytosterols and phytic acid—essential bioactive compounds providing health benefits (Ortega, 2006). The polyunsaturated fatty acids found in fish effectively regulate haemostatic factors, protect against cardiac arrhythmias, cancer and hypertension, and play a vital role in the maintenance of neural functions and the prevention of certain psychiatric disorders as well as skin aging. Accumulating evidence suggests that olive oil, an integral component of the MD, may have health benefits, including the reduction of the risk of coronary heart disease, the prevention of several types of cancer and the modification of the immune and inflammatory responses. Olive oil is known for its high levels of monounsaturated fatty acids and is a good source of phytochemicals, such as polyphenolic compounds, squalene and alpha-tocopherol (Ortega, 2006). Many studies have shown that a "Mediterranean" diet improves the chances of living longer.

The aim of the Martinez-Gonzales et al. (2010) study was to evaluate the association between the adherence to the MD and the incidence of fatal and non-fatal cardiovascular events (CVD) among initially healthy middle-aged adults from the Mediterranean area. The study concluded that there is an inverse association between adherence to the Mediterranean diet and the incidence of fatal and non-fatal CVD in initially healthy middle-aged adults. Besides, the MD is significantly inversely associated with both systolic and diastolic blood pressure. It also has benefits in relation to the prevention of cardiovascular events, reduces the risk of mortality after myocardial infarction, and reduces peripheral arterial disease. The risk of obesity decreases with increasing adherence to the traditional MD. The MD also has a preventive effect on cancer, through its antiproliferative and pro-apoptotic effects, mostly due to the components of virgin olive oil and vegetables. There is some evidence of the benefits of the MD in relation to bone metabolism, rheumatoid arthritis, and neurodegenerative age-related diseases (cognitive deficit, Alzheimer's disease, Parkinson's disease) (Perez-Lopez et al., 2009). The review from Sofi et al. (2008) reveals that greater adherence to a Mediterranean diet is associated with a significant improvement in health status, as seen by a significant reduction in overall mortality (9%), mortality from cardiovascular diseases (9%), incidence of or mortality from cancer (6%), and incidence of Parkinson's disease and Alzheimer's disease (13%). Authors conclude that results seem to be clinically relevant for public health, in particular for encouraging a Mediterranean-like dietary pattern for primary prevention of major chronic diseases. Some positive associations with quality of life and inverse associations with the risk of certain cancers and with overall mortality were also reported for MD in the review by Roman et al. (2008). Additionally, it was reported and later confirmed that a greater adherence to a traditional Mediterranean diet was associated with a significant reduction of the total causes of mortality by Trichopoulou et al. (2003). A group of researchers from Boston and Greece have investigated the importance of individual diet components and their impact on longevity (Trichopoulou et al., 2003). The researchers reviewed data collected from the European Prospective Investigation into Cancer and Nutrition, a study that included 23,349 healthy Greek men and women. Adherence to the traditional Mediterranean diet was assessed by a ten-point Mediterranean-diet scale that incorporated the salient characteristics of this diet (range of scores, 0 to 9, with higher scores indicating greater adherence). Authors used proportional-hazards regression to assess the relation between adherence to the Mediterranean diet and total mortality, as well as mortality due to coronary heart disease and mortality due to cancer, with adjustment for age, sex, body-mass index, physical-activity level, and other potential confounders. They followed participants for 8.5 years, specifically looking at their diets and how closely they adhered to a traditional Mediterranean diet. For both men and women, people who more closely followed the Mediterranean Diet had lower chances of dying from cancer or from other causes. They also found that specific aspects of the diet may be more strongly linked to longevity. These include high consumption of vegetables and olive oil, low consumption of meat, and moderate consumption of alcohol. However, the study also claimed that following a Mediterranean diet high in fish, seafood and cereals, and low in dairy products, was not indicative of longevity. Long-term effect of Mediterranean-style diet and calorie restriction on biomarkers of longevity and oxidative stress in overweight men was investigated in the recent study of Esposito et al. (2010). Study concludes that prolonged adherence to a Mediterranean-style diet, with or without calorie restriction, in overweight or obese men is associated with significant amelioration of multiple risk factors, including a better cardiovascular risk profile, reduced oxidative stress, and improved insulin sensitivity. Another recent study found out that increased physical activity and greater adherence to the Mediterranean diet was associated with increased total antioxidant capacity (Kavouras et al., 2010). Similar results were previously published by Pitsavos et al. (2005) where greater adherence to the Mediterranean diet was associated with elevated total antioxidant capacity (TAC) levels and low oxidized LDL-cholesterol concentrations. To sum up, the Mediterranean diet consists of vegetables, legumes, fruits, nuts, whole grains, fish, moderate alcohol, a high ratio of monounsaturated fats to saturated fats (ample olive oil) and lean meat (chicken), with dairy and red meat used more as a side dish. Tourlouki et al. (2009) conclude their study on the secrets of the elderly on Mediterranean islands with the statement: "A favorable adherence to the Mediterranean diet, midday naps and smoking cessation with an increase in age was characteristic of our elderly population." MD could have beneficial effects also on the skin. Dietary antioxidant vitamins, minerals, and phytochemicals in addition to n-3 polyunsaturated fatty acids, n-9 monounsaturated fatty acids, and low pro-inflammatory n-6 polyunsaturated fatty acids, have demonstrated protective properties in reducing photooxidative damage. The presence of these elements in the traditional Greek-style Mediterranean diet may have contributed to the low rates of melanoma in the Mediterranean region despite high levels of solar radiation (Shapira, 2010). The study by Fortes et al. (2008) suggests that some dietary factors present in the Mediterranean diet might protect from cutaneous melanoma. Authors have found a protective effect for weekly consumption of fish, shellfish, fish rich in n-3 fatty acids, daily tea drinking and high consumption of vegetablesin particular carrots, cruciferous and leafy vegetables and fruits, in particular citrus fruits. No association was found for alcohol consumption and any other food items.

At Least Five Portions of Fruits and Vegetables Per Day

Consumption of vegetables and plant-derived foods and beverages has positive effect on the prevention of age associated diseases like coronary heart disease and atherosclerosis as well as for longevity (Hertog et al., 1993; Corder et al., 1998; Sahyoun et al., 1996) and skin aging. Many other plant extracts have potential application as anti-aging substances for the body. Based on the analysis of available epidemiological data, a daily intake of at least 400 g of fruits and vegetables has been recommended by the World Health Organization (www.who.int). Many animal studies have shown that an increased intake of antioxidants in the diet can increase average lifespan and prevent degenerative diseases in humans (Block et al., 1992; Frankel et al., 1993; Goldberg, 1995; Renaud and de Lorgeril, 1992; Steinmetz and Potter, 1991). However, detailed analysis of protective foods and drinks shows that they contain different amounts of *total*antioxidants. Researchers have found a lower occurrence of cancer, heart and vein diseases only in people who consume sufficient quantities of fruits and vegetables, but not in people who consume supplements of vitamins (Halliwell, 2000). The positive effects of the protective substances that originate from food are greater because of the synergic activity between individual antioxidant substances, nutritional fibrin and secondary vegetal substances in food, mainly in vegetables and fruits. Correlation between the high antioxidant capacity of fruits and vegetables and the positive impact of diets high in fruits and vegetables is believed to play an important role in the free-radical theory of aging. Each part of a cell is protected by a different antioxidant nutrient, which is why only a comprehensive intake of nutrients can protect you. For example, some nutrients defend against free radical attack in the blood surrounding the cell, others defend inside the cell, and still other nutrients protect the cell mitochondria. Some nutrients can activate genes responsible for cell repair and protection(Rietjens et al., 2001).

The Problem of ORAC Units

ORAC is the Oxygen Radical Absorbance Capacity of food. ORAC provides us with a measure of the overall antioxidant power of foods and supplements. ORAC values measure the time an antioxidant takes to react to free radicals, as well as the amount of antioxidants in the specific food. It combines these elements into one measurement. The higher the ORAC value of a food, the more antioxidant power it contains. In theory, the higher the ORAC number, the greater the amount of antioxidants in the food. Foods with a higher ORAC value have a greater antioxidant potential than those with low values. A wide variety of foods have been tested using this methodology, and certain spices, berries and legumes have been rated very highly.

Table 10. Data on foods with high ORAC scores

Food	Serving size	Antioxidant capacity per serving size[*]
Small Red Bean	½ cup dried beans	13727
Wild blueberry	1 cup	13427
Red kidney bean	½ cup dried beans	13259
Pinto bean	½ cup	11864
Blueberry	1 cup (cultivated berries)	9019
Cranberry	1 cup (whole berries)	8983
Artichoke hearts	1 cup, cooked	7904
Blackberry	1 cup (cultivated berries)	7701
Prune	½ cup	7291
Raspberry	1 cup	6058
Strawberry	1 cup	5938
Red Delicious apple	1 apple	5900
Granny Smith apple	1 apple	5381
Pecan	1 oz	5095
Sweet cherry	1 cup	4873
Black plum	1 plum	4844
Russet potato	1, cooked	4649
Black bean	½ cup dried beans	4181
Plum	1 plum	4118
Gala apple	1 apple	3903

[*]Units are Total Antioxidant Capacity per serving in units of micromoles of Trolox equivalents. Table taken from: http://en.wikipedia.org/wiki/Oxygen_radical_absorbance_capacity.

In 2007, scientists with the United States Department of Agriculture published an updated list of ORAC values for 277 foods commonly consumed by the U.S. population (fruits, vegetables, nuts, seeds, spices, grains, etc.) (Nutrient Data Laboratory, Agriculture Research Service, U.S. Department of Agriculture, Oxygen Radical Absorbance Capacity (ORAC) of Selected Foods, 2007). Values were expressed as the sum of the lipid-soluble (e.g., carotenoid) and water-soluble (e.g., phenolic) antioxidant fractions (i.e., "total ORAC") reported in micromole Trolox equivalents (TE) per 100 gram sample.

The problem with ORAC values as shown in the above table is the fact that these measured values cannot be directly extrapolated to determine the effect of these food components on human health. Information is lacking regarding how absorbable and functional these concentrated antioxidants are in the human body. The *in vitro* antioxidant capacity of fruits and vegetables cannot be linearly related to the *in vivo* capacity once these foods are ingested. Besides, supplement companies manipulate the figures to make their products look more powerful by using different sets of measurements—either dry weight, liquid measures, or typical serving sizes, etc.

Health-promoting nutrition involves the daily intake of five to ten vegetables and fruits, fruit juices, red wine and tea that are rich sources of micronutrients with antioxidant properties. According to Willcox et al. (2006), prudent food choices that maximize nutritional properties of foods while minimizing caloric density would be the favored strategy for anyone who attempts a CR regimen. Simply avoiding calorie-dense refined sugars, saturated fats and processed foods and replacing them with nutrient-dense but calorie-poor vegetables, fruits and legumes will not only likely lead to spontaneous weight loss through lower calorie intake but would also result in a vastly increased intake of health-enhancing phytonutrients, including key vitamins and minerals, antioxidants and flavonoids needed for our skin cells to work properly.

Skin Aging, Immunotoxicity and Inflammation

Inflammation and the resulting accumulation of reactive oxygen species (ROS) play an important role in the intrinsic and photoaging of human skin in vivo. Environmental insults such as ultraviolet (UV) rays from the sun, cigarette smoke exposure and pollutants, and the natural process of aging contribute to the generation of free radicals and ROS that stimulate the inflammatory process in the skin (Pillai, 2005). Inflammation can be determined with in vivo and in vitro studies. In vitro studies of inflammation, including monitoring the release of pro-inflammatory mediators such as cytokines, chemokines, nitric oxide, upregulation of transcription factors such as nuclear factor kappaB (NF-κB) and activator protein 1 (all known to be important in initiating inflammatory responses), is possible in different cellular sources.

For the proper homeostatic functioning of the skin immune system, the multiple pro-inflammatory signals that can be generated by skin cells must eventually be counterbalanced by mechanisms capable of promoting resolution of a cutaneous inflammatory process. Failure of these mechanisms may predispose skin to the development of chronic inflammatory process (Williams and Kupper, 1996; Katiyar and Mukhtar, 2001). The cells that make up the skin immune system are distributed on both sides of the basement membrane separating epidermis and dermis and include several populations of nonleukocytes. Most of the attention has been focused on epidermal components (i.e., keratinocytes, Langerhans cells, and dendritic epidermal T-cells in mice). However, the dermal components of the skin immune system, including dermal fibroblasts, microvascular endothelial cells, dermal dendritic cells, mast cells, and resident perivascular T-cells, also participate in the cutaneous immune response (Williams and Kupper, 1996; Katiyar and Mukhtar,2001).

The pro-inflammatory mediators increase the permeability of capillaries leading to infiltration and activation of neutrophils and other phagocytic cells into the skin. The net result of all these effects is inflammation and free radical generation (both reactive oxygen and nitrogen species). Furthermore, elastsases and other proteases (cathepsin G) released from neutrophils cause further inflammation, and activation of matrix metalloproteases. The inflammation further activates the transcription of various matrixes degrading metalloproteases, leading to abnormal matrix degradation and accumulation of non-functional matrix components. In addition, the inflammation and ROS cause oxidative damage to cellular proteins, lipids and carbohydrates, which accumulates in the dermal and epidermal compartments, contributing to the etiology of photoaging (Pillai, 2005).

Nutrition and Inflammation

Inflammation is an important determinant of longevity. Aging is associated with a greater risk of dysfunction of the immune system and with development of a chronic inflammatory state. Inflammation is an endogenous source of free radicals. The inflammation theory of aging states that toxic materials of whatever source (e.g., free radicals and others) are thought to initiate pre-inflammatory changes in target tissues and in immune cells, as well as other contiguous target tissues such as vascular epithelium. The major pro-inflammatory cytokines involved appear to be tumor necrosis factor-α (NTF- α) and interleukin-6 (IL-6) (Visser et al., 2002), although other pro-inflammatory cytokines are also likely to be involved. ROS can activate harmful genes, and this can be even more damaging in the long run (Arking, 2006). All the proinflammatory cytokines are activated by the NFκB transcription factor, which is very sensitive to ROS levels. Interactions that selectively inhibit the NFκB pathway may provide a useful intervention for inflammation-related senescent diseases.

When an infection occurs, immune cells secrete large amounts of free radicalsto combat the invader. But, these inflammatory chemicals also attack normal tissue surrounding the infection and damage critical components of cells, including DNA. During chronic inflammation, that damage may lead to mutations or cell death and even to cancer and other diseases. The most likely sources of these oxidizing radicals are the phagocytic leukocytes (e.g., neutrophils, monocytes, macrophages, and eosinophils) that invade the tissue. Granulocytes and mononuclear phagocytes reducemolecular O_2 to superoxide radicals and H_2O_2, both states of oxygen being intended for the killing and destruction of the phagocytosed material.Although ROS produced were intended for intracellular killing, they may escape into the extracellular milieu and harm phagocytes and body's own macromolecules. Chronic infections also cause chronic inflammatory bystander damage through ROS and other free radicals. Among many examples, infections by the enterobacter *Helicobacter pylori*cause local inflammatory responses that increase DNA oxidation, cell proliferation and the mutational load and are a major cause of gut cancer. For this reason, inflammation, free radical damage and oxidative stresshave become major health issues in recent years, the subject of much research and concern. Inflammation, free radical damage and oxidative stress are not "diseases." In fact, they are often the by-product of normal cellular processes. Different food can influence the formation of ROS, oxidative stress and inflammatory processes.

All foods could be set in three categories: pro-inflammatory, neutral, and anti-inflammatory. Aging at the cellular level could be decreased by consuming foods that are anti-inflammatory and rich in antioxidants. Interventions using nutrients with anti-inflammatory properties such as vitamin E and ω-3 polyunsaturated fatty acids may reduce levels of inflammation and improve cell and tissue function (Grimble, 2003).Age-related changes may be abrogated by taking foods and drinks that are rich in a great number of components, including antioxidants, and are anti-inflammatory, like *cold-water fish and richly colored fruitsand vegetables*. On the other hand, pro-inflammatory foods can quicken aging. If we consume large amounts of *saturated or trans-fatty acids, starches, and sugars,* insulin levels surge quicken the process of aging.

Acute Inflammation - Free Radicals

Help in Fighting Infection
Some free radicals are important components in biological systems, and they are, in fact, essential for the maintenance of life. Free radicals perform many critical functions in our bodies from controlling the flow of blood through our arteries, to fighting infection, to keeping our brains alert and in focus.

Free Radicals as "Good Guys"
The direct role of free radicals in microbial killing is well established. During phagocytosis, cells consume high amounts of oxygen, a process termed as a respiratory burst, producing: superoxide anion radical, hydrogen peroxide, hydroxyl radical, hypochlorus acid, which are capable of damaging cell membranes and biomolecules. The ability of ROS to activate transcription is now recognized. Low doses of ROS stimulate the growth of fibroblasts and epithelial cells. Thus free radicals can play the positive role in early inflammation by promoting fibrosis and wound healing.

Is the use of antioxidants in acute inflammation contraindicatory? In theory, yes. However, antioxidants (like vitamin C) can also improve our immune system. Certain antioxidants (e.g., phenols) also have antibactericidal properties.

The Problem of Chronic Inflammation
While in the short term, inflammation-derived free radical damage is not a problem, in the long term, it causes progressive damage. Chronic inflammation is a pathological condition characterized by continued active inflammation response and tissue destruction. Many of the immune cells including macrophages, neutrophils and eosinophils are involved directly or by production of inflammatory cytokine in the pathology of chronic inflammation. In chronic inflammation, the inflammation becomes the problem rather than the solution to infection, injury or disease. The chronic inflammatory response can break down healthy tissue in a misdirected attempt at repair and healing. Diseases characterized by chronic inflammation include, among others, diabetes, coronary artery disease (atherosclerosis), rheumatoid arthritis, asthma, solid organ transplant rejection, etc. Laneet al. (2003) described a mechanism whereby old cells lose the capability to reduce inflammation through the initiation of transcription factors for stress-reduction genes, and, therefore, the chronic inflammatory response disturbs gene regulation and expression (Schweitzer and Alessio, 2006). Many studies suggest that chronic inflammation could have an important role in a wide variety of age-related diseases, including skin aging.

Chronic inflammation takes place also in photodamaged skin (Lavker and Kligman, 1988). While intrinsically aged skin shows reduction in cell numbers, photoaged skin shows increase in the number of dermal fibroblasts, mast cells, histiocytes and mononuclear cells (Krutmann and Gilchrest, 2006).

Chronic Inflammation and Protective Role of Antioxidants
In addition to scavenging free radicals, there are antioxidants that actually block inflammation. The antioxidant effect (the blocking of certain oxidizing proteins) lowers the activation of inflammatory signals. Scientists have also found that combinations of certain

antioxidants have greater effect than single antioxidants on certain types of inflammation. There have been many studies investigating the role of antioxidants on the inflammation process:

- The most consistent evidence of modulation of inflammation from dietary intervention studies involves antioxidants and polyunsaturated fatty acids (Forsey et al., 2009). α-toccopherol suplemented at 1200 IU/day in type 2 diabetics with/without microvascular complications and matched controls leads to decreases in CRP and IL-6 (Deveraj and Jialal, 2000). Vitamin C or vitamin C and E combinations have been shown to reduce exercise-induced inflammation (Thompson et al., 2001; Vassilakopoulus et al., 2003; Fischer et al., 2004). Vitamin E administered to older volunteers at 900 mg/day for four months potentiated insulin-mediated glucose disposal (Paolisso et al., 1994) and high doses of vitamin E and C supplementation immediately before a meal challenge attenuated the postprandial inflammatory responses (Esposito et al., 2003). ω-3 polyunsaturates may provide some protection against cardiovascular diseases in older men by lowering plasma triglycerides, decreasing lipoprotein peroxidation and the ratio of reduced to total glutathione, and decreasing soluble adhesion molecule 1 levels (marker of vascular inflammation) (Yaqoob and Calder, 2003; Cazzola et al., 2007). Dietary fish oil suppresses the production of pro-inflammatory cytokines and expression of adhesion molecules. ω-3 polyunsaturates can downregulate NFkB activity. Clinical trials have shown oral fish oil to have beneficial effects in rheumatoid arthritis and asthma patients (Calder, 2002).
- Oxidative stress triggersthe production of the inflammatory cytokine interleukin-6 (IL-6), and antioxidant micronutrients playa critical role in decreasing this inflammatory response. Theresearch sought to identify the relations between serum levelsof antioxidant nutrients and IL-6 and mortality in older women.Levels of α- and ß-carotene, lycopene, lutein/zeaxanthin,α -cryptoxanthin, total carotenoids, retinol, α -tocopherol, zinc,and selenium were measured at baseline in 619 participants in*Women's Health and Aging Study I* (Baltimore, Maryland, 1992 to 1998). Participants with the highest serum levels of ß-carotene,total carotenoids, and selenium were significantly less likelyto be in the highest tertile of serum IL-6 at baseline. Those with the lowest levels of α- and ß-carotene,lutein/zeaxanthin, and total carotenoids were significantlymore likely to have increasing IL-6 levels over a period oftwo years. Those with the lowest selenium levels had a significantlyhigher risk of total mortality over a period of five years. These findingssuggest that specific antioxidant nutrients may play an importantrole in suppressing IL-6 levels in disabled older women.
- In the study of Singh et al. (1995), the role of free radical intermediates in the inflammation (in human synovial tissue) was studied. The specimens from rheumatoid arthritis and osteoarthritis patients demonstrated increased production of ROS. This change was reduced by both inhibitors of the endothelial-based enzymexanthine oxidase.
- In the study of Colbart et al. (2004), the use of multivitamin supplements, beta-carotene, vitamin C and/or vitamin E was associated with lower levels of C-reactive

protein and interleukin-6, regardless of whether the participant reported high or low exercise levels.
- The study by Fuchs and Milbradt (1994)concluded that several natural antioxidants such as catalase, superoxide dismutase and dihydrolipoate have anti-inflammatory properties in dermatitis induced by ROS.
- The study of Esteban et al. (1999) investigated oxidative stress and pulmonary oxidation. An increased oxidative stress accompanied by reduced endogenous antioxidant defenses may have a role in the pathogenesis of a number of inflammatory pulmonary diseases, including asthma.
- Connere and Grisham (1996) reported that essential nutrients such as vitamins C and Emay protect against oxidant-mediated inflammation and tissue damage by their ability to scavenge free radicals and by their ability to inhibit the activation of NF-kB (and possibly other oxidant-sensitive transcription factors).

Foods to Calm Inflammation

The body manufactures its own antioxidants. Some of them are in the form of enzymes, such as glutathione peroxidase, superoxide dismutase, and catalase—all of which require selenium and zinc for their proper functions. Lipoic acid, N-acetylcysteine, and glutathione are substances that rely on sulfur. Supplemental lipoic acid, in conjunction with L-Carnitine, works in the mitochondria to reduce the harmful effects of free radicals and diminish the actions of inflammatory signals. The best sources of antioxidants are vegetables, fruits, tea and wine. It is a good idea to get antioxidants from a variety of sources. The more colorful natural foods are the better—yellow, orange, green, red, brown and blue-purple plant foods provide a variety of antioxidants, and the more brightly colored, the richer the food is in antioxidants. There are thousands of antioxidants found in fruits, vegetables, whole grains, nuts, legumes, poultry, fish, chocolate, coffee, and red wine. There is growing number of antioxidants being discovered (so far, there are more than 4,000 known flavonoids, and that's only one class of antioxidants).All eukaryotes, including plants, encode sirtuins in their genomes (Frye, 2000; Pandey et al., 2002). The plant polyphenols that activate sirtuins in yeast and animals are produced by plants in response to various types of environmental stress, including drought, nutrient deprivation and UVirradiation (Dixon and Paiva, 1995). It seems, therefore, reasonable to suggest that some plant polyphenols might function as endogenous regulators of plant sirtuins and other stress responses. Plants were, for millions of years, exposed to sun and other free radical generators from the environment. Because plants cannot walk away or hide, they had to make their own protection against free radicals.

Slowing aging at the cellular level could be affected by consuming foods that are anti-inflammatory and rich in antioxidants. On the other hand, pro-inflammatory foods can quicken aging. If we consume large amounts of saturated or trans fatty acids, starches, and sugars, insulin levels surge and quicken the process of free radical formation.

Preventative anti-inflammatory treatments are numerous and may be applied at various levels of care.

The following plants are rich sources of antioxidants and anti-Inflammatory phytochemicals:

Blueberries

Blueberries are the fruit of a shrub native to North America. Much research has shown that blueberries provide health benefits in the areas of anti-aging, antioxidant action, disease prevention, treatment of urinary tract infection, improving eyesight and controlling cholesterol. Blueberries are powerful antioxidants. Anthocyanin, which is the pigment that makes the blueberry blue, is the key antioxidant responsible for these benefits (Prior et al., 1998). Researchers believe that the phytochemicals in blueberries may reduce inflammatory processes in tissues by increasing cell membranes' ability to allow vital nutrients and chemical signals to pass in and out of the cell (Smith et al., 2000). There are currently no scientific recommendations as to the amount of blueberries to consume to achieve positive health benefits. Blueberries can be purchased in capsule form or extracts, teas, or in their natural state. If using the capsule form, follow the dosage advice on the container.

Mexican Red Beans

Mexican red beans are similar to red kidney beans, only smaller, darker and rounder. Also called the small red bean, the Mexican red bean holds both shape and firmness when cooked. It is most often used in soups, salads, chili and Creole dishes. Besides, Mexican red beans have very high oxygen radical absorbance capacity (ORAC). The flavonoids that give Mexican red beans their bright-red color are powerful antioxidants. These beans are also a good source of fiber, folic acid, and carbohydrates.

Prunes

Prunes are actually the dried version of European plums. The name was recently officially changed to dried plum. They contain an unusually high concentration of unique phytonutrients called *neochlorogenic* and *chlorogenic acid*. These substances found in prunes and plums are classified as phenols, and their function as antioxidants has been well documented. They are especially good at neutralizing *superoxide anion radical*, and they have also been shown to help prevent oxygen-based damage to fats. The ability of prunes to fight free radicals is boosted by beta-carotene. Beta-carotene acts as a fat-soluble antioxidant, eliminating free radicals that would otherwise cause a lot of damage to our cells and cell membranes (Cho et al., 2004).

Milk Thistle Extract

Milk thistle is a plant native to the Mediterranean. It usually grows in dry, sunny areas. It is a stout thistle that grows to a height of four to ten feet and has red-purple flowers. The active ingredient is called silymarin. Consisting of a group of compounds known as flavonolignands, silymarin helps repair liver cells that have been damaged by alcohol and other toxins. Silymarin also has potent antioxidant and anti-inflammatory effects. Most milk thistle-based products are standardized to contain 70% to 80% silymarin (Agency for Healthcare Research and Quality, 2000).

Curcumin

Curcumin, a biphenol with a remarkable range of activities, is the active ingredient of the Indian spice turmeric, a preservative from the herb *Curcuman longa*. Over the last few decades, hundreds of small-scale studies have proven scientifically what Indian people have known for centuries: that curcumin has the ability to halt or prevent certain types of cancer, stop inflammation, improve cardiovascular health, prevent cataracts and kill or inhibit the toxic effects of certain microbes including fungi and dangerous parasites (Arora et al., 1971). Curcumin has been shown to protect against the deleterious effects of injury by attenuating oxidative stress and suppressing inflammation (Heng, 2010). Curcumin is a naturally occurring source of cyclooxygenase-2 (COX-2) inhibitors, which can be artificially obtained through some commercially available supplements. People who take COX-2 inhibitors are statistically less likely to develop cancer thanthose who do not (Reddy and Rao, 2002).

Curcumin, a component of the spice turmeric, was tested for its potential hormetic anti-aging effects as an inducer of mild stress in the study of Lima et al. (Lima et al., 2010). Early-passage young human skin fibroblasts treated with low doses of curcumin (below 20 µM) showed a time- and concentration-dependent induction of heme oxygenase-1 (HO-1), followed by compensatory increase in glutathione-S-transferase activity, GSH levels and GSH/GSSG ratio. These effects were preceded by induction of oxidative stress (increased levels of reactive oxygen species and DNA damage) and impairment of cells' GSH redox state. The induction of stress responses by curcumin in human cells led to protective hormetic effects to further oxidant challenge. Curcumin-induced hormetic stimulation of cellular antioxidant defenses can be a useful approach toward anti-aging intervention.

Ginkgo Biloba Extract

The Ginkgo tree is the oldest living tree on the planet. Over the past three decades, hundreds of clinical studies have focused on the health benefits that Ginkgo leaf extract can bring to the human body. Ginkgo acts as a booster of blood flow to the brain and throughout the entire body. It increases metabolism efficiency, regulates neurotransmitters, and boosts oxygen levels in the brain, which uses 20% of the body's oxygen. Ginkgo has two groups of active substances, flavonoids and terpene lactones, including ginkgolides A, B, and C, bilobalide, quercetin, and kaempferol. The ginkgolides have been shown to control allergic inflammation, anaphylactic shock and asthma. In addition, Ginkgo is a powerful antioxidant (Coates et al., 2005).

Propolis

The pharmacologically active molecules in propolis are flavonoids and phenolic acids and their esters. These components have proven antibiotic effects on bacteria, fungi, and viruses (Mirzoeva and Calder, 1996; Borelli et al., 2002; Rossi et al., 2002; Ozturk et al., 2000; Gregory et al., 2002).

Resveratrol

Resveratrol, a flavonoid found in red wine, is an effective inhibitor of inflammatory cytokine release from macrophages. The other possible mechanism of polyphenols-mediated inhibition of inflammatory response is by quenching oxidants and aldehydes and inhibiting histone deacetyltransferase activity. See also the chapter on Mediterranean diet.

Green Tea

Catechins present in green tea (epigallocatechin-3-gallate) may be effective in decreasing oxidative stress and inflammatory response.

Synthetic Antioxidants

The results of clinical trials with antioxidant supplements have yet to provide conclusive indication of health benefits. We still do not properly understand how antioxidants integrate their function within the tissues and cells and how they adjust to physiological and pathological challenges.

Foods to Avoid

The anti-inflammatory diet is strict avoidance of foods that contain high amounts of arachidonic acid (AA), the main precursor of the negatively associated inflammatory cascade process. Metabolites of AA include platelet-activating factors (prostaglandins (PGs), LTs, and thromboxanes), which are closely involved in both acute and chronic inflammatory responses. Another source of dietary inflammation is hydrogenated foods, which often have an increased amount of linoleic acid (LA) and a decreased amount of the beneficial alphalinolenic acid (ALA). Dietary gluten and lectins are also recognized as common triggers of inflammation.

Eating for Optimal Nutrition

After all, we are what we eat. The changes in skin aging are dependent not only on genetics and lifestyle, but also on nutrition. The foods you eat make a huge difference in how your body responds as you get older. Severe vitamin deficiencies (scurvy or pellagra) are very rare in the developed world. Nevertheless, diet in developed countries is energetically too dense but is usually deprived of essential micronutrients and phytochemicals. A balanced diet is also recommended for optimal wound healing since poor nutrition has adverse impact on wound healing. Experts agree—while there's no formal recommendation for the amount of antioxidants we need, the best way to obtain antioxidants is from a varied diet. Foods rich in antioxidants include all fresh and seasonal fruit and vegetables (peppers, apples, onions, pineapple, dark leafy vegetables, flaxseeds, walnuts, pumpkin seeds, olives, etc.), olive oil and fish. Antioxidants work synergistically. Unlike many other nutrients, antioxidants in the body (water-soluble antioxidants) cannot be stored for a longer time, so we have to keep replenishing the supply of antioxidants each day. Optimal intake is five to ten small portions of fruit and vegetables per day.

The study of Purba et al. (2001) addressed whether food and nutrient intakes were correlated with skin wrinkling in a sun-exposed site. One hundred and seventy-seven Greek-born subjects living in Melbourne (GRM), 69 Greek subjects living in rural Greece (GRG), 48 Anglo-Celtic Australian (ACA) living in Melbourne and 159 Swedish subjects living in Sweden (SWE) participating in the International Union of Nutritional Sciences IUNS "Food Habits in Later Life" study had their dietary intakes measured and their skin assessed. Skin wrinkling was measured using a cutaneous microtopographic method. SWE elderly had the least skin wrinkling in a sun-exposed site, followed by GRM, GRG and ACA. Correlation analyses on the pooled data and using the major food groups suggested that there may be less actinic skin damage with a higher intake of vegetables, olive oil, fish and legumes and with lower intakes of butter and margarine, milk products and sugar products. In particular, a high intake of vegetables, legumes and olive oil appeared to be protective against cutaneous actinic damage; a high intake of meat, dairy and butter appeared to be adverse. Prunes, apples and tea explained 34% of variance amongst ACA. This study illustrates that skin wrinkling in a sun-exposed site in older people of various ethnic backgrounds may be influenced by the types of foods consumed.

People with genetic predispositions to reduce low levels of inflammatory cytokines seem to be more likely to live to an old age, and so it has been suggested that control of the pro-inflammatory response to aging may provide a route to healthy aging. The most consistent evidence to date concerns long chain ω-3 fatty acids, antioxidants such as vitamin C and E, weight loss and increased physical activity, but much more research is required before conclusions can be drawn (Stanner et al., 2009).

Overweight and Inflammation

During aging, lean tissue tends to be lost and be replaced by fat so that for a given body mass index, older persons will tend to have higher body fat content. Since obesity is characterized by mild chronic inflammation (Trayhurn, 2005), the increase in prevalence of being overweight and being obese (until about age 75 years) is likely to exacerbate any age-related increase in inflammation.

Also, exercise can be very anti-inflammatory by increasing muscle-derived IL−6 production (which is independent of TNF−α) and reducing C-reactive protein (*CRP)* (Evans et al., 2005). Besides exercise, also adequate sleep is important in inflammatory process control because it can reduce TNF−α and IL−6 secretion (both of which induce sleepiness and fatigue).

Modern nutritional science is now developing new insights intothe relation between food intake and health, and interest inthe role of diet, specific food ingredients, and supplementsin reducing the risk of skin disorders is growing. Specificpositive effects of food ingredients on skin conditions mayprove to be biologically relevant and may consequently allowfor claims on products containing these functional ingredients,resulting in the development of new functional foods for optimalskin condition (Boelsma et al., 2001).

The Importance of Eating Habits

Number of Meals withRegard to Electron Transport in Mitochondria

The "three-meals-a-day-plus-snacks" diet is typical of many modern industrialized countries. In contrast to the continuous availability of food that we currently enjoy, our ancestors were often forced to endure extended periods from many hours to days without food (Mattson et al., 2003). When food supplies are plentiful, individuals consume more calories than necessary for the maintenance of health.

When overeating, high amounts of energy become available and mitochondria do not operate very efficiently and generate more superoxide. The electron transport always proceeds as fast as energy is removed from the gradient.

Electron transport is *driven* by the free energy that is available from the energy carriers,,which, in turn, is obtained from substrates such as glutamate or Krebs intermediates. It is *restricted* by the chemiosmotic gradient. Electron transport can proceed only in a manner that is proportional to the extent that the energy in the gradient is dissipated (David R. Caprette, Rice University, http://www.ruf.rice.edu/ ~bioslabs/studies/mitochondria/mitotheory.html). Electron transport is driven by the increasing affinities of successive carriers for electrons and by the availability of substrates to provide electrons and free energy. It is restricted by the chemiosmotic gradient, such that electron transport can only go as fast as energy is lost from the gradient. Anything that increases the turnover of energy from the gradient increases the rate of electron transport proportionally. ROS production thus plummets when ATP demand is high. Decreased proton concentration or membrane potential brings about a nonlinear and striking decrease in the level of inadvertent electron leaks, and this likely accounts for ROS decrease (Arking, 2006).

For this reason, it is important to have many small amounts of food per day and not one large amount that would provide too much free energy (electrons) at once to the mitochondrial electron transport system. Besides, glucose in the blood increases after consuming a meal, and for this reason, work instead of resting should be performed in order to maintain an appropriate electron flow and avoid electron leaks.

Additionally, recent research has revealed that eating quickly increases the risk of weight gain. The research team of Dr. Kokkinos et al. (2009) concluded that "Eating at a physiologically moderate pace leads to a more pronounced (satiety) gut peptide response than eating very fast." The study of Arble et al. (2009) showed that eating at irregular times—the equivalent of the middle of the night for humans, when the body wants to sleep—influences weight gain.

The regulation of energy by the body's circadian rhythms may play a significant role. This study also provides the first causal evidence linking meal timing and increased weight gain. For more information on circadian rhythm, see next paragraph.

8.7. The Importance of Lifestyle

Sleeping and Melatonin Production

A circadian rhythm roughly represents a 24-hour cycle in the biochemical, physiological or behavioral processes of living entities, including plants, animals, fungi and cyanobacteria. The primary role of these cell-autonomous clocks is to maintain their own 24-hour molecular rhythm and to drive the rhythmic expression of genes involved in physiology, metabolism and behavior. Photosensitive proteins and circadian rhythms are believed to have originated in the earliest cells with the purpose of protecting the replication of DNA from free radicals, as in guarding against high ultraviolet radiation during the daytime. As a result, cell replication was relegated to the dark.

The pineal gland secretes the hormone melatonin. Secretion of melatonin peaks at night and ebbs during the day. In all organisms, melatonin is produced primarily during the daily period of darkness, with only small amounts being synthesized during the day. For this reason, people should sleep in complete darkness in order to produce necessary amounts of the endogenous powerful antioxidant melatonin (Tan et al., 1993; Hardeland, 2005) and benefit from its particular role in the protection of nuclear and mitochondrial DNA (Reiter et al., 2001). Melatonin is an antioxidant that can easily cross cell membranes and the blood-brain barrier (Hardeland, 2005). Melatonin is a direct scavenger of OH, O_2^- and NO (Poeggeler et al., 1994). Unlike other antioxidants, melatonin does not undergo redox cycling, the ability of a molecule to undergo reduction and oxidation repeatedly. Lack of sleep has been associated with contributing to oxidative stress.

In man and other mammals, melatonin is produced and secreted from the pineal gland during the night; however, the night-time production of melatonin falls markedly with aging such that a night-time melatonin rise in senescent animals is barely measurable. This may be significant for aging in the light of recent observations thatshow that melatonin is a highly efficient free radical scavenger and antioxidant both *in vitro* and *in vivo*. The loss of this potent antioxidant during aging may have consequences for cellular and organismal aging, as well as for the onset of age-related diseases.

Experimental results from a variety of sources suggest that a more determined approach to the study of melatonin as an anti-aging factor is warranted (Reiter, 1995). Nevertheless, when people get less than six or seven hours of sleep each night, their risk for developing diseases begins to increase. For more on melatonin, see also the chapter Hormones and skin aging.

Melatonin also has a significant effect on skin cells. Skin represents one of the extrapineal sites of melatonin synthesis. In the skin, melatonin plays, for example, the role of an antioxidantthatscavenges and inactivates free radicals arising due to UV irradiation. Melatonin protects skin cells from the action of UVA and UVB. The protective effect of different melatonin concentrations might result from variable expression of melatonin receptors (Izykowska et al., 2009). Fisher et al. (2008) reported that melatonin could act as a major skin protectant: from free radical scavenging to DNA damage repair.Melatonin also manifests strong potency of inhibiting growth of dermal melanoma cells both under in vitro and in vivo conditions. Although the mechanism of the phenomenon has not been fully clarified yet, melatonin receptors seem to play a key role in the inhibition (Danielczyk and Dziegiel, 2009).

Avoidance of Polluted Environments

Free radicals and reactive oxygen species are involved in the toxic mechanisms of many environmental pollutants, such as certain air pollutants, metals, ionizing and non-ionizing radiation, alcohols, pesticides, etc. The most efficient preventive step to avoid exogenous free radical exposure would be to avoid as much as possible exposure to certain environmental pollutants. But since this is not always possible, protection could be obtained by an adequate antioxidant balance. There is a growing body of evidence suggesting that the involvement of antioxidants could prevent or decrease the damage generated by environmental sources of oxidizing species.

Environmental pollutants with known oxidizing properties include nitrogen oxide, ozone, sulfur oxides, particulate matter, etc. Tobacco smoke is one of the most exposed air pollutants that is high in ROS. Cigarette smoke is a complex mixture of toxic agents, some of which are free radicals and others are free-radical-generating agents. Besides free radicals, there are many other carcinogenic compounds in smoke. The combustion of cigarette tobacco produces many smoke free-radical species in the tar and gas phases. One puff of cigarette smoke has been estimated to contain as many as 10^{15} gas-phase radicals and 10^{14} tar-phase radicals. Moreover, smokers have been shown to have decreased levels of protective antioxidants in their bodies.

Besides human-emitted pollutants, UV radiation from the sun is a significant source of free radicals to which our eyes and skin are exposed. Exposure of human skin to UV radiation leads to depletion of cutaneous antioxidants, impaired regulation of gene expression, and ultimately to the development of skin diseases. Both UVA and UVB have been shown to lead to oxidative damage and ROS production by the direct interaction of photons with target molecules like DNA, the generation of ROS, and the formation of proinflammatory molecules inducing the physiological production of ROS. Evidence of the harmful effects on the skin associated with overexposure to UV has been demonstrated in many studies.

Enhanced UVB radiation suppresses antioxidant systems and causes some active oxygen species to accumulate in irradiated cells, such as superoxide anion radical (O_2^-.) production and the concentration of hydrogen peroxide (H_2O_2) and malodiadehyde (MDA). Many studies suggest that exogenous supplementation of antioxidants prevents UVR-induced photooxidative damage. On the other hand, moderate UV exposure is necessary for the production of Vitamin D and might have many positive effects regarding our psycho-physical stress reduction and the generation of serotonin (for further reading, see also paragraph entitled "Antioxidant prevention of damage induced by entrinsic factors").

Avoid Excessive Psycho-Physical Stressful Situations

In this paragraph, the question of whether emotional stress contributes to increased oxidative stress will be attempted to be answered. Psychological stress is becoming common in modern society and is known to predispose individuals to several diseases, since stress can diminish the effectiveness of the immune system (Halliwell and Gutteridge, 1999) and possibly also the effectiveness of the antioxidant system and repair processes. It is known that adrenalin is released into the blood when a person faces a stressful situation. If adrenalin is not used for either fight or flight (as it was in the past), it slowly oxidizes in the presence of O_2 to yield superoxide (Halliwell and Gutteridge, 1999) and increases oxidative stress. Emotional stress in humans associates with higher biomarkers for oxidative stress. Emotional stress increases catecholamine metabolism, which increases oxidative stress by increasing the production of free-radicals. Similarly, academic stress (stress due to academic commitments, financial pressures, and lack of time management skills among students) (Eskiocak and Gozen, 2005) or sleep deprivation (Everson and Laatsch, 2004) associate with lower protective antioxidant levels in blood. Eskiocak and Gozen (2005) demonstrated that glutathione and free sulphydryl levels in seminal plasma decreased in subjects undergoing examination stress. Everson and Laatsch (2004) found out that recovery sleep normalized antioxidant content in liver and enhanced enzymatic antioxidant activities in both the liver and the heart. Results of their study link uncompensated oxidative stress to health effects induced by sleep deprivation and provide evidence that restoration of antioxidant balance is a property of recovery sleep.

Higher scores for Tension-Anxiety and perceived work-load correlate with higher oxidized nucleic acid levels in the blood of female workers (Irie and Asami, 2002). Their study investigated whether the formation of 8-hydroxydeoxyguanosine (8-OH-dG), a known oxidative DNA damage relevant to carcinogenicity, can be associated with psychological factors. Male subjects who had self-blame coping strategies displayed significantly high levels of 8-OH-dG. Moreover, the worse the subjective closeness to parents in childhood, the higher the levels of 8-OH-dG became in male subjects. The levels of 8-OH-dG increased reliably in subjects who had experienced the loss of a close family member within three years, when compared with non-bereaved subjects. Women under high psychological stress have higher levels of oxidative damage and significantly shorter telomeres than do nonstressed controls (Epel et al., 2004; Sapolsky, 2004). On the other hand, higher protective antioxidant enzyme levels (Sharma and Sen, 2003) and lower oxidized lipid levels (Schneider and Nidich, 1998) were found in blood samples of meditation practitioners. Since psychosocial stress increases oxidative stress, Sharma and Sen (2003) conducted an exploratory study to investigate the effects of stress reduction with the Sudarshan Kriya (SK) (specific form of yoga) program, on superoxide dismutase (SOD), catalase, glutathione and blood lactate levels in practitioners and non-practitioners of SK. Significantly lower levels of blood lactate and higher levels of SOD, glutathione and catalase were found in practitioners as compared to non practitioners of SK. Immobilization-stress approximates emotional stress in animals, and associates with greater oxidative stress: increased free-radical production, decreased antioxidant enzyme levels, and increased oxidized lipids in tissues, including brain (Oishi and Yokoi, 1999; Liu et al., 1996; Olivenza et al., 2000; Fontella et al., 2005). Sleep-deprivation of animals produces similar oxidative changes (Silva et al., 2004; D'Almeida et al., 1998; Ramanathan et al., 2002). Prolonged sleep deprivation significantly decreases Cu/Zn-SOD activity in the hippocampus and brainstem, suggesting an alteration in the metabolism of ROS resulting in oxidative stress. Lui et al. (1996) showed that eight hours of immobilization stress in rats led to significant increases in DNA damage (8-OHdG) in the cerebral cortex. Other brain areas showed nonsignificant increases. There were no increases in oxidative DNA damage in the liver or kidney. The stress induced in rats by immobilization leads to falls in glutathion and increases in protein carbonyls, lipid peroxidation and 8-OHdG in various regions of the brain and liver (Liu et al., 1996). Adachi, Kawamura, and Takemoto (1993) measured 8-OH-dG in rats exposed to psychologically conditioned stress. Experimental animals were placed in a 30-chamber communication box along with animals that were intermittently shocked. While the experimental animals were not shocked, they were exposed to visual, auditory, and olfactory signals from the shocked animals. Six studies have directly examined the contribution of stress to oxidative damage of DNA. Three of the studies have been conducted with rats (Adachi et al., 1993; Irie et al., 2000; Liu et al., 1996), and three have been conducted with humans (Irie et al., 2001a; Irie et al., 2001b; Nakajima Takeuchi, Takeshita, & Morimoto, 1996). Other studies (e.g., Forlenza, et al., 2000; Cohen et al., 2000) did not measure DNA damage directly, but rather examined effects of stress on measures of DNA repair. Studies in both animals (Adachi et al., 1993; Liu et al., 1996) and humans (Irie et al., 2001a; Irie et al., 2001b) demonstrate that stress is related to oxidative damage of DNA as measured by 8-OHdG from nuclear DNA. Above-mentioned studies involved in the role of stress on oxidative DNA damage were reviewed by Forlenza (2002). Forlenza (2002) concluded that based on the findings of increased DNA repair during stress, it is hypothesized that stress will increase levels of oxidative DNA damage.

Excessive psycho-physical stress should be avoided, and we should take time to relax and enjoy the things we like doing. Besides, social support and the feeling of belonging are important to human beings, especially to older individuals.

A study led by Erik Giltay of the Psychiatric Center GGZ Delfland, Delft, in the Netherlands recently found that people possessing higher levels of optimism were 55 percent less likely to die from any cause, and 23 percent were less likely to die from a heart-related illness as compared to the pessimistic group (Giltay et al., 2004). Results of the study provide support for a graded and independent protective relationship between dispositional optimism and all-cause mortality in old age. Besides, dispositional optimism in elderly men is associated with healthy lifestyle and dietary habits. A low level of optimism may indirectly affect proneness to cardiovascular death via unhealthy behavioral choices (Giltay et al., 2007).

Another research team led by Dr. Hilary Tindle from the University of Pittsburgh found similar results (Tindle et al., 2009; Tindle et al., 2010). Their results showed that eight years into the study, women who scored the highest in optimism were 14 percent more likely to be alive than those with the lowest, most pessimistic scores, with pessimists more likely to have died from any cause, including heart disease and cancer. In addition, pessimistic black women were 33 percent more likely to have died after eight years than optimistic black women, while white pessimists were only 13 percent more likely to have died than their optimistic counterparts. Optimistic people tend to have more friends and a larger social network on which they can rely during crises. They are also better able to handle stress, a risk factor highlighted in previous studies for its association with high blood pressure, heart disease and early death. Authors conclude that optimism and cynical hostility are independently associated with important health outcomes in black and white women.

Evidence continues to accumulate that strongly suggests that the state of a human being's mind, which associates psychosocial factors with emotional states such as depression, and with behavioral dispositions that include hostility and psychosocial lifestyle stresses, can directly and significantly influence human physiological function and, in turn, health outcomes (Vitetta and Anton, 2007).

In modern society, we are faced with excessive psychological stress, as well as an epidemic of overeating, and the two together appear to have synergistic effects according to Epel (2009). Chronic stress can lead to overeating, co-elevation of cortisol and insulin, and suppression of certain anabolic hormones. This state of metabolic stress, in turn, promotes abdominal adiposity. Increased cortisol accelerates aging. Both the direct stress response and the accumulation of visceral fat can promote a milieu of systemic inflammation and oxidative stress. Epel et al. (2004) provide evidence that psychological stress—both perceived stress and chronicity of stress—is significantly associated with higher oxidative stress, lower telomerase activity, and shorter telomere length, which are known determinants of cell senescence and longevity, in peripheral blood mononuclear cells from healthy premenopausal women. Women with the highest levels of perceived stress have telomeres shorter on average by the equivalent of at least one decade of additional aging compared to low stress women.

Physiological status has also great effect on tumor development. Physical and emotional stressors have been found to mediate a wide variety of biological changes including the facilitation of tumor progression.

Table 11. Measures for reducing ROS-induced damage

Prevention of ROS formation	• calorie restriction and calorie restriction mimetics • sequestration of transition metal ions • uncoupling (and heat production; living in moderate lower ambient temperatures) • regular performing of work (increasing cellular energy demand, decreasing mitochondrial membrane potential and proton leak) • avoiding exposure to environmental ROS through air, water and food pollutants • avoiding psycho-physical stress • reducing moderate chronic inflammatory conditions and avoiding chronic infections • maintaining low plasma glucose and insulin levels
Neutralization (quenching) of ROS	• increased intake of exogenous antioxidants from food • increasing activity of endogenous enzymatic and non-enzymatic antioxidant defense systems (hormesis and hormesis mimetics, sleeping and melatonin secretion)
Increasing repair and replacement mechanisms to remove (replace) ROS-induced damage	• hormesis effect and hormesis mimetics (nutritional hormesis) • etc.

Studies have shown that chronic stress or UV radiation independently suppresses immunity. For example, exposure to stress (fox urine) reduces the latency of UV-induced SCC from 21 weeks to 8 weeks in mice (Parker et al., 2004). Similar study by Saul et al. (2005) showed that chronic stress increased susceptibility to UV-induced squamous cell carcinoma in the mouse model by suppressing type 1 cytokines and protective T cells and increasing regulatory/suppressor T cell numbers. Cortisol increase in stressful situations is well documented. Increased endogenous glucocorticoid production adversely affects barrier homeostasis (Denda et al., 2000) and epidermal cell proliferation (Tsuchiya and Horri, 1996). A large number of skin diseases, including atopic dermatitis and psoriasis, appear to be precipitated or exacerbated by psychological stress (Muizzuddin et al., 2009). Psychological stress inhibits epidermal lipid synthesis, which results in decreased lamellar bodies formation and secretion compromising both cutaneous permeability barrier homeostasis and stratum corneum (SC) integrity (Choi et al., 2005). There is also a reduction in the density of corneodesmosomes in the lower SC (Choi et al., 2005). Short periods of rest or vacation drastically improve the appearance of concerned individuals suffering from psychological stress or anxiety (Muizzuddin et al., 2009). If psychological stress directly or indirectly increases oxidative stress and leads to increased damage, then stress reduction and prevention strategies may be important also in skin anti-aging prevention. It was reported that stress seems to affect the integrity of skin collagen through glucocorticoid-mediated processes that alter its synthesis and degradation. Glucocorticoids also affect skin quality through modulation of the immune system (Kahan 2009).

Chapter 9

The Role of Telomeres in Skin Aging

Telomeres are protective DNA-protein complexes that promote chromosomal stability. A telomere is a repeating DNA sequence (for example, TTAGGG) at the end of the cell's chromosomes. The intrinsic aging is mainly controlled by progressive telomere shortening (Kosmadaki and Gilchrest, 2004). At the end of a chromosome is a telomere, which acts like a bookend. Telomeres keep chomosomes protected and prevent them from fusing into rings or binding with other DNA. Telomeres function by preventing chromosomes from losing base pair sequences at their ends. They also stop chromosomes from fusing to each other. Telomeres play an important role in cell division. Telomerase is a ribonucleoprotein that synthesizes the repeated sequences at chromosome ends and helps DNA polymerases to complete the replication. Telomerase enzyme is normally present only in the epidermal basal layer, but is elevated in sun-exposed skin, skin precancers, and cancers (Brash et al., 2010). The telomere can reach a length of 15,000 base pairs. However, each time a cell divides, some of the telomere is lost (usually 25 to 200 base pairs per division). When a cell stops replicating, it enters into a period of decline known as "cell senescence," which is the cellular equivalent of aging. It has been suggested that cell senescence may be good because it is a defense against cancer, which is marked by uncontrolled cell division. Cells unable to regrow their telomeres stop dividing before they can cause too many mistakes. As there is no telomerase in many somatic tissues, telomere erosion may well be a major factor in cell aging (Boukamp, 2001).When the telomere becomes too short, the chromosome reaches a "critical length" and can no longer replicate. This means that a cell becomes "old" and dies by a process called *apoptosis*.

The majority of cells have the capacity for about 60 to 70 postnatal doublings during their lifecycles, and thereafter they reach senescence, remaining viable but incapable of proliferation. This event facilitates end-to-end chromosomal fusions resulting in karyotype disarray with subsequent apoptosis, thus serving as the "biological clock" (Glogau, 2003). Even in fibroblasts of quiescent skin, more than 30% of the telomere length is lost during adulthood (Allsopp et al., 1992).

Telomeres are important so their steady shrinking with each mitosis might impose a finite lifespan on cells. Normal (non-cancerous) cells do not grow indefinitely when placed in culture. Since telomerase is not expressed in human somatic cells (like skin cells), their telomeres become 50 to 100 nucleotides shorter with every cell division. For example, studies on keratinocytes, fibroblasts, and melanocytes have revealed that they all show an age-associated decrease in cumulative doublings. Fibroblasts, for instance, taken from a normal human tissue go through only about 25 to 50 population doublings when cultured in standard medium. More than 30% of the telomere length is lost during adulthood in skin fibroblasts (Allsop et al., 1992). Towards the end, proliferation slows down and finally stops, and the cell enter a state from which it never recover (Makrantonaki and Zouboulis, 2010). Researchers can use the length of a cell's telomeres to determine the cell's age and how many more times it will replicate. This is important in anti-aging research and in determination of biological skin age. Age-adjusted telomere length is a method to assess biological age using structural analysis of chromosomal change in the telomere. Serial evaluation of telomere length is an indicator of how rapidly one ages relative to a normal population (www.spectracell.com).

On the other hand, some cells are able to maintain the length of their telomeres. They do so with the aid of the enzymetelomerase. Telomerase, also called telomere terminal transferase, is the enzyme made of protein and *RNA* subunits that elongates chromosomes by adding TTAGGG sequences to the end of existing chromosomes. Telomerase is found in fetal tissues, adult *germ cells*, and also tumor cells. Telomerase activity is regulated during development and has a very low, almost undetectable activity in *somatic* (body) cells. Because these somatic cells do not regularly use telomerase, they age. The result of aging cells is an aging body. Telomerase adds telomere repeat sequences to the 3' end of DNA strands. By lengthening this strand, DNA polymerase is able to complete the synthesis of the "incomplete ends" of the opposite strand. The regulation of telomerase in mammalian cells is multifactorial, involving telomerase gene expression, post-translational protein-protein interactions, and protein phosphorylation. Several proto-oncogenes and tumor-suppressor genes are involved in the regulation of telomerase activity (Liu, 1999). Several physiological factors, like EGF and/or amphiregulin, and growth factors, can also influence telomerase (Matsui et al., 2000).

Cellular aging is the process by which a cell becomes old and dies. One of the reasons is also due to the shortening of chromosomal telomeres to the point that the chromosome reaches a critical length. Oxidative stress is linked to telomere length. Hyperoxia accelerates telomere shortening by causing oxidative stress. A reduction of stress, for example by the action of free radical scavengers, delays replicative senescence. A telomere acts as a "sentinel" for oxidative damage to the genome and replicative senescence may be triggered by telomeres as a consequence of DNA damage. It is thus very important to ensure that cells have sufficient telomerase (Lorenz et al., 2001). Guanine of the telomerase 3' overhang (TTAGGG) can be considered as a target for reactive oxygen species or UV irradiation (Yaar et al., 2002). It was reported that UV irradiation disturbs the telomerase activity in human keratinocytes (Kurfürst et al., 2000) and mutations of the p53 gene are considered to be UV specific (Ueda, 1997) and are linked to telomerase activity. Besides, there may be hormonal control of telomerase activity. Sex steroids may thus influence cell senescence and aging (Kyo, 1999). Estrogen activates telomerase via direct and indirect effects.

Telomerase therapy might one day help generate a new supply of cells to treat age-related diseases. It has been shown that there is a telomerase activity in the skin. Telomeres are central to cellular proliferative capacity and gene expression in the skin. When telomeres become critically shortened, skin cells may enter proliferative senescence or change expression of genes in close proximity to the DNA terminus (Ning et al. 2003; Jenkins et al., 2009). After approximately 60 postnatal doublings, telomeres reach a critically short length, cells stop dividing and enter into the state of proliferative senescence (Harley et al., 1990). Intrinsic skin aging is strongly associated with progressive telomere shortening, the result of cumulative cell division (Sugimoto et al., 2006).

On the other hand, post-mitotic cells never divide, such as nerve, muscle and fat cells. Mitotic cells, such as keratinocytes and fibroblasts, divide, and this fact plays an important role in skin aging. Replicative senescence is the process that limits the number of cell divisions. As senescent fibroblasts and keratinocytes accumulate with age in human skin, this could explain the deterioration of the appearance and properties of the skin. Senescent cells secrete degrading enzymes that modify the cytokine/interleukin balance, causing the loss of functional integrity (Campisi, 1998).

Several authors have calculated that humans have a theoretical maximum of 125 years. Many scientists believe that this limit on lifespan and decline in health is imposed by the gradual shortening of telomeres. The study of Ornish et al. (2008) addressed whether improvements in nutrition and lifestyle are associated with increases in telomerase activity. Authors aimed to assess whether three months of intensive lifestyle changes increased telomerase activity in peripheral blood mononuclear cells (PBMC). Comprehensive lifestyle changes significantly increase telomerase activity and consequently telomere maintenance capacity in human immune-system cells (Ornish et al., 2008). Given this finding and the pilot nature of this study, larger randomized controlled trials are warranted to confirm the findings of this study.

Also, diet can have an impact on the telomere length. An inflammatory diet, or one that increases oxidative stress, will shorten telomeres faster. This includes refined carbohydrates, fast foods, processed foods, sodas, artificial sweeteners, trans fats and saturated fats. A diet with a large amount and variety of antioxidants that improves oxidative defense and reduces oxidative stress will slow telomere shortening. Consumption of ten servings of fresh and relatively uncooked fruits and vegetables, mixed fiber, monounsaturated fats, omega-3 fatty acids, cold-waterfish, and high-quality vegetable proteins will help preserve telomere length (www.spectracell.com).

In January, 2007, a commercial health-maintenance program, PattonProtocol-1, was launched that included a natural product-derived telomerase activator (TA-65((R)), 10 to 50 mg daily), a comprehensive dietary supplement pack, and physician counseling/laboratory tests at baseline and every three to six months thereafter. Harley et al. (2010) report analysis of the first year of data focusing on the immune system. Low nanomolar levels of TA-65((R)) moderately activated telomerase in human keratinocytes, fibroblasts, and immune cells in culture; similar plasma levels of TA-65((R)) were achieved in pilot human pharmacokinetic studies with single 10- to 50-mg doses. The most striking in vivo effects were declines in the percent senescent cytotoxic (CD8(+)/CD28(-)) T cells and natural killer cells at 6 and 12 months (Harley et al., 2010). The article reports that TA-65 can cause telomerase to become active in human cells. Although TA-65 is probably not the single important factor to arrest the aging process, it is the first telomerase activator recognized as safe for human use.

The effects of social status on biological aging were measured by white-blood-cell telomere length in the study of Cherkas et al. (2006). Authors studied 1,552 female twins. A venous blood sample was taken from each twin and isolated white-blood-cells used for extraction of DNA. Terminal restriction fragment length was measured. According to this study, low socio-economic status, in addition to the harmful effects of smoking, obesity and lack of exercise, appears to have an impact on telomere length (Cherkas et al., 2006).

Loss of division potential due to the telomere shortening does not likely seem to be a primary aging mechanism because the rate of aging appears to be the same in both dividing and non-dividing cells of an organism (Klapper et al., 2001; Slagboom et al., 2000). It seems that oxidative stress and damage plays a major role in cell's senescence. Nevertheless, telomere shortening plays an important role in skin aging.

Chapter 10

Hormones and Skin Aging

Hormones also play an important role in skin functioning and aging. The importance of the endocrine environment in the initiation of the aging process has been elucidated in several in vivo and in vitro studies. Changes in endocrine pathways accompany healthy aging, and these include the growth hormone/insulin-like growth factor-I axis (somatopause) and that of sexual hormones, namely estradiol (menopause), testosterone (andropause), and dehydroepiandrosterone and its sulphate (adrenopause) (Makrantonaki et al., 2010). The clinical significance of these changes is variable and results in morphological and functional alterations of all organ systems, including the skin.

Intrinsic skin aging is determined primarily by genetic factors and hormonal status. Skin has the ability to produce hormones by itself and fulfills all the criteria for the independent peripheral endocrine organ (Zouboulis 2000; 2004). Evidence for the role of hormones in oxidative stress and aging is slowly emerging. The hormonal influences include reduced pituitary, adrenal and gonadal secretion.

The hormonal changes of aging lead to the development of a specific body and skin phenotype as well as behavior patterns. Zouboulis et al. (2006) reported that hormones are decisively involved in intrinsic aging, which is accompanied by reduced secretion of the pituitary and adrenal glands and the gonads (Zouboulis, 2000; Phillips et al., 2001; Thiboutot, 1995).

ROS and Hormones

As reviewed by Brown-Borg and Harman (2003) there are numerous mechanisms by which hormones can affect the process of oxidative stress and oxidative damage. First, hormones may alter the rate at which oxygen free radicals are produced by the mitochondrial cytochrome system (e.g., upregulation of genes involved in oxidative metabolism by thyroid hormones (Jameson and DeGroot, 1995)). Second, hormones may modulate the production or activation state of enzymes and other compounds involved in quenching ROS (e.g., growth hormonedownregulates the production of Cu and Zn SOD and CAT in some tissues in mice (Brown-Borg et al., 1999)). Third, hormones may themselves act as antioxidants or oxidants, as has been shown for estrogens (Persky et al., 2000; Green et al., 1998) and dehydroepiandrosterone (DHEA) (Tamagno et al., 1998). Fourth, hormones may influence rates of repair of oxidized tissue components (e.g., reduction in activity of the heat shock protein HSP70 by glucocorticoids) (Udelsman et al., 1994). ROS can also alter receptor function. For example, oxidase stress caused by hydrogen peroxide rapidly inhibits the internalization of receptor-bound EGF in human fibroblasts, so that the breakdown of the EGF-receptor complex is inhibited. Hydrogen peroxide also alters negative feedback within the cell, and attenuates growth factor-induced signal transduction, leading to altered cell metabolism (De Wit et al., 2000).

Hormone Decline with Age

Skin aging is affected by growth-factor modifications and hormone activity that declines with age (Puizina-Ivic, 2008). The best-known decline is that of sex steroids such asestrogen, testosterone, dehydroepiandrosterone (DHEA), and its sulfate ester (DHEAS) (Wespes and Schulman 2002; Phillips et al., 2001; Arlt and Hewison, 2004). Other hormones such as melatonin, insulin, cortisol, thyroxine, insulin-like growth factor-I (IGF-I) and growth hormone decline, too.

At the same time, induced levels of certain signaling molecules such as cytokines and chemokines decline as well, leading to the deterioration of several skin functions (Swift et al., 2001). Also, the levels of their receptors decline as well (Avratet al., 2000). The levels of receptors for vitamin D (Bell and Jackson, 1995), beta-adrenergic compounds (Schutzer and Mader, 2003), neurotransmitters (Peters, 2002) and dopamine (Ingram 2000) decrease with age. In the epidermis, there is a decline in the expression and synthesis of receptors for the interleukin-1 cytokine family. At the same time, some signaling molecules increase with age. One of these is a cytokine called transforming growth factor beta1, which induces fibroblast senescence (Puizina-Ivic, 2008).

Fat Distribution and Hormones

Hormone changes linked to aging may also cause difference in body fat distribution. With aging, fat is depleted from certain facial areas including the forehead, preorbital, buccal, temporal and perioral regions. In contrast, there is an increase in the bulk of fatty tissue in other areas including the submental regions, the jowls, the nasolabial folds and the lateral malar areas (Yaar, 2006). In a youth's face, fat is diffusely dispersedbut in aging facial skin fat tends to accumulate in pockets, and due to gravity, sagging and drooping of the skin occurs (Donofrio 2000).

Energy metabolism is also regulated via leptin, a fat cell-derived hormone, in adults (Rocquet and Bonte 2002). The concentration of leptin in the blood varies during the menstrual cycle. Leptin binding activity is low at birth and high in the pre-pubertal years, but it is stable during adult life and does not vary with aging (Quinton et al., 1999a; Quinton et al., 1999b; Chehab, 2000). The adipocytes also act as estradiol stores. The circulating concentration of this hormone varies with age and is most important in mature skin.

Sex Hormones, Andro- and Menopause

The skin locally synthesizes significant amounts of sexual hormones with intracrine or paracrine actions. The local level of each sexual steroid depends upon the expression of each of the androgen- and estrogen-synthesizing enzymes in each cell type, with sebaceous glands and sweat glands being the major contributors (Zouboulis et al., 2007).

Androgens affect several functions of the human skin, such as sebaceous gland growth and differentiation, hair growth, epidermal barrier homeostasis and wound healing. Their effects are mediated by binding to nuclear androgen receptors. Androgen activation and deactivation are mainly intracellular events. Testosterone in women and 5alpha-dihydrotestosterone in both genders are also synthesized in the skin. Skin cells express all androgen-metabolizing enzymes required for the independent cutaneous synthesis of androgens (Zouboulis 2004). Estrogens clearly have an important function in many components of human skin, including the epidermis, dermis, vasculature, hair follicle and the sebaceous, eccrine and apocrine glands, having significant roles in skin aging, pigmentation, hair growth, sebum production and skin cancer (Thornton 2002).

Localization of sex steroid receptors in human skin was investigated by Pelletier and Ren (2004). To determine the sites of action of estrogens, androgens and progestins, studies have been performed during the recent years to accurately localize receptors for each steroid hormone in human skin. Androgen receptors (AR) have been localized in most keratinocytes in epidermis. In the dermis, AR was detected in about 10% of fibroblasts. In sebaceous glands, AR was observed in both basal cells and sebocytes. In hair follicles, AR expression was restricted to dermal papillar cells. Estrogen receptor (ER) alpha was poorly expressing, being restricted to sebocytes. In contrast, ERbeta was found to be highly expressed in the epidermis, sebaceous glands (basal cells and sebocytes) and eccrine sweat glands. In the hair follicle, ERbeta is widely expressed with strong nuclear staining in dermal papilla cells, inner sheath cells, matrix cells and outer sheath cells including the buldge region. Progesterone receptors (PR) staining was found in nuclei of some keratinocytes and in nuclei of basal cells and sebocytes in sebaceous glands. PR nuclear staining was also observed in dermal papilla cells of hair follicles and in eccrine sweat glands.

Sex hormones manifest a variety of biological and immunological effects in the skin (Pierard et al., 1995). Individuals in developed lands spend up to a third of their lives (women-post-menopausal) or perhaps 20 years (men-partial androgen deficiency of the aging man, PADAM) with estrogen or androgen deficiency (Zouboulis, 2003). The fall in hormone levels at menopause induces numerous physiological changes in the skin, including a reduction in the biosynthesis of collagen and hyaluronic acid. It also effects the secretion of the sebaceous glands. The finding that male rats have more malodialdehyde in their livers than do females could indicate that estrogens may be involved in oxidative process (Huh et al., 1994). Menopause, the physiological cessation of menstruation caused by decreased function of the ovaries, leads to thinning of the dermis, mainly due to a decrease in the collagen content, atrophy of subcutaneous tissues and increased skin dryness (Broniarczyk-Dyla and Joss-Wichman, 1999; Bonté, 2001). The significant changes sustained by the skin during the menopause are due to the effect sustained on the skin's individual components. The estrogen receptor has been detected on the cellular components of the skin. Accordingly, dermal cellular metabolism is influenced by the hypoestrogenoemic state of menopause leading to changes in the collagen content, alterations in the concentration of glycoaminoglycans and most importantly the water content. Consequently, changes in these basic components lead to an alteration in function compatible with skin aging. Changes in the skin collagen lead to diminished elasticity and skin strength (Raine-Fenning et al., 2003).All of the changes lead to a loss of skin elasticity and strength and increased skin dryness (Shah and Maibach 2001). There is a strong correlation between skin collagen loss and estrogen deficiency due to the menopause. Skin aging, especially in the face, is associated with a progressive increase in extensibility and a reduction in elasticity. With increasing age, the skin also becomes more fragile and susceptible to trauma, leading to more lacerations and bruising. Furthermore, wound healing is impaired in older women (Calleja-Agius et al., 2007). The physiologic and pharmacologic role of estrogen's protective effects against oxidative damage is the subject of intense investigation. In responsive women, estrogen, alone or together with progesterone, has been reported to prevent or reverse skin atrophy, dryness, and wrinkles due to chronological aging or photoaging (Pierardet al., 2010). Systemic substitution of estrogens in females and growth hormone in males has been shown to lead to positive effects on several organs including signs of skin rejuvenation in both cases and to prevention of the further aging process in controlled studies (Callens et al., 1996; Rudmen et al., 1990). Postmenopausal women who utilize estrogen supplementation tend to have lower wrinkle scores, less xerosis, and relatively thicker skin than women not receiving hormone replacement therapy (Hall and Philips, 2006). Estrogen and progesterone in responsive women stimulate proliferation of keratinocytes, while estrogen suppresses and prevents epidermal atrophy. Estrogen also enhances collagen synthesis and both estrogen and progesterone suppress collagenolysis by reducing MMP activity in fibroblasts. Estrogen additionally maintains skin moisture by increasing hyaluronic acid levels in the dermis (Pierard et al., 2010).

Additionally, side levels of serum total and free testosterone in males gradually decline as well (Sternbach, 1998). Men show a decrease in testosterone levels of up to 1.6% per year (Yuul and Skakkebaek, 2002). It also seems that estrogen and progesterone contribute to elastic fiber maintenance (Bologna et al., 1989).Somatopause is characterized by a progressive decrease of growth hormone production starting as soon as in the third decade.It is still unknown to what extent estrogens can influence skin quality and age-associated diseases in men (Katz 2000).The exact effect of testosterone deficiency on the skin is also not known; however, animal research has shown negative influence of testosterone on the epidermal barrier and wound healing (Kao et al., 2001; Gilliver et al., 2003).Epidermal lamellar body formation and secretion both decrease, resulting in decreased extracellular lamellar bilayers in testosterone-replete animals. Studies of Kao et al. (2000) demonstrate that fluctuations in testosterone modulate barrier function and that testosterone repletion can have negative consequences for permeability barrier homeostasis. The androgen receptor is expressed by inflammatory cells, keratinocytes and fibroblasts during wound healing, suggesting that androgens may regulate inflammatory and/or repair processes. Although estrogens accelerate healing, the actions of the "male" sex hormones 5alpha-dihydrotestosterone and testosterone are primarily deleterious. The shift that occurs in the balance between serum estrogen and androgen levels as a normal feature of human aging may, therefore, have important consequences for fundamental tissue repair processes (Gilliver et al., 2007). According to Gilliver et al. (2003), it appears that endogenous testosterone inhibits wound healing and promotes inflammation since castration of male miceor systemic treatment with the androgen receptor antagonist flutamide accelerates cutaneous wound healing and reduces the inflammatory response. Androgens affect several functions inhuman skin, such as sebaceous gland growth and differentiation, hair growth, epidermal barrier homeostasis and wound healing. Their effects are mediated by binding to the nuclear androgen receptor. Estrogens, besides being implicated in skin aging, are also connected with pigmentation, hair growth, sebum production and skin cancer (Zouboulis et al., 2007).

Pituitary Thyroid-Stimulating Hormone

During aging, a slight decrease in pituitary thyroid-stimulating hormone is observed. Like most hormones in our bodies, as we age, less and less thyroid hormone is available. Glands, which produce these hormones, become sluggish or irregular. The thyroid gland is no exception. Thyroid hormone is a prime regulator of intermediary metabolism in nearly every cell type in the body. It accelerates the rate at which cells oxidize fuel, leading to increased thermogenesis (see also chapter on uncoupling proteins). Thyroid hormone upregulates enzymes and cytochromes involved in mitochondrial function. Thyroid-stimulating hormone (also known as TSH or thyrotropin) is a peptide hormone synthesized and secreted by thyrotrope cells in the anterior pituitary gland, which regulates the endocrine function of the thyroid gland (Sacher and McPherson, 2000). TSH stimulates the thyroid gland to secrete the hormones thyroxin (T_4) and triiodothyronine (T_3). Both, T4 and T3 concentrations decline with age. T3 is an important regulator of growth and development of different body systems and is involved in acceleration of cell proliferation of the skin and wound healing (Safer et al., 2005). The endocrine function of the skin was reported by Kaplan et al. (1988); authors observed that human epidermal keratinocytes in culture convert thyroxine to 3,5,3'-triiodothyronine by type II iodothyronine deiodination, and this function may be impaired with age.

It has been an open question whether the thyroid hormone-induced increase in mitochondrial membrane proton leak might be associated with accelerated generation of ROS and increase in the rate of oxidative damage to mitochondria. Thyroid hormone appears to increase mitochondrial production of ROS in a variety of cells and tissues, an effect variably associated with compensatory increases in antioxidant defenses (Brown-Borg and Harman, 2003).

DHEA and Melatonin

Dehydroepiandrosterone (DHEA) and its ester sulfate metabolite, DHEAS, are steroids mainly secreted by the adrenal cortex, but also within the brain where they are considered as neurosteroids. DHEA and its sulfate (DHEA-S) are the most abundant steroids in humans whose low levels are related to aging, greater incidence of various cancers, immune dysfunction, atherosclerosis, and osteoporosis. No receptor was identified for DHEA or DHEAS. Although the exact roles of DHEA and melatonin in human skin are still under scrutiny, researchers have identified several mechanisms through which these hormones protect against aging, maintain the health of skin, and affect how sunlight reacts with skin cells. The sleep hormone (melatonin) and the anti-stress hormone (DHEA) are both found in human skin. Both are converted to other entities with important jobs to do. DHEA is converted into estrogen- and androgen-type metabolites found only in skin (Labrie et al., 2000). The consequences of decreased DHEA production are still matter of debate. DHEA/DHEAS putative effects are mediated by their conversion into active sexual steroids, estradiol and testosterone, but their role is not clarified. In humans, DHEA is a crucial precursor of sex steroid biosynthesis and exerts indirect endocrine and intracrine actions following conversion to androgens and estrogens. DHEA levels decline monotonously with age from puberty to senescence. Decreased serum levels of DHEA\DHEAS are associated with aging and have also been found in age-associated diseases. However, the results of epidemiological studies are contradictory and few therapeutic trials were published. A positive effect was found on the libido, bone status and skin in women over 70 years of age (Pitti-Ferrandi, 2003). Besides, decreased free radical damage in response to DHEA has been seen in number of in vitro as well as in vivo studies (reviewed in Brown-Borg and Harman, 2003).

Estrogen's skin-enhancing effects are wellknown (Dunn et al., 1997; Shah et al., 2001). It provokes collagen and a moisture factor known as hyaluronic acid. Aging decreases both estrogen and collagen. Enzymes that convert DHEA to estrogen also decline. Not surprisingly, women who take synthetic estrogen have scientifically proven thicker skin. Women who take both estrogen and testosterone have really thick skin (48% thicker than women who don't take either hormone) (Brincat et al., 1983). DHEA administration in elderly women seems to be associated with favorable effects on physical and psychological well-being. Modulation of collagen metabolism by the topical application of dehydroepiandrosterone to human skin has been reported (Shin et al., 2005). DHEA may be related to the process of skin aging through the regulation and degradation of extracellular matrix protein (Lee et al., 2000). The study of Mills et al. (2005) suggests that exogenous application of DHEA accelerates impaired wound repair, results thatmay be applicable to the prophylaxis and treatment of human impaired wound-healing states (Mills et al., 2005). Topical DHEA tends to improve skin brightness, to counteract papery appearance of skin and epidermal atrophy, a characteristic feature of hormone-related skin aging. Topical DHEA could also act on skin process related to wrinkles (Nouveau et al., 2008). Two hundred and eighty healthy individuals (women and men 60 to 79 years old) were given DHEA, 50 mg, or placebo, orally, daily for a year in a double-blind, placebo-controlled study. No potentially harmful accumulation of DHEAS and active steroids was recorded. Besides the reestablishment of a "young" concentration of DHEAS, a small increase of testosterone and estradiol was noted (Baulieu et al., 2000). A significant increase in most libido parameters was also found in these older women. Improvement of the skin status was observed, particularly in women, in terms of hydration, epidermal thickness, sebum production, and pigmentation (Baulieu et al., 2000). In contrast, no effect of DHEA administration was observed in healthy man after oneyear of DHEA replacement (50 mg/day) (Percheron et al., 2003).

Daily oral administration of DHEA (25/50 mg) is safe in elderly subjects (Legrain et al., 2000). Besides, giving DHEA to postmenopausal women thickened their bones and skin. A study in the *Journal of Surgical Research* demonstrates the extraordinary ability of topically applied DHEA to protect skin's delicate blood vessels. Researchers found that if DHEA was applied after a serious burn, the blood vessels underlying the burned area are protected (Araneo et al., 1995).

Melatonin is a hormone produced in the glandula pinealis under the influence of β-adrenergic receptors. To melatonin we already dedicated a paragraph on the importance of sleeping, focusing mainly on melatonin's antioxidant properties and circadian clock. Melatonin follows a circadian rhythm of secretion, with low serum levels during day and an increase at night (Fischer and Elsner, 2000). The first hormone whose serum levels change with age is melatonin. Its levels decrease as early as from 5th up to 20th year of life and stay at a low plateau until the age of 75 (Phillips et al., 2001; Zouboulis and Makrantonaki, 2006). A group at the University of Zurich has shown that topical melatonin gives excellent protection against sunburn if applied before sun exposure (Bangha et al., 1997). A double-blind randomized study was designed to examine the influence of the antioxidant, melatonin, on the anti-erythema effect. Topical treatment of the skin with melatonin 15 min before UV irradiation proved to almost completely suppress the development of an UV-induced erythema. In contrast, no significant protective effects of melatonin were observed when it was applied after UV irradiation. The researchers concluded that topically applied melatonin has a clear-cut protective effect against UV-induced erythema. Free radical scavenging of UV-generated hydroxyl radicals and interference with the arachidonic acid metabolism are possible mechanisms of the melatonin action (Bangha E. et al, 1997). Melatonin also appears to have a role in repairing burned skin. In a study in *Brain Research Bulletin*, melatonin levels rose sixhours after burn injury, then fell to normal (Scott et al., 1986).

Glucocorticoids

Glucocorticoids are naturally produced steroid hormones, or synthetic compounds, that inhibit the process of inflammation. Glucocorticoids are stress hormones with actions causing increased glucose in the blood, maintenance of vascular tone and blood pressure, and protection of cells against various kinds of stress. Glucocorticoids also modulate immune function, tending to decrease inflammation and thus modulate free radical production since ROS generation is an important component of the response of a variety of the immune cells after contact with foreign antigens.

Conclusion

The role of hormones in oxidative stress and aging is slowly emerging. All cells present within the skin (keratinocytes, Langerhans cells, melanocytes, fibroblasts) are under hormonal influence. Changes in the endocrine system are thought to play a significant role in age-related physiological function decline. Since the skin not only fulfills a protective function for the organism but is also an active peripheral endocrine organ, which even releases effective hormones in the circulation, local hormone substitution could become interesting in the future.

With aging, there is a decrease in the level of hormones, such as estrogen, testosterone, dehydroepiandrosterone sulfate, and growth hormone. The effect of this decrease on the skin has been poorly documented, although more data are available for estrogen than for other hormones. Treatments administered for menopause, in particular hormone replacement therapy, appear to alter its effects on the basic components of the skin as well as the more complex structures residing in the skin, consequently retarding the skin-aging process (Raine-Fenning et al., 2003).Estrogen treatment in postmenopausal women has been repeatedly shown to increase collagen content, dermal thickness and elasticity, and data on the effect of estrogen on skin water content are also promising. Further, physiologic studies on estrogen and wound healing suggest that hormone replacement therapy (HRT) may play a beneficial role in cutaneous injury repair. Results on the effect of HRT on other physiologic characteristics of skin, such as elastin content, sebaceous secretions, wrinkling and blood flow, are discordant. Given the responsiveness of skin to estrogen, the effects of HRT on aging skin require further examination, and careful molecular studies will likely clarify estrogen's effects at the cellular level (Brincat et al., 2005). Makrantonaki et al. (2006) studied human hormonal aging in an in vitro model. Human skin cells cultured under hormone-substituted conditions showed altered lipid synthesis and metabolism and affected expression of genes involved in processes, such as DNA repair and stability, mitochondrial function, oxidative stress, transcriptional regulation and apoptosis, indicating that these processes could be hormone-dependent.

Growth hormone therapy has favorable effects on lean body mass, skin atrophy as well on body fat reduction. However, numerous side effects and the theoretical increased risk of cancer limit the use of growth hormone therapy in the elderly. Experimental data suggest that growth hormone and its downstream effector, Insulin-like Growth Factor I (IGF-I), may alter cellular oxidative process, thereby contributing to oxidative stress and actually promoting aging. Treatments with testosterone and DHEA risk to induce the growth of an occult prostate cancer and a long-term treatments with estrogen can increase the risk of breast cancer. There is a strong association between circulating IGF-I levels and the relative risks of breast and prostate cancer (Martin-Du Pan,1999). The relationship of the endocrine system physiology to oxidative damage processes are complex, sometimes incompletely understood, and variable, depending on the hormone in question. Hormones are important modulators and mediators of oxidative stress. Hormonally active molecules play significant roles both in protecting cells against oxidative stress and in generation of free radical damage or sensitizing cells to such damage (Brown-Borg Harman, 2003).

Chapter 11

Topical Treatment of Skin Aging

Cosmetic

Cosmetic Ingredients

According to Article 1 (76/768/EEC): A "cosmetic product" shall mean any substance or preparation intended to be placed in contact with the various external parts of the human body (epidermis, hair system, nails, lips and external genital organs) or with the teeth and the mucous membranes of the oral cavity with a view exclusively or mainly to cleaning them, perfuming them, changing their appearance and/or correcting body odors and/or protecting them or keeping them in good condition.

Cosmeceuticals are agents that are marketed as cosmetic products, contain biologically active ingredients, and are available without a prescription (Helfrich, 2008). Since the term "cosmeceutical" was coined over twodecades ago, the number of products in this category that claim to combat dermal aging has grown dramatically.Cosmetic products containing peptides, antioxidants, botanicals, phytonutrients, etc., are examples of cosmeceuticals. Due to the purpose of the book, this chapter will focus mainly on antioxidants as cosmetic ingredients. Despite advertising claims, almost all available topical formulations contain very low concentrations of antioxidants that are not well absorbed by the skin. Cosmeceuticals do not undergo the rigorous testing required for drug approval, and there are few clinical controlled trials of these products. Drugs exert a biologic effect, are dispensed by prescription, and are regulated by the U.S. Food and Drug Administration.

With the rise of the cosmeceutical industry, numerous formulations have surfaced with claims of reducing the clinical manifestations of aging and photoaging. Many of these products capitalize on the positive connection the public makes with vitamins, especially with respect to their antioxidant capabilities. An impressive amount of basic science and clinical research has been conducted in both an attempt to discover novel strategies for preventing detrimental sun damage and to validate the addition of vitamins to skin care products (Zussman et al., 2010).

The lack of controlled studies confirming the efficacy of dermocosmetic products as well as the superiority of the preparation incorporating the active agent over the corresponding base is a problem yet to be solved. Retinol and antioxidant agents such as vitamin C and coenzymes that positively act via several mechanisms on collagen biosynthesis can be considered evidence-based substances for the management of aging skin (Pavicic et al., 2009).

Vitamins are a natural constituent of human skin and are part of a system of antioxidants that protect the skin from oxidative stress. There has been an increased interest in the use of natural antioxidants in the form of vitamins to help restore dermal antioxidant activity. A variety of ingredients with antioxidative potential (e.g., retinoic acid, vitamins, flavonoids) are incorporated into cosmetic products claiming to delay/reverse premature aging. Controversy exists as to whether topical antioxidants can be effective in protecting against and reversing photodamage to the skin. Some of these have a scientifically proven effect; others lack a scientifically confirmed efficacy. Vitamins A, C, E, B3 and many other compounds have been shown to have potent antioxidant and anti-inflammatory properties, but to achieve optimal effectiveness, products must be delivered in appropriate formulations and absorbed into the skin. Topical vitamins C and E, as well as topical selenium, protect skin against sunburn, suntan and skin cancer and also reverse the mottled pigmentation and wrinkles of photoaging according to some studies. However, only certain forms of these labile antioxidants are stable and active after percutaneous absorption. Some products are further limited in their efficacy by the fact that the incorporated active ingredients are either not contained in an adequate concentration, or not stable in the cream base, or do not penetrate through the stratum corneum. Products containing alpha-tocopherol (vitamin E), L-ascorbic acid (vitamin C), retinol (vitamin A), and niacinamide (vitamin B3), are effective for the treatment of photoaging (for further reading, see also chapter on exogenous antioxidants). These compounds have also shown effectiveness in the treatment of inflammatory dermatoses, acne, pigmentation disorders and wound healing. There is emerging evidence that combinations of vitamins have additive or even synergistic effects that provide enhanced efficacy compared with individual compounds (Burgess, 2008).

There are two great advantages in applying an active formulation of topical antioxidants to the skin. First, the skin attains far higher levels of each antioxidant than can be achieved by only taking these vitamins orally. For example, the level of vitamin C attained in the skin by topical application is 20 to 40 times that achievable with oral vitamin C. With topical application, the concentration of vitamin E in the skin increases by a factor of 10.6 and selenium by a factor of 1.7. Second, topical application arms the skin with a reservoir of antioxidants that cannot be washed or rubbed off, a protectionthatstays in the skin for several days after application (Burke 2004). Besides well-known antioxidants, there are other active ingredients for skin treatment. Functional agents currently include alpha hydroxy acids (AHAs), poly-AHAs, complex poly-AHAs, retinoids, fish polysaccharides, anti-enzymatic agents,and antioxidants (including pycnogenol, ursolic acid, vegetable isoflavones, coenzyme Q10, lipoic acid, resveratrol, l-carnosine and taurine), as well as agaricic acid and various plant extracts and many others.

Some of the active ingredients found in topical cosmetics possess antioxidative properties and are useful in prevention and treatment of premature aging. Below we will discuss some of them:

Vitamin A (retinol) and retinoic acid: One of the few anti-aging-pharmaceuticals with a scientifically proven efficacy. Retinol is a cosmetic ingredient that is structurally similar to all-trans-retinoic acid, which has been shown to be effective in the treatment of photodamage. Since skin keratinocytes are reported to metabolize retinol to retinoic acid, investigators have hypothesized that retinol may also be helpful in improving skin photodamage. When applied topically, it is transformed to retinoic acid by human keratinocytes. Retinol stimulates collagen production in the skin, and its application can result in a reduction of wrinkles and skin pigmentation (Tucker-Samaras etal., 2009; Lee et al., 2006). Additionally, topical retinol significantly induces glycosaminoglycan, which is known to retain substantial water, and increased collagen production are most likely responsible for wrinkle effacement. With greater skin matrix synthesis, retinol-treated aged skin is more likely to withstand skin injury and ulcer formation along with improved appearance (Kafi et al., 2007).

Topical administration of tretinoin has proved to be effective in treating clinical signs of photodamaged skin (Gilchrest, 1997). In the research of Samuel et al. (2005),randomized controlled trialsthatcompared drug or surgical interventions with no treatment, placebo or another drug, in adults with mild, moderate or severe photodamage were reviewed. Authors concluded that there is conclusive evidence that topical tretinoin improves the appearance of mild to moderate photodamage on the face and forearms, in the short term. However, erythema, scaling/dryness, burning/stinging and irritation may be experienced initially. There is limited evidence that tazarotene and isotretinoin benefit patients with moderate photodamage on the face: both are associated with skin irritation and erythema. The effectiveness of other interventions remains uncertain according to Samuel et al. (2005). Topical tretinoin (all-trans retinoic acid) is the agent approved so far for the treatment of photoaging but also works to prevent it (Kang et al., 2001).

Randomized, double-blind, vehicle-controlled, left and right arm comparison study performed by Kafi et al. (2007) concluded that topical retinol improves fine wrinkles associated with natural aging. Significant induction of glycosaminoglycan, which is known to retain substantial water, and increased collagen production are most likely responsible for wrinkle effacement. With greater skin matrix synthesis, retinol-treated aged skin is more likely to withstand skin injury and ulcer formation along with improved appearance.

Studies have shown that topical all-trans-RA can prevent UV-induced skin responses that lead to degradation and downregulation of type I collagen in human skin in vivo. The study of Fisher and Voorhees (1998) reported all-trans retinoic acid acts to inhibit induction of c-Jun protein by ultraviolet irradiation, thereby preventing increased matrix metalloproteinases and ensuing dermal damage. The ability of retinoids to restore collagen is thought to be the main underlying mechanism by which the appearance of photodamaged skin is improved (Rittie et al., 2006; Griffiths et al., 1993).

Vitamin C: It stimulates collagen production and has a photoprotective effect. Its wrinkle-improving effect has been proven in clinical studies (Fitzpatrick and Rostan, 2002). One problem is its instability in various topical products, as vitamin C is prone to oxidation, and may lose its efficacy this way. For effective topical application, vitamin C has to be non-esterified, acidic and optimally at 20% concentration (Burke, 2004).

Oxidation of vitamin C leads to its fast degeneration even before the vitamin C-containing product can be applied to the skin. Furthermore, some topical products do not penetrate through the stratum corneumand thus are not able to render the desired effects. As already mentioned, vitamin C should be non-esterified, acidic and optimally at 20% concentration.

Transdermal administration of a vitamin C derivative, which can permeate through the membrane, completely reversed the skin thinning and deterioration of collagen and elastin in the mutant CuZn-SOD-deficient mice. These indicate that the vitamin C derivative is a powerful agent for alleviating skin aging through regeneration of collagen and elastin (Murakami et al., 2009).

Alpha-lipoic acid: It has antioxidative effects and has been shown to significantly reduce symptoms of skin aging and skin roughness in clinical studies. A-lipoic acid also known as thioctic acid has generated considerable clinical interest as a thiol-replenishing and redox-modulating agent. Lipoic acid is the only thiol-replenishing safe human nutrient known so far that is readily taken up by cells and promptly reduced by cellular enzymes to dihydrolipoic acid (Sen et al., 2003).

Flavonoids: Group of substances found in many foods. Flavonoids also have a photoprotective effect. Anthocyanins have received much attention as agents with potentials preventing chronic diseases, e.g., anthocyanins from edible bog blueberry were reported to be protective against UV-induced skin photoaging (Bae et al., 2009). In addition to single polyphenols, plant extracts have been assessed for their photoprotective potential (grape seeds, ginkgo biloba and green tea).

Green tea extracts: In vitro and in vivo animal and human studies suggest that green tea polyphenols are photoprotective in nature and can be used as pharmacological agents for the prevention of solar UVB light-induced skin disorders including photoaging, melanoma and nonmelanoma skin cancers after more clinical trials in humans. Topical treatment or oral consumption of green tea polyphenols (GTP) inhibit chemical carcinogen- or UV radiation-induced skin carcinogenesis in different laboratory animal models. Topical treatment of GTP and EGCG (Epigallocatechin Gallate) resulted in prevention of UVB-induced inflammatory responses, immunosuppression and oxidative stress, which are the biomarkers of several skin disease states. Topical application of GTP and EGCG prior to exposure of UVB protects against UVB-induced local as well as systemic immune suppression in laboratory animals, which was associated with the inhibition of UVB-induced infiltration of inflammatory leukocytes (Katiyar, 2003). Another study of Vayalil et al. (2003) demonstrated that topical application of green tea polyphenols reduced UVB-induced oxidation of lipids and proteins and depletion of antioxidant enzymes. Also, topically applied silymarin and apigenin are both reported to be beneficial (Birt et al., 1997; Katiyar et al., 1997). The review from Vaid and Katiyar (2010) suggested that silymarin may favorably supplement sunscreen protection and may be useful for skin diseases associated with solar UV radiation-induced inflammation, oxidative stress and immunomodulatory effects (Vaid and Katiyar 2010). Other protective effects include the reduced production of ROS and lipid peroxidation products, a reduced depletion of Langerhans cells and of endogenous antioxidant systems as reported by Afaq and Mukhtar (2002).

Selenium: Selenium (Se) is also an important micronutrient for the skin cells. Selenium is only percutaneously absorbed and active when applied topically as l-selenomethionine, optimally at 0.02-0.05% (Burke, 2004).

Copper: Copper peptides seem to have effects on skin aging. Clinical studies showed wrinkle reduction and improvement of elasticity. Copper is essential to wound healing and in skin aging. Wound healing and skin aging are facilitated by matrixmetalloproteinases (MMP), which remodel the extracellular matrix, and interleukin-8 (IL-8), linked with copper. Copper can be thus essential micronutrient for the skin as well as damaging (Philips et al., 2010).

Sleeping on fabrics containing copper-impregnated fibers was reported to have a positive cosmetic effect on the skin. Consistent sleeping for fourweeks on copper oxide-containing pillowcases caused a significant reduction in the appearance of facial wrinkles and crow's feet/fine lines and significant improvement in the appearance of facial skin (Borkow et al., 2009). Additionally, results from the study of Mahoney et al. (2009) suggest that the bi-metal, 0.1% copper-zinc malonate-containing cream has the propensity to increase elastin synthesis in human skin in vivo and that regeneration of elastic fibers may contribute to wrinkle effacement in female patients with photoaged facial skin.

A combination of agents were used in the recent study by Leyden and Parr (2010). The clinical effects of treating photodamaged skin with a proprietary copper zinc malonate lotion and a proprietary 4% hydroquinone cream, plus tretinoin cream, were evaluated in 42 females in a 24-week investigator-blind randomized study. Treatment was associated with early and significant improvements in mean scores on an overall integrated assessment of photodamage and for multiple signs of photodamage—tactile roughness; mottled hyperpigmentation, lentigines and fine wrinkling; laxity; crepiness and coarse wrinkling. Treatment was generally well tolerated, and 94% of subjects were satisfied or very satisfied.

Vitamin E: Data on the antioxidant effects of Vitamin E from clinical studies indicate a reduced wrinkle depth and a decrease in skin roughness. Vitamin E is found in various cosmetic products; however, in some of these, its concentration is so low that no effects on the skin can be expected. For effective topical application, vitamin E must be the non-esterified isomer d-alpha-tocopherol at 2% to 5% concentration (Burke, 2004).

Topically applied vitamin E (1%) can reduce phototoxic damage. UV-induced erythema, sunburn cell formation and skin wrinkling were reduced to some extent (Dreher et al., 1998; Lin et al., 2003, 2005). Topical application of vitamin E has been shown to decrease the incidence of ultraviolet (UV)-induced skin cancer in mice. A study revealed that topical application of alpha-tocopherol inhibits ultraviolet (UV) B-induced photocarcinogenesis and DNA photodamage in C3H mice in vivo. This study also suggests that incorporation of tocopherol compounds into sunscreen products confers protection against procarcinogenic DNA photodamage and that cellular uptake and distribution of tocopherol compounds is necessary for their optimal photoprotection (McVean and Liebler, 1999).

Vitamin E provides protection against UV-induced skin photodamage through a combination of antioxidant and UV-absorptive properties. Topical application of alpha-tocopherol on mouse skin inhibits the formation of cyclobutane pyrimidine photoproducts. However, topically applied alpha-tocopherol is rapidly depleted by UVB radiation in a dose-dependent manner (Krol et al., 2000).

Tocopherol carrier systems were tested for skin penetration and intracellular delivery. Skin penetration experiments showed that 55% of the applied α-tocopherol accumulated in full thickness skin after 24h (Ainbinder and Touitou, 2010). Tocopherol acetate is very often the antioxidant used in sunscreen products. It is usually present at concentrations in the range 0.2% to 1.5%, and concentrations of less than 0.5% probably have no antioxidative effect in human skin.

Coenzyme Q10: The processes of aging and photoaging are associated with an increase in cellular oxidation. This may be in part due to a decline in the levels of the endogenous cellular antioxidants, among them lipophilic antioxidant coenzyme Q10 (ubiquinone, CoQ10), which is significantly reduced in aging humans. After the age of 35 to 40, the organism begins to lose its ability to synthesize Co Q10 from food and its deficiencydevelops. Aging, poor eating habits, stress and infection—they all affect our ability to provide adequate amounts of Co Q10. It was reported that levels of CoQ10 are reduced also in skin cells from aging donors, and that topical supplementation can ameliorate processes involved in skin aging (Blatt et al., 2005).

Recent data reveal that CoQ10, besides being important in mitochondrial bioenergetics, also affects expression of genes involved in human cell signaling, metabolism, and transport, and some of the effects of exogenously administered CoQ10 may be due to this property (Littarru and Tiano, 2007).

Coenzyme Q10 has been reported as a powerful antioxidant in plasma. However, CoQ10 was barely satisfactory in topical drug delivery because of its lipid solubility. To improve the antioxidative efficiency of CoQ10 in skinphotoaging, Yue et al. (2010) prepared a novel CoQ10 nano-structured lipid carrier (CoQ10-NLC). In UVA-irradiated fibroblasts, the protection of CoQ10-NLC was more effective than the CoQ10-emulsion as demonstrated by cell viability and morphological changes of the cell body and nucleus. In addition, malondialdehyde (product of lipid peroxidation) concentration decreased by 61.5% in the group treated with CoQ10-NLC compared to the group subjected to general CoQ10-emulsion. In the presence of CoQ10-NLC, the activities of the antioxidative enzymes superoxide dismutase (SOD) and glutathione peroxidase (GSH-px) were reinstated to 81% and 75%, respectively, of the control group. In vivo, the CoQ10-NLC displayed a stronger capability to penetrate the stratum corneum and permeate the dermis after a topical skin application. This study revealed that CoQ10-NLC has greater antioxidant properties and topical skin penetration than the CoQ10-emulsion (Yue et al., 2010).

The research team by Hoppe et al. (1999) hasinvestigated whether topical application of CoQ10 has the beneficial effect of preventing photoaging. Authors of the study were able to demonstrate that CoQ10 penetrated into the viable layers of the epidermis and reduced the level of oxidation measured by weak photon emission. Furthermore, a reduction in wrinkle depth following CoQ10 application was also shown. CoQ10 was determined to be effective against UVA-mediated oxidative stress in human keratinocytes in terms of thiol depletion, activation of specific phosphotyrosine kinases and prevention of oxidative DNA damage. CoQ10 was also able to significantly suppress the expression of collagenase in human dermal fibroblasts following UVA irradiation.

In another study, CoQ10 was reported to reduce ROS production and DNA damage triggered by UVA irradiation in human keratinocytes in vitro. Further, CoQ10 was shown to reduce UVA-induced MMPs in cultured human dermal fibroblasts and UVB wrinkle formation in vitro and in vivo (Inui et al., 2008). Protection of epidermis against oxidative stress and enhancement of production of epidermal basement membrane components were reported to be involved in the anti-aging properties of CoQ10 in skin (Muta-Takada et al., 2009).

The combination of CoQ10 as a component of the respiratory chain in mitochondria, and creatine, as another important component of the cellular energy system clearly depicts their beneficial effects as active ingredients in topical formulations by improving signs of skin aging (Blatt et al., 2005). As a zwitter-ion, creatine is able to penetrate skin remarkably well and is able to replenish energy stores of epidermal cells.

Phyto-oestrogens: These are plant-derived substances with a hormone-like effect on the skin, such as isoflavones. They are found in soy products, grapes, and many different fruits. Studies showed positive effects on skin tightness and wrinkle reduction after topical application of isoflavones in postmenopausal women.

N-acetyl cysteine and genistein: The study of Kang et al. (2003) investigated genistein, which possesses both tyrosine kinase inhibitory and antioxidant activities, and N-acetyl cysteine, which can be converted into the endogenous antioxidant glutathione, to impair responses to ultraviolet light that eventuate in photoaging in human skin in vivo. Topical N-acetyl cysteine and genistein prevented ultraviolet-light-induced signaling that leads to photoaging in human skin in vivo. Their data indicate that compounds similar to genistein and N-acetyl cysteine, which possess tyrosine kinase inhibitory and/or antioxidant activities, may prevent photoaging.

Melatonin: Also, topical melatonin in combination with vitamins E and C protects skin from ultraviolet-induced erythema in a human study in vivo (Dreher et al., 1998). The study of Fischer et al. (1999) also showed suppression of UV-induced erythema by topical treatment of a 0.5% melatonin nanocolloid gel.

Synergistic Effect between Topical Antioxidants

The synergistic effect between antioxidants and their ability to regenerate was already presented in previous chapters of the book. Since also when applied topically, the synergism between different antioxidants is observed, we will briefly present some of the facts:

Although many cosmeceutical formulations contain vitamin C and/or vitamin E, very few are actually effective in topical application. First, because there is only a low concentration; second, because the stability is compromised as soon as the product is opened and exposed to air and light; and third, because the form of the molecule (an ester or a mixture of isomers) is not absorbed or metabolized effectively by the skin. However, when a stable formulation delivers a high concentration of the nonesterified, optimal isomer of the antioxidant, vitamins C and E do, indeed, inhibit the acute ultraviolet (UV) damage of erythema, sunburn, and tanning as well as chronic UV photoaging and skin cancer. Both are highly effective depigmenting agents. Because vitamin C regenerates oxidized vitamin E, the combination in a cosmeceutical formulation is synergistic—particularly in UV protection (Burke, 2007).

Another study was performed to see if a combination of topical vitamins C and E is better for UV protection to skin than an equivalent concentration of topical vitamin C or E alone. It was concluded that appreciable photoprotection can be obtained from the combination of topical vitamins C and E. Authors suggest that these natural products may protect against skin cancer and photoaging (Lin et al., 2003). Many other studies were published where the synergistic effect between two or more antioxidants was observed, if compared to the same antioxidants applied alone.

ConclusionIt is important to pretreat the skin with antioxidants before sun exposure. Animal and human studies have convincingly demonstrated pronounced photoprotective effects of "natural" and synthetic antioxidants when applied topically before UVR exposure. No significant protective effect of melatonin or the vitamins when applied alone or in combination were obtained when antioxidants were applied after UVR exposure. No improved photoprotective effect was obtained when multiple applications were done. UVR-induced skin damage is a rapid event, and antioxidants possibly prevent such damage only when present in relevant concentration at the site of action beginning and during oxidative stress (Dreher et al., 1999). Treatment of the skin with antioxidants after the damage was caused by UVR might cause additional harmful effects on cell cycle control and apoptosis process. The photoprotective effects of antioxidants are significant when applied in distinct mixtures in appropriate vehicles. Topical application of such combinations may result in a sustained antioxidant capacity of the skin, possibly due to antioxidant synergisms. UVA-induced skin alterations are believed to be largely determined by oxidative processes; topical administration of antioxidants might be particularly promising (Dreher and Maibach 2001). However, topical delivery of antioxidants to the skin has several obstacles, e.g., antioxidants must penetrate through the cell to reach its site of action, and they are very unstable, which makes them difficult to formulate. Antioxidants like tocopherols, vitamin C, and flavonoids are now being added as protective agents to skin creams. However, their ability to penetrate deep into the skin is limited, and an additional way of raising antioxidant levels in the dermis is to consume more of them in the diet.

Nevertheless, the use of topical antioxidants is gaining favor among dermatologists because of their broad biologic activities. Many are not only antioxidants but also possess anti-inflammatory and anticarcinogenic activities. These cosmeceuticals thus have many potential applications. In general, topical antioxidants exert their effects by downregulating free radical mediated pathways that damage skin (Farris 2007).

Additionally, there is no widely accepted method to choose antioxidant anti-aging products, like sunscreens, which have an SPF-rating system to guide consumers in their purchases. ORAC (Oxygen Radical Absorbance Capacity) and ABEL-RAC (Analysis By Emitted Light-Relative Antioxidant Capacity), are both accepted worldwide as a standard measure of the antioxidant capacity of foods and are rating systems that could be applied to all antioxidant skincare products according to a recent article by Palmer and Kitchin (2010). The standardization of antioxidant creams could revolutionize the cosmeceutical market and give physicians and consumers the ability to compare and choose effectively.

Certain exogenous antioxidants may exert an anti-aging effect as well as by preventing and even reversing sun damage. Many other antioxidants and botanicals that are popular on the market but were not discussed are: Rosmarinus officinalis, Vitis vinifera (grapeseed extract), Citronellol, Limonene, Oenothera biennis (evening primrose), Glycyrrhiza glabra (licorice extract), Aframomum angustifolium seed extract, Diosgenin (wild yam), N6 furfuryladenine (kinetin), and Ergothioneine (Cronin and Draelos, 2010).

Skin Moisturizing

The altered skin texture and structure of elderly people is caused by changes in proteins, lipids and water, leading to altered mechanical properties, such as wrinkling, sagging, loss of elasticity and apparent dryness. Dry skin remains the most common of human skin disorders. The incidence of atopic skin conditions (which is not equal to normal dry skin condition) in adults is estimated to be between 2% and 10% (Bath-Hextall and Williams, 2007). In general, the degree of skin hydration, as well as the level of natural moisturizing factor (NMF), were found to decrease as a function of age (Rawlings et al., 1994; Tagami, 1994; Rogiers et al., 1990), although this observation was sometimes contradicted by other scientists (Wilhelm et al., 1991; Conti et al., 1995).

Dry skin is a consequence of both intrinsic and extrinsic factors (Laloeuf and Byrne, 2009). Extrinsic factors include climate, environment, exposure to soaps, detergents, chemicals or medications (Pons- Guirard 2007). Intrinsic factors include genetics, diseases, hormone imbalance and aging (Engelke et al., 1999).

Since other factors affecting the skin were already discussed, this paragraph will be dedicated to skin moisturizing. One of the most important functions of the epidermis is the creation of a highly water-impermeable barrier in the stratum corneum (Elias, 2005). Stratum corneum (SC) is composed of fibrous-enriched corneocytes and a lipid-enriched intracellular matrix (Proksch et al., 1993). Our major protection against body water loss as well as toward penetration of toxic substances, allergens and microorganisms, is an ultrathin (~ 0.05μm) lipid structure situated in the stratum corneum extracellular space (Norlen, 2009). The water impermeable multi-lamelar lipids are located in the stratum corneum and are composed of three main non-polar lipid classes: fatty acids, cholesterol and ceramides (Elias, 2005). The strength of the water barrier depends on specific lipid composition and proportions of cholesterol, ceramides and free fatty acids (Jackson et al., 1996), especially linoleic acid (Elias, 1996). Also, hyaluronic acid and glycerol contribute to maintain skin hydration (Farage et al., 2010). These intracellular lipids, as well as sebum, natural moisturizing factor, organic acids and inorganic ions, impart the water-holding capacity of stratum corneum (Tagami, 2008). Disturbance of the lipid ratios results in a reduction in barrier function and an increase in the water flux across the skin, the so-called transepidermal water loss (Ghadially et al., 1996). In stratum spinosum, overlaying the stratum basale, the synthesis of characteristic organelles such as lamellar bodies is initiated. Lamelar bodies serve as carriers of precursors of stratum corneum barrier lipids. The main lipid classes in lamellar bodies are polar lipids, such as glycosphingolipids, free sterols, and phospholipids. Glucosylceramides and sphyngomyelin are converted into ceramides, while phospholipases are responsible for the generation of free fatty acids from the phospholipids (Bouwstra, 2009). As already mentioned, the major lipid classes in stratum corneum are ceramides, cholesterol and free fatty acids. Maintenance of an optimal level of hydration by the stratum corneum is according to Muizzuddin et al. (2009) dependent on several factors: intracellular lammellar lipids, which provide an effective barrier to the passage of water through the tissue; the diffusion path length, which retards water, since water must traverse the tortuous path created by the SC layers and corneocyte envelopes; and the amount of natural moisturizing factor, which is a complex mixture of low-molecular-weight, water-soluble compounds, first formed within the corneocytes by degradation of the histidine-rich protein filaggrin. The skin barrier function is efficient when correct balanced lipid lamellae are present in combination with intact superficial hydrolipidic film (Brod, 1991; Wertz and van den Bergh, 1998).

An increased transepidermal water loss elicits a pro-inflammatory response in the epidermal keratinocytes with an increased production of the pro-inflammatory cytokines IL-1α, TNF, and GM CSF, while manual occlusion of the perturbed barrier abrogated these events (Wood et al., 1994; Wood et al., 1992). Global reduction in SC lipids (about one-third less than in young SC) explains the paucity of membrane structures that underlie the barrier deficit in aged SC. The decline in ceramide, cholesterol and fatty acid content/synthesis is attributable to reduced activities of key enzymes for each of these lipids, including SPT, HMGCoAreductase, and acetyl CoA carboxylase (ACC) (Ghadially et al., 1996). Aged skin is unable to synthesize the longer chain ή-6 fatty acids required for proper barrier function and desquamation, and the precursor to these, the so-called essential fatty acid linoleic acid, must be supplied from the diet(Jenkins et al., 2009).

Collagen and elastin are the skin proteins responsible for elasticity, tone and texture. Water structure is important because water can bind to various proteins and is important for maintaining the structural and mechanical properties of proteins. Their natural interaction is diminished in photoaged skin, leading to decreased collagen stability and the fragmentation of collagen fibrils (Gniadecka et al., 1998). The distribution of glycosaminoglycans (GAG) in the dermis seems to be modified in sun-damaged skin and could be linked to alterations of deep protein. Glycosoaminoglycans (GAG's or mucopolysaccharides) and proteoglycans hold water in the skin (these are very similar to mucus proteins) and are the true skin moisturizers. GAGs contain special sugars such as glucosamine hydrochloride, N-acetyl glucosamine, and glucosamine sulfate that have high water-holding properties. These are built into larger water-holding chains of sugars such as hyaluronic acid, keratin sulfate, heparin, heparin sulfate, dermatin sulfate, and chondroitin sulfate. Proteoglycans are larger molecules with many attached GAGs. Proteoglycans are linear GAGs made up of repeating disaccharide units composed of sugars (glucuronic or iduronic acid) and hexosamines (glucosamine or galactosamine) that are bound to a protein core. The abundance of hydroxyl, carboxyl and sulfate groups makes the GAGs intensely hydrophilic (water-loving) molecules able to form porous, hydrated gels. Hydrated GAG's cushion and provide mechanical support to tissues (http://www.skinbiology.com/skinhealth&aging.html). Since SC is located in the superficial layer of the skin and is continuously exposed to oxidative stimuli via direct oxidation of lipid peroxides, it is likely that proteins in the SC may be targets of oxidative modification (Hirao, 2009; Stadtman et al., 1992).

As a person ages, the epidermal cells become thinner and less sticky. The thinner layer of cells make the skin look noticeably thinner. The decreased stickiness of the cells decreases the effectiveness of the barrier function allowing moisture to be released instead of being kept in the skin. This causes dryness. In contrast, cosmetic moisturizers cover the skin with a water-impermeable barrier such as petrolatum or a heavy oil. This artificially slows the loss of moisture from the skin and gives the skin a temporary appearance of plumpness and fullness.

SC moisturization is essential not only for keeping or obtaining a smooth and supple skin with a pleasing appearance but also for its normal functioning (De Paepe and Rogiers, 2009; De Polo, 1998; Rawlings and Harding, 2004; Rawlings and Matts, 2005). According to De Paepe and Rogiers (2009) "distinction should be made between temporarily dry skin and constantly dehydrated skin. For the first group, it is usually sufficient to eliminate the causing factor responsible for the barrier damage provoking dry skin and to advise restriction of detergents and cleansing products. In the second group, the occurrence of dry skin has a genetic predisposition and, therefore, it is essential to keep up the SC moisture content and to prevent further aggravation of the skin conditions. This can be achieved by frequent application of moisturizing creams and by lotions in sufficient amounts" (Breternitz et al., 2008; Proksch, 2008). According to De Paepe and Rogiers (2009), moisturizing products that either limit water loss from the skin or rehydrate the upper skin layers can be used to improve skin conditions. A combination of both targets may result in a more ideal skin care product that enhances both the barrier function and the moisturization of the SC.

Methods to improve skin hydration:

Water homeostasis depends on several factors, for example, the supply of water from the body, water diffusion through the viable layers of the epidermis, transepidermal water loss, and water-holding capacity of the stratum corneum (Brandner, 2009).

Aged skin often feels dry to the touch; its dryness is worsening in cold climates. For this reason, it is important to consume lots of water to keep the body and the skin hydrated. Many people's health problems and aging signs would improve if they would just drink more good water.

However, chlorine is added to drinking water to kill or inactivate harmful organisms that cause various diseases. When Cl_2 is added to water, hypochlorous acid (HOCl) is formed. This acid is highly reactive and able to oxidize many biological molecules. Besides, HOCl reacts with O_2^- to give OH^- and with H_2O_2 to form singlet O_2. Also, skin cells can be damaged by chlorine if ingested or by the dermal contact.

According to dermatologists at the University of Maryland Medical Center, tap water strips skin of its natural barrier oils and moisture that protect against wrinkles. If we wash them off too often, we wash away also the protection. Unless our soap contains skin-protecting moisturizers, it is better to use a facial cleanser instead of soap.

Cleansing and moisturizing are the key components to maintaining healthy, youthful skin. Cleansing removes dirt, grime, and dead skin cells, but cleansers also have a harmful effect on the skin by drying it out. The irritancy potential of cleansing agents is dependent on a number of factors, which include pH, and soaps are known to increase skin surface pH. Acidic cleansers are less irritating than neutral or alkaline ones, and people prone to dry skin are advised to use acidic cleansers. Agents with slightly acidic or neutral pH, nonionic surfactants, may be preferable for patients who are at increased risk for irritating skin reactions. Therefore, advise patients with skin conditions to choose a mild cleaning agent with a low pH (Yosipovitch and Hu, 2003).

Moisturizers not only increase the skin's water content, but they also protect the skin and encourage an orderly desquamation (shedding) process that makes the skin appearsmoother. Moisturizers are recommended as a means to relieve feelings of dryness and itching. They should be applied on a daily basis to ensure maximum benefit. Successful treatment of dry skin with appropriate moisturizers leads to smoother, softer and firmer skin. In the article of Rawlings et al. (2004), it is explained what kind of different ingredients are added to cosmetic products to prevent skin dehydration:

- Humectants attract water from the dermis into the epidermis, increasing the water content in the epidermis. Humectants are small hygroscopic molecules that penetrate the stratum corneum where they subsequently act as humectants. When humidity is higher than 70 percent, humectants can also attract water from the atmosphere into the epidermis. Corneocytes contain a reservoir of the natural moisturizing factor (NMF), hydrating substances that have the capacity to attract and bind water. Widely used humectant is Glycerine or glycerol.
- Occlusives increase the water content of the skin by slowing the evaporation of water from the surface of the skin. These ingredients are often greasy and are most effective when applied to damp skin.
- Emollients are ingredients that remain in the stratum corneum to act as lubricants. They help maintain the soft, smooth, and pliable appearance of the skin (e.g., mineral oils, fats, waxes, and plant oils).
- Chemicals that slow oxidation by reacting with free radicals.

- Moisturizers that are products for the skinthatincrease the water content of the upper skin layers.

Also, pH of the creams is very important. pH is a key feature of epidermal barrier function and, therefore, crucial in understanding topical skin treatment. "Skin pH" means "Skin Potential of Hydrogen," and it is used to measure the degree of acidity or alkalinity in the outer layers of the skin.

Normal skin surface pH is between 4 and 6.5 in healthy people, though it varies among the different areas of the skin. It's important to protect the stratum corneum because if it's damaged, skin surface pH has been shown to increase, creating susceptibility to bacterial skin infections or skin damage and disease (Yosipovitch and Hu, 2003).The acid mantle, the combination of sebum (oil) and perspiration, on the skin's surface protectsthe skin and renders the skin less vulnerable to damage and attack by environmental factors such as sun and wind and less prone to dehydration.

Creams primarily slow the rate of water loss from the skin and help keep the skin supple. It should be stressed that collagen creams work only on the skin surface. A moisturizer with or without collagen cannot penetrate the skin and is not designed to be absorbed. No moisturizer can undo the cumulative effect of collagen loss. Additionally, nutrition can also have beneficial effects on skin-barrier function.

Crowther and Matts (2009) pointed out that "different moisturizer formulations can have different effects on the SC and the epidermis. In the short term, moisturizers will increase SC hydration, and in the medium term, they improve desquamation, however, in the longer term, it has become apparent that some can actually compromise SC barrier function, while others can strengthen it.

In vitro and in vivo studies have also demonstrated the ability of some moisturizing ingredients to influence SC thickness" (Crowther and Matts, 2009, and the references therein).

Protection of the Skin from SunDamage and the Use of Sunscreen Blocks

It is well established that sun exposure is the main cause for the development of skin cancer and other skin damage leading to skin aging. Chronic continuous UV radiation and intermittent high-dose UV exposure is believed to induce malignant melanoma and contribute to the occurrence of actinic keratoses as precursor lesions of squamous cell carcinoma as well as basal cell carcinoma. Not only photocarcinogenesis but also the mechanisms of photoaging have recently become apparent. In this respect, the preventive measures aimed at avoiding direct sun exposure and the use of sunscreens seemed to prove to be more and more important and popular within the last decades (Maier and Korting, 2005).

First of all, it is advised to avoid sunburn or excessive exposure by staying out of direct sunlight as the primary defense. When possible, avoidance of outdoor activities during the hours between 10 AM and 4 PM, when the sun's rays are the strongest, is advised.

However, it is not always possible to stay out of direct sunlight, and on those occasions, we should protect our skin from the inside and from the outside.

1. Skin Outside Protection: The Use of Sunscreen Blocks

The skin is equipped with two endogenous photoprotective mechanisms: the melanin in the lower layer of epidermis and the urocanic acid barrier of the stratum corneum, which reflects and absorbs a significant amount of UVB radiation. *Trans*-urocanic acid, produced in keratinocytes from the metabolism of histidine, is a potent absorber of UV radiation and protects DNA in keratinocyte nuclei from UV-induced damage. However, isomerization of *trans*-urocanic to the *cis* isoform by UVB radiation renders the compound a potent immunosuppressor (DeFabo and Noonan, 1983). The thickness of the stratum corneum also appears to be highly significant for photoprotection (Gniadecka et al., 1996). Additionally, skin contains chromophores. Chromophores absorb energy and become transformed into their excited state: they quickly undergo chemical changes (photochemistry), transfer their energy to other molecules, or give off the extra energy as light (fluorescence) or heat. Indeed, it is mainly the UVA range with its less energetic potential that reacts with chromophores; UVB radiation directly penetrates the barrier (keratin layer) and causes mutations on DNA bases, lipids, proteins, and other cell molecules (Laurent-Applegate and Schwarzkopf, 2001). The formation of ROS during exposure to UVR is initiated following absorbtion by endogenous or exogenous chromophores in the skin, e.g., trans-uronic acid, melanins, flavins, porphyrins, quinones, tryptophan moieties, and glycation end products (Cross et al., 1998; Thiele, 2001). Following absorbtion, the activated chromophore may react in two ways (Thiele et al., 2006), as was explained by Laurent-Applegate and Schwarzkopf (2001) "In type I photoreactions, the excited chromophore directly reacts with a substrate molecule via electron or hydrogen atom transfer, giving rise to free radicals. In the presence of molecula O2 superoxide anion radical can be formed, which dismutates to H2O2. Alternatively, in the presence of metal ions such as Fe(II) and Cu(II), H2O2 can be converted to the OH˙. In major type II reactions, reactive single oxygen (1O2) is formed from UVR-excited chromophores in the presence of triplet oxygen (3O2) (Theile et al., 2006). ROS species can then react with all cellular macromolecules. The major cellular chromophores absorbing in the UVB (290 to 320 nm) wavelength range are nucleic acids and proteins. There are many chromophores in the UVA (320 to 400 nm) region, but they are usually present in low concentrations when compared to those absorbing in the shorter wavelengths. Because they have low extinction coefficients, the relationship for specific UVA-absorbing molecules and the effect of UVR on cells is more difficult to establish. There are a variety of biomolecules absorbing UVB radiation, including nicotinamide adenine dinucleotide (NADH), quinones, flavins, and other heterocyclic cofactors. In the UVA range, protein cofactors and soluble metabolites may be responsible for UVA-induced responses in cells. The actual amount of UVR absorbed by each tissue is proportional to its concentration and absorption coefficient, and each endogenous chromophore has its range of wavelengths absorbed and the maximum peak of absorption" (Laurent-Applegate and Schwarzkopf, 2001).

On the other hand ,the use of sunscreen offers exogenous skin protection.

Broad-spectrum (including UVB and UVA and other protection) sunscreens should be used when other means of protection are not feasible. These sunscreens should be used to reduce exposure rather than lengthen the period of exposure to the sun, as is wrongly believed by many sunscreen users.

Sunscreens' way of defense is based on reflecting or absorbing UV light on skin surface. The absorbed energy is then released from the sunscreen molecules mostly as fluorescence or heat. Sunscreens protect by absorbing or reflecting UV on the skin surface. Physical sunscreens mostly reflect light, whereas chemical sunscreens mostly absorb light. In general, UV filters can be divided into physical and chemical filters, and most modern sunscreens contain a mixture of both. Additionally, chemical filters can be divided into molecules that absorb primarily in the UVB region, such as p-aminobenzoic acid and derivatives and zinc acid esters, and molecules that primarily absorb in the UVA region, e.g., butyl-methoxydibenzoylmethane. In addition, some filter molecules absorb both UVA and UVB photons, e.g., benzophenone (Krutmann and Yarosh, 2006). The most frequently used chemical filters are ethylhexyl-methoxycinnamate and butyl-methoxydibenzoylmethane (Lowe et al., 1997). Chemical UV filters have the capacity to absorb short wavelength UV and transform photons into heat-emitting long-wavelength (infrared) radiation. Most of them absorb a small wavelength range. They can be divided into three groups. The first group consists of molecules that primarily absorb the UVB spectrum (p-aminobenzoic acid derivatives and zincacid esters), and second of molecules that primarily absorb the UVA spectrum (butyl- methoxydibenzoylmethane). The third group consists of molecules that absorb UVA and UVB photons (benzophenone). A combination of different filters in the same product renders the whole filter system photo-unstable (Puizina-Ivic, 2008). That means that UV exposure causes photochemical reactions that generate ROS with subsequent phototoxic and photoallergic reactions. Great efforts have been made to stabilize molecules in UV filters, which has improved the efficacy of photoprotection with chemical UV filters. There is a growing need for standardization and evaluation of UVA photoprotection, while for UVB, there is already consensus on the international level (Gilchrest and Krutmann, 1999).

Besides reflection and absorption of UV light by sunscreens, also quenching and neutralization of free radicals and other ROS can offer additional protection against UVR damage. The addition of antioxidants to sunscreen provides protection by quenching UV-induced reactive oxygen species inside skin.

The study conducted by Oresajo et al. (2010) demonstrated that a combination of antioxidants and sunscreens complement each other, resulting in superior photoprotection. The formula containing sunscreens + the antioxidant complex was the most protective in reducing UV-induced skin damage, followed by the formula with the antioxidant alone.

The study performed by Agrawal and Kaur (2010) provides the first preclinical evidence for the use of topically delivered curcumin to attenuate photoaging. Authors demonstrated inhibitory effect of encapsulated curcumin on ultraviolet-induced photoaging in mice.

The study done by Oresajo et al. (2008) confirms the protective role of a unique mixture of antioxidants containing vitamin C, ferulic acid, and phloretin on human skin from the harmful effects of UV irradiation. Authorspropose that antioxidant mixture will complement and synergize with sunscreens in providing photoprotection for human skin.

Ultraviolet (UV) radiation induces also immunomodulatory effects that may be involved in skin cancer. As a result, sunscreens, which mainly absorb UVB, may be less effective in preventing UV radiation-induced immunosuppression than broad-spectrum products. The study done by Moyal and Fourtainier (2008)revealed that broad-spectrum sunscreens provide better protection from solar ultraviolet-simulated radiation and natural sunlight-induced immunosuppression in human beings (Moyal and Fourtanier, 2008).

The study ofVielhaber et al (2006) indicates that UVA1 filters with a maximum absorption at > or =360 nm are most effective in preventing UVA1 radiation-induced MMP-

1, IL-1alpha, and IL-6 expression pointing towards a critical role for effective filtering beyond > or =360 nm for protection against UVA1-induced photoaging.

UV filters not only protect against acute skin injury, such as sunburn, but also against long-term and chronic skin damage, including cellular DNA damage, photo-induced immune suppression, and, by extension, skin cancer. The protection provided by modern sunscreens against UV-induced skin cancer was shown in animal photocarcinogenicity studies and confirmed by numerous in vitro, animal, and human investigations. Additional benefits of ultraviolet filters include prevention of photodermatoses, such as polymorphic light eruption, and, possibly, photoaging.

Thus, strategies to prevent photodamage caused by this cascade of reactions initiated by UV include (Pillai, 2005): prevention of UV penetration into skin by physical and chemical sunscreens; prevention/reduction of inflammation using anti-inflammatory compounds (e.g., cyclooxygenase inhibitors, inhibitors of cytokine generation); scavenging and quenching of ROS by antioxidants; inhibition of neutrophil elastase activity to prevent extracellular matrix damage and activation of matrix metalloproteases (MMPs); and inhibition of MMP expression (e.g., by retinoids) and activity (e.g., by natural and synthetic inhibitors). Additionally, a modern UV filter should be heat and photostable, water resistant, nontoxic, and easy to formulate. It should absorb and/or reflect UV radiation and provide absorption over a wide spectrum of UV; it must be stable on the human skin despite exposure to heat and sunlight; it must remain on skin surface without penetrating into and through the skin; it should be also water resistant. Identification of a substance that meets these criteria is as difficult as discovering a new drug; hundreds of new molecules are synthesized and screened before a lead candidate is identified. The most important aspect in the development of a new UV filter should be its safety (Nohynek and Schaefer, 2001). Prior to human use, all new skin products should be evaluated by in vitro screening; including photostability, cytotoxicity, photocytotoxicity, genotoxicity, and photogenotoxicity tests. The safety and efficacy of UV filters are regulated and approved by national and international health authorities. Safety standards in the European Union, United States, or Japan stipulate that new filters pass a stringent toxicological safety evaluation prior to approval. The safety dossier of a new UV filter resembles that of a new drug and includes acute toxicity, irritation, sensitization, phototoxicity, photosensitization, subchronic and chronic toxicity, reproductive toxicity, genotoxicity, photogenotoxicity, carcinogenicity, and, in the United States, photocarcinogenicity testing (Nohynek and Schaefer, 2001). Prior to marketing, new UV filters undergo stringent human testing to confirm their efficacy as well as the absence of irritation, sensitization, photoirritation, and photosensitization potential in man. In Europe, 27 active sunscreen agents are permitted, while only 16 UV filters are approved for use by FDA. This discrepancy could be explained by the fact that sunscreen ingredients are treated like drugs in USA and as cosmetic products in EU.

There is a need for new strategies to ensure sunscreen safety by minimizing its penetration into cells and systemic absorbtion. Until recently, metal oxides have been promoted as safer alternatives to organic sunscreens, based on the fact that they do not penetrate beyond the stratum corneum. Serpone et al. (2001) showed that titanium dioxide nanoparticles can induce free radical formation in the presence of UV. On the other hand, a recent review by Nohynek et al. (2007) concluded that there is no evidence that metal nanoparticles penetrate into human skin. Additionally, the Scientific Committee on Consumer Products (SCCP) published their opinion that there is no conclusive evidence for skin penetration into viable tissues by 20 nm or larger nanoparticles, which are used in metal oxide sunscreens (SCCP, 2007). A nanoparticle is a particle with one or more dimensions at the nanoscale and is defined as a particle with at least one dimension<100nm. Nanoparticles can be divided into two groups: i) soluble and/or biodegradable nanoparticles thatdisintegrate upon application to skin into their molecular components (e.g., liposomes, microemulsions, nanoemulsions), and ii) insoluble particles (e.g., TiO2, fullerenes, quantum dots). At present, the *in vitro* diffusion cell chamber is the standard device for estimating percutaneous absorption. However, because mechanical factors may be important in potential penetration/absorption of nanoparticles, the standard model may not be ideal. Classic skin permeability techniques do not take into account possible mechanical effects that may be relevant for the penetration of insoluble nanoparticles or nanomaterials. Therefore, new methodologies to assess percutaneous penetration pathways are urgently needed. All *in vivo*and *in vitro* risk-assessment methods for nanomaterials are still in the research phase. Although some validated *in vitro* methods do exist, they have never been validated with nanomaterials as reference compounds. Many studies have demonstrated the reactivity of nanoparticles and their capacity to produce reactive oxygen species (ROS), inducing oxidative stress. Review of the safety of the insoluble nanomaterials presently used in sunscreens is required according SCCP (SCCP 2007).

The use of sunscreen helps to prevent the damage to the skin caused by UVR. Special attention is dedicated also to the use of DNA-repair enzymes as additional strategy to increase repair of DNA damage after it occurs but before it can cause biological consequences. Many DNA-repair enzymes have been identified. With the development of liposomes engineered for delivery into skin, the use of DNA-repair enzymes for photoprotection became practically possible (Yarosh et al., 1994).Liposomes are colloidal particles, typically consisting of phospholipids and cholesterol, with other possible ingredients. The lipid molecules form bilayers surrounding an aqueous core. Both the bilayer and the core can be used to entrap and present ingredients to the skin.

2. Skin inside Protection: The Use of Antioxidants

Another skin damage preventive approach could be obtained by the use of diet-derived antioxidants. As already discussed in previous chapters, antioxidants could provide protection against UVR damage. The use of fruit and vegetables as rich sources of antioxidants or the use of antioxidant supplements should be always done some hours or days BEFORE the sun exposure. Exposure of the human skin to UV radiation leads to depletion of antioxidants in our skin and ultimately to the development of skin diseases.

UV radiation to skin might cause a large degree of depletion of antioxidants immediately after irradiation. Enhanced UVB radiation suppressed the enzymatic antioxidant systems and caused some active oxygen species to accumulate in irradiated cells, e.g., superoxide anion radical ($O_2^-.$) production and the concentration of hydrogenperoxide (H_2O_2) and malodiadehyde (MDA). Many studies suggest that exogenous supplementation of antioxidants prevents UVR-induced photooxidative damage. In recent years, there has been much interest in the use of oral and topical antioxidants as photoprotective agents. This topic was extensively described already in previous chapters.

Conclusion

Skin contains many defenses against UVR and other harmful compounds. Nevertheless, with the use of topical compounds, we can offer extra protection mostly from UVR and some other environmental insults. According to Rona and Berardesca (2008), "the rationale of a combined approach for the anti-aging treatment of skin is based on the synergic effect between functional substances applied locally, where the problem arises, and other agents working from the inside to correct a need, to restore altered functions or conditions and to guarantee the correct intake of nutrients or active substances" (Rona and Berardesca, 2008). It should be stressed that sunscreens are placed only on the third place of sun protection mechanisms. On the first place, our behavior is located. This means that we should not exaggerate with intentional sun exposure, should not take sun between 10 a.m. and 4p.m., should not use sun beds. On the second place, protective clothes and sunglasses are located.

Promoting sunscreen use is an integral part of preventionprograms aimed at reducing ultraviolet (UV) radiation-induced skin damage and skin cancers. Protection against both UVB and UVA radiation is advocated. At present, the sun protection factor (SPF) is the most reliable information for the consumer as a measure of sunscreen filter efficacy. Recently, combinations of UV filters with agents active in DNA repair have been introduced in order to improve photoprotection. Always wear a broad-spectrum (protection against both UVA and UVB) sunscreen with an SPF of 30 or higher. It is important that the sunscreen blocks both UVA and UVB rays. Most sunscreens combine chemical UV-absorbing sunscreens and physical inorganic sunscreens, which reflect UV, to provide broad-spectrum protection. SPF is affected by application density, water resistance and other factors. An adequate SPF for an individual should be balanced to skin phenotype and exposure habits. The correct use of sunscreens should be combined with the avoidance of midday sun and the wearing of protective clothing and glasses, as part of an overall sun protection regimen. (Moloney et al., 2002).There is still much research necessary before the perfect sunscreen is developed. In the meantime, people using sunscreens should use only those with the highest SPF and be aware that they are for their protection from the sun and not for tanning purposes (WHO, Ultraviolet radiation, Environmental Health Criteria: 160).

Children need extra protection from the sun. One or two blistering sunburns before the age of 18 dramatically increase the risk of skin cancer. Children should be encouraged to play in the shade, wear protective clothing and apply sunscreen regularly.

Published research indicates that both children and adults are still spending considerable time in the sun during peak UV exposure periods (Kozarev, 1998).A survey conducted on 51 physician volunteers of various specialties showed that 33% spent more than twopeak UV hours outdoors every day, and another 33.33% are regularly sun exposed for at least fivehours. Only 39% of the survey groupregularly used sunscreen, and those that did used an inadequate amount for full body protection. A majority of the respondents did not believe that sunscreens protected against skin cancer, but they did believe that sunscreens could slow the aging process. Common reasons for not using sunscreen were the amount of time involved in application and the relative high cost. The researcher concluded that participants lacked well-formed sun protection habits and that there continues to be a poor understanding of the need for sun protection despite worldwide campaigns warning of the dangers. Special attention should be dedicated also to the appropriate thickness (or amount) of the sunscreen applied on the skin.

As it was already pointed out previously in this book, it is estimated that ¾ of sun exposure is not intentional. This means that our skin is exposed to majority of UVradiation when we are outdoors working and not when we are intentionally exposed to the sun on the beach. At this time, we also do not use sun-creams with UVA/UVB protection. The only protection of our skin is its endogenous protection (melanine and enzymatic antioxidants) and antioxidants we consume from the food (vitamin A, C, E, etc.).

Chapter 12

Skin Curative Approaches

The study of skin aging focuses on two main streams of interest: On the one hand, the esthetic problem and its management; on the other, the biological problem of aging in terms of microscopic, biochemical, and molecular changes (Trüeb, 2005). Primary skin-aging prevention encompasses measures that are taken before the aging process has started, whereas secondary prevention starts when the first signs of aging have come into sight. Eventually, tertiary measures are aimed at correcting established signs of aging (Trüeb, 2005). Until now mostly primary preventive approaches or methods to retard the process of skin aging were discussed with the focus on molecular and biochemical pathways. In the last chapter some paragraphs werealso dedicated to curative methods—to improve the cutaneous changes and the appearance of the skin. It should be stressed that by most of thesemethods, skin cells are not rejuvenated, just the appearance or the esthetic look of the skin is improved. As a result, people look younger and more self-confident, which provides better quality of life thanks to their appearance. However, by the application of the aesthetic methods, the health, vitality and youth cannot be restored. People who take care of themselves, live a healthy way, recreate regularly, and do not ingest exaggerated amounts of calories are, as the result, thin with less fat tissue. With years, the amount of collagen in their skin is decreased. And since they do not possess elevated amounts of fat tissue, their face looks tired and "flaccid." Here the paradox appears—people are vital and active, feel good, are perhaps ten years younger in their biological age compared with their chronological age but nevertheless might need some of the aesthetic medicine approaches.Nevertheless, first the change of lifestyle (e.g., sun exposure, smoking, and nutrition) has to take place. Only then, other tertiary anti-aging methods can be used.These measures include minimally invasive cosmetic procedures such as chemical peels, microdermabrasion, soft-tissue fillers, non-ablative laser rejuvenation, radiofrequency techniques and botulinum toxin, as well as laser skin resurfacing and corrective surgical procedures, including autologous hair transplantation. Dermatologic options for revitalization range from nonsurgical modalities (Botox, filler substances, and nonablative lasers), more aggressive resurfacing procedures (chemical peels, dermabrasion, and ablative lasers), to more traditional surgical procedures (liposuction, blepharoplasty, face and neck lifting) (Scarborough et al., 2010). The five top cosmetic non-surgical procedures are botulinum toxin injection, microdermabrasion, filler injection, laser hair removal, and chemical peeling, whereas important cosmetic surgical procedures include liposuction, breast augmentation, eyelid surgery, nose reshaping, and breast reduction. Various noninvasive to minimally invasive techniques can be used for the improvement of cutaneous changes seen with photoaging. These include dermabrasion, chemical peels, ablative and nonablative lasers, and filler agents such as hyaluronic acid. Modern technologies of skin rejuvenation include many physical and chemical intervention tools, e.g., laser irradiation, oxygen and ozone therapy, chemical peels, plastic surgery operations, all of them affecting by different mechanisms the sensitive physiological free radical/antioxidant balance in the skin. All these interventions induce from mild to severe tissue damage, providing beneficial biochemical stimuli for skin re-epithelization. Paradoxically, free radical production in the course of tissue inflammation helps to combat free radical damage consequent to the aging process (de Luca et al.,2007).

There are many "skin aging" treatments available in the market. Let us take a look at some of these possibilities.

Botox

The most common nonsurgical cosmetic procedure performed in the treatment of rhytides or facial wrinkles is injection with botulinum toxin (Yamauchi, 2010). Botox is the brand name of a toxin produced by the bacterium *Clostridium botulinum*. In large amounts, this toxin can cause botulism. Despite the fact that one of the most serious complications of botulism is paralysis, scientists have discovered a way to use it to human advantage. Small, diluted amounts can be directly injected into specific muscles causing controlled weakening of the muscles. Botox® works by neuromuscular inhibition, and the effects last from three to six months. Purified botulinum toxin type A (Botox®, Allergan Inc., Irvine, CA) is a neurotoxin used to paralyze various muscle groups of the face for cosmetic improvement of wrinkles. Botox can inhibit muscular contraction and diminish the excess, undesirable lines that communicate fatigue or negative expressions. The toxin binds on the receptor sites of motor nerve terminals and blocks neuromuscular conduction by inhibiting the release of acetylholin (Scarborough et al., 2010). Injection of Botox® is easily one of the most popular procedures for aesthetic enhancement. Botox® is most commonly used to treat wrinkles of the glabella (the space between the eyebrows and above the nose), forehead, and periocular regions. Paralysis of these small muscle groups of the face results in a more youthful appearance. With time and repeated injections, many patients will note softening or disappearance of particular facial lines (Helfrich et al., 2008). In April 2002, Botox gained FDA approval for treatment of moderate-to-severe frown lines between the eyebrows. However, Botox is often used for other areas of the face as well.

Side effects of Botox® injections include pain, bruising, and paralysis of the nerves that control eyelid function (Helfrich et al., 2008).

Fillers

Over the last decade, injectable soft tissue fillers have become an integral part of facial plastic surgery practice. The types of materials approved for dermal fillers vary from biologic to synthetic materials and absorbable to nonabsorbable compounds.

The vast choice of new products being brought to the market, improved safety profile, lower costs in the current economic climate and high street availability mean that demand for nonsurgical rejuvenation treatments are increasing at an exponential rate and are no longer the preserve of the affluent (Bray et al., 2010). In contradiction to neurotoxins, which are injected into the muscle that causes the rhytides, fillers are placed in the dermis directly beneath the line of depression and typically last from sixmonths to oneyear or more (Donath, 2010). In choosing the appropriate filler for a given individual, there are many considerations that should be examined. Temporal combinations refer to the use of different fillers at different times, whereas anatomic combinations refer to the use of different fillers in different parts of the face. In general, fillers can be classified biodegradable (12 to 18 months), slow biodegradable (two to five years), or permanent. Based on their duration, some of the most commonly used injectables can be categorized: temporary biodegradables (autologous fat, human collagen, bovine collagen, and hyaluronic acid), long-lasting biodegradables (calcium hydroxylapatite, poly-lactic acid) and permanent (polymethylmethacrylate) (Scarborough, 2010).

In the late 1980s, plastic surgeons and the public were introduced to a new concept, filling in wrinkles with collagen. Collagen came from cows and was treated to make it inert so that it could be safely injected into humans. First approved in 1981, bovine collagen was the gold standard for soft tissue augmentation, but in recent years, non-animal stabilized hyaluronic acid gel marketed as Restylane® has gained tremendous popularity among patients and physicians and is currently the most widely used filler in the United States and Canada (Helfrich et al.,2008; Coleman and Carruthers, 2006). Currently available dermal fillers include bovine, human and porcine collagens, hyaluronic acids of animal and biosynthetic origin, poly-L-lactic acid, calcium hydroxylapatite, and polymethylmethacrylate.

Contraindications for use:
All dermal fillers are contraindicated for patients with

- known sensitivities to the filler material; and
- history of severe allergy or anaphylaxis; and
- bleeding disorders.

Chemical Peels

Chemical peel is one of the most popular treatments for an aging face. In the United States, 1.03 million chemical peels were performed in 2007 (American Society of Plastic Surgeons, October 2008).

Chemical peels can be classified by their depth of skin penetration (superficial, medium, deep). During the procedure, the chemical solution is applied to the affected area. The chemical agents then work to separate and "peel" the outer surface layers of the skin. These layers often contain dead skin, which is removed during the process. The chemical agents stimulate the generation of new skin cells through the healing process. As the skin regrows after injury, new collagen and glycosaminoglycans are produced.

The result is increased skin elasticity and volume, tighter and firmer skin, which minimizes the appearance of wrinkles (Clark and Lawrence, 2008). The main clinical indications in the cosmetic field are photoaging, dyschromias, and acne scars, which are classified according to the histologic depth of the clinical changes. Proper patient selection, skin priming, and postpeel care are of utmost importance in ensuring a satisfactory outcome (Clark and Lawrence, 2008).

Microdermabrasion

Dermabrasion and microdermabrasion are facial resurfacing techniques that mechanically ablate aged or damaged skin to promote reepithelialization. Although the act of physically abrading the skin is common to both procedures, dermabrasion and microdermabrasion employ different instruments and are distinct in their technical executions. Dermabrasion completely removes the epidermis and penetrates to the level of the papillary or reticular dermis, inducing remodeling of the skin's structural proteins. Microdermabrasion only removes the uppermost layer of the epidermis, accelerating the natural process of exfoliation (Alkhawam and Alam, 2009).

Microdermabrasion is an effective and nonsurgical method for younger, smoother looking skin. The microdermabrator contains aluminum oxide or sodium chloride crystals that strike the skin and produce superficial trauma. It is theorized that the repetitive intraepidermal injury causes gradual improvement in damaged skin by stimulating fibroblast proliferation and collagen production, leading to new collagen deposition in the dermis (Shpall et al., 2004). In contrast to lasers that thermally ablate the skin, dermabrasion is a "cold" form of ablating that minimizes the vascular stimulation throughout the healing phase (Lawrence 2000)

Laser Treatment

Laser procedures for the aging face are numerous and emerging rapidly (Helfrich et al. 2008). Today, laser therapy is standard treatment for a wide variety of dermatologic complaints. From skin rejuvenation to the management of complex vascular malformations, laser treatment has proved to be an effective, innovative solution to once-challenging dilemmas (Cole et al., 2009). Ablative laser resurfacing is considered to be the gold standard to improve clinical features of the aging face.

It improves fine and some coarse wrinkles and overall dyspigmentation, lightens dark under-eye circles, and generally improves the texture of skin. Non-ablative laser resurfacing procedures are much less invasive than ablative lasers. There is much interest in these techniques because of the intense wound care, high cost, and recovery time immediately associated with ablative laser resurfacing (Helfrich et al., 2008). When using lasers, side effects have been observed frequently.

A recently developed photorejuvenation method using non-thermal stimulation of skin cells with low energy and narrow band light has been termed photomodulation. Light-emitting diodes are the ideal source of this kind of light that stimulates mitochondrial cell organelles leading to upregulation of cytochrome electron transport pathway leading to mitochondrial DNA gene modulation (Helbig et al., 2010).

Facelifts

A facelift, technically known as a rhytidectomy, is a type of cosmetic surgery procedure used to give a more youthful appearance. During a traditional facelift, an incision that typically begins around the hairline from the temple and curves around the earlobe, ending at the bottom of the hairline is made. The incisions may extend into the scalp. Once the incisions are made, various degrees of undermining of the skin are performed, and the deeper layers of the face are "lifted." Excess skin is removed, and some fat may be removed with liposuction. In other cases, the skin and muscle tissues are reshaped.

Growth Factors

Rangarajan and Dreher (2010) reported about the use of topical growth factors for skin rejuvenation. Growth factors are believed to reduce signs of aging due to their capacity to promote epidermal keratinocyte and dermal fibroblasts proliferation, as well as to stimulate extracellular matrix formation including collagen and hyaluronic acid. While the role of growth factors and cytokines in cutaneous wound healing is well documented, about their use for skin rejuvenation only very few studies exist and only a few products containing a mixture of growth factors are currently available.

Stem Cells

Stem cells could be used in the therapy for skin anti-aging. Dermal multipotent stem cells may be applied in skin photoaging by activating transforming growth factor-beta TGF-β/Smad and p38 mitogen-actived protein kinase (MAPK) signaling pathways, and then stimulating fibroblasts to secrete and synthesize collagen or elastin, heightening the extracellular matrix, finally eliminating wrinkles and strengthening skin elasticity (Zhong et al., 2010). These would provide a novel approach for anti-skin photoaging.

Conclusion

Life is like a hot bath. It feels good while you are in, but the longer you stay, the more wrinkled you get.

Jim Davis

Current knowledge tells us that aging is not entirely a programmed process. A recent report shows that extrinsic, environmental forces and lifestyle may play major roles in determining the course of the aging process. Regardless of our genetic inheritance, we can accelerate or retard the aging by lifestyle choices and environmental conditions to which we expose our genes. Currently, studies of oxidative stress-related modifications in cellular components with age are most popular among researchers because they provide testable cellular and molecular mechanisms. According to the tenets of the Oxidative Stress Theory of Aging, imbalances and dysregulation in the cellular redox process are responsible for oxidatively damaged homeostasis (Yu, 1999). At the moment, the oxidative damage is the major senescence process, and the mitochondria are the major source of endogenous reactive oxygen species formation while UVR, air pollution and smoking are the main exogenous sources.

Overall, antioxidant defense seems to be in approximate balance with oxygen-derived species generation *in vivo*. There appears to be no great reserve of antioxidant defenses in mammals, perhaps because some oxygen-derived species perform useful metabolite roles. It also seems that by additional intake of synthetic antioxidants, total antioxidant activity in the blood/cells cannot be further increased, or it cannot offer additional protection if one is having an optimal nutrition and lifestyle. Epidemiological studies on synthetic antioxidants failed to completely confirm the beneficial intake of these compounds into our diet. A healthy adult person thus should not need additional vitamin and mineral supplements if he eats varied and diverse foods with a sufficient energy intake. Nevertheless, during aging, the oxidative stress of the organism is increasing and approaches to lower the increased ROS formation in our cells should be implemented.

There are approaches an individual can take to decrease oxidative stress. Some of the presented approaches are necessary but not a sufficient condition for retarding the aging process. It is important to consider the synergistic effects of different methods described in this book. We have so far considered a number of distinct mechanisms that can contribute to aging. For each of these, there is evidence supporting the hypothesis that it is indeed an agent affecting senescence. However, the extent of contribution to senescence almost always appears too small for the individual mechanism to be sufficient contributor for aging prevention or delay. The obvious solution to this problem is that cellular aging is multi-causal and that various mechanisms must be applied in fighting aging since each plays its part in the battle. These mechanisms can react in the synergistic way between different anti-aging pathways. For instance, accumulation of mitochondrial DNA mutations will reduce the cell-energy production needed for damage repair and building of free radical protection. Mitochondrial mutations can also interfere with signalling pathways regulating cell cycle control and apoptosis and thus allow survival of severely damaged cells. Another effective example of the synergistic effect is the combinations of dietary restriction with appropriate nutrition and exercise, which is particularly effective at improving insulin sensitivity.

The most efficient preventive step to avoid exogenous free radical exposure would be to avoid, as much as possible, exposure to endogenous and exogenous ROS-generating compounds, including oxygen species, cigarette smoke and UVR. But since this is not always possible, protection could be obtained by adequate antioxidant protection, decreasing the formation of free radicals (e.g., CR), or increasing damage-repair systems (e.g., CR and hormesis mimetics) of the cells. Antioxidants are necessary for organisms living with a high $^3O_2$ concentration because they lessen the intensity and frequency of oxidative stress. Diet-derived antioxidants might be important agents in aging and disease risk reduction and might be beneficial for skin health as well, especially in the second part of life, when some of the endogenous antioxidant defense systems fail to offer appropriate protection against elevated oxidative stress. Oxidative stress is produced during the normal metabolism of a cell. Since radicals are a normal component of life, antioxidative protection should also be a part of life. Only the presence of an antioxidant in all cell compartments will offer efficient protection. However, a single antioxidant cannot fulfill this task. For this reason, different water- and fat-soluble antioxidants should be used synergistically for this purpose. To achieve this goal, we should eat fresh seasonal fruits and vegetables of many different colors, at least five to ten times per day. Dietary antioxidants and essential micronutrient vitamins and trace elements, primarily present in fresh fruits and vegetables, could play an important preventive role in combating exposure to elevated environmental oxidative stress or opposing aging and aging-related diseases. Researchers have found a lower occurrence of cancer, heart and vein diseases only in people that consume sufficient quantities of fruits and vegetables, but not in people that consume vitamin supplements. For this reason, health-promoting nutrition involves the daily intake of five to ten vegetables and fruits, fruit juices, red wine and tea that are rich sources of micronutrients with antioxidant properties, including the antioxidant vitamins C, E, β-carotene and many others. Since endogenous free radical protection cannot be deliberately increased sufficiently (untilnow), all we can do is increase the level of exogenous antioxidant protection of our bodies to fight the toxic effects of ROS. Some researchers claim that additional synthetic antioxidant supplement intake does not prolong lifespan by decreasing the accumulation of free radical-induced damage. It also seems that additional antioxidant intake by a healthy person with appropriate eating habits does not lead to an additional increase of total antioxidant capacity in the blood. Further increases in antioxidant intake thus offer little additional protection. Since free radicals are not guided missiles, the mutations they cause occur at random locations inside the cell. The randomness of this genetic damage explains, in part, why people with ideal lifestyles can also develop cancer (or other ROS-induced diseases) early in life, while other people with poor lifestyles(e.g., smokers) can sometimes live to extreme old age (Olshansky and Carnes,

2001). The intake of synthetic antioxidants could be beneficial only for people with poor nutrition or severe oxidative stress (see also chapter "Should supplements of antioxidants be taken").

However, it is estimated that there is more than a 50% decline in endogenous antioxidant (ubiquinon, etc.) and cell repair defenses after 50 years of age. At this age, mitochondria have accumulated a lot of oxidative damage, which results in increased ROS formation and leakage. The current methods of processing food have led to a point where food products are greatly impoverished in terms of minerals and vitamins. Additionally, soils are lacking minerals due to intense farming, and the fact that unripe fruit is picked and transported to markets prior to consumption is less than ideal since it is known that antioxidants are synthesized only at ripening due to the fact thatplants use them as protection against environmental effects (UV radiation), diseases, pests, and other stressful factors.Furthermore, fruits are sprayed with pesticides that can extinguish the beneficent characteristics of protective substances found in the fruit.Unsuitable mechanical preparation and heat treatment can greatly decrease the nutritive value of a food product and affect the antioxidant potential of the food.Data from research concerning "Risk factors for contagious diseases between adult residents of Slovenia" show that 31.6% of adults in Slovenia do not eat vegetables daily, and 43.0% do not eat fruit daily.Of participants in this research,21.9%eat vegetables several times a day, and 31.1% eat fruit several times a day. All of these observations support the need for additional antioxidant and mineral intake. This trend is similar in almost all developed countries.

Approximately 40 micronutrients (vitamins, antioxidants, minerals) have been reported as essential components in the diet (Alvarez-Leon et al., 2006). But the daily intake of thesemacro and micro nutrients is often inadequate, especially in the elderly population (Ames, 2006) due to their poor socio-economic situation, loss of appetite, lack of teeth and intestinal malabsorbtion (Candore et al.,2010). These facts point to the conclusion that additional intake of vitamins and minerals is necessary in certain circumstances.

Although many studies performed could not conclude for certain if the intake of synthetic antioxidants has any effect on lifespan, there will be continuous interest in the use of antioxidants for the treatment of skin aging, as well as in the antioxidant-induced prevention of disease development. Herbert (1994) suggests that antioxidants are mischaracterized by describing them solely as "antioxidants." They, in fact, are redox agents, antioxidants in some circumstances (like the physiological quantities found in food), and pro-oxidants (producing billions of harmful free radicals) in other circumstances (often so in the pharmacologic quantities found in ill-designed supplements). Positive effects of the protective substances that originate from food are greater because of the synergistic activity between individual antioxidant substances (Rietjens et al., 2001), nutritional fibers and secondary vegetal substances. Another mechanism of antioxidant action involves activation of genes encoding proteins involved in the antioxidant defense.

There have been many studies confirming the protective use of antioxidants on prevention of skin-induced free radical formation. It would be advantageous to increase skin reservoir of antioxidants in order to improve defense against UV-induced damage. This could be achieved through diet or by topical application. Topical application of antioxidants and other phytonutrients could target the chemicals directly at the skin, thus decreasing the amount of antioxidants needed for effective protection as compared to oral administration.

As it was already mentioned, endogenous antioxidants and the repair system cannot be deliberately increased. Paradoxically, the efficiency of defense and repair may be enhanced following exposure to ROS since expression of many DNA repair enzymes is upregulated following oxidative stress (Wani, 1998; Bases, 1992). There are, however, promising studies in the field of antioxidant mimetics and investigation of the effects of CR and hormesis. However, we should wait for some more conclusive results from these fields. To date, only caloric restriction (with adequate vitamin and mineral intake) has obtained scientifically based results for the prolonging of life. The mean and maximum lifespan of a range of mammals can be increased by up to 50% simply by reducing their caloric intake as long as nutrition (minerals, vitamins, essential amino acids) is maintained (Weindruch and Sohal, 1997; Mattison et al., 2003).

Of course, there is obviously a limit to how much caloric intake can be reduced without causing tissue wasting and death from starvation (Mattson et al., 2003). Physiological changes in primates undergoing CR have been studied extensively and include reduced body size, lower body temperature, and decreases in the levels of plasma growth hormone and insuline-like growth factor. Restricted animals also show lower levels of glucose and insulin in their plasma. A delay in sexual maturation and reduction of fertility has also been observed (Gredilla and Barja, 2003). The Baltimore Longitudinal Study of Aging revealed that individuals with lower body temperature and insulin levels (changes observed also in CR rodents and monkeys) live longer (Roth et al., 2002).

It could be concluded that prevention of mitochondrial ROS generation is a more efficient approach to decreasing oxidative stress (e.g., by CR) than quenching any already formed free radicals with antioxidants, since the lifetime of most aggressive free radicals is very short (e.g., OH$^-$) and they react with the first compound encountered (e.g., protein, DNA). Thus, avoiding UVR exposure is far more efficient than using methods to prevent or cure UVR damage.

In general, inhibition of electron flow causes electron leaks from the complexes and consequently leads to the generation of more ROS. On the other hand, the reduction of energy metabolism may actually reduce ROS generation from mitochondria and consequently extend lifespan (Ishii and Hartman, 2003). In either case, avoiding electron leakage from electron transport and the resultant ROS production seems to be essential for a normal life. To achieve this and further decrease oxidative stress, we should sleep enough in total darkness, avoid excessive exposure to particular environmental pollutants (e.g., ozone, particulate matter, tobacco smoke, etc.), avoid UVR exposure, avoid excessive intake of fat and "junk" food, practice regular fitness, maintain a high level of activity whilst not engaging in excessive sporting activities, decrease infections and chronic inflammations, drink enough non-chlorinated water, avoid excessive psycho-physical stress, reduce caloric intake, eat smaller amounts of food comprising at least fiveservings per day (with an additional five to ten servings of fruits and vegetables), and avoid overeating. Avoiding oxidative stress can only lower the probability/risk of accumulating oxidative damage to susceptible components of the DNA architecture (e.g., tumor suppressor or promoter genes).

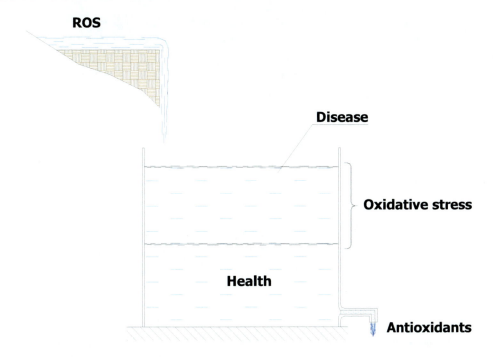

Figure 40. Health can be represented as a barrel of water, where normal level of water represents health, water influx is represented by the amount of ROS, and antioxidants are the pipe, which is the outflow of the water from the barrel. Disease manifests when the water level critically increases and pours over the edge of the barrel.

Our growth in knowledge of endogenous and exogenous formation of reactive oxygen species, oxidative damage, and the role of protection against ROS suggests that factors in our diet and lifestyle can be effective in preventing or retarding the disease/damage accumulation process. New and detailed research efforts aimed at enhancing our understanding of the role of hormesis, mitochondrial uncoupling, caloric restriction, exogenous and endogenous antioxidants, eating habits and lifestyle in modifying oxidative damage should be undertaken. Since we do not know to what extent some of the proposed methods decrease oxidative stress, it would be ideal to perform all methods that are practically possible in order to obtain a potential synergistic effect in fighting aging of our cells.

There is substantial evidence from a variety of speciesdemonstrating that *in vivo* oxidative damage is highly correlatedwith biological aging. However, to date, interventions aimedat reducing oxidative damage in mammals, primarily through manipulationsof antioxidant enzyme systems, have yielded disappointing results. The biology of living things can be altered by natural or artificial selection over extended periods of time or directly by the direct manipulation of genes. It is difficult, however, to imagine how any technology or any genetic intervention could address genetic damage occurring randomly within trillions of our cells at any moment. Besides, we should not wait forthe symptoms of an age-related disease. Oxidative stress formation and damage should be avoided rather than cured. The time has come to shift the attention of modern medicine to attacking the seeds of aging that are sown early in the lifespan of every person (Olshansky and Carnes, 2001).

It may be possible to increase cell viability or delay their aging by methods of modification/repair of genotype, but there are restrictions in their practical achievement. Anti-aging manipulations like telomere shortening, cell cycle control, interfering with oncogene/anti-oncogene balance, etc., are, in theory, possible but still far from being applicable. Genetic repair and therapy, by putting suitably modified copies of the mitochondrial genes into the cell nucleus and all mitochondrial proteins that would then be imported into the mitochondria or by potential use of the stem cells, or any other strategy for engineered negligible senescence, could be used as suggested by Aubrey de Grey. Doctor de Grey has suggested also that genes taken from bacteria could be transmitted into the genome of human cells to produce enzymes that dissolve and eliminate lipofuscin, thereby rejuvenating the cells. It is difficult to change genes in every cell of the body and to do this without inducing any deleterious side effects. Years or even decades will pass before attempts at genetic repair and gene therapy will be possible, safe accessible and efficient for everybody.Until molecular repair technologies are available, anti-aging approaches aimed not to rejuvenate but to delay the aging processshould be applied. Approaches presented in this book could be implemented into everyday life in order to decrease the oxidative stress of an organism and delay the aging process.Enormous immediate benefit can be gained from almost inexpensive approaches like reducing caloric intake (while maintaining adequate nutrition), avoiding environmental pollutants, tobacco smoke, UVR exposure and alcohol, exercising, eating low-fat/high-fiber diets, protecting skin with appropriate moisturisers, etc. On the other hand, health policy is focused on expensive investments of money into treating age-related diseases and almost no money is spent onaging prevention and oncampaigns of disease prevention strategies. Many different aspects regarding aging and oxidative stress were considered in the book. Some are speculations, some are supported with experiments *in vitro*, on cell lines, and some are done on animal models. All of them cannot be directly extrapolated on humans. Many researches presented are even conflicting and contradictory. There are missing data provided by different clinical trials on humans, etc. Thinkers, philosophers and scientists just try to explain the phenomena, but there is missing the need for implementation of the changes into the system. Problem-based approach would focus not just on problem definition and search for reasons, consequences and explanations of the phenomena but also onapproaches for solutions thatwould change the problem, eliminate the cause and not just deal with the buffering of the consequences. The main question remains about what are the practical suggestions for decreasing oxidative stress and thus avoiding chronical degenerative diseases and retarding the aging process of the human skin and other cells. In order to reduce endogenous oxidative stress levels and its damage, it would be ideal first to perform clinical trials on human volunteers, where different approaches would be estimated in order to quantify their impacts on oxidative stress. Since this was not done and most probably in the near future the results will not be available (it would take more than 50 years to get the results from human trials), all we can do at the moment is to try to form some conclusions with the data and knowledge available; for example: protect your skin from UVA and UVB light, protect dry skin with appropriate moisturizers, maintain a well-balanced diet by eating plenty of fruits and vegetables (at least five portions per day), with as many different colors of fruit and vegetable as possible (white, red, yellow/orange, blue and green), and preferably those that are organic and seasonable. Not destroying the nutrients in our foods by overcooking and increasing the consumption of raw or lightly cooked foods. Increase starches and other complex carbohydrates by eating a combination of breads, cereals and legumes. Eat less but varied food (withno malnutrition and with sufficient nutrients intake), do not overeat, have moderate nutrition with many portions of food per day, ingest low-fat, nutrient-dense diets. Practice regular but moderate physical activity. Do not participate in any sport or physical activity to an excessive degree. Take some time for physical and mental activities every day; maintain a healthy weight and body shape. Avoid fatty, fried and processed foods, excessive red meet, sugar and salt intake (> 5g per day), and avoid the high intake of iron, copper, lead and chromium and chlorinated water, while increasing the intake of food rich in selenium, magnesium and zinc. Consume cold-pressed oils such as olive, flax and walnut oil (rich in chemically stable saturated and mono-unsaturated fats). Eliminate "junk" food from our diets. Drink enough water (maintain adequate hydration) and tea (green tea) and less coffee and alcoholic beverages (only a moderate red wine consumption), at least tenglasses of pure water every day for basic hydration. Avoid chronic infections and chronic, low-grade inflammations. Many antioxidants (e.g., CoQ10, epigallocatechin-3-gallate from green tea and carotenoids) possess anti-inflammatory effects (Fuller et al., 2006). Avoid excessive psycho-physical stressful situations. Learn techniques to relax (e.g., yoga). Challenge your mind by learning new things. Build a strong social network. Mild heat stress (e.g., sauna once per month) could have anti-aging and life-prolonging effects, although acute heat exposure is not beneficial and could be even mutagenic (Kligman and Kligman, 1994). Follow a healthy sleeping pattern, and get enough sleep. Go to sleep before midnight. Lack of sleep has been highlighted as a contributing factor to oxidative stress. And finally, regularly monitor your oxidative stress status. It is important to start the preventive steps to reduce oxidative damage already early in life, preferably during or soon after adolescence. Do not smoke and avoid passive smoking. It is important to avoid intake of toxins and exposure to tobacco smoke especially during pregnancyin order to minimize the risk of genetic damage and thus to provide healthy future for the children.In order to reduce exogenous oxidant damage, it is important to avoid polluted environments (e.g., elevated concentrations of ozone, particulate matter, SO_2, NO_x, etc.). Avoid prolonged exposure to UV rays or sun beds, and always use adequate protection when exposed to this radiation. Aging is a complex system, and its cause is not possible to attribute to any single source. The optimal health and appearance of the skin is the result of several factors: extrinsic aging (e.g., UV damage, environmental pollution), intrinsic aging (lifestyle, genetics), and hormonal aging (e.g., estrogen loss) (Pontius and Smith, 2011). The phenotypic appearance of aged skin results from the accumulation of functional alterations from chronological aging and additive morphological/physiological changes from chronic photodamage (Thiele et al., 2006; Fisher et al., 2002; Yaar et al., 2002). There are many indications from the scientific studies that mitochondrial damage mediated by ROS plays a significant role in the aging process. The reader of the book was first introduced to the aging process in general. Then, the various aging theories were explained, but none were able to explain the complex aging process in all the details. Intracellular biochemical reactions with impact onthe aging process were presented with the focus on oxidative stress formation as the most important single contributor on aging, since the unifying factor in determining skin aging is the increased generation of ROS from endogenous as well as from the exogenous sources.

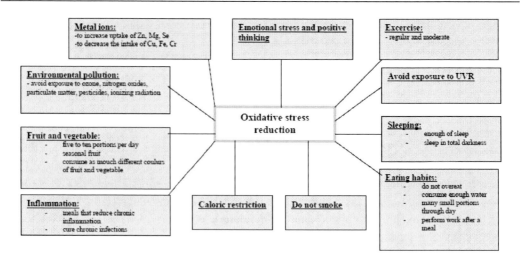

Figure 41. Summary of factors affecting the oxidative stress.

After investigation through causes and consequences of aging in general as well as on skin aging, the existing and potential methods for defense against ROS formation and ROS damage were introduced on two levels: 1) antioxidants as ROS quenchers and 2) various defenses thatdecrease ROS formation or increase ROS damage repair systems. As already discussed, skin aging is influenced by various external and internal processes with different origins: on molecular level, telomere shortening, the mitochondrial dysfunction and free radicals, respectively, account for the characteristic structural and functional changes of chronologically aged skin, while on a cellular level, apoptosis and decreased proliferative capacity affect epidermal structure and function (Fisher et al., 2002; Yaar et al., 2002). All of them have one thing in common. They are all linked with the increased oxidative stress formation as a common underlying mechanism. Oxidative damage plays a central role in cellular aging. For example, cellular responses to growth signals and oxidative stress are mediated, in part, by growth-factor-activated and stress-activated MAP kinases.It is probable that oxidative damage is the single-most damaging contributor to skin aging leading to DNA and mtDNA damage, telomere shortening, protein glycolsylation and protein oxidation, collagen and elastin degradation, downregulation of collagen synthesis, increased expression of matrix metalloproteinases, neovascularization, etc. Increasing evidence exists that cellular redox status is an important regulator of various cellular events including aging. Preventable environmental factors that amplify extrinsic aging include sun exposure and smoking. Long-term UVA radiation exposure accelerates aging via the formation of reactive oxygen species (ROS) and direct DNA damage. ROS lead to inflammatory cytokines and the upregulation of matrix metalloproteinases, which result in the breakdown of collagen. ROS are able todirect oxidation of cellular macromolecules. UVB radiation can also contribute to this aging process by causing direct DNA mutations or direct oxidation of cellular components. Decreased amount of ROS could be achieved by decreased formation from the endogenous or exogenous sources or from the quenching by antioxidants and other compounds. Antioxidants could have additional influence on increased repair systems.Measuring the in vivo antioxidant status would assist in the evaluation of health and aging status of an individual, since maximum lifespan potential in the animal kingdom has been demonstrated to be directly associated with the level of several endogenous antioxidant defense systems, including SOD, CAT, as well as some exogenous vitamins like C and E, and inversely with oxidative stress.

It is not possible to estimate how much each skin aging factor—for example intrinsic (electron transport leake in mitochondria, telomere shortening, hormone disruption) and extrinsic factors like UVR, smoking, environmental pollution, etc.,—contribute to the total skin aging. These factors might have different roles on skin aging at different age periods; as well, there might be a synergistic effect between them that makes it impossible to estimate the share of a particular role of each individual factor on skin aging. Nevertheless, several methods were presented in this book in order to help our bodies and skin cells to fight with consequences of increased oxidative stress with the aim of preventing its formation inthe first place.

At this point, the logical question would be "Why did mother nature not provide our bodies or cells (during evolution) with better protection against damaging effects of free radicals?" It was explained previously that normal metabolism is associated with unavoidable mild oxidative stress resulting in biomolecular damage that cannot be totally repaired or removed by cellular degradative systems. Besides, UVR causes permanent damage to our skin cells, and endogenous antioxidants, melanin and repair processes cannot offer us total protection.

Approximately 2,500 million years ago, blue-green algae started producing O_2 as by-product formed during photosinthesis. The concentration of O_2 in the atmosphere was about one percent1,300 million years ago. Five hundrend million years ago, the concentration of O_2 in the atmosphere was about 10%, and fivemillion years ago, when ancestors of humans apeared, the concentration of O_2 in the atmosphere reached 21%.Also during this period, ozone (O3) was formed and offered protection to early life forms against damaging effects from UVC. In this way, the first organisms could leave water and settle on the land. Of course, oxygen is essential for life. Humans and other aerobes need O_2 because they evolved electron transport chains and other enzyme systems utilizing O_2 and can tolerate its toxic by-products by antioxidant defense. But even present-day aerobes suffer oxidative damage. Why? Why during the evolution of the reaction of O_2 reduction to water in the mitochondriadidn't there become more "perfect"—in the aspect of producing less "harmful"—by-products. According to de Grey (2007), "Evolution is, over the long term, an extremely clever engineer, and has learned ways of making the best of a bad job, e.g., harnessing hydrogen peroxide for its own purposes." The beneficial physiological cellular use of ROS is now being demonstrated in different areas, including intracellular signaling and redox regulation. Thus, our cells also generate some hydrogen peroxide on purpose, for use as a chemical signal that regulates everything from glucose metabolism to cellular growth and proliferation (Rhee,1999). Let us discuss Theodosius Grygorovych Dobzhansky's famous statement*"Nothing in Biology Makes Sense Except in the Light of Evolution"* in the aspect of ROS formation and evolution.

First, it is important to highlight the fact the all the time of human history, the average life expectancy was around 30 years or even less. Next, the problem of famine through human and animal history should be stressed. Most organisms in our biosphere have had to evolve mechanisms that allow them to adapt to episodic and often extended periods of nutrient deprivation. Nature is a highly competitive place, and almost all animals in nature die before they attain old age. It was similar in the history of humans. Most of them died before they reached old age. Since most animals rarely reach their maximum lifespan in the wild

(Kirkwood and Mathers(2009), there is no evolutionary drive to keep the body fit for the long haul—not much selection pressure for traits that would maintain viability past the time when most animals or humans would most likely be dead, killed by predators or disease, accident or famine. It has recently been argued that during years of famine, it may be evolutionarily desirable for an organism to avoid reproduction and to upregulate protective and repair enzyme mechanisms in an effort to ensure that it is fit for reproduction in future years (Charlie Rose—Caloric restriction). For this reason, energy minimization is a favourite tool from an evolutionary perspective. The body uses energy from food for metabolism, reproduction, repair and maintenance. Thus, mechanisms that protect cells from oxidative stress (e.g., endogenous antioxidants, DNA repair processes) are consuming significant amounts of energy when being activated in all compartments of a cell all of the time. It would require too much energy to build enough defenses to prevent all oxidative damage all the time throughout the life of an organism. Kowald and Kirkwood (1994, 1996) have done a quantitative MARS (mitochondria, abberant proteins, radicals, and scavengers) model. Using this simulation, they predicted that a virtual immortality might be achieved if 55% of the total energy of the simulated cell were devoted to repair and/or prevention of free-radical and oxidative damage. Similarly, due to energy minimization, the amount of pigment (UVprotection) decreased in individuals of cultures living further away from the equator, and it is only stress (UV exposure) that activates melanocytes to produce pigment. During a time of famine, an organism should choose between investment in either producing offspring or maintaining the soma. With a finite supply of food, the body must compromise and will not perform any of these functions quite as well as it would under different food conditions. It is the compromise in allocating (less) energy to the repair function that causes the body to gradually deteriorate with age (Kirkwood, 1977). Limited food supply influences lifespan. Among mammals, the long-lived species are generally those that are most highly evolved and, therefore, possess the most sophisticated mechanisms for competing for food.

If famine is the first leading cause of death throughout human evolution, infectious and parasitic diseases are not far behind. A small amount of oxidative stress might be beneficial in signaling events and protection against pathogenic microorganisms, the second leading cause of death in almost all of human history. Life expectancy just 100 years ago was only 45 to 49 years, mostly due to death from infectious diseases in childhood. Increased oxidative stress might prevent the development and spread of some pathogenic microorganism diseases in childhood since increased oxidative potential is a hostile environment for the reproduction of microorganisms. The direct role of free radicals in microbial killing is well established. During phagocytosis, cells consume high amounts of oxygen, a process termed as a respiratory burst, producing: superoxide anion radical,hydrogen peroxide, hydroxyl radical, hypochlorus acid, which are capable of damaging cell membranes and biomolecules.The ability of ROS to activate transcription is now recognized. Low doses of ROS stimulate the growth of fibroblasts and epithelial cells. Thus, free radicals can play a positive role in early inflammation by promoting fibrosis and wound healing.

The antagonistic pleiotropy theory (Williams, 1957) states that one of the effects is beneficial and another is detrimental. In essence, this refers to genes that offer benefits early but not later in life. An individual gene product can perform more than one function at any moment in time. Nature would favor genes with beneficial roles early in life, even though they may be harmful later on because of their advantages in young individuals. Chronic inflammation is a source of cellular damage. When an infection occurs, immune cells secrete large amounts of free radicalsto combat the invader. But, these inflammatory chemicals also attack normal tissue surrounding the infection and damage critical components of cells, including DNA. During chronic inflammation, that damage may lead to mutations or cell death and even to cancer and other diseases. But interfering with inflammation might impair immune defenses against pathogens. Defending free radicals with antioxidants might as well impair the battle against pathogen microorganisms when an infection is present or could even help cancer cells to prevent apoptosis and to protect themselves against chemotherapy and radiotherapy.

ROS play a significant role in cell signaling processes. Once regarded as simply toxic metabolites, free radicals are now recognized as important signaling molecules mediating a wide range of biological phenomena such as vasodilatation, neurotransmission, neuronal plasticity, cardiac preconditioning, only to name a few. The beneficial physiological cellular use of ROS is now being demonstrated in different areas, including intracellular signaling and redox regulation. ROS induce various biological processes that include a transient elevation of intracellular Ca^{2+} concentration, phosphorylation of specific proteins, activation of specific transcription factors, modulation of eicosanoid metabolism, and stimulation of cell growth (Kaul and Forman, 2000). Nitric oxide was identified as a signaling molecule as early as 1987 (Palmer et al., 1987), and is now well known as a regulator of transcription factor activities and other determinants of gene expression. Hydrogen peroxide and superoxide have similar intracellular effects (Kimata and Hirata, 1999). ROS can directly affect conformation and/or activities of all sulfhydryl-containing molecules, such as proteins or GSH, by oxidation of their thiol moiety. Among many other enzymes and membrane receptors, this type of redox regulation affects many proteins important in signal transduction and carcinogenesis, such as protein kinase C, Ca^{2+}-ATPase, collagenase, and tyrosine kinase (Dalton et al., 1999). For several transcription factors, ROS are physiological mediators of transcription control (Nordberg and Arner 2001). The well-known examples of redox-sensitive transcription factors are nuclear factor-kB (NF-kB) and Activator Protein-1 (AP-1). Thus, increased oxidative stress is not beneficial for the cell, and an increase in cellular reducents might impact redox regulation and signal transduction. The complete elimination of free radicals would thus disrupt, rather than extend, the normal functioning of the body.

To control these reactive species with "two faces" cells evolved complex and critical regulatory mechanisms thatbecome disrupted with age (Gilca et al. 2007). Senescence is just one example of pathophysiological implications of redox dysregulations (Valkoet al., 2007). The initiation of aging is marked by a shift from redox regulation to redox dysregulation (Humphries et al., 2006). Why this shift takes place is yet not clear.

From the perspective of an individual, free radical damage accumulation leads to the development of chronic diseases and aging. When free radicals interact with nuclear DNA, they can cause a mutation. Most of the mutations are harmful, and selection operates to reduce these alterations. However, once in a while, a mutation offers a survival advantage. Thus, looking from the perspective of a species, small amounts of mutations are beneficial, especially if nature operates to preserve the individual just untilthe end of its reproduction period, when the oxidative damage is not yet devastating. The central idea of Dawkins' message is that nature does not care much about the health and longevity of organisms. In the language of the layman, we could say that nature is more "stepmother" than "mother" and that "she" cares more about others (the descendants of genes) than us. The main tendency of genes is to make their own copies before environmental influences cause damage. The duplication is successful if the copies are the same as the original (the principle of fidelity) and if they are numerous (the principle of fecundity) (Dawkins, 1982, 1999). The main tendency of the body (phenotype), on the other hand, is to remain functional for as long as possible. According to Dawkins, without taking the effects of genes into account, an organism would take good care of its own health and longevity (to live as long as possible) (Dawkins, 1976, 2006). Each organism has both types of tendencies. But, as Dawkins states, multiplication is not survival. He stresses the serious tension between genes and the individual's body, with multiplication usually prevailing over survival (Dawkins, 1976, 2006). In biology, it is well known that the desire for multiplication is the strongest instinct in nature (Bryson 2003, 2006; Ridley, 1999, 2002). Although the tendency for longevity is also genetically based, for genes it is enough to delay the death of the body for as long as it is needed for multiplication (Dawkins, 1976, 2006). Therefore, relatively good health and relative longevity of the body are sufficient for the successful gene transfer. For further reading on "Nutrition of the sefish gene," see review done by Ostan et al. (2009).

Is selection for advantage at the species' level more effective than selection among individuals for the advantages of a longer life? Kirkwood and Mathers(2009) reported that aging makes negligible contribution to mortality in wild populations of animals. For example, 90% of wild mice are dead by the age of tenmonths, although the same animals might live for three years in protective environment (Austad, 1997). Survial in the wild is limited by high levels of death from extrinsic factors (predation, accident, starvations or disease). This has an important bearing on how far the mouse genome should invest in mechanisms for the long-term maintenance and repair of its somatic (non-reproductive) cells. If 90% of wild mice is dead by tenmonths, any investment in maintenance to keep the body in good condition much beyond this point can benefit 10% of the population at most. From a Darwinianpoint of view, the mouse will benefit more from investing any spare resources into thermogenesis or reproduction than into better DNA-repair capacity that it needs to ensure adequate function for a limited time period (Kirkwood and Mathers, 2009). This immediately suggests that there will be little evolutionary advantage in building long-term survival capacity into a mouse (Kirkwood and Mathers, 2009). There was no pressure to evolve the high levels of maintenance and to repair that might be required for biological immortality. The argument is further strengthened when we observe that nearly all of the survival mechanisms required by the mouse to combat intrinsic deterioration (e.g., oxidative damage) require metabolic resources. These are scarce, as is evidenced by the fact that the major cause of mortality for wild mice is cold, due to insufficient energy to maintain body temperature (Berry and Bronson, 1992). For nature, it is important that reproductive or germ cell lineage are maintained at the level that preserves viability across the generations, whereas the some needs only to support the survival of a single generation. Evolutionary processes evolved to favor investing more energy in the germline at the expense of the soma. From this perspective, having the somatic cells that protect the germline periodically replaced is a small price to pay for the evolutionary advantages that together sum to drastically increased fitness (Smelick, 2003).

A short-lived organism would waste metabolic energy by over-investing in antioxidant or DNA-repair enzymes (it was calculated by Kowald and Kirkwood (1994, 1996) that 55% of energy must be invested into repair and ROS defense in order to prevent oxidative stress and damage) when the energy could be spent on rapid growth and reproduction. When a species has fewer predators, evolution invests fewer resources into speedy reproduction and more into genetic resources (DNA repair, etc.), namely into a longer reproductive period (longer life). In the case of birds, the mitochondrial membranes contain more unsaturated fatty acids, making them less vulnerable to lipid peroxidation. The protein complexes of the respiratory chain of mitochondria generate fewer free radicals in birds than in mammals. It is conceivable that an animal with well-engineered cells could live many centuries. Human germ cells have arguably lived for millions of years through an investment in DNA-repair enzymes, antioxidant enzymes and telomerase (Best, accessed 2009).

As mentioned already, from an individual point of view, it is good to possess an efficient damage-repair mechanism to avoid accumulation of oxidative damage, which increases the probability of developing mutations. The speed of aging, the amount of endogenous free radical formation, and the efficacy of the repair processes differ between animals. Species like Blanding's Turtle (*Emydoidea blandingii*) and the painted turtle (*Chrysemys picta*) have not shown signs of aging in studies lasting decades (Congdon et al., 2001, 2003). This phenomenon seems to occur due to the uniqueness of telomere biology in turtles (Girondot and Garcia, 1999), and some evidence suggests that the cells of turtles have enhanced mechanisms to protect against reactive oxygen species formation and damage (Lutz et al. 2003).

On the other hand, if looking from the perspective of an individual and not that of the whole species, an enhanced protective system against ROS-induced cellular damage and an increased repair system might be an obstacle for the evolution of the species. Species of turtles have, therefore, remained the same since the era of the dinosaurs. These species have thus almost stopped developing over the course of evolution.

To sum up, a long life in the hostile world of our ancestors would have been an extravagant waste of precious physiological resources better spent producing babies (Olshansky and Carnes, 2001).If humans did not age and continued to multiply, we would soon consume available food resources. In order to survive in such a scenario, we would have to reproduce less (e.g., the effect of CR on reproduction). However, this would result in diminished variability within the species (Missirlis, 2003) because reproduction allows recombination and genetic shuffling. Aging as a consequence of constant free radical-induced accumulation of damage might have evolved exactly to tune such problems of ecological balance and, in this respect, might be a programmed event (Missirlis 2003).

We should not forget that the average life expectancy throughout the human history was less than 40 years. Humans probably experienced very high mortality by age 50 in our ancestral environment. According to de Grey and Rae (2007), the organism had the choice during evolution between doing a quick and dirty job of its growth, leading to early fertility but sloppy construction, or a more perfectionist job that delays sexual maturity but creates a more smooth-running machine in the end.

It can be concluded that ROS has played an important role during the evolution of aerobic organisms indeed, and it should not be considered (during evolution) as just"bad guys" that increase the probability of senescent degenerative diseases and as accelerators in the aging process. ROS formation"had an important role during human history, e.g., ROS protected infants from dying due to infections and other pathogenic microorganisms related to diseases. However, the current role of ROS has changed. People live for many more years, and hygiene has developed to the point where the spreading of diseases no longer represents the leading cause of death in the developed world. Also, food shortage is a rare event in western countries today. For this reason, the role of ROS in the modern lifestyle has changed.

Natural selection is interested in preserving the individual just untilthe end of its reproduction period. After this period, protection against oxidative stress and damage-repair declines. However, each individual has the right to continue to live and delay ROS-related degenerative damage for as long as possible. It is up to us how effective we will be in fighting ROS-induced damage and thus in retarding our aging process. For this reason, the strategies to reduce the formation of oxidative stress in an organism should be the priority of studies in the field of oxidative stress and longevity research.

In the end, we learned that living in the atmosphere rich in oxygen and other pollutants can have side effects resulting in free radical production and damage. Breathing air has an impact on aging process. Number of breaths could be correlated with lifespan. But on the other hand, even more important than for how long we will breathe and how many breaths we will take in our lives, it is important how many breathtaking moments will we face during our life. In the words ofOlhansky and Carnes (2001): "Fear of tomorrow can cause you to miss the moments of happiness that can be shared today."

There are many other studies regarding the skin aging and skin damage, but they were not mentioned in the book. We would like to recommend some of the very good publications for those interested in further reading from the field of skin aging:

References

Fuchs J, Packer L, (eds). Oxidative Stress in Dermatology. Marcel Dekker, Inc, New York. 1993.

Farage MA, Miller KW, Maibach HI, (Eds). Textbook of aging skin. Springer-Verlag, Berlin, 2010.

Gilchrest, B; Krutmann, J. (Eds.). Skin aging. Springer-Verlag, Berlin 2006.

Stanner, S; Thompson, R; Buttriss, J, (eds.): Healthy aging—The role of nutrition and lifestyle. Wiley-Blackwell, 2009.

Jenkins, G; Wainwright, LJ; Green, M. Healthy aging: The skin. In: Healthy aging. The role of nutrition and lifestyle (Ed: Stanner, S; Thompson, R; Buttriss, JL.). Wiley-Backwell, 2009.

Alessio, HM and Hagerman, AE. (Eds.). Oxidative stress, exercise and aging. Imperial College Press, London, 2006.

Fuchs, J; Packer, L. Environmental stressors in health and disease Marcel Dekker, Inc., 2001

Cutler, RG; Rodriguez, H. (Eds.) Critical Reviews of oxidative stress and aging. World Scientific, 2003.

Baumann, L. Cosmetic dermatology. New York: McGraw-Hill, 2002.

Halliwell, B; Gutteridge, J. M.C. (2005): Free Radicals in Biology and Medicine.—Oxford: Oxford University Press.

Rawlings, AV; Leyden, JJ. (Eds.). Skin moisturization. Infotma Healthcare, New York, 2009.

Acknowledgments

The author would like to thank Dr. Mateja Dolenc–Voljc, Dr. Raja Gosnjak Dahmane and Dr. Irina Milisav Ribaric for their valuable comments and suggestions when reviewing the manuscript. Thanks to all authors involved in oxidative stress, aging and skin disease research whose important results and publications were cited in this book. The author is thankful to Ana Benedicic, Tanja Planinšek Ručigaj and Florian Probst for their photographs and figures as well as to Katja Gorjanc and Petra Ricchobon and Tilen Lovrecic for his help with graphical design. Thanks to Lana Ceh for language corrections. Special thanks go to my parents for their support.

Share of the earnings from this book will be invested in future oxidative stress research.

Medical Disclaimer

In the book there are no claims or representations regarding treatment, cure, or mitigation of any specific disease or condition. The information in this book is not intended to diagnose and/or treat any health-related issues and is provided solely for informational and educational purposes only. Please consult your own doctor, healthcare practitioner, and/or pharmacist for any health problem or before making any changes to your healthcare regime (before deciding to self-treat or making any changes to your prescribed medications). Even what may seem like simple changes in the diet for example, can interact with and alter the efficiency of medications and/or the body's response to the medications. Many herbs and supplements exert powerful medicinal effects. The author does not assume any responsibility for the reader's use or misuse of the presented information. If you are ill, we recommend you see a qualified health professional.

References

Abdel-Galil, AM; Wrba H; El-Mofty MM. (1984). Prevention of 3-methylcholanthrene-induced skin tumors in mice by simultaneous application of 13-cis-retinoic acid and retinyl palmitate (vitamin A palmitate).*Exp. Pathol.*, 25(2), 97-102.

Adachi, S; Kawamura, K; Takemoto, K. (1993). Oxidative damage of nuclear DNA in liver of rats exposed to psychological stress. *Cancer Research*, 53, 4153-4155.

Afanas'ev, IB; Dorozhko, AI; Brodskii, AV; Kostyuk, VA; Potapovitch, AI. (1998). Chelating and free radical scavenging mechanisms of inhibitory action of rutin and quercetin in lipid peroxidation. *Biochem. Pharmacol.*, 38, 1763-9.

Afaq, F; Mukhtar, H. (2002). Photochemoprevention by botanical antioxidants. *Skin Pharmacol. Appl. Skin Physiol*, 15, 297-306.

Agar, NS; Halliday, GM; Barnetson, RS. et al. (2004). The basal layer in human squamous tumors harbors more UVA than UVB fingerprint mutations:a role for UVA in human skin carcinogenesis. *Proc. Natl. Acad. Sci. USA*, 101, 4954-4959.

Agarwal, R; Mukhtar, H. Oxidative stress in skin chemical carcinogenesis. In: Fuchs J, Packer L, Eds.. *Oxidative Stress in Dermatology*. New York: Marcel Dekker, Inc, 1993; 207–241.

Age-Related Eye Disease Study Research Group. (2001). "A randomized, placebo-controlled, clinical trial of high-dose supplementation with vitamins C and E and beta-carotene for age-related cataract and vision loss: AREDS report no. 9," *Arch. Ophthalmol*, 119, 1439-52.

Aggarwal, BB; Shishodia, S. (2006). Molecular targets of dietary agents for prevention and therapy of cancer." *Biochem. Pharmacol.*, 71, 1397–421.

Ahmad, N; Gali, H; Javed, S; Agarwal R. (1998). Skin cancer chemopreventive effects of a flavonoid antioxidant silymarin are mediated via impairment of receptor tyrosine kinase signaling and perturbation in cell cycle progression. *Biochem. Biophys. Res. Commun.*, 18, 247(2):294-301.

Ainbinder, D; Touitou, E. Skin photodamage prevention: state-of-the-art and new prospects. In: *Textbook of aging skin* (Farage MA, Miller KW, Maibach HI (Eds). Springer-Verlag; Berlin; 2010.

Akimichi M. (2007). Tobacco smoke causes premature skin aging. *Journal of dermatological scien*ce., 48(3), 169-175.

Albanes, D; Heinonen, OP; Taylor, PR; Virtamo, J; Edwards, BK; Rautalahti, M; Hartman, AM; Palmgren, J; Freedman, LS; Haapakoski, J; Barrett, MJ; Pietinen, P; Malila, N; Tala, E; Liippo, K; Salomaa, ER; Tangrea, JA; Teppo, L; Askin, FB; Taskinen, E; Erozan, Y; Greenwald, P; Huttunen, JK. (1996). Alpha-Tocopherol and beta-carotene supplements and lung cancer incidence in the alpha-tocopherol, beta-carotene cancer prevention study: effects of base-line characteristics and study compliance. *J. Natl. Cancer Inst.*, 88(21), 1560-70.

Aldini, G; Orioli, M; Rossoni, G; Savi, F; Braidotti, P; Vistoli, G; Yeum, KJ; Negrisoli, G; Carini, M. (2010). The carbonyl scavenger carnosine ameliorates dyslipidemia and renal function in zucker obese rats. *J. Cell Mol. Med.* [Epub ahead of print]).

Allen, RG; Sohal, RS. (1982). Life-lengthening effects of gamma-radiation on the adult housefly, Musca domestica. *Mech. Ageing Dev.*, 20(4), 369-75.

Allen, RG; Farmer, KJ; Newton, RK; Sohal, RS. (1984). Effects of paraquat administration on longevity, oxygen consumption, lipid peroxidation, superoxide dismutase, catalase, glutathione reductase, inorganic peroxides and glutathione in the adult housefly. *Comp. Biochem. Physiol C.*, 78(2), 283-8.

Alessio, HM. Oxidative stress across the exercise continuum. In: *Oxidative stress, exercise and aging.* (Eds: Alessio HM and Hagerman, AE.). Imperial College Press; London; 2006.

Alessio, HM; Goldfarb, AH. (1988). Lipid peroxidation and scavenger enzymes during exercise. Adaptive response to training. *J. Appl. Physiol*, 64, 1333-1336.

Alessio, HM; Hagerman, AE; Fulkerson, BK; Ambrose, J; Rice, RE; Wiley, RL. (2000). Generation of reactive oxygen species after exhaustive aerobic and isometric exercise. *Med. Sci. Sports Exerc.*, 32(9):1576-81.

Alessio, HM. Exercise. In: *Critical Reviews of oxidative stress and aging.* Cutler RG, Rodriguez H. (Eds.) World Scientific, 2003.

Alkhawam, L; Alam, M. (2009). Dermabrasion and microdermabrasion. *Facial. Plast. Surg.*, 25(5), 301-10.

Allsopp, RC; Vaziri, H; Patterson, C; Goldstein, S; Younglai, EV, et al. (1992). Telomere length predicts replicative capacity of human fibroblasts. *Proc. Natl. Acad. Asci.* USA,89, 10114-10118.

Allsopp, RC; Vaziri, H; Patterson, C; Goldstein, S; Younglai, EV; Futcher, AB; Greider, CW; Harley, CB. (1992). Telomere length predicts replicative capacity of human fibroblasts. *Proc. Natl. Acad. Sci.* USA, 89, 10114–8.

Allsopp, RC; Patterson, C; Goldstein, S; Younglai, EV; Futcher, AB; Greider, CW; Harley, CB. (1992). Telomere length predicts replicative capacity of human fibroblasts. *Proc. Natl. Acad. Sci.* USA, 89, 10114–8.

Alvarez-León, EE; Román-Viñas, B; Serra-Majem, L. (2006). Dairy products and health: a review of the epidemiological evidence. *Br. J. Nutr.*, 96, S94-S99.

Amara, CE;Shankland, EG;Jubrias, SA;Marcinek, DJ;Kushmerick, MJ;Conley, KE. (2007). Mild mitochondrial uncoupling impacts cellular aging in human muscles in vivo. *Proc. Natl. Acad. Sci.*, 104(3), 1631-1635.

American Academy of Dermatology. (2005). "Turning Back the Hands of Time." Last accessed June 20, 2005.

Ames, BN. (2006). Low micronutrient intake may accelerate the degenerative diseases of aging through allocation of scarce micronutrients by triage. *Proc. Natl. Acad. Sci. USA*, 103, 17589-17594.

Ames, BN; Gold, LS. (1998). The causes and prevention of cancer: the role of environment. *Biotherapy*, 11, 105.

Ames, BN. (1998). Micronutrients prevent cancer and delay aging. *Toxicol. Lett.*, 102-103, 5-18.

Ames, BN. (1983). Dietary carcinogens and anticarcinogens. *Science*, 221, 1256–1264.

Ames, B.N; Liu, J. (2004). Delaying the Mitochondrial Decay of Aging with Acetyl Carnitine. *Ann. NY Acad. Sci.*, 1033, 108-116.

Ames, BN; Shigenaga, M; Hagen, MT. (1993). Oxidants, antioxidants and the degenerative diseases of aging. *Proc. Natl. Acad. Sci. USA*, 17, 7915-22.

Ames, BN. (2004). A Role for Supplements in Optimizing Health: the Metabolic Tune-up. *Archives of Biochemistry and Biophysics*, 423, 227-234.

Ames, BN. (2001). DNA damage from micronutrient deficiencies is likely to be a major cause of cancer. *Mutat. Res.*, 475(1-2), 7-20.

Andersen, WK; Labadie, RR; Bhawan, J. (1997). Histopathology of solar lengitines of the face: a quantitative study. *J. Am. Acad. Dermatol*, 36, 444-7.

Anderson, D; Phillips, BJ. (1999). Comparative in vitro and in vivo effects of antioxidants. *Food Chem. Toxicol*, 37, 1015-1025.

Anderson, RM; Bitterman, KJ; Wood, JG; Medvedik, O; Sinclair, DA. (2003). Nicotinamide and Pnc 1 govern lifespan extension by calorie restriction in S. cerevisiae, *Nature*, 432, 181-185.

Anderson, RM; Bohr, V. (2000). Mitochondria, oxidative DNA damage and aging. *J. Amer. Aging Assoc.*, 23, 1999-218.

Anderson, S; Bankier, AT; Barrell, BG; de Bruijn, MH; Coulson, AR; Drouin, J; Eperon, IC; Nierlich, DP; Roe, BA; Sanger, F; Schreier, PH; Smith, AJ; Staden, R; Young, IG. (1981). Sequence and organization of the human mitochondrial genome. *Nature*. 290(5806), 457-65.

Anderson, L. (2006). Looking Good, the Australian guide to skin care, cosmetic medicine and cosmetic surgery. AMPCo. Sydney. ISBN 0-85557-044-X.

Andreassi, K; Simoni, S; Fiorini, P; Fiamiani, M. (1987). Phenotypic characters related to skin type and minimal erythema dose. *Photodermatology*, 4, 43-6.

Antell, D; Taczanowski, E. (1999). How environmental and lifestyle choices influence the aging process. *Ann. Plast. Surg*, 43, 585-588.

Anson, RM; Guo, Z; de Cabo, R; Iyun, T; Rios, M; Hagepanos, A; Ingram, DK; Lane, MA; Mattson, MP. (2003). Intermittent fasting dissociates beneficial effects of dietary restriction on glucose metabolism and neuronal resistance to injury from calorie intake. *Proc. Natl. Acad. Sci.* USA,100(10), 6216-20.

Anupam, B. (2009). Cancer Prevention and Treatment with Resveratrol: From Rodent Studies to Clinical Trials, *Cancer Prevention Research*, 2, 58-60.

Applegate, LA; Frenk, E. (1995). Oxidative defense in cultured human skin fibroblasts and keratinocytes from sun-exposed and non-exposed skin. *Photodermatol. Photoimmunol. Photomed*,11, 95–101.

Applegate, LA; Luscher, P; Tyrrell, RM. (1991). Induction of heme oxygenase: a general response to oxidant stress in cultured mammalian cells. *Cancer Res*, 51, 974–978.

Applegate, LA; Noel, A; Vile, G; Frenk, E; Tyrrell, RM. (1995). Two genes contribute to different extents to the heme oxygenase enzyme activity measured in cultured human skin fibroblasts and keratinocytes: implication for protection against oxidant stress. *Photochem. Photobiol*, 61, 285–291.

Applegate, LA; Scaletta, C; Panizzon, RG; Niggli, H; Frenk, E. (1999). In vivo induction of pyrimidine dimers in human skin by UVA radiation: Initiation of cell damage and/or intercellular communication? *Int. J. Mol. Med*, 3, 467–472.

Applegate, LA; Scaletta, C; Panizzon, RG; Niggli, H; Frenk, E. (1999). In vivo induction of pyrimidine dimers in human skin by UVA radiation: Initiation of cell damage and/or intercellular communication? *Int. J. Mol. Med*, 3, 467–472.

Arble, DA; Bass, J; Laposky, AD; Vitaterna, MH, Turek, FW. (2009). Circadian Timing of Food Intake Contributes to Weight Gain. *Obesity*, 17(11), 2100-2.

Arck, PC; Overall, R; Spatz, K; Liezman, C; Handjiski, B; Klapp, BF; Birch-Machin, MA; Peters, EM. (2006). Towards a "free radical theory of graying": melanocyte apoptosis in the aging human hair follicle is an indicator of oxidative stress-induced tissue damage. *FASEB J.*, 20(9), 1567-9.

Arking, R. *The biology of aging, observations and principles*. Third edition. Oxford University Press, New York, 2006.

Arlt, W; Hewison, M. (2004). Hormones and immune function: implications of aging. *Aging Cell.*,3, 209–16.

Armstrong, BK. (1988). Epidemiology of malignant melanoma: intermittent or total accumulated exposure to the sun? *J. Dermato., Surg. Oncol.*, 14, 835-49.

Arora, RB; Basu, N; Kapoor, V; Jain, AP. (1971). Anti-inflammatory studies on Curcuma-longa (turmeric). *Ind. J. Med. Res.*, 59, 1289-95.

Ashburner, M; Bonner, JJ. (1979). The induction of gene activity in Drosophila by heat shock. *Cell*, 17, 241-254.

Ashcroft, GS; Horan, MA; Herrick, SE; Tarnuzzer, RW; Schultz, GS; Ferguson, MW. (1997). Age-related differences in the temporal and spatial regulation of matrix metalloproteinases (MMPs) in normal skin and acute cutaneous wounds of healthy humans. *Cell Tissues Res*, 29, 581-91.

Asif, M; Egan, J; Vasan, S; Jyothirmayi, GN; Masurekar, MR; Lopez, S; Williams, C; Torres, RL; Wagle, D; Ulrich, P; Cerami, A; Brines, M; Regan, TJ. (2000). An advanced glycation end product cross-link breaker can reverse age-related increases in myocardial stiffness. *Proc Natl Acad Sci* USA, 14, 97(6), 2809-13.

Aust, O; Stahl, W; Sies, H; Tronnier, H; Heinrich, U. (2005). Supplementation with tomato-based products increases lycopene, phytofluene, and phytoene levels in human serum and protects against UV-light-induced erythema. *Int J. Vitam Nutr Res.*, 75(1), 54-60.

Austad, SN. (1997). Comparative aging and life histories in mammals. *Exp Gerontol*, 32(1-2): 23-38.

Austad, SN. *Why We Age: What Science Is Discovering about the Body's Journey through Life*. John Wiley & Sons, New York, 1997.

Avrat, E; Broglio, F; Ghigo, E. (2000). Insulin-like growth factor I: implications in aging. *Drugs Aging.*, 16, 29–40.

Azizi, E; Lusky, A; Kushelevsky, AP; Schewach-Millet, M. (1988). Skin type, haircolor, and freckles are predictors of decreased minimal erythema ultraviolet radiation dose *J. Am. Acad. Dermatol.*, 19, 32-8.

Azzi, A. (2007). "Molecular mechanism of alpha-tocopherol action." *Free Radic. Biol. Med.*, 43, 16–21.

Babior, BM; Woodman, RD. (1990). Chronic granulomatous disease. *Semin. Hematol*, 27, 247-259.

Bae, JY; Lim, SS; Kim, SJ; Choi, JS; Park, J; Ju, SM; Han, SJ; Kang, IJ; Kang, YH. (2009). Bog blueberry anthocyanins alleviate photoaging in ultraviolet-B irradiation-induced human dermal fibroblasts. *Mol Nutr Food Res.*, 53(6), 726-38.

Balantine, J. *Pathology of oxygen toxicity*. Academic press: New York, 1982.

Balin, AK; Allen, RG. Oxidative stress and skin cancer. In: *Critical reviews of oxidative stress and aging*. Cutler RG and Rodriguez H. (eds.). World Scientific, 2003.

Bain, C; Green, A; Siskind, V; Alexander, J; Harvey, P. (1993). Diet and melanoma. An exploratory case-control study.*Ann Epidemiol.*, 3(3), 235-8.

Bandy, B; Davison, AJ. (1990). Mitochondrial mutations may increase oxidative stress: implications for carcinogenesis and aging? *Free Radical Biol. Med.*, 8, 523-539.

Barger, JL; Kayo, T; Vann, JM; Arias, EB; Wang, J; Hacker, TA; Wang, Y; Raederstorff, D; Morrow, JD; Leeuwenburgh, C; Allison, DB; Saupe, KW; Cartee, GD; Weindruch, R; Prolla, TA. (2008). A Low Dose of Dietary Resveratrol Partially Mimics Caloric Restriction and Retards Aging Parameters in Mice, *Plose One*, 3, 1-10.

Barja, G. (2002). Endogenous oxidative stress: relationship to aging, longevity and caloric restriction. *Ageing Res. Rev.*, 1, 397–411.

Barja, G. (1999). Mitochondrial oxygen radical generation and leak: sites of production in states 4 and 3, organ specificity, and relation to aging and longevity. *J.Bioenerg Biomembr.*, 31(4), 347-66.

Barros, MH; Bandy, B; Tahara, EB; Kowaltowski, AJ. (2004). Higher Respiratory Activity Decreases Mitochondrial Reactive Oxygen Release and Increases Lifespan in Saccharomyces cerevisiae. *J. Biol. Chem*, 279, 49883-8.

Bartke, A.; Wright, J.C.; Mattison, J.A.; Ingram,D.K.; Miller, R.A.; Roth, G.S. (2001). Extending the Lifespan of Long-lived Mice. *Nature*, 414, 412.

Barysch, MJ; Hofbauer, GF; Dummer, R. (2010). Vitamin D, *Ultraviolet Exposure, and Skin Cancer in the Elderly. Gerontology.*, 56(4), 410-413. [Epub ahead of print].

Bases, R; Franklin, WA; Moy, T; Mendez, F. (1992). Enhanced expression repair activity in mammalian cell after ionizing radiation. *Int. J. Radiat. Biol*, 62, 427-441.

Basu-Modak, S; Gordon, MJ; Dobson, LH; Spencer, JP; Rice-Evans, C; Tyrrell, RM. (2003).Epicatechin and its methylated metabolite attenuate UVA-induced oxidative damage to human skin fibroblasts. *Free Radic Biol Med.*, 35(8), 910-21.

Bates, EJ; Johnson, CC; Lowther, DA. (1985). Inhibition of proteoglycan synthesis by H2O2 in cultured bovine articular cartilage. *Biochim. Biophys. Acta*, 838, 221-228.

Bath- Hextall, F;Williams, H. (2007). Skin disorders: Eczema (atopic). *BMJ Clin Evid*, 12, 1716.

Baulieu, EE; Thomas, G; Legrain, S; Lahlou, N; Roger, M; Debuire, B; Faucounau, V; Girard, L; Hervy, MP; Latour, F; Leaud, MC; Mokrane, A; Pitti-Ferrandi, H; Trivalle, C; de Lacharrière, O; Nouveau, S; Rakoto-Arison, B; Souberbielle, JC; Raison, J; Le Bouc, Y; Raynaud, A; Girerd, X; Forette, F. (2000). Dehydroepiandrosterone (DHEA), DHEA sulfate, and aging: contribution of the DHEAge Study to a sociobiomedical issue.*Proc Natl Acad Sci USA*, 97(8), 4279-84.

Baumann L. *Cosmetic dermatology*. New York: McGraw-Hill, 2002, 226 p.

Baur, JA; Pearson, KJ; Price, NL. (2006). Resveratrol improves health and survival of mice on a high-calorie diet. *Nature*, 444, 337-342.

Bayne, S; Liu, JP. (2005). Hormones and growth factors regulate telomerase activity in aging and cancer. *Mol. Cell Endocrinol.*, 240, 11-22.

Beard, J. (2002). Dietary iron intakes and elevated iron stores in the elderly: is it time to abandon the set-point hypothesis of regulation of iron absorption? *Am. J. Clin. Nutr.*, 76, 1189-90.

Beckman, KB; Ames, BN. (1998). The free radical theory of aging matures. *Physiol. Rev*, 78, 547–581.

Beehler, BC; Przybyszewski, J; Box, HB; Kulesz-Martin, MF. (1992). Formation of 8-hydroxydeoxyguanosine within DNA of mouse keratinocytes exposed in culture to UVB and H2O2. *Carcinogenesis* (Lond), 13, 2003–2007.

Beligni, VM; Fath, A; Bethke, PC; Lamattina, L; Jones, JR. (2002). Nitric Oxide Acts as an Antioxidant and Delays Programmed Cell Death in Barley Aleurone Layers. *Plant Physiol,* 129, 1642-1650.

Bell, MN;Jackson, AG. (1995). Role of vitamin D in the pathogenesis and treatment of osteoporosis. *Endocr Pract*, 1:44-47.

Berge, U; Behrens, J; Rattan SI. (2007). Sugar-induced premature aging and altered differentiation in human epidermal keratinocytes. *Ann. N Y Acad. Sci.*, 1100, 524-9.

Berlett, BS; Stadtman, ER. (1997). Protein oxidation in ageing, disease and oxidative stress. *J. Biol. Chem*, 272, 20313-6.

Berneburg, M; Plettenberg, H; Medve-König, K; Pfahlberg, A; Gers-Barlag, H; Gefeller, O; Krutmann, J. (2004).Induction of the photoaging-associated mitochondrial common deletion in vivo in normal human skin. *J. Invest. Dermatol.*, 122, 1277-1284.

Berneburg, M; Gremmel, T; Kürten, V; Schroeder, P; Hertel, I; von Mikecz, A; Wild, S; Chen, M; Declercq, L; Matsui, M; Ruzicka, T; Krutmann, J. (2005). Creatine supplementation normalizes mutagenesis of mitochondrial DNA as well as functional consequences. *J. Invest. Dermatol.*, 125(2), 213-20.

Berneburg, M; Grether-Beck, S; Kürten, V; Ruzicka, T; Briviba, K; Sies, H; Krutmann, J. (1999). Singlet oxygen mediates the UVA-induced generation of the photoaging-associated mitochondrial common deletion. *J. Biol. Chem.*, 274(22), 15345-9.

Bernstein, EF; Chen, YQ; Kopp, JB; Fisher, L; Brown, D.,B; Hahn, PJ; et al. (1996). Long-term sun exposure alters the collagen of the papillary dermis. Comparison of sun-protected and photoaged skin by northern analysis, immunohistochemical staining, and confocal laser scanning microscopy. *Journal of the American Academy ofDermatology*, 34(2 Pt 1), 209-218.

Berton, TR; Mitchell, DL; Fischer, SM; Locniskar, MF. (1997). Epidermal proliferation but not the quantity of DNA photodamage is correlated with UV-induced mouse skin carcinogenesis. *J. Invest. Dermatol*, 109, 340–347.

Berry, RJ; Bronson, FH. (1992). Life history and bioeconomy of the house mouse. *Biol. Rev. Cambridge Philos. Soc.*, 67, 519–550.

Best, B. (2009). Mechanisms of aging. http://www.benbest.com/lifeext/aging.html accessed December, 2009.

Beyer, W; ImLay, J; Fridovich, I. (1991). Superoxide dismutases. *Prog. Nucl. Acid Res*, 40, 221-253.

Bhattacharyya, TK. Skin Aging in animal models: histological perspective. In: *Textbook of skin aging*. Farage MA, Miller KW, Maibach (Eds). Springer-Verlag, Berlin, 2010.

Bhuvaneswari, V; Nagini, S. (2005). Lycopene: a review of its potential as an anticancer agent. *Curr. Med. Chem. Anticancer. Agents.*, 5(6), 627-35.

Bielenberg, DR; Bucana, CD; Sanchez, R; Donawho, CK; Kripke, ML; Fidler, IJ. (1998). Molecular regulation of UVB-induced cutaneous angiogenesis. *J. Invest. Dermatol.*, 111(5), 864-72.

Biesalski, HK; Obermueller-Jevic, UC. (2001). UV light, beta-carotene and human skin—beneficial and potentially harmful effects. *Arch. Biochem. Biophys.*, 389(1), 1-6.

Birch-Machin, MA; Tindall, M; Turner, R; Haldane, F; Rees, JL. (1998). Mitochondrial DNA deletions in human skin reflect photo- rather than chronologic aging. *J. Invest. Dermatol.*, 110(2), 149-52.

Bjelakovic, G; Nikolova, D; Gluud, L; Simonetti, R; Gluud, C. (2007). "Mortality in Randomized Trials of Antioxidant Supplements for Primary and Secondary Prevention: Systematic Review and Meta-analysis." *Jama*, 8, 842–57.

Bjelakovic, G; Nikolova, D; Simonetti, RG; Gluud, C. (2004). Antioxidant supplements for prevention of gastrointestinal cancers: a systematic review and meta-analysis. *Lancet* 2004, 36, 1219-28.

Blair, SN; Wei, M. (2000). Sedentary habits, health, and function in older women and men. *Am. J. Health Promot.*, 15(1), 1-8. Review.

Blank, IH. (1953).Further observations on factors which influence the water content of the stratum corneum. *J. Invest. Dermatol*, 21(4), 259-271.

Blatt, T; Lenz, H; Koop, U; Jaspers, S; Weber, T; Mummert, C; Wittern, KP; Stäb, F; Wenck, H. (2005).Stimulation of skin's energy metabolism provides multiple benefits for mature human skin. *Biofactors.*, 25(1-4), 179-85.

Blatt, T; Wenck, H; Wittern, KP. Alterations of energy metabolism in cutaneous aging. In: *Textbook of aging skin*. Farage, MA; Miller, KW; Maibach, HI. (Eds). Springer-Verlag, Berlin, 2010.

Blumthaler, M; Ambach, W, (1985). Neure Messugen der Albedo verschiedener Oberflaechen fur erythemwirksame Strahlung Annal. *Meteorol.*,22, 114-5.

Bodkin, NL, Ortmeyer, HK; Hansen, BC. (1995). Long-term dietary restriction in older-aged rhesus monkeys: effects on insulin resistance. *J. Gerontol. A Biol. Sci. Med. Sci.*, 50(3), B142-7.

Bodkin, NL; Alexander, TM; Ortmeyer, HK; Johnson, E; Hansen, BC. (2003). Mortality and Morbidity in Laboratory-maintained Rhesus Monkey and Effects on Long-term Dietary Restriction. *J. Gerontol. A Biol. Sci. Med. Sci.*, 58, 212-219.

Boelsma, E; Hendriks, HF; Roza L. (2001). Nutritional skin care: health effects of micronutrients and fatty acids. *Am. J. Clin. Nutr.*, 73(5):853-64.

Boelsma, E; van de Vijver, LP; Goldbohm, RA; Klöpping-Ketelaars, IA; Hendriks, HF; Roza, L. (2003). Human skin condition and its associations with nutrient concentrations in serum and diet. *Am. J. Clin. Nutr.*, 77(2), 348-55.

Bolognia, JL; Braverman, IM; Rousseau, ME; Sarrel, PM. (1989). Skin changes in menopause. *Maturitas.*, 11, 295–304.

Bolognia, JL. (1993).Dermatologic and cosmetic concerns the older women. *Clinic in Geriatric Medicine*, 9, 209-29.

Bolognia, JL. (1995). Aging skin. *Am. J. Med.*, 98(1A), 99S-103S.

Bonina, F; Lanza, M; Montenegro, L; Puglisi, C; Tomaino, A; Trombetta, D; Castelli, F; Saija, A. Flavonoids as potential protective agents against photooxidative skin damage. (1996).*International Journal of Pharmaceutics* 145(1-2), 87-94.

Bonnefoy, M; Drai, J; Kostka, T. (2002). Antioxidants to slow aging, facts and perspectives. *Presse Med.,* 31, 1174-84.

Bonté, F; Pinguet, P; Saunois, A; Meybeck, A; Beugin, S; Ollivon, M; Lesieur, S. (1997). Thermotropic phase behavior of in vivo extracted human stratum corneum lipids, *Lip*, 32, 653-60.

Bonté, F; Saunois, A; Pinguet, P; Meybeck, A. (1997). Existence of a lipid gradient in the upper stratum corneum and its possible biological significance. *Ach. Dermatol. Res*, 289, 78-82.

Bonté, F. (2001). Régulations hormonales cutanées et utilization d'extraits végétaux correcteurs par voie topique. *Phytothérapie*, 25-8.

Bonté, F. (1999). Skin lipids: their origin and function. *Recent Res. Devel. Lipids Res*, 3, 43-62.

Boothby, LA; Doering, PL. (2005). "Vitamin C and vitamin E for Alzheimer's disease." *Ann. Pharmacother*, 39, 2073–80.

Borkow, G; Gabbay, J; Lyakhovitsky, A; Huszar, M. (2009). Improvement of facial skin characteristics using copper oxide containing pillowcases: a double-blind, placebo-controlled, parallel, randomized study. *Int. J. Cosmet. Sci.* 31(6), 437-43.

Bougnoux, P; Giraudeau, B; Couet, C. (2006). Diet, cancer, and the lipidome. *Cancer Epidemiol. Biomarkers Prev.*, 15(3), 416-21.

Boukamp, P. (2001). Ageing mechanisms: the role of telomere loss. *Clin. Exp. Dermatol*, 26, 562-5.

Bouwstra, JA. Lipid organization of the skin barrier. In: Skin moisturization. (Eds.: Rawlings, AV; Leyden, JJ). *Infotma Healthcare*, New York, 2009.

Bowler, C; Slooten, L; Vandenbranden, S; De Rycke, R; Botterman, J; Sybesma, C; Van Montagu, M; Inze, D. (1991). Manganese superoxide dismutase can reduce cellular damage mediated by oxygen radicals in transgenic plants. *Embo J.*, 10, 1723-32.

Boyd, S; Stasko, T; King, LE Jr; Cameron, GS; Pearse, AD; Gaskell, SA. (1999). Cigarette smoking-associated elastotic changes in the skin. *J. Am. Acad. Dermatol.*, 41, 23–6.

Braeckman, BP; Houthoofd, K; Vanfleteren, JR. (2001). Insulin-like signaling, metabolism, stress resistance and aging in Caenorhabditis elegans. *Mechanisms of Aging & Development*, 122, 673-693.

Brand, MD. (2000). Uncoupling to survive? The role of mitochondrial inefficiency in ageing. *Exp. Gerontol.*, 35(6-7), 811-20.

Brand, MD; Pamplona, R; Portero-Otín, M; Requena, JR; Roebuck, SJ; Buckingham, JA; Clapham, JC; Cadenas, S. (2002). Oxidative damage and phospholipid fatty acyl composition in skeletal muscle mitochondria from mice underexpressing or overexpressing uncoupling protein 3. *Biochem. J.*, 368(Pt 2), 597-603.

Brash, D. (1997). Sunlight and the onset of skin cancer. *Trends Genet.*, 13, 410-414.

Brash, DE; Heffernan, TP; Nghiem, P. Carcinogenesis: UV Radiation. In: Farage, MA; Miller, KW; Maibach, HI. *Textbook of aging skin*. Berlin: Springer-Verlag, 2010.

Brash, DE; Ziegler, A; Jonason, AS; Simon, JA; Kunala, S; Leffell, DJ. (1996). Sunlight and sunburn in human skin cancer: p53, apoptosis, and tumor promotion. *J. Invest. Dermatol Symp. Pro*c, 1, 136-142.

Braverman, IM; Fonferko, E. (1982). Studies in cutaneous aging. The elastic fiber network. *J. Invest. Dermatol*, 78, 434-443.

Bravo, L. (1998). Polyphenols: chemistry, dietary sources, metabolism, and nutritional significance. *Nutrition Reviews*, 56, 317-333.

Bray, D; Hopkins, C; Roberts, DN. (2010). A review of dermal fillers in facial plastic surgery. *Curr. Opin. Otolaryngol. Head Neck Surg.*, 18(4), 295-302.

Brennan, RJ; Swoboda, BE; Schiestl, RH. (1994). Oxidative mutagens induce intrachromosomal recombination in yeast. *Mutat Res.*, 308(2), 159-67.

Breternitz, M; Kowatzki, D; Langenauer, M, et al. (2008). Placebo-controlled, double-blind, randomized, prospective study of a glycerol-based emollient on eczematous skin in atopic dermatitis: Biophysical and clinical evaluation. *Skin. Pharmacol. Physiol,* 21, 39-45.

Brincat, MP; Baron, YM; Galea, R. (2005). Estrogens and the skin. *Climacteric.*, 8(2), 110-23.

Brinckmann, J; Acil, Y; Wolff, HH; Müller, PK. (1995). Collagen synthesis in (sun)-aged human skin and in fibroblasts derived from sun-exposed and sun-protected body sites. *J. Photochem. Photobiol*, 27, 33-8.

Brod, J. (1991). Characterization and physiological role of epidermal lipids. *Int. J. Dermatol*, 30, 84-90.

Bryson, B. *A Short History of Nearly Everything*. Ljubljana: Mladinska knjiga, 2003/ 2006.

Broniarczyk-Dyla, G; Joss-Wichman, E. (1999). Aging of the skin during menopause. *Med. Sci. Monit*, 5, 1024-9.

Bonté, F. (2001).Régulations hormonales cutanées et utilization d'extraits végétaux correcteurs par voie topique. *Phytothérapie*, 25-8.

Brown-Borg HM and Harman. Hormones and oxidative stress. In: Critical reviews of oxidative stress and aging. Cutler RG and Rodriguez H (Eds.). *World Scientific*, 2003.

Brown-Borg, HM; Bode, AM; Bartke, A. (1999). Antioxidative mechanisms and plasma growth hormone levels: potential relationship in the aging process. *Endocrine*, 11, 41-48.

Bruce, S. (2008).Cosmeceuticals for the attenuation of extrinsic and intrinsic dermal aging. *J. Drugs Dermatol.*, 7(2 Suppl):s17-22.

Bruls, WAG; Slaper, H; van der Leun, JC; Berrins, L. (1984). Transmission of human epidermis and stratum corneum as a function of thickness in the ultraviolet and visible wavelengthsPhotochem. *Photobiol.*, 40, 485-94.

Brunk, UT; Jones, CB; Sohal, RS. (1992). A novel hypothesis of lipofuscinogenesis and cellular aging based on interaction between oxidative stress and autophagocitosis. *Mutat. Res*, 275, 395-403.

Brunk, UT; Terman, A. (2002). The mitochondrial-lysosomal axis theory of aging: accumulation of damaged mitochondria as a result of imperfect autophagocytosis. *Eur. J. Biochem.*,269, 1996-2002.

Bucala, R; Cerami, A. (1992). "Advanced glycosylation: chemistry, biology, and implications for diabetes and aging."*Adv. Pharmacol.*,23, 1–34.

Bulteau, AL; Petropoulos, I; Friguet, B. (2000). Age-related alterations of proteasome structure and function in aging epidermis. *Exp. Gerontol.*, 35(6-7), 767-77.

Bunout, D; Garrido, A; Suazo, M; Kauffman, R; Venegas, P; de la Maza, P; Petermann, M; Hirsch, S. (2000). Effects of supplementation with folic acid and antioxidant vitamins on homocysteine levels and LDL oxidation in coronary patients. *Nutrition.*, 16(2), 107-10.

Burgess, C. (2008). Topical vitamins. *J. Drugs Dermatol.*, 7(7 Suppl), s2-6.

Burke, KE; Wei, H. (2009). Synergistic damage by UVA radiation and pollutants. *Toxicol. Ind. Health.*, 25(4-5), 219-24.

Burke, KE. (2007). Interaction of vitamins C and E as better cosmeceuticals. *Dermatol. Ther.*, 20(5), 314-21.

Burke, KE. (2004). Photodamage of the skin: protection and reversal with topical antioxidants. *J. Cosmet. Dermatol.*, 3(3), 149-55.

Bürkle, A; Beneke, S; Brabeck, C; Leake, A; Meyer, R; Muiras, ML; Pfeiffer, R. (2002).Poly(ADP-ribose) polymerase-1, DNA repair and mammalian longevity. *Exp. Gerontol.*, 37(10-11), 1203-5.

Burr, GO; Burr, MM; Miller, E. (1930). "On the nature and role of the fatty acids essential in nutrition" (PDF). *J. Biol. Chem.*, 86, 587.

Bykov, VJ; Marcusson, JA; Hemminki, K. (2000). Effect of constitutional, pigmentation on ultraviolet B-induced DNA damage in fair-skinned people, *J. Invest. Dermatol*, 114, 40-3.

Bykov, VJ. (1999). *UV-induced DNA damage in humans*. Stockholm: Thesis Karolinska Institute, 1999:28.

Cadet, J; Berger, M; Douki, T; Morin, B; Raoul, S; Ravanat, JL; Spinelli, S. (1997). Effects of UV and visible radiation on DNA-final base damage. *Biol Chem.*, 378(11), 1275-86.

Cai, J; Jones, DP. (1998). Superoxide in apoptosis. Mitochondrial generation triggered by cytochrome c loss. *J. Biol. Chem.*, 273(19), 11401-4.

Cai, J; Yang, J; Jones, DP. (1998). Mitochondrial control of apoptosis: the role of cytochrome c. *Biochim. Biophys. Acta.*, 1366(1-2), 139-49.

Callaghan, TM; Wilhelm, KP. (2008). A review of ageing and an examination of clinical methods in the assessment of ageing skin. Part I: Cellular and molecular perspectives of skin ageing. *Int. J. Cosmet. Sci.*, 30(5), 313-22.

Calleja-Agius, J; Muscat-Baron, Y; Brincat, MP. (2007). *Skin ageing*. Menopause Int. 13(2), 60-4.

Callens, A; Vaillant, L; Lecomte, P; Berson, M; Gall, Y; Lorette, G. (1996). Does hormonal skin aging exist? A study of the influence of different hormone therapy regimens on the skin of postmenopausal women using non-invasive measurement techniques. *Dermatology.*, 193(4), 289-94.

Cámara, Y; Duval, C; Sibille, B; Villarroya, F. (2007). Activation of mitochondrial-driven apoptosis in skeletal muscle cells is not mediated by reactive oxygen species production. *Int. J. Biochem. Cell Biol.*, 39(1), 146-60.

Campisi, J. (1998). The role of cellular senescence in skin ageing. *J. Invest. Dermatol. Symposium Proceedings*, 3: 1-5.

Candore, G; Scapagnini, G; Caruso, C. Aging and anti-aging strategies. In: *Textbook of aging skin*. Farage MA, Miller KW, Maibach HI (Eds). Springer-Verlag, Berlin, 2010.

Caraballoso, M; Sacristan, M; Serra, C; Bonfill, X. (2003). Drugs for preventing lung cancer in healthy people. *Cochrane Database Syst. Rev*, 2. CD002141.

Carlisle, DL; Pritchard, DE; Singh, J; Owens, BM; Blankenship, LJ; Orenstein, JM; Patierno, SR. (2000). Apoptosis and P53 induction in human lung fibroblasts exposed to chromium(VI): effect of ascorbate and tocopherol. *Toxicol. Sci.*,55, 60-68.

Carr, A; Frei, B. (1999). Does vitamin C act as a pro-oxidant under physiological conditions? *Faseb. J.*, 13, 1007-1024.

Castiella, L; Rigoulet, M; Penicaud, L. (2001). Mitochondrial ROS metabolism: modulation by uncoupling proteins. *Iubmb. Life*, 52, 181–188.

Cefalu, WT; Bell-Farrow, AD; Wang, ZQ; Sonntag, WE; Fu, MX; Baynes, JW; Thorpe, SR. (1995). Caloric restriction decreases age-dependent accumulation of the glycoxidation products, N epsilon-(carboxymethyl)lysine and pentosidine, in rat skin collagen. *J. Gerontol. A Biol. Sci. Med. Sci.*, 50(6), B337-41.

Cellini, L; Di Campli, E; Masulli, M; Di Bartolomeo, S; Allocati, N. (1996). Inhibition of Helicobacter pylori by garlic extract (Allium sativum). *FEMS Immunol. Med. Microbiol.*, 13(4), 273-7.

Cerutti, PA. (1985). Pro-oxidant states and promotion. *Science*, 227, 375–381.

Césarini, JP; Michel, L; Maurette, JM; Adhoute, H; Béjot, M. (2003). Immediate effects of UV radiation on the skin: modification by an antioxidant complex containing carotenoids. *Photodermatol. Photoimmunol. Photomed.*, 19(4), 182-9.

Chan, R; Woo, J; Suen, E; Leung, J; Tang, N. (2009). Chinese tea consumption is associated with longer telomere length in elderly Chinese men. *Br. J. Nutr.*, 12, 1-7.

Cheeseman, KH; Slater, TF. (1993). An introduction to free radical biochemistry. *Br. Med. Bull*, 49, 481-493.

Chehab, FF. Leptin as a regulator of adipose mass and reproduction. *Trends in Pharmacological Sciences*, 21, 309-14.

Chen, D; Guarente, L. (2007). SIR2: a potential target for calorie restriction mimetics. *Trends in Molecular Medicine*, 13, 64-71.

Chen, LH; Lowry, SR. (1989). Cellular antioxidant defense system. In: *Dietary restriction and Aging*, Alan, RL, Inc. New York, 247-256.

Chen, M; Goyal, S; Cai, X; O'Toole, EA; Woodley, DT. (1997). Modulation of type VII collagen (anchoring fibril) expression by retinoids in human skin cells. *Biochim. Biophys. Acta.*, 1351(3), 333-40.

Cheng, KC; Cahill, DS; Kasa, H; Nishimura, S; Loeb, LA. (1992). 8-Hydroxyguanosine, an abundant form of oxidative DNA damage, causes G-T and A-C substitutions. *J. Biol. Chem.*, 267, 166–172.

Cherkas, LF; Aviv, A; Valdes, AM; Hunkin, JL; Gardner, JP; Surdulescu, GL; Kimura, M; Spector TD. (2006). The effects of social status on biological aging as measured by white-blood-cell telomere length. *Aging Cell.*, 5(5), 361-5.

Cherubini, A; Vigna, G; Zuliani, G; Ruggiero, C; Senin, U; Fellin, R. (2005). "Role of antioxidants in atherosclerosis: epidemiological and clinical update." *Curr. Pharm. Des*, 11, 2017–32.

Chesney, JA; Eaton, JW; Mahoney J. (1996). Bacterial glutathione: a sacrificial defense against chlorine compounds. *J. Bacteriol.*, 178 (7), 2131–2135.

Childs, A; Jacobs, C; Kaminski, T; Halliwell, B; Leeuwenburgh, C. (2001). Supplementation with vitamin CandV-acetyl-cysteine increases oxidative stress in humans after an acute muscle injury induced by eccentric exercise. *Free Radic. Biol. Mcd.*, 31, 745-153.

Cho, E; Seddon, JM; Rosner, B; Willett, WC; Hankinson, SE. (2004). Prospective study of intake of fruits, vegetables, vitamins, and carotenoids and risk of age-related maculopathy. *Arch. Ophthalmol.*, 122, 883-92.

Cho, HS; Lee, MH; Lee, JW; No, KO; Park, SK; Lee, HS; Kang, S; Cho, WG; Park, HJ; Oh, KW; Hong JT. (2007). Anti-wrinkling effects of the mixture of vitamin C, vitamin E, pycnogenol and evening primrose oil, and molecular mechanisms on hairless mouse skin caused by chronic ultraviolet B irradiation. *Photodermatol. Photoimmunol. Photomed.*, 23(5), 155-62.

Cho, S; Lee, DH; Won, CH; Kim, SM; Lee, S; Lee, MJ; Chung, JH. (2010). Differential Effects of Low-Dose and High-Dose Beta-Carotene Supplementation on the Signs of Photoaging and Type I Procollagen Gene Expression in Human Skin in vivo.*Dermatology*., Ahead of print.

Cho, S; Won, CH; Lee, DH; Lee, MJ; Lee, S; So, SH; Lee, SK; Koo, BS; Kim, NM; Chung, JH. (2009). Red ginseng root extract mixed with Torilus fructus and Corni fructus improves facial wrinkles and increases type I procollagen synthesis in human skin: a randomized, double-blind, placebo-controlled study. *J. Med. Food.*, 12(6), 1252-9.

Choi, BS; Song, HS; Kim, HR; Park, TW; Kim, TD; Cho, BJ; Kim, CJ; Sim, SS. (2009). Effect of coenzyme Q10 on cutaneous healing in skin-incised mice. *Arch. Pharm. Res.*, 32(6), 907-13.

Chondrogianni, N; Kapeta, S; Chinou, I; Vassilatou, K; Papassideri, I; Gonos, ES. (2010). Anti-ageing and rejuvenating effects of quercetin. *Exp. Gerontol.*, 45(10), 763-71.

Chung, HY; Sung, B; Jung, KJ; Zou, Y; Yu, BP. (2006). The molecular inflammatory process in aging. *Antioxid. Redox. Signal.*, 8, 572–581.

Chung, JH; Kang, S; Varani, J; Lin, J; Fisher, GJ; Voorhees, JJ. (2000). Decreased extracellular-signal-regulated kinase and increased stress-activated MAP kinase activities in aged human skin in vivo. *J. Invest. Dermatol.*, 115(2), 177-82.

Cibin, TR; Gayathri Devi, D; Abraham A. (2010). Chemoprevention of skin cancer by the flavonoid fraction of Saraca asoka (Chemoprevention of skin cancer by the flavonoid fraction of Saraca asoka). *Phytotherapy Research*, 24(5), 666—672.

Cinque, B; Palumbo, P; La Torre, C,et al., Probiotics in aging skin. In: Farage, MA; Miller, KW; Maibach HI. (Eds.). *Textbook of aging skin*. Berlin: Springer-Verlag, 2010.

Clark, E; Lawrence, S. (2008). Superficial and medium-depth chemical peels. *Clin Dermatol*, 26, 209-218.

Clement, MV; Ramalingam, J; Long, LH; Halliwell B. (2001). The in vitro cytotoxicity of ascorbate depends on the culture medium used to perform the assay and involves H2O2. *Antioxid Redox Signal.*, 3(1), 157-63.

Cobarg, CC. (1995).Physikalische Grundlagen der wassergefilterterten Infrarot-A-Strahlung. In: Vaupel, P. und Krüger, W. (Hrsg.) Wärmetherapie mit wassergefilterter Infrarot-A-Strahlung, Grundlagen und Anwendungsmöglichkeiten, 2 Auflage: 19-28, 1995, Hippokrates, Stuttgart.

Cobo, JM; Castiñeira, M. (1997). Oxidative stress, mitochondrial respiration, and glycemic control: clues from chronic supplementation with Cr3+ or As3+ to male Wistar rats. *Nutrition.*, 13(11-12), 965-70.

Cole, PD; Hatef, DA; Kaufman, Y; Pozner, JN. (2009). Laser therapy in ethnic populations. *Semin Plast Surg.*, 23(3), 173-7.

Coleman, KR; Carruthers, J. (2006). Combination therapy with Botox® and fillers: The new rejuvenation paradigm. *Dermatologic Therapy*, 19, 177-188.

Comfort, A. (1971). Effect of ethoxyquin on the longevity of C3H mice. *Nature*, 229, 254-255.

Composition of Foods Raw, Processed, Prepared USDA National Nutrient Database for Standard Reference, Release 20 USDA, Feb. 2008.

Congdon, JD; Nagle, RD; Kinney, OM; van Loben Sels, RC. (2001). Hypotheses of aging in a long-lived vertebrate, Blanding's turtle (Emydoidea blandingii). *Exp. Gerontol*, 36, 813–827.

Congdon, JD; Nagle, RD; Kinney, OM; van Loben Sels, RC; Quinter, T; Tinkle, DW. (2003). Testing hypotheses of aging in long-lived painted turtles (Chrysemys picta). *Exp. Gerontol*, 38, 765–772.

Connor, MJ; Wheeler, LA. (1987). Depletion of cutaneous glutathione by ultraviolet radiation. *Photochem. Photobiol.*, 46(2), 239-45.

Conti, A; Schiavi, ME; Seidenari, S. (1995). Capacitance, transepidermal water loss and causallevel of sebum in healthy subjects in relation to site, sex and age. *Int. J. Cosmet. Sci*, 17, 77-85.

Cook, CI; Yu, BP. (1998). Iron accumulation in aging: modulation by dietary restriction. *Mechanisms of Ageing and Development*, 102, 1-13.

Cook, NC; Samman, S. (1996). Flavonoids - Chemistry, metabolism, cardioprotective effects, and dietary sources. *Journal of Nutritional Biochemistry*, 7, 66-76.

Cook, R; Calabrese, E.J. (2006). "The Importance of Hormesis to Public Health." *Environmental Health Perspectives*, 114, 1631-1635.

Cooke, MS; Evans, MD; Podmore, ID; Herbert, KE; Mistry, N; Mistry, P; Hickenbotham, PT; Hussieni, A; Griffiths, HR; Lunec J. (1998). Novel repair action of vitamin C upon in vivo oxidative DNA damage. *FEBS Lett.*, 439(3), 363-7.

Coquette, A; Berna, N; Poumay, Y; Pittelkow, MR. The keratinocyte in cutaneous irritation and sensitization. In: Kydonieus AF, Wille JJ, (eds). *Biochemical Modulations of Skin Reactions*. Boca Raton: CRC Press, 2000:125–143.

Corder, EH; Saunders, AM; Strittmatter, WJ; Schmechel, DE; Gaskell, PC; Small, GW. (1993). Gene dose of apolipoprotein E type allele and the risk of Alzheimer's disease in late onset families. *Science*, 261, 921-3.

Corder, R; Mullen, W; Khan, NQ; Marks, SC; Wood, EG; Carrier, MJ; Crozier, A. (2006). Oenology: Red wine procyanidins and vascular health. *Nature*. 2006 Nov 30;444(7119):566.

Cordero, A. Jr. (1983). La vitamina a acida en la piel senile. *Actualizaciones TerDermatologica,* 6, 49-54.

Cortopassi, GA; Wang, E. (1996). "There is substantial agreement among interspecies estimates of DNA repair activity." *Mechanisms of Aging and Development*, 91, 211–218.

Cosgrove, MC; Franco, OH; Granger, SP; Murray, PG; Mayes, AE. (2007). Dietary nutrient intakes and skin-aging appearance among middle-aged American women. *Am J. Clin Nutr.*, 86(4), 1225-31.

Cosmetic Ingredient Review Expert Panel. (2007). Final report on the safety assessment of Aloe Andongensis Extract, Aloe Andongensis Leaf Juice,aloe Arborescens Leaf Extract, Aloe Arborescens Leaf Juice, Aloe Arborescens Leaf Protoplasts, Aloe Barbadensis Flower Extract, Aloe Barbadensis Leaf, Aloe Barbadensis Leaf Extract, Aloe Barbadensis Leaf Juice,aloe Barbadensis Leaf Polysaccharides, Aloe Barbadensis Leaf Water, Aloe Ferox Leaf Extract, Aloe Ferox Leaf Juice, and Aloe Ferox Leaf Juice Extract. *Int. J. Toxicol.,* 26 Suppl 2, 1-50.

Choi, CM; Berson, DS. (2006). Cosmeceuticals. *Semin. Cutan. Med. Surg.*, 25(3), 163-8.

Cho, HS; Lee, MH; Lee, JW; No, KO; Park, SK; Lee, HS; Kang, S; Cho, WG; Park, HJ; Oh, KW; Hong, JT. (2007). Anti-wrinkling effects of the mixture of vitamin C, vitamin E, pycnogenol and evening primrose oil, and molecular mechanisms on hairless mouse skin caused by chronic ultraviolet B irradiation. *Photodermatol. Photoimmunol. Photomed.*, 23(5), 155-62.

Costa, V; Moradas-Ferreira, P. (2001). Oxidative stress and signal transduction in Saccharomyces cerevisiae: insights into ageing, apoptosis and diseases. *Mol. Aspects Med.*, 22, 217-246.

Costello, RB; Moser-Veillon, PB. (1992). A review of magnesium intake in the elderly. A cause for concern? *Magnes. Res.*, 5(1), 61-7.

Craven, NM; Helbling, I; Chadwick, CA; Ferguson, JE; Potten, CS; Griffiths, CEM. (1998).Photoageing is associated with persistence of thymine dimers in epidermis and dermis. *Brit. J. Dermatol*, 138, 724-53.

Crawford, D; Zbinden, I; Amstad, P; Cerutti, P. (1988). Oxidant stress induces the proto-oncogenes cfos and c-myc in mouse epidermal cells. *Oncogene*, 3, 27–32.

Cripps, DJ; Rankin, J.(1973). "Action Spectra of Lupus Erythematosus and Experimental Immunofluorescence," *Arch. Dermatol.*, 107, 563-567.

Cronin, H; Draelos, ZD. (2010). Top 10 botanical ingredients in 2010 anti-aging creams. *J. Cosmet. Dermatol.*, 9(3), 218-25.

Cross, CE; van der Vliet, A; Louie, S; Thiele, JJ; Halliwell, B. (1998). Oxidative stress and antioxidants at biosurfaces: plants, skin, and respiratory tract surfaces. *Environ. Health Perspect.*, 5, 1241-51.

Cross, AJ; Sinha, R. (2006). Impact of Food Preservation, Processing and Cooking on Cancer Risk. In: *Carcinogenic and Anticarcinogenic Food Components*. Baer-Dubowska, W.; Bartoszek, A.; Malejka- Giganti, D. (Eds.).—CRC Press, Taylor & Francis Group, USA, 97-112.

Crowther, JM; Matts, PJ. Measuring water gradients using confocal raman microspectroscopy. In: *Skin moisturization.* (Eds.: Rawlings, AV; Leyden, JJ). Infotma Healthcare, New York, 2009.

Cunningham, ML; Johnson, JS; Giovanazzi, SM; Peak, MJ. (1985).Photosensitized production of superoxide anion by monochromatic (290–405 nm) ultraviolet irradiation of NADH and NADPH coenzymes. *Photochem. Photobiol.*, 42, 125–128.

Cunningham, ML; Krinsky, NI; Giovanazzi, SM; Peak, MJ. (1985). Superoxide anion is generated from cellular metabolites by solar radiation and its components. *Free Radic. Biol. Med.*, 5, 381–385.

Cutchis, P. (1980). A formula for comparing annual damaging ultraviolet (DUV) radiation doses at tropical and mid-latitude sites Final Report FAA-EE 80-21. Washington, DC: U.S. Department of Transportation, Federal Aviation Administration Office of Environment and Energy.

Cutler, RG. Genetic stability, dysdifferentiation, and longevity determinant genes. In: *Critical reviews of oxidative stress and damage.* Cutler RG, Rodriguez H (Eds.). World Scientific, 2003.

Cutler and Mattson. Measuring oxidative stress and interpreting its relevance in humans. In: *Oxidative stress and Aging* (Eds: Cutler RG and Rodriguez, H.). World Scientific, 2003.

Cypser, JR; Johnson, TE. J. (2002). Multiple stressors in Caenorhabditis elegans induce stress hormesis and extended longevity. *J. Gerontol. A Biol. Sci. Med. Sci.*, 57, B109–B114.

Czochralska, B; Bartosz, W; Shugar, D. (1984). Oxidation of excited-state NADH and NAD dimer in aqueous medium - involvement of O2- as a mediator in the presence of oxygen. *Biochim Biophys Acta*, 801, 403-409.

D'Agostini, F; Fiallo, P; Pennisi, TM; De Flora, S. (2007). Chemoprevention of smoke-induced alopecia in mice by oral administration of L-cystine and vitamin B6. *J. Dermatol. Sci.*, 46(3), 189-98.

D'Agostini, F; Balansky, R; Pesce, C; Fiallo, P; Lubet, RA; Kelloff, GJ; De Flora, S. (2000). Induction of alopecia in mice exposed to cigarette smoke. *Toxicol. Lett.*, 114(1-3), 117-23.

D'Almeida, V; Lobo, LL; Hipólide, DC; de Oliveira, AC; Nobrega, JN; Tufik, S. (1998). Sleep deprivation induces brain region-specific decreases in glutathione levels. *Neuroreport.*, 9(12), 2853-6.

Dalle Carbonare, M; Pathak, MA. (1992). Skin photosensitizing agents and the role of reactive oxygen species in photoaging. *J. Photochem. Photobiol. B.*, 14(1-2), 105-24.

Dalton, TP; Shertzer, HG; Puga, A. (1999). Regulation of gene expression by reactive oxygen. *Annu. Rev. Pharmacol. Toxicol.*, 39, 67-101.

Damian, DL. (2010). Photoprotective effects of nicotinamide. *Photochem. Photobiol. Sci.*, 9(4), 578-85.

Danby, FW. (2010). Nutrition and aging skin: sugar and glycation. *Clin. Dermatol.*, 28(4), 409-11.

D'Andrea, G. (2010). Pycnogenol: A blend of procyanidins with multifaceted therapeutic applications? *Fitoterapia*. [Epub ahead of print].

Danielczyk, K; Dziegiel, P. (2009). The expression of MT1 melatonin receptor and Ki-67 antigen in melanoma malignum. *Anticancer Res.*, 29(10), 3887-95.

Darr, D; Fridovich, I. (1994). Free radicals in cutaneous biology. *J. Invest. Dermatol*, 102, 671–675.

Darvin, ME; Fluhr, JW; Meinke, MC; Zastrow, L; Sterry, W; Lademann, J. (2011). Topical beta-carotene protects against infra-red-light-induced free radicals. *Exp. Dermatol.*, 20(2):125-9. doi: 10.1111/j.1600-0625.2010.01191.x.

Date, A; Hakozaki, T. In vitro method to visualize UV-induced reactive oxygen species in a skin equivalent model. In: *Textbook of aging skin* (Farage, MA; Miller, KW; Maibach, HI. (Eds). Springer-Verlag, Berlin, 2010.

Date, A; Hakozaki, T; Yoshii, T; Yasui, H; Sakurai, H. (2006). Detection and identification of reactive oxygen species and followed free radicals generated in the UVB-exposed three-dimensional human epidermal cells-EpidermTM as measured by spin-trapping method. In: The 126th annual meeting of pharmaceutical society of Japan, Sendai, Japan (2006), pp 28.

Dayan, D; Abrahami, I; Buchner, A; Gorsky, M; Chimowitz, N. (1988). Lipid pigment (lipofuscin) in humanperioral muscles with aging. *Exp. Gerontol.*, 23, 97–102.

Daynes, RA; Spellman, CW; Woodward, JG; Stewart, DA. (1977). Studies into the Transplantation Biology of Ultraviolet-Induced Tumors." *Transplantation*, 23, 343-348.

Davies, KJ. (1995). Oxidative stress: the paradox of aerobic life. *Biochem. Soc. Symp.*, 61, 1-31.

Dawkins, R. *The Selfish Gene*. Oxford: Oxford University Press, 1976.

Dawkins, R. *The Extended Phenotype*. Oxfordshire: Oxford University Press, 1999.

Dawkins, R. *The Extended Phenotype: The long Reach of the Gene.* Oxford, New York: Oxford University Press, 1982/1999.

Dawkins, R. *The Selfish Gene.* Sebični gen. Ljubljana: Mladinska knjiga, 1976/2006

DeFabo, EC; Noonan, FP. (1983). Mechanism of immune suppression by ultraviolet irradiationin vivo. I. Evidence for the existence of a unique photoreceptor in skin and its role in photoimmunology. *J. Exp. Med.,*158, 84-98.

De Grey, ADNJ. (2005). Reactive Oxygen Species Production in the Mitochondrial Matrix: Implications for the Mechanism of Mitochondrial Mutation Accumulation. *Rejuvenation Res.*, 8(1), 13-7.

De Grey, ADNJ; Rae, M. *Ending Aging.* New York, St. Martin's Griffin,2007.

de Luca, C; Deeva, I; Mikhal'Chik, E; Korkina, L. (2007). Beneficial effects of pro-antioxidant-based nutraceuticals in the skin rejuvenation techniques. *Cell Mol. Biol.* (Noisy-le-grand), 53(1), 94-101.

De Magalhaes, JP; Church, GM. (2006). Cells discover fire: employing reactive oxygen species in development and consequences for aging. *Exp. Gerontol.*, 41, 1-10.

Demin, OV; Kholodenko, BN; Skulachev, VP. (1998). A model of O2.-generation in the complex III of the electron transport chain. *Mol. Cell Biochem.*, 184(1-2), 21-33.

De Paepe, K; Rogiers, V. Glycerol as humectant in cosmetic formulations. In: *Skin moisturization.* (Eds.: Rawlings AV and Leyden JJ). *Infotma Healthcare*, New York, 2009.

De Polo, KF. Moisturizers and humectants. In: De Polo, KF (ed). *A short textbook of cosmetology.* Augsburg: Verlag fur Chemische Industrie, H. Ziolkowsky GmbH, 1998, 134-148.

De Wit, R; Capello, A; Boonstra; Verkleij, AJ, Post, JA. (2000). Hydrogen proxide inhibits epidermal growth factor receptor internalization in human fibroblasts. *Free Rad. Biol.Med*, 28, 28-38.

Delehedde, M; Cho, SH; Sarkiss, M; Brisbay, S; Davies, M; El-Naggar, AK; McDonnell, TJ. (1999). Altered expression of bcl-2 family member proteins in nonmelanoma skin cancer. *Cancer.*, 85(7),1514-22.

Demaison, L; Sergiel, JP; Moreau, D; Grynberg, A. (1994). Influence of the phospholipid n-6/n-3 polyunsaturated fatty acid ratio on the mitochondrial oxidative metabolism before and after myocardial ischemia. *Biochim. Biophys. Acta*, 1227, 53.

Demetrius, L. (2006). Aging in mouse and human systems: a comparative study. *Ann. N.Y. Acad. Sci.*, 1067, 66-82.

Demierre, MF; Brooks, D; Koh, HK; Geller, AC. (1999). "Public knowledge, awareness, and perceptions of the association between skin aging and smoking." *Journal of the American Academy of Dermatology*, 41(1), 27-30.

Demmig-Adams, B; Adams, WW. (2002). Antioxidants in photosynthesis and human nutrition. *Science*, 298(5601), 2149-2153.

Denda, M; Tsuchiya, T; Elias, PM. et al. (2000). Stress alters cutaneous permeability barrier homeostasis. *Am. J. Physiol. Regul. Integr. Comp. Physiol*, 278(2), R367-R372.

Dhahbi, JM; Kim, HJ; Mote, PL; Beaver, RJ; Spindler, SR. (2004). Temporal linkage between the phenotypic and genomic responses to caloric restriction. *Proc. Natl. Acad. Sci. U.S.A.*, 101, 5524-5529.

Dietary Reference Intakes for Vitamin A, Vitamin K, Arsenic, Boron, Chromium, Copper, Iodine, Iron, Manganese, Molybdenum, Nickel, Silicon, Vanadium, and Zinc, Chapter 4, Vitamin A.Food and Nutrition Board of the Institute of Medicine, 2001.

Diffey, BL. (2010). Is casual exposure to summer sunlight effective at maintaining adequate vitamin D status?*Photodermatol. Photoimmunol. Photomed.*, 26(4), 172-6.

Diffey, BL; Farr, PM. (1988). The action spectrum in drug-induced photosensitivityPhotochem.*Photobiol.*, 47, 49-54.

Diffey, BL. (1991). Solar ultraviolet radiation effects on biological systems. *Review in Physics in Medicine and Biology*, 36(3), 299-328.

Diplock, AT; Charleux, JL; Crozier-Willi, G; Kok, FJ; Rice-Evans, C; Roberfroid, M; Stahl, W; Viña-Ribes, J. (1998). Functional food science and defense against reactive oxidative species. *Br. J. Nutr.*, 80(1), S77-112.

Dirks, AJ; Leeuwenburgh, C. (2006). Calorie restriction in humans: potential pitfalls and health concerns. *Mech. Ageing Dev.*, 127,1–7.

Doda, DD; Green, AE. (1981). Surface reflection measurements in the UV from an airborne platform. Part 2 *Appl. Opt.*, 20, 636-42.

Donath, AS. Facial rejuvenation: a chronology of procedures. In: Farage, MA;, Miller, KW; Maibach, HI. *Textbook of aging skin*. Berlin: Springer-Verlag, 2010.

Dong, KK; Damaghi, N; Picart, SD; Markova, NG; Obayashi, K; Okano, Y; Masaki, H; Grether-Beck, S; Krutmann, J; Smiles, KA; Yarosh, DB. (2008). UV-induced DNA damage initiates release of MMP-1 in human skin.*Exp Dermatol.*, 17(12):1037-44.

Donofrio, LM. (2000). Fat distribution: a morphologic study of the aging face. *Dermatol Surg*,26, 1107-1112.

Doshi, D; Hanneman, K; Cooper, K. (2007). Smoking and skin aging in identical twins. *Arch Dermatol*, 143, 1543-1546.

Draelos, ZD. (2009). Cosmeceuticals: undefined, unclassified, and unregulated. *Clin Dermatol.*, 27(5), 431-4.

Dreher, F; Denig, N; Gabard, B; Schwindt, DA; Maibach, HI. (1999). Effect of topical antioxidants on UV-induced erythema formation when administered after exposure. *Dermatology.*, 198(1), 52-5.

Dreher, F; Gabard, B; Schwindt, DA; Maibach, HI. (1998). Topical melatonin in combination with vitamins E and C protects skin from ultraviolet-induced erythema: a human study in vivo. *Br. J. Dermatol.*, 139(2), 332-9.

Dreher, F; Maibach, H. (2001). Protective effects of topical antioxidants in humans. *Curr. Probl. Dermatol.*, 29, 157-64.

Duan, W; Guo, Z; Jiang, H; Ware, M; Mattson, MP. (2003). Reversal of behavioral and metabolic abnormalities, and insulin resistance syndrome, by dietary restriction in mice deficient in brain-derived neurotrophic factor. *Endocrinology.*, 144(6), 2446-53.

Duan, W; Guo, Z; Jiang, H; Ware, M; Li, XJ; Mattson, MP. (2003). Dietary restriction normalizes glucose metabolism and BDNF levels, slows disease progression, and increases survival in huntingtin mutant mice. *Proc. Natl. Acad. Sci.* USA,100(5), 2911-6.

Duan, W; Lee, J; Guo, Z; Mattson, MP. (2001). Dietary restriction stimulates BDNF production in the brain and thereby protects neurons against excitotoxic injury. *J. Mol. Neurosci.*, 16(1), 1-12.

Duan, W; Mattson, MP. (1999). Dietary restriction and 2-deoxyglucose administration improve behavioral outcome and reduce degeneration of dopaminergic neurons in models of Parkinson's disease. *J. Neurosci. Res.*, 57(2), 195-206.

Duffy, P; Feuers, RJ; Leaky, JFA; Hart, RW. (1987). Chronic caloric restriction in old female mice: changes in the circadian rhythms and physiological and behavioral parameters. In: *Biological effects of caloric restriction.* Fishbein, L. Ed. New York: Springer, 1987.

Dumas, M; Berville, R; Barré, P; Bonté; Meybeck, A. (1994). *In vitro processing of melanosomes by normal human keratinosytes.* 18th IFSCC Congress, Venice, 1994.

Dunn, AL; Marcus, BH; Kampert, JB; Garcia, ME; Kohl, HW 3rd; Blair, SN. (1999). Comparison of lifestyle and structured interventions to increase physical activity and cardiorespiratory fitness: a randomized trial. *JAMA.*, 281(4), 327-34.

Early Detection and Treatment of Skin Cancer. American Family Physician. July 15, 2000. http://www.aafp.org/afp/20000715/357.html. Retrieved 2010-02-08.

Eberlein-König, B; Placzek, M; Przybilla, B. (1998). Protective effect against sunburn of combined systemic ascorbic acid (vitamin C) and d-alpha-tocopherol (vitamin E). *J. Am. Acad. Dermatol*, 38, 45–8.

Echtay, KS; Murphy, MP; Smith, RA; Talbot, DA; Brand, MD. (2002). Superoxide activates mitochondrial uncoupling protein 2 from the matrix side. *J. Biol. Chem.*, 277, 47129-47135.

Elias, PM; Feingold, KR. (1992). Lipids and the epidermal water barrier: metabolism, regulation, and pathophysiology. *Semin. Dermatol*, 11, 176–182.

Elias, PM; Ghadially, R. (2002). The aged epidermal permeability barrier: basis for functional abnormalities. *Clin. Geriatr. Med*, 18, 103-120.

Elias, PM. (1996). Stratum corneum architecture, metabolic activity and interactivity with subjacent cell layers. *Exp. Dermatol*, 5, 191–201.

Elmore, AR. (2005). Final report of the safety assessment of L-Ascorbic Acid, Calcium Ascorbate, Magnesium Ascorbate, Magnesium Ascorbyl Phosphate, Sodium Ascorbate, and Sodium Ascorbyl Phosphate as used in cosmetics. *Int. J. Toxicol.*, 24(2), 51-111.

Elosua, R; Demissie, S; Cupples, LA; Meigs, JB; Wilson, PW; Schaefer, EJ; Corella, D; Ordovas, JM. (2003). Obesity modulates the association among APOE genotype, insulin, and glucose in man. *Obes. Res.*, 11, 1502-1508.

Enerbäck, S. (2009). The origins of brown adipose tissue. *N. Engl. J. Med.*, 360 (19): 2021–2023.

Engelke, M; Jensen, JM; Ekanayake-Mudiyanselage, S; et al. (1997). Effects of xerosis and ageing on epidermal proliferation and differentiation. *Br. J. Dermatol*, 137, 219-225.

Epel, ES; Blackburn, EH; Lin, J; Dhabhar, FS; Adler, NE; Morrow, JD; Cawthon, RM. (2004). Accelerated telomere shortening in response to life stress. *Proc. Natl. Acad. Sci. USA*,101(49), 17312-5.

Epel, ES. (2009). Psychological and metabolic stress: a recipe for accelerated cellular aging? *Hormones* (Athens)., 8(1), 7-22.

Esposito, K; Di Palo, C; Maiorino, MI; Petrizzo, M; Bellastella, G; Siniscalchi, I; Giugliano, D. (2010). Long-term effect of Mediterranean-style diet and calorie restriction on biomarkers of longevity and oxidative stress in overweight men. *Cardiol. Res. Pract.*, 2011, 293916.

Epstein, J; Gershon, D. (1972). Studies on aging in nematodes, IV. The effect of antioxidants on cellular damage and lifespan. *Mech. Ageing Dev.*, 1, 257-264.

Ernster, LF; Orsmark-Andree, P. (1993). Ubiquinol-10: an endogenous antioxidant in aerobic organisms. *Clin. Invest*, 71, S60-S65.

Ernster, VL; Grady, D; Miike, R; Black, D; Selby, J; Kerlikowske, K. (1995) Facial wrinkling in men and women, by smoking status. *Am. J. Public Health*, 85, 78–82.

Errera, M. (1952). Etude photochemique de l'acide désoxyribonucleique I. Mesures énergétiques Biochim. *Biophys. Acta*, 8, 30-7.

Eskiocak, S; Gozen, AS; Yapar, SB; Tavas, F; Kilic, AS; Eskiocak, M. (2005). Glutathione and free sulphydryl content of seminal plasma in healthy medical students during and after exam stress. *Hum. Reprod.*, 20(9), 2595-600.

Evans, EM; Racette, SB; Peterson, LR; Villareal, DT; Greiwe, JS; Holloszy, JO. (2005). Aerobic power and insulin action improve in response to endurance exercise training in healthy 77–87 yr olds. *J. Appl. Physiol.*, 98, 40 - 45.

Evans, MD; Dizdaroglu, M; Cooke, MS. (2004). Oxidative DNA damage and disease: induction, repair and significance. *Mutat. Res.*, 567, 1–61.

Facchini, FS. (1998). Effect of phlebotomy on plasma glucose and insulin concentrations. *Diabetes Care.*, 21(12), 2190.

Facchini, FS; Saylor, KL. (2002). Effect of iron depletion on cardiovascular risk factors: studies in carbohydrate-intolerant patients. *Ann N Y Acad Sci.,* 967, 342-51.

Fagot, D; Asselineau, D; Bernerd, F. (2002). Direct role of human dermal fibroblastsand indirect participation of epidermal keratinocytes in MMP-1 production after UVB irradiation. *Arch. Dermatol Res*, 293, 576-83.

Fang, YZ; Yang, S; Wu, GY. (2002). Free radicals, antioxidants, and nutrition. *Nutrition*, 18, 872-879.

Farage, MA; Miller, KW; Elsner, P; Maibach, HI. (2008). Intrinsic and extrinsic factors in skin ageing: a review. *Int. J. Cosmet. Sci.*, 30(2), 87-95.

Farage, MA; Miller, KW; Maibach, HI. Degenerative changes in aging skin. In: *Textbook of skin aging*. Farage, MA; Miller, KW; Maibach, HI. (Eds). Springer-Verlag, berlin, 2010.

Farkas, B; Csete, B; Magyarlaki, M; Bernath, S; Sümegi, B. (2002).Topical poly(ADP-ribose) polymerase (PARP) regulator and its prospects for use, *Ann. Dermatol. Venerol*, 129, 1S91.

Farman, JC; Gardiner, BG; Shaklin, JD. (1985). Large losses of total ozone in Antarctica reveal seasonal ClOx/NOx interaction.*Nature*, 315, 207-10.

Farris, P. (2007). Idebenone, green tea, and Coffeeberry extract: new and innovative antioxidants. *Dermatol. Ther.*, 20(5), 322-9.

Feig, DI; Reid, TM; Loeb, LA. (1994). Reactive oxygen species in tumorigenesis. *Cancer Res.*, 54(7), 18902–18904.

Feldman, D; Bryce, GF; Shapiro, SS. (1990). Mitochondrial inclusions in keratinocytes of hairless mouse skin exposed to UVB radiation. *J. Cutan. Pathol.*, 17(2), 96-100.

Felton, JS; Knize, MG; Bennett, LM; Malfatti, MA; Colvin, ME; Kulp, KS. (2004). Impact of environmental exposures on the mutagenicity/carcinogenicity of heterocyclic amines. *Toxicology.*, 198(1-3), 135-45.

Fenske, NA; Lober, CW. (1986). Continuing and functional changes of normal aging skin*J. Amer. Dermatol*, 15, 571-85.

Fernández-Real, JM; López-Bermejo, A; Ricart, W. (2002). Cross-talk between iron metabolism and diabetes. *Diabetes.*, 51(8), 2348-54.

Filipe, P; Silva, JN; Haigle, J; Freitas, JP; Fernandes, A; Santus, R; Morlière, P. (2005). Contrasting action of flavonoids on phototoxic effects induced in human skin fibroblasts by UVA alone or UVA plus cyamemazine, a phototoxic neuroleptic. *Photochem. Photobiol. Sci.*, 4(5), 420-8.

Finch, CE. *The biology of human longevity*. Elsevier, Amsterdam, 2007.

Finkel, T; Nikki, J. Holbrook. (2000). Oxidants, oxidative stress and the biology of ageing. *Nature*, 408, 239-247.

Fischer, T; Bangha, E; Elsner, P; Kistler, GS. (1999). Suppression of UV-induced erythema by topical treatment with melatonin. Influence of the application time point.*Biol. Signals Recept.*, 8(1-2), 132-5.

Fischer, TW; Slominski, A; Zmijewski, MA; Reiter, RJ; Paus, R. (2008). Melatonin as a major skin protectant: from free radical scavenging to DNA damage repair. *Exp. Dermatol.*, 17(9), 713-30.

Fisher, GJ; Kang, S; Varani, J; Bata-Csorgo, Z; Wan, Y; Datta, S; Voorhees, JJ. (2002). Mechanisms of photoaging and chronological skin aging. *Arch. Dermatol.*, 138(11), 1462-70.

Fisher, GJ. (2005). "The Pathophysiology of Photoaging of the Skin." *Cutis*, 75(2S), 5-9.

Fisher, MS; Kripke ML. (1977). Systemic Alteration Induced in Mice by Ultraviolet Light Irradiation and its Relationship to Ultraviolet Carcinogenesis," *Proc. Natl. Acad. Sci. USA,*74, 1688-1692.

Fisher, GJ; Voorhees, JJ. (1998). Molecular mechanisms of photoaging and its prevention by retinoic acid: ultraviolet irradiation induces MAP kinase signal transduction cascades that induce Ap-1-regulated matrix metalloproteinases that degrade human skin in vivo. *J. Investig. Dermatol. Symp. Proc.*, 3(1), 61-8.

Fisher, GJ; Wang, ZQ; Datta, SC; Talwar, HS; Wang, ZQ; Varani, J; Kang, S; Voorhees, JJ. (1996). Molecular basis of sun-induced premature skin ageing and retinoid antagonism. *Nature*, 379, 335-9.

Fisher, GJ; Wang, ZQ; Datta, SC; Varani, J; Kang, S; Voorhees, JJ. (1997). Pathophysiology of premature skin aging induced by ultraviolet light. *N. Engl. J. Med*, 337, 1419-28.

Fisher,TW; Elsner, P. (2001). The antioxidative potential of melatonin in the skin. *Curr. Probl. Dermatol*, 29, 165-174.

Fisher, GJ; Datta, SC; Talwar, HS; Wang, ZQ; Varani, J; Kang, S., et al. (1996). Molecular basis of sun-induced premature skin ageing and retinoid antagonism. *Nature*, 379(6563), 335-339.

Fitzpatrick, RE; Rostan, EF. (2002). Double-blind, half-face study comparing topical vitamin C and vehicle for rejuvenation of photodamage. *Dermatol. Surg.*, 28(3), 231-6.

Fitzpatrick, TB. (1975). Soleil et peau. *J. Med. Esthet.*, 2, 33-4.

Fitzpatrick, TB; Szabo, G; Wick MW. (1983). *Biochemistry and physiology of melanin pigmentationBiochemistry and Physiology of the Skin*. Goldsmith, LA (Ed.). Oxford: Oxford University Press, 1983, pp 687-712.

Fitzpatrick, TB. (1988). The validity and practicality of sun-reactive skin types I through VI. *Arch. Dermatol*, 124(6), 869-71.

Fleming, DJ; Tucker, KL; Jacques, PF; Dallal, GE; Wilson, PW; Wood, RJ. (2002). Dietary factors associated with the risk of high iron stores in the elderly Framingham Heart Study cohort. *Am. J. Clin. Nutr.*, 76, 1375-84.

Floyd, RA. Measurement of oxidative stress in vivo. In: *The Oxygen paradox*. Cleup University Press. Padova, 1995, 89-103.

Fonager, J; Beedholm, R; Clark, BF; Rattan, SI. (2002). Mild stress-induced stimulation of heat-shock protein synthesis and improved functional ability of human fibroblasts undergoing aging in vitro. *Exp. Gerontol.*, 37(10-11), 1223-8.

Fontana, L; Klein, S. (2007). Aging, Adiposity, and Calorie Restriction.*Jama*, 297, 986-994.

Fontella, FU; Siqueira, IR; Vasconcellos, AP; Tabajara, AS; Netto, CA; Dalmaz, C. (2005). Repeated restraint stress induces oxidative damage in rat hippocampus. *Neurochem. Res.*, 30(1), 105-11.

Forlenza, MJ. (2002). Relationship between psychological stress and oxidative stress in victims of motor vehicle accidents. Doctor's dissertation. University of Pittsburgh, 2002.

Forlenza, MJ; Latimer, JJ; Baum, A. (2000). The Effects of Stress on DNA Repair. *Psychology and Health: An International Journal*, 15, 881-981.

Forman, HJ; Boveris, A. Superoxide radical and hydrogen peroxide in mitochondria. In: Pryor, E. *Free Radicals in Biology*. New York: Academic Press, 1982, 65-90.

Fortes, C; Mastroeni, S; Melchi, F; Pilla, MA; Antonelli, G; Camaioni, D; Alotto, M; Pasquini, P. (2008). A protective effect of the Mediterranean diet for cutaneous melanoma. *Int. J. Epidemiol.*, 37(5), 1018-29.

Fox, GN; Sabovic, Z. (1998). Chromium picolinate supplementation for diabetes mellitus. *J. Fam. Pract.*, 46(1), 83-6.

Fraga, CG; Motchnik, PA; Shigenaga, MK; Helbock, HJ; Jacob, RA; Ames, BN. (1991). Ascorbic acid protects against endogenous oxidative DNA damage in human sperm. *Proc. Natl. Acad. Sci.* USA, 88(24), 11003-6.

Fraga, CG; Oteiza, PI. (2002). Iron toxicity and antioxidant nutrients. *Toxicology*, 180, 23-32.

Frankenberg, D; Frankenberg-Schwager, M; Harbich, R. (1993). Mechanisms of oxygen radiosensitization in irradiated yeast. I. DNA double-strand breakage. *Int. J. Radiat. Biol.*, 64(5), 511-21.

Franzoni, F; Plantinga, Y; Femia, FR; Bartolomucci, F; Gaudio, C; Regoli, F; Carpi, A; Santoro, G; Galetta, F. (2004). Plasma antioxidant activity and cutaneous microvascular endothelial function in athletes and sedentary controls. *Biomed. Pharmacother.*, 58(8), 432-6.

Frances, C. (1998) Smoker's wrinkles: epidemiological and pathogenic considerations. *Clin. Dermatol,* 16, 565–570.

Frederick, JE. (1990). Trends in atmospheric ozone and ultraviolet radiation: mechanisms and observations for the Northern Hemisphere. *Photochem. Photobiol.*, 51, 757-63.

Frederick, JE; Snell, HE; Haywood, EK. (1989). Solar ultraviolet radiation at the earth's surface Photochem. *Photobiol.*, 50, 443-50.

Frei, B. (1999). On the role of vitamin C and other antioxidants in atherogenesis and vascular dysfunction. *Proc. Soc. Exp. Biol. Med.*, 222, 196-204.

Frei, B; England, L; Ames, BN. (1989). Ascorbate is an outstanding antioxidant in human blood plasma. *Proc. Natl. Acad. Sci. USA*, 86, 6377–6381.

Freifelder, D. (1987). Molecular Biology 2nd edn. Boston: Jones and Bartlett, pp 277-92.

Friedberg, EC; McDaniel, LD; Schultz, RA. (1995). *DNA repair and mutagenesis*. ASM Press, Washington, 1995.

Frye, RA. (2000). Phylogenetic classification of prokaryotic and eucaryotic Sir2-like proteins. *Biochemical & Biophysical Research Communications*, 273, 793-798.

Fu, MX; Wells-Knecht, KJ; Blackledge, JA; Lyons, TJ; Thorpe, SR; Baynes, JW. (1994).Glycation, glycoxidation, and cross-linking of collagen by glucose. Kinetics, mechanisms, and inhibition of late stages of the Maillard reaction. *Diabetes.*, 43(5), 676-83.

Fuch, J;Podda, M;Zollner, T. Redox Modulation and Oxidative Stress in Dermatotoxicology. In: *Environmental stressors in health and disease* (Ed. Fuchs, J; Packer, L.). Marcel Dekker, Inc.,2001.

Fuchs, J. (ed.) *Oxidative Injury in Dermatopathology. Heidelberg*: Springer Verlag, 1992.

Fuchs, J; Huflejt, M; Rothfuss, L; Carcamero, G; Packer, L. (1989). Impairment of enzymic and nonenzymic antioxidants in skin by UVB irradiation. *J. Invest. Dermatol.*, 93, 769-773.

Fuchs, J; Huflejt, ME; Rothfuss, LM; Wilson, DS; Carano, G; Packer, L. (1989). Acute effects on near ultraviolet and visible light on the cutaneous antioxidant defense system. *Photochem. Photobiol.*, 50(6), 739–744.

Fuchs, J; Kern, H. (1989). Modulation of UV-light-induced skin inflammation by D-alpha-tocopherol and L-ascorbic acid: a clinical study using solar simulated radiation. *Free Radic. Biol. Med.*, 25, 1006–12.

Fuchs, J.Dermatotoxicology of Environmental and Occupational Chemical Hazards: Agents and Action. In: *Environmental stressors in health and disease* (Ed. Fuchs J and Packer L.). Marcel Dekker, Inc.,2001

Fuchs, J; Milbradt, R. (1994). Antioxidant inhibition of skin inflammation induced by reactive oxidants. *Skin. Pharmacol.*, 7, 278-84.

Fuller, B; Smith, D; Howerton, A; Kern, D. (2006). Anti-inflammatory effects of CoQ10 and colorless carotenoids. *J. Cosmet. Dermatol.*, 5(1), 30-8.

Gaetke, LM; Chow, CK. (2003). Copper toxicity, oxidative stress, and antioxidant nutrients. *Toxicology.*, 189(1-2), 147-63.

Gallagher, RP; Spinelli, JJ; Lee, TK. (2005).Tanning beds, sunlamps, and risk and risk of cutaneous malignant melanoma. *Cancer Epidemiol. Biomarkers Prev*, 14, 562-566.

Gao, P. (2007). HIF-dependent antitumorigenic effect of antioxidants in vivo. *Cancer Cell*, 12, 230–238.

Garmyn, M; Ribaya-Mercado, JD; Russel, RM; Bhawan, J; Gilchrest, BA. (1995). Effect of beta-carotene supplementation on the human sunburn reaction. *Exp. Dermatol*, 4, 104–11.

Gems, D; Partridge, L. (2008). "Stress-Response Hormesis and Aging: 'That which Does Not Kill Us Makes Us Stronger.'" *Cell Metabolism*, 7, 200–203.

Gerritsen, ME; Carley, WW; Ranges, GE; Shen, CP; Phan, SA; Ligon, GF; Perry, CA. (1995).Flavonoids inhibit cytokine-induced endothelial cell adhesion protein gene expression. *Am. J. Pathol.*, 147(2), 278-92.

Gensler, HL; Watson, RR; Moriguchi, S; Bowden, GT. (1987). Effects of dietary retinyl palmitate or 13-cis-retinoic acid on the promotion of tumors in mouse skin. *Cancer Res.*, 47(4), 967-70.

Ghadially, R; Brown, BE; Hanley, K; Reed, JT; Feingold, KR; Elias, PM. (1996). Decreased epidermal lipid synthesis accounts for altered barrier function in aged mice. *J. Invest. Dermatol.*,106, 1064–1069.

Ghadially, R; Brown, BE; Sequeira-Martin, SM; Feingold, KR; Elias, PM. (1995). The aged epidermal permeability barrier. Structural, functional, and lipid biochemical abnormalities in humans and a senescent murine model. *J. Clin. Invest.*, 95, 2281–2290.

Giacomoni, PU; Rein, G. Skin aging: a generalization of the micro-inflammatory hypothesis. In: Farage, MA; Miller, KW; Maibach, HI. (eds). *Textbook of aging skin*. Berlin: Springer-Verlag, 2010.

Gibbons, LW; Mitchell, TL; Wei, M; Blair, SN; Cooper, KH. (2000). Maximal exercise test as a predictor of risk for mortality from coronary heart disease in asymptomatic men. *Am. J. Cardiol.*, 86(1), 53-8.

Gilbert, DL. *Oxygen and living processes: an interdisciplinary approach*. Springer Verlag: New York, 1981.

Gilca, M; Stoian, I; Atanasiu, V; Virgolici, B. (2007). The oxidative hypothesis of senescence. *J. Postgrad. Med.*, 53(3): 207-213.

Gilchrest, BA; Krutmann, *J. Skin aging*. Heidelberg: Springer; 2006. 198 p;

Gilchrest, BA. (1998). Overview of skin aging. *J. Cut. Aging & Cos. Derm*, 1(1), 1-2

Gilchrest, BA. (1997). Treatment of photodamage with topical tretinoin: an overview. *J. Am. Acad. Dermatol.*, 36(3 Pt 2), S27-36.

Gilchrest, BA. (1990). Skin aging and photoaging. *Dermatology Nursing*, 2 (2), 79-82.

Gilchrest, P; Schieke, S; Morita, A. Premature skin aging by infrared radiation, tobacco smoke and ozone. In: *Skin aging*. (Gilchrest, B; Krutmann, J. (Eds.). Springer-Verlag, Berlin 2006.

Green, LJ. *The dermatologist's guide to looking younger*. Freedom, CA: Crossing Press; 1999. 134 p.

Giles, RE; Blanc, H; Cann, HM; Wallace, DC. (1980). Maternal inheritance of human mitochondrial DNA. *Proc. Natl. Acad. Sci.* USA, 77(11), 6715-9.

Gilliver, SC; Ashworth, JJ; Ashcroft, GS. (2007). The hormonal regulation of cutaneous wound healing. *Clin. Dermatol.*, 25(1), 56-62.

Gilliver, SC; Wu, F; Ashcroft, GS. (2003). Regulatory roles of androgens in cutaneous wound healing. *Thromb Haemost.*, 90(6), 978-85.

Giltay, EJ; Geleijnse, JM; Zitman, FG; Buijsse, B; Kromhout, D. (2007). Lifestyle and dietary correlates of dispositional optimism in men: The Zutphen Elderly Study. *J. Psychosom. Res.*, 63(5), 483-90.

Giltay, EJ; Geleijnse, JM; Zitman, FG; Hoekstra, T; Schouten, EG. (2004). Dispositional optimism and all-cause and cardiovascular mortality in a prospective cohort of elderly Dutch men and women. *Arch. Gen. Psychiatry.*, 61(11), 1126-35.

Girondot, M; Garcia, J. Senescence and longevity in turtles: What telomeres tell us. In.: Miaud C, Guye´tant R. 9th Extraordinary Meeting of the Europea Societas Herpetologica, Chambe´ ry, France, 1999, 25–29.

GISSI-Prevenzione Investigators. (1999). Dietary supplementation with n-3 polyunsaturated fatty acids and vitamin E after myocardial infarction: results of the GISSI-Prevenzione trial. *Lancet*, 354, 447-55.

Glauce Socorro de Barros, V; Luzia Kalyne A; Leal M; Juvenia Bezerra Fontenele. Role of plant extracts and polyphenolic compounds in oxidative stress-related diseases. In: *Handbook of Free Radicals: Formation, Types and Effects*. Kozyrev, D; Slutsky, V. (eds.) New York: Nova Science Publishers, Inc., 2010.

Glick, JL. (1990). Dementias: the role of magnesium deficiency and a hypothesis concerning the pathogenesis of Alzheimer's disease. *Med. Hypotheses.*, 31(3), 211-25.

Glogau, RG. (2003). Systemic evaluation of the aging face. In: Bolognia JL, Jorizzo JL, Rapini RP, editors.*Dermatology*. Edinburgh: Mosby, 2003, p. 2357–60.

Glogau RG. Chemical peeling and aging skin. *J. Geriatr. Dermatol.* 1994.

Gniadecka, M; Nielsen, OF; Wessel, S; Heidenheim, M; Christensen, DH; Wulf, HC. (1998). Water and protein structure in photoaged and chronically aged skin, *J. Invest. Dermatol*, 111, 1129-33.

Gniadecka, M; Wulf, HC; Mortensen, NN; Poulsen T. (1996). Photoprotection in vitiligo and normal skin. A quantitative assessment of the role of stratum corneum viable epidermis and pigmentation. *Acta Derm. Venereol.*, 76, 429–32.

Godar, DE. (2005). UV doses worldwide. *Photochem. Photobiol.*, 81(4), 736-49.

Golden, T; Morten, K; Johnson, F; Samper, E; Melov, S. Mitochondria: A critical role in aging. In: *Handbook of the biology of aging*. Sixthedition. Ed: Masoro, EJ; Austad, S. Elsevier, 2006.

Goldhammer, E; Tanchilevitch A, Maor, I; Beniamini, Y; Rosenchein, U; Sagiv, M. (2005). Exercise training modulates cytokinesactivity in coronary heart disease patients. *Int. J. Cardiol.*, 100, 93-99.

Goldstein, S; Moerman, EJ; Porter, K. (1984). High-voltage electron microscopy of human diploid fibroblasts during ageing in vitro. Morphometric analysis of mitochondria. *Exp Cell Res.*, 154(1), 101-11.

Gollnick, HPM; Hopfenmuller, W; Hemmes, C; et al. (1996). Systemic beta-carotene plus topical UVsunscreen are an optimal protection against harmful effects of natural UV sunlight: results of the Berlin-Eilath study. *Eur. J. Dermatol.*, 6, 200–5.

Goodrick, CL. (1980). Effects of long-term voluntary wheel exercise on male and female Wistar rats. *Gerontology*, 26, 22-23.

Goswami, A; Dikshit, P; Mishra, A; Mulherkar, S; Nukina, N; Jana, NR. (2006). Oxidative stress promotes mutant huntingtin aggregation and mutant huntingtin-dependent cell death by mimicking proteasomal malfunction. *Biochem. Biophys. Res. Commun.*, 342, 184–190.

Goto, S; Radak, Z; Takahasi, R. Biological implications of protein oxidation. In: *Critical review of oxidative stress and aging* (Eds: Cutler, R and Rodriguez, H). World Scientific, New Jersey, 2003

Goukassian, D; Gad, F; Yaar, M; Eller, MS; Nehal, US; Gilchrest, BA. (2000). Mechanisms and implications of age-associated decrease in DNA repair capacity. *FASEB J.*,14, 1325-1334.

Grady, D; Ernster, V. (1992). Does cigarette smoking make you ugly and old? *Am. J. Epidemiol.* 135, 839–842.

Graedel, TE; Crutzen, Paul J; Freeman, WH. (1993). Atmospheric Change: An Earth System Perspective. *J. Chem. Educ.*, 70 (9), p A252.

Grant, WB; Garland CF; Holick, MF. (2005). Comparisons of estimated economic burdens due to insufficient solar ultraviolet irradiance and vitamin D and excess solar UV irradiance for the United States. *Photochem. Photobiol.*, 81, 1276-1286.

Greco, M; Villani, G; Mazzucchelli, F; Bresolin, N; Papa, S; Attardi, G. (2003). Marked aging-related decline in efficiency of oxidative phosphorylation in human skin fibroblasts. *FASEB J.*, 17(12), 1706-8.

Gredilla, R; Barja, G. (2003). Mitochondrial oxidative stress and caloric restriction. *Advances in cell aging and gerontology*, 14, 105-122.

Gredilla, R; Sanz, A; Lopez-Torres, M; Barja, G. (2001). Caloric restriction decreases mitochondrial free radical generation at complex I and lowers oxidative damage to mitochondrial DNA in the rat heart. *Faseb J.,* 15, 1589-1591.

Green, GA. (2008). "Review: antioxidant supplements do not reduce all-cause mortality in primary or secondary prevention." *Evid. Based Med.,* 2008 13 (6): 177.

Green, PS; Gridley, KE; Simpkins, JW. (1998). Nuclear estrogen receptor-independent neuroprotection by estratrienes: a novel interaction with glutathione. *Neuroscience.,* 84(1), 7-10.

Green, A; MacLennan, R; Youl, P; Martin, N. (1993). Site distribution of cutaneous melanoma in Queensland. *Int. J. Cancer.,* 53(2),232-6.

Green, A; McCredie, M; Giles, G; Jackman, L. (1996). Occurrence of melanomas on the upper and lower limbs in eastern Australia. *Melanoma Res.,* 6(5),387-94.

Green, A; Williams, G; Neale, R; Hart, V; Leslie, D; Parsons, P; Marks, GC; Gaffney, P; Battistutta, D; Frost, C; Lang, C; Russell, A. (1999). Daily sunscreen application and beta-carotene supplementation in prevention of basal-cell and squamous-cell carcinomas of the skin: a randomized controlled trial. *Lancet.,* 354(9180), 723-9.

Greenberg, ER; Baron, JA; Stukel, TA; Stevens, NM; Mandel, JS; Spencer, SK; Elias, PM; Lowe, N; Nierenberg, DW; Bayrd, G; Vance, JC; Freeman, DH; Clendenning, WE; Kwan, T; The alpha-tocopherol, beta-carotene cancer prevention study group. (1990). A clinical trial of beta-carotene to prevent basal-cell and squamous-cell cancer on the skin. *N. Engl. J. Med,* 323, 789–795.

Greenwald, RA; Zucker, S; Golub, LM. (1999). Inhibition of matrix metalloproteinases: therapeutic applications. New York Acad Sci, 878:1-761. Proceedings of a conference. Tampa, Florida, USA. October 21-24, 1998.

Gregory, SR; Piccolo, N; Piccolo, MT; Piccolo, MS; Heggers, JP. (2002).Comparison of propolis skin cream to silver sulfadiazine: A naturopathic alternative to antibiotics in treatment of minor burns. *J. Altern. Complement. Med.,* 8, 77–83.

Greul, AK; Grundmann, JU; Heinrich, F; Pfitzner, I; Bernhardt, J; Ambach, A; Biesalski, HK; Gollnick, H. (2002). Photoprotection of UV-irradiated human skin: an antioxidative combination of vitamins E and C, carotenoids, selenium and proanthocyanidins. *Skin. Pharmacol. Appl. Skin Physiol.,* 15(5), 307-15.

Grether-Beck, S; Wlaschek, M; Krutmann, J; Scharffetter-Kochanek, K. (2005). Photodamage and photoaging-prevention and treatment.*J. Dtsch. Dermatol. Ges.,* 3(2), S19-25.

Griffiths, CE;Russman, AN; Majmudar, G; Singer, RS; Hamilton, TA; Voorhees, JJ. (1993). Restoration of collagen formation in photodamaged human skin by tretinoin (retinoic acid).*N. Engl. J. Med.,* 329(8), 530-5.

Griffiths, HR; Rayment, SJ. Effects of antioxidant vitamins C and E on gene expression in the vasculature. In: *Critical reviews of oxidative stress and aging,* World Scientific, 2003.

Grootveld, M; Silwood, C; Claxson, AWD. NMR evaluation of thermally induced peroxidation in culinary oils. In: *Rhodes CJ. Toxicology of the human environment.* Tylor & Francis, London, 2000.

Grube, K; Bürkle, A. (1992). Poly(ADP-ribose) polymerase activity in mononuclear leukocytes of 13 mammalian species correlates with species-specific lifespan, *Proc. Natl. Acad. Sci. USA*,89, 11759–11763.

Grune, T; Reinheckel, T; Davies, KJ. (1997). Degradation of oxidized proteins in mammalian cells. *Faseb. J.*, 11, 526-34.

Guan, X; Matte, JJ; Ku, PK; Snow, JL; Burton, JL; Trottier, NL. (2000). High chromium yeast supplementation improves glucose tolerance in pigs by decreasing hepatic extraction of insulin. *J. Nutr.*, 130(5), 1274-9.

Guarente, L; Picard, F. (2005). Calorie restriction—the SIR2 connection. *Cell*, 120, 473-482.

Gugliucci, A. *Sour Side of Sugar*, A Glycation Web Page.

Guinot, C; Malvy, DJ; Ambroisine, L; Latreille, J; Mauger, E; Tenenhaus, M; Morizot, F; Lopez, S; Le Fur, I; Tschachler, E. (2002). Relative contribution of intrinsic vs. extrinsic factors to skin aging as determined by a validated skin age score. *Arch. Dermatol.*, 138(11), 1454-60.

Guitton, C; Gros, P; Comtat, M; Tarroux, R; Bordat, P. (2005). Evaluation of antioxidant properties of dermocosmetic creams by direct electrochemical measurements. *J. Cosmet. Sci.*, 56(2), 79-90.

Gunn, DA; Rexbye, H; Griffiths, CE; Murray, PG; Fereday, A; Catt, SD; Tomlin, CC; Strongitharm, BH; Perrett, DI; Catt, M; Mayes, AE; Messenger, AG; Green, MR; van der Ouderaa, F; Vaupel, JW; Christensen, K. (2009). Why some women look young for their age. *PLoS One.* 4(12), e8021.

Guo, Q; Packer, L. (2000). Accorbate dependent recycling of the vitamin E homologue Trolox by dihydrolipoate and glutathione in murine skin homogenates. *Free Radic. Biol.Med*, 29, 368-374.

Gutteridge, JMC. (1985). Superoxide dismutase inhibits the superoxide-driven Fenton reaction at two different levels. *FEBS Lett*, 185, 19-23.

Guyton, KZ; Kensler, TW. (1993). Oxidative mechanisms in carcinogenesis. *Br. Med. Bull*, 49, 523–544.

Guyuron, B; Rowe, DJ; Weinfeld, AB; Eshraghi, Y; Fathi, A; Iamphongsai, S. (2009). Factors contributing to the facial aging of identical twins. *Plast. Reconstr. Surg.*, 123(4),1321-31.

Haddad, LS; Kelbert, L; Hulbert, AJ. (2007). Extended longevity of queen honey bees compared to workers is associated with peroxidation-resistant membranes. *Exp. Gerontol.*, 42(7), 601-9.

Hagen, JL; Krause, DJ; Baker, DJ; Fu, MH; Tarnopolsky, MA; Hepple, RT. (2004). Skeletal muscle aging in F344BN F1-hybrid rats: I. mitochondrial dysfunction contributes to the age-associated reduction in CO2max. *J. Gerontol.A. Biol. Sci. Med. Sci.*, 59, 1099–1110.

Hagen, TM. (2003). Oxidative stress, redox imbalance, and the aging process. *Antioxid. Redox Signal*, 5, 503–506.

Hagen, TM; Liu, J; Lykkesfeldt, J; Wehr, CM; Ingersoll, RT; Vinarsky, V; Bartholomew, JC; Ames, BN. (2002). Feeding acetyl-L-carnitine and lipoic acid to old rats significantly improves metabolic function while decreasing oxidative stress.*Proc. Natl. Acad. Sci. U.S. A.*, 99(4), 1870-5.

Hakim, A; Petrovich H; Burchfiel, CM; Ross, GW; Rodriguez, BL; White, LR; Yano, K; Curb, JD; Abbott, RD. (1998). Effects of walking on mortality among non-smoking men. *N. Engl. J. Med.*, 388, 94-99.

Hakozaki, T; Swanson, CL; Bissett, DL. Hyperpigmentation in aging skin. In: Farage MA, Miller KW, Maibach HI. *Textbook of aging skin.* Berlin: Springer-Verlag, 2010.

Hall, GK; Philips, TJ. Hormone replacement therapy and skin aging. In: *Skin aging,* Gilchrest B, Krutmann J (Eds.). Springer-Verlag, Berlin 2006.

Halliwell, B. (1987). Oxidants and human disease: some new concepts. *Faseb J.*, 1, 358-3649.

Halliwell, B. (2000). Vitamin C and genomic stability. *Mutat Res.*, 475, 29-35.

Halliwell, B; Cross, CE. (1994). Oxygen-derived species: their role in human disease and environmental stress. *Environ. Health Perspect.*, 102, 5-12.

Halliwell, B; Gutteridge, J MC. (2005).*Free Radicals in Biology and Medicine.* Oxford: Oxford University Press, 2005.

Halliwell, B; Gutteridge, JM. (1985). The importance of free radicals and catalytic metal ions in human diseases. *Mol. Aspects Med.*, 8(2):89-193. Review.

Halliwell, B; Rafter, J; Jenner, A. (2005). Health promotion by flavonoids, tocopherols, tocotrienols, and other phenols: direct or indirect effects? Antioxidant or not? *Am. J. Clin. Nutr.*, 81(1 Suppl), 268S-276S.

Halliwell, B; Gutteridge, J. (1984). Oxygen toxicity, oxygen radicals, transition metals and disease. *Biochemical J*, 219(1), 1-14.

Halliwell, B; Gutteridge, J. (1999). *Free radicals in biology and medicine* (3rd edn). Oxford: Clarendon Press, 1999.

Halliwell, B; Gutteridge, J. (2007). *Free radicals in biology and medicine*(4th edn). Oxford: University Press, 2007.

Halliwell, B; Whiteman, M. (1997). Antioxidant and pro-oxidant properties of vitamin C. In: Packer L, Fuchs J, Eds.. *Vitamin C in Health and Disease.* New York: Marcel Dekker. Pp. 59–73.

Halvorsen, B. L; Holte, K; Myhrstad, M. C; Barikmo, I; Hvattum, E; Remberg, S. F; Wold, A. B; Haffner, K; Baugerod, H; Andersen, L. F; Moskaug, O; Jacobs, D. R; Blomhoff, R. (2002). A systematic screening of total antioxidants in dietary plants. *J. Nutr.*, 132, 461-71.

Hamilton, ML; Van Remmen, H; Drake, JA; Yang, H; Guo, ZM; Kewitt, K; Walter, CA; Richardson, A. (2001). Does oxidative damage to DNA increase with age? *Proc. Natl. Acad. Sci. USA*, 98, 10469-10474.

Hammett, CJ; Oxenham, HC; Baldi, JC; Doughty, RN; Ameratunga, R; French, JK; White, HD; Stewart, RA. (2004). Effect of six months' exercise training on C-reactive protein levels in healthy elderly subjects. *J. Am. Coll. Cardiol.*, 44(12), 2411-3.

Hansford, RG; Hogue, BA; Mildaziene, V. (1997). Dependence of H2O2 formation by rat heart mitochondria on substrate availability and donor age. *J. Bioenerg. Biomembr.*, 29(1), 89-95.

Hanson, K; Clegg, R. (2002). Observation and quantification of UV-induced reactive oxygen species in ex vivo human skin. *Photochem. Photobiol*, 76, 57-63.

Hanson, KM; Simon, JD. (1998) Epidermal trans-urocanic acid and the UVA-induced photoaging of the skin. *Proc. Natl. Acad. Sci. USA*, 95, 10576–10578.

Hanson, KM; Li, B; Simon, JD. (1997). A spectroscopic study of the epidermal chromophore trans-urocanic acid. *J. Am. Chem. Soc.*, 119, 2715–2721.

Hardeland, R. (2005). "Antioxidative protection by melatonin: multiplicity of mechanisms from radical detoxification to radical avoidance." *Endocrine*, 27, 119–30.

Harley, CB; Futcher, AB; Greider, CW. (1990). Telomeres shorten during ageing of human fibroblasts. *Nature*, 345, 458-60.

Harley, CB; Liu, W; Blasco, M; Vera, E; Andrews, WH; Briggs, LA; Raffaele, JM. (2010). A Natural Product Telomerase Activator as Part of a Health Maintenance Program. *Rejuvenation Res.* [Epub ahead of print].

Harman, D. (1972). "A biologic clock: the mitochondria?" *Journal of the American Geriatrics Society*, 20, 145–147.

Harman, D. (1956). "Aging: a theory based on free radical and radiation chemistry." *Journal of Gerontology*, 11, 298–300.

Harman, D. (2001). Aging: overview. *Ann. N.Y. Acad. Sci.*,928, 1–21.

Harman, D. (1968). Free radical theory of aging: effect of free radical inhibitors on the mortality rate of male LAf1 mice. *Gerontol.*, 23, 476-482.

Harrison, DE; Archer, JR. (1988). Natural-selection for extended longevity from food restriction. *Growth Dev. Aging*, 52, 65.

Hattori, H; Kawashima, M; Ichikawa, Y; et al. (2004). The epidermal stem cell factor is over-expressed in lentigo senilis: Implication for the mechanism of hyperpigmentation. *J. Invest. Dermatol.* 122, 1256-1265.

Havsteen, BH. (2002). The biochemistry and medical significance of the flavonoids. *Pharmacol. Ther.*, 96, 67-202.

Hawkes, J; Wang, E; Cochran, GM; Moyzis, R. (2007). *Recent Acceleration of Human Adaptive Evolution.—Proceedings of the National Academy of Sciences of the United States of America*, 104, 20753-20758.

Hayflick, L. (2004). The not-so-close relationship between biological aging and age-associated pathologies in humans. *J. Gerontol. Bio. Sci.*, 59, 547–550.

Hearing, VJ.(1999). Biochemical control of melanogenesis and melanosomal organization. *J. Invest Dermatol Symp Proc.*, 4, 24-28.

Heart Protection Study Collaborative Group (2002). "MRC/BHF Heart Protection Study of antioxidant vitamin supplementation in 20,356 high-risk individuals: a randomized placebo-controlled trial" *Lancet*, 360(9326), 23-33.

Heck, DE; Gerecke, DR; Vetrano, AM; Laskin, JD. (2004). Solar UV radiation as a trigger of cell signal transduction. *Toxycol. Appl. Pharmacol.*, 195, 288-297.

Heilbronn, LK; de Jonge, L; Frisard, MI; DeLany, JP. (2006). Effect of six-month calorie restriction on biomarkers of longevity, metabolic adaptation, and oxidative stress in overweight individuals. *Jama*, 295, 1539-1548.

Heinrich, U; Neukam, K; Tronnier, H; Sies, H; Stahl, W. (2006). Long-term ingestion of high flavanol cocoa provides photoprotection against UV-induced erythema and improves skin condition in women. *J. Nutr.*, 136(6), 1565-9.

Heinrich, U; Wiebusch, M; Tronnier, H. (1998). Photoprotection from ingested carotenoids. *Cosm. Toilet.*, 113, 61–70.

Heinrich, U; Gärtner, C; Wiebusch, M; Eichler, O; Sies, H; Tronnier, H; Stahl, W. (2003). Supplementation with beta-carotene or a similar amount of mixed carotenoids protects humans from UV-induced erythema.*J. Nutr.*, 133(1), 98-101.

Helbig, D; Simon, JC; Paasch, U. (2010). Epidermal and dermal changes in response to various skin rejuvenation methods. *Int. J. Cosmet. Sci.* [Epub ahead of print].

Helfrich, YR; Sachs, DL; Voorhees, JJ. (2008). Overview of skin aging and photoaging. *Dermatol. Nurs.*, 20(3), 177-83.

Helfrich, YR; Yu, L; Ofori, A; Hamilton, TA; Lambert, J; King, A; Voorhees, JJ; Kang, S. (2007). Effect of smoking on aging of photoprotected skin: evidence gathered using a new photonumeric scale. *Arch. Dermatol.*, 143(3), 397-402.

Helland, DE; Doetsch, PW; Haseltine, WA. (1986). Substrate specificity of a mammalian DNA repair endonuclease that recognizes oxidative base damage. *Mol. Cell Biol*, 6, 1983–1990.

Hellerstein, MK. (1998). Is chromium supplementation effective in managing type II diabetes? *Nutr. Rev.*, 56(10), 302-6.

Henderson, ST. (1977). *Daylight and its Spectrum*(Bristol: Adam Hilger) p33.

Heng MC. (2010). Curcumin targeted signaling pathways: basis for anti-photoaging and anti-carcinogenic therapy. *Int. J. Dermatol.*, 49(6), 608-22.

Hennekens, CH; Buring, JE; Manson, JE; Stampfer, M; Rosner, B; Cook, NR; Belanger, C; LaMotte, F; Gaziano, JM; Ridker, PM. (1996). Lack of effect of long-term supplementation with beta-carotene on the incidence of malignant neoplasms and cardiovascular disease. *N. Engl. J. Med.*, 334, 1145–1149.

Heppell, HCN. (2002). "Nutritional losses and gains during processing: future problems and issues." *Proc. Nutr. Soc.*, 61, 145–8.

Herbert, V. (1994). The antioxidant supplement myth. *Am. J. Clin. Nutr.*, 60, 157–158.

Herman, D. (1993). Free radical involvement in aging: pathophysiology and therapeutic implications. *Drugs Aging*, 3, 60-80.

Herrero, A;Barja, G. *(*1997a*)*. ADP-regulation of mitochondrial free radical production is different with complex I- or complex II-linked substrates: implications for the exercise paradox and brain hypermetabolism. *J. Bioenerg. Biomembr.*, 29, 241–249.

Hertog, MG; Feskens, EJ; Hollman, PC; Katan, MB; Kromhout, D. (1993). Dietary antioxidant flavonoids and risk of coronary heart disease: the Zutphen Elderly Study, *Lancet*, 342, 1007–1011.

Hibatallah, J; Carduner, C; Poelman, MC. (1999). In-vivo and in-vitro assessment of free radical scavenger activity of ginkgo flavone glycosides at high concentration. *J. Pharm. Pharmacol.*, 51, 1435–40.

Higami, Y; Pugh, TD; Page, GP; Allison, DB; Prolla, TA; Weindruch, R. (2004). Adipose tissue energy metabolism: altered gene expression profile of mice subjected to long-term caloric restriction. *Faseb. J.*, 18, 415-417.

Hillebrand, GG; Demirli, R. (2009). Method and apparatus for realistic simulation of wrinkle aging and de-aging, 2009, U.S. Patent Application 20090028380A1.

Hillebrand, GG; Levine, MJ; Miyamoto, K. (2001). The age-dependent changes in skin condition in African Americans, Caucasians, East Asians, Indian Asians and Latinos. *IFSCC Mag.*, 4, 259-266.

Hillebrand, GG. Facial wrinkling: The Marquee clinical sign of skin aging. In: Farage MA, Miller KW, Maibach HI. *Textbook of aging skin*. Berlin: Springer-Verlag, 2010.

Hindhede, M. (1921). The effects of food restriction during war on mortality in Copenhagen. *Jama*, 74, 381-382.

Hipkiss, AR; Brownson, C; Carrier, MJ. (2001). "Carnosine, the anti-ageing, antioxidant dipeptide, may react with protein carbonyl groups," *Mech. Ageing Dev.*, 122(13), 1431-45.

Hipkiss, AR. (2009). Carnosine and its possible roles in nutrition and health. *Adv. Food Nutr. Res.*, 57, 87-154.

Hipkiss, AR. (2006). Would carnosine or a carnivorous diet help suppress aging and associated pathologies? *Ann. N Y Acad. Sci.*, 1067, 369-74.

HiraoT. Cornified envelope. In: *Skin moisturization*. (Eds.: Rawlings AV and Leyden JJ). *Infotma Healthcare*, New York, 2009.

Hirota, K; Matsui, M; Iwata, S; Nishiyama, A; Mori, K; Yodoi, J. (1997). AP-1 transcriptional activity is regulated by a direct association between thioredoxin and Ref-1. *Proc. Natl. Acad. Sci. USA.*, 94(8), 3633-8.

Ho, E. (2004). Zinc deficiency, DNA damage and cancer risk. *J. Nutr. Biochem.*, 15(10), 572-8. Review.

Hockenbery, DM; Oltvai, ZN; Yin, XM; Milliman, CL; Korsmeyer, SJ. (1993). Bcl-2 functions in an antioxidant pathway to prevent apoptosis. *Cell.*, 75(2), 241-51.

Hodges, GJ; Sharp, L; Stephenson, C; Patwala, AY; George, KP; Goldspink, DF; Tim, Cable N. (2010). The effect of 48 weeks of aerobic exercise training on cutaneous vasodilator function in post-menopausal females. *Eur. J. Appl. Physiol.*, 108(6), 1259-67.

Hohmann, S; Mager, HRG. Landes Company, 1997, 171-204.

Hollander, J; Fiebig, R; Gore, M; Bejma, J; Ookawara, T; Ohno, H; Ji, LL. (1999). Superoxide dismutase gene expression in skeletal muscle: fiber-specific adaptation to endurance training. *Am. J. Physiol.*, 277, R856-R862.

Holley, AE; Cheeseman, KH. (1993). Measuring free radical reactions in vivo. *British Medical Bulletin*, 49(3), 494-505.

Holliday, R. (1989). Food, reproduction and longevity: is the extended lifespan of calorie-restricted animals an evolutionary adaptation? *Bioessays*, 10, 125–127.

Holick, MF. (2004). Vitamin D: importance in the prevention of cancers, type 1 diabetes, heart disease and osteoporosis. *Am. J. Clin. Nutr.*, 79, 362-371.

Holloszy, JO. The biology of aging. *Mayo Clin. Proc.*, 2000, 75, 3-8.

Holloszy, JO; Smith, EK; Vining, M; Adams, S. (1985). Effect of voluntary exercise on longevity of rats. *J. Appl. Physiol.*, 59(3), 826-31.

Holloszy, JO; Smith, EK. (1986). Longevity of cold-exposed rats: a reevaluation of the "rate-of-living theory."*J. Appl. Physiol.*, 61(5), 1656-60.

Hoppe, U; Bergemann, J; Diembeck, W; Ennen, J; Gohla, S; Harris, I; Jacob, J; Kielholz, J; Mei, W; Pollet, D; Schachtschabel, D; Sauermann, G; Schreiner, V; Stäb, F; Steckel, F. (1999). Coenzyme Q10, a cutaneous antioxidant and energizer. *Biofactors.*, 9(2-4), 371-8.

Hourigan, R. Cellular energy metabolism and oxidative stress. In: Farage MA, Miller KW, Maibach HI. *Textbook of aging skin*. Berlin: Springer-Verlag, 2010

Houthoofd, K; Braeckman, BP; Vanfleteren, JR. (2003). Metabolism and lifespan determination in C. elegans; in Mattson, Mark P. (editor). Energy metabolism and Lifespan Determination; *Advances in cell aging and gerontology*, Vol. 14, 143-175.

Howard, EW; Benton, R; Ahern-Moore, J; Tomasek, J. (1996). Cellular contraction of collagen lattices is inhibited by nonenzymatic glycation. *Exp. Cell Res*, 228, 132-7.

Howes, RM. (2006). The free radical fantasy: A panoply of paradoxes. *Ann. N.Y. Acad. Sci.*, 1067, 22-6.

http://www.ehealthmd.com/library/skincancer.
http://www.fda.gov/Food/DietarySupplements/default.htm.
http://www.skinbiology.com/skinhealth&aging.html.
http://www.who.org.

https://www.who.int/uv/publications/UVEHeffects.pdf.
http://www.nas.nasa.gov.
http://www.melanomaawareness.org/spring2008.pdf.
http://www.aad.org/RaysYourGrade/.
http://www.census.gov; U.S. Census Bureau, Population Division.
Hua, NW; Stoohs, RA; Facchini, FS. (2001). Low iron status and enhanced insulin sensitivity in lacto-ovo vegetarians. *Br. J. Nutr.*, 86(4), 515-9.
Huh, K; Shin, US; Choi, JW; Lee, SI. (1994). Effect of sex hormones on lipid peroxidation in rat liver. *Arch. Pharm. Res.*, 17(2), 109-14.
Hulbert, AJ. (2008). Explaining longevity of different animals: is membrane fatty acid composition the missing link? *Age (Dordr)*, 30(2-3), 89-97.
Hulbert, AJ; Turner, N; Storlien, LH; Else, PL. (2005). Dietary fats and membrane function: implications for metabolism and disease. *Biol. Rev. Camb. Philos. Soc.*, 80(1), 155-69.
Humbert, PG; Haftek, M; Creidi, Lapière, C; Nusgens, B; Richard, A., et al. (2003). Topical ascorbic acid on photoaged skin. Clinical, topographical and ultrastructural evaluation: Double-blind study vs. placebo. *ExperimentalDermatology*, 12, 237-244.
Humphries, KM; Szweda, PA; Szweda, LI. (2006). Aging: A shift from redox regulation to oxidative damage. *Free Radic. Res.*, 40, 1239-43.
Hutchinson, F. (1985). Chemical changes induced in DNA by ionizing radiation. *Prog. Nucleic Acid Res. Mol. Biol*,. 32, 115-154.
Ibbotson, SH; Moran, MN; Nash, JF; Kochevar, IE. (1999). The effects of radicals compared with UVB as initiating species for the induction of chronic cutaneous photodamage. *J. Invest. Dermatol.*, 112(6), 933-8.
Ikeda, M; Schroeder, KK; Mosher, LB; Woods, CW; Akeson, AL. (1994). Suppressive effect of antioxidants on intracellular adhesion molecule-1 (ICAM-1) expression in human epidermal keratinocytes. *J. Invest. Dermatol.*, 103, 791–796.
Imai, S. (2010). A possibility of nutriceuticals as an anti-aging intervention: activation of sirtuins by promoting mammalian NAD biosynthesis. *Pharmacol. Res.*, 62(1), 42-7.
Imlay, J. (2003). Pathways of oxidative damage. *Annu. Rev. Microbiol.*, 57, 395–418.
Imlay, JA; Chir, SM; Linn, S. (1988). Toxic DNA damage by hydrogen peroxide through the Fenton reaction in vivo and in vitro. *Science*, 240, 640-642.
Ingram, DK. (2000). Age-related decline in physical activity: Generalization to nonhumans. *Med. Sci. Sports Exerc.*, 32, 1623-1629.
Ingram, DK; Zhu, M; Mamczarz, J. (2006). Calorie restriction mimetics: an emerging research field. *Aging Cell.*, 5, 97-108.
International programme on chemical safety, Environmental Health Criteria, 160, Ultraviolet radiation (EHC 160, 1994, 2nd edition), accessed: www.inchem.org/documents/ehc/ehc/ehc160.htm.
Inui, M; Ooe, M; Fujii, K; Matsunaka, H; Yoshida, M; Ichihashi, M. (2008). Mechanisms of inhibitory effects of CoQ10 on UVB-induced wrinkle formation in vitro and in vivo. *Biofactors.*, 32(1-4), 237-43.
Ionescu, JG; Merk, M; Dowes, F. (1998). Clinical application of redox potential testing in the blood. Syllabus of 33rd AAEM Annual Meeting, Baltimore, USA, 503-512.
Ionescu, JG; Novotny, JS; Latsch, V; Blaurock-Busch, A; Eisenmann-Klein, M. (2006). Increased levels of transition metals in breast cancer tissue. *Neuro Endocrinol. Lett.*, 27, 1, 36-9.

Ionescu, J; Poljsak, B. (2010).Metal Ions Mediated Pro-Oxidative Reactions with Vitamin C: Possible Implications for Treatment of Different Malignancies, *Int. J. Canc. Prev*, 149-174.

Ionescu, G. *Anti-aging for professionals*. 2005.

Irie, M; Asami, S; Nagata, S; Ikeda, M; Miyata, M; Kasai, H. (2001a). Psychosocial factors as a potential trigger of oxidative DNA damage in human leukocytes. *Japanese Journal of Cancer Research*, 92, 367-375.

Irie, M; Asami, S; Nagata, S; Miyata, M; Kasai, H. (2000). Classical conditioning of oxidative DNA damage in rats. *Neuroscience Letters*, 288, 13-16.

Irie, M; Asami, S; Nagata, S; Miyata, M; Kasai, H. (2002). Psychological mediation of a type of oxidative DNA damage, 8-hydroxydeoxyguanosine, in peripheral blood leukocytes of non-smoking and non-drinking workers. *Psychother. Psychosom.*, 71(2), 90-6.

Irie, M; Asami, S; Nagata, S; Miyata, M; Kasai, H. (2001b). Relationships between perceived workload, stress and oxidative damage. *International Archives of Occupational and Environmental Health*, 74, 153-157.

Iscovich, J; Howe, GR. (1998). Cancer incidence patterns (1972-91) among migrants from the Soviet Union to Israel. *Cancer Causes Control.*, 9 (1), 29-36.

Ishii, N. (2000). Oxidative stress and aging in Caenorhabditis elegans. *Free Radical Research*,33, 6, 857–64.

Ishii, N; Hartman, PS. (2003). Electron transport and lifespan in C. elegans; in Mattson, Mark P. (editor). Energy metabolism and Lifespan Determination; *Advances in cell aging and gerontology*Vol. 14, 177-195.

Ismail, F; Willows, A; Khurana, M; Tomlins, PE; James, S; Mikhalovsky, S; Vadgama, P. (2008). A test method to monitor in vitro storage and degradation effects on a skin substitute. *Med. Eng. Phys.*, 30(5), 640-6.

Ivshina, AV. (2006). Genetic reclassification of histologic grade delineates new clinical subtypes of breast cancer. *Cancer Res.*, 66, 10292–10301.

Iwasaki, K; Gleiser, CA; Masoro, EJ; McMahan, CA, Seo, EJ; Yu, BP. (1988). The influence of the dietary protein source on longevity and age-related disease processes of Fischer rats. *Journal of gerontology*, 43, B5-B12.

Izawa, S; Inoue, Y; Kimura, A. (1995). Oxidative stressresponse in yeast: effect of glutathione on adaptation to hydrogen peroxide stress in Saccharomyces cerevisiae. *Fabs Lett*, 368, 73-76.

Izykowska, I; Cegielski, M; Gebarowska, E; Podhorska-Okolow, M; Piotrowska, A; Zabel, M; Dziegiel, P. (2009). Effect of melatonin on human keratinocytes and fibroblasts subjected to UVA and UVB radiation In vitro. *In Vivo.*, 23(5), 739-45.

Jackson, SM; Williams, ML; Feingold, KR, et al. (1993). Pathobiology of the stratum corneum. *West J. Med.*, 158, 279-285.

Jacob, S; Ruus, P; Hermann, R; Tritschler, HJ; Maerker, E; Renn, W; Augustin, HJ; Dietze, GJ; Rett, K. (1999). Oral administration of RAC-alpha-lipoic acid modulates insulin sensitivity in patients with type-2 diabetes mellitus: a placebo-controlled pilot trial. *Free Radic. Biol. Med.*, 27(3-4), 309-14.

Jacobs, HT. (2003). The mitochondrial theory of aging: dead or alive? *Aging cell*, 2, 11.

Jägerstad, M; Skog, K. (2005). Genotoxicity of heat-processed foods. *Mutat. Res.*, 574(1-2), 156-72.

Jameson, J; DeGroot, LJ. (1995). Mechanisms of tyroid hormone action. In: *Endocrinology* (DeGroot LJ, ed). Harcourt Brace Co, Philadelphia.

Jamnik, P; Goranovic, D; Raspor, P. (2007). Antioxidative action of royal jelly in the yeast cell. *Exp. Gerontol.*, 42, 594-600.

Jamnik, P; Raspor, P. (2003). Stress response of yeast Candida intermedia to Cr(VI). J. Biochem. *Mol. Toxicol.*, 17, 316-23.

Jarmuszkiewicz, W; Woyda-Płoszczyca, A. (2008). Mitochondrial uncoupling proteins: regulation and physiological role. *Postepy Biochem.*, 54(2), 179-87.

Jasin, HE (1993). Oxidative modofocation of inflammatory synovial fluid IgG. *Inflammation*, 17, 167.

Jeanmaire, C; Danoux, L; Pauly, G. (2001). Glycation during human dermal intrinsic and actinic ageing: an in vivo and in vitro model study. *Brit. J. Dermatol*, 145, 10-8.

Jemed, GBE; Selvaag, E; Agren, M; Wulf, HC. (2001). Measurement of the mechanical properties of skin with ballistometer and suction cup. *Skin Res. Technol*, 7, 122-126.

Jenkins, G; Wainwright, LJ; Green, M. Healthy aging: The skin. In: *Healthy aging. The role of nutrition and lifestyle.* (Ed: Stanner, S; Thompson, R; Buttriss, JL.). Wiley-Backwell, 2009

Fang, Ji; Pierre, Z; Liu, S; Hwang, B; Hill, ZH; Hubbard, K; Steinberg, M. (2006).Novel mitochondrial deletions in human epithelial cells irradiated with an FS20 ultraviolet source in vitro. *J. Photochem. Photobiol.*, 184: 340-346.

Jablonski, NG; Chaplin, G. (2000). The evolution of human skin coloration. *J. Hum. Evol.*, 39(1), 57-106.

Ji, LL. (1993). Antioxidant enzyme response to exercise and aging. *Med. Sci. Sport Exerc*, 25, 225-231.

Jin, Y; Koizumi, A. (1994). Decreased cellular proliferation by energy restriction is recovered by increasing housing temperature in rats. *Mech. Ageing and Development*, 75, 59-67.

Johnson, AW; Demple, B. (1988). Yeast DNA 3'-repair diesterase is the major cellular apurinic/apyrimidinic endonuclease: substrate specificity and kinetics. *J. Biol. Chem*, 263, 18017–18022.

Johnson, TE. (2006). Recent results: biomarkers of aging. *Exp. Gerontol.*, 41, 1243-1246.

Johnson, GE. (1963). The effect of cold exposure on the catecholamine excretion of adrenalectomized rats treated with reserpine. *Acta Physiol. Scand.*, 59, 438-44.

Jonak, C; Klosner, G; Trautinger, F. (2009). Significance of heat shock proteins in the skin upon UV exposure. *Front Biosci.*, 14, 4758-68.

Jones, TE; Baar, K; Ojuka, E; Chen, M; Holloszy, JO. (2003). Exercise induces an increase in muscle UCP3 as a component of the increase in mitochondrial biogenesis. *Am. J. Physiol. Endocrinol. Metab.*, 284(1), E96-101.

Jurkiewicz, BA; Buettner, GR. (1996). EPR detection of free radicals in UV-irradiated skin: mouse versus human. *Photochem. Photobiol.*, 64, 918–922.

Juul, A; Skakkebaek, NE. (2002). Androgens and the ageing male. *Hum. Reprod. Update*, 8, 423-433.

Juvan, S; Bartol, T; Boh, B. (2005). Data structuring and classification in newly emerging scientific fields. *Online Information Review*, 29(5): 483-498.

Juzeniene, A; Setlow, R; Porojnicu, A; Steindal, AH; Moan, J. (2009). Development of different human skin colors: a review highlighting photobiological and photobiophysical aspects. *J. Photochem. Photobiol. B.*, 96(2), 93-100.

Kadono, S; Manaka, I; Kawashima, M, et al. (2001). The role of the epidermal endothelin cascade in the hyperpigmentation of lentigo senilis. *J. Invest. Dermatol.*, 116, 571-577.

Kadunce, DP; Burr, R; Gress, R; Kanner, R; Lyon, JL; Zone, JJ. (1991), Cigarette smoking: risk factor for premature facial wrinkling. *Ann. Intern. Med.*, 114, 840–844.

Kafi, R; Kwak, HS; Schumacher, WE; Cho, S; Hanft, VN; Hamilton, TA; King, AL; Neal, JD; Varani, J; Fisher, GJ; Voorhees, JJ; Kang, S. (2007). Improvement of naturally aged skin with vitamin A (retinol). *Arch. Dermatol.*, 143(5), 606-12.

Kagawa, Y. (1978). Impact of Westernization on the nutrition of Japanese: changes in physique, cancer, longevity and centenarians. *Prev. Med.*, 7, 205-217.

Kahan, V; Andersen, ML; Tomimori, J; Tufik, S. (2009). Stress, immunity and skin collagen integrity: evidence from animal models and clinical conditions. *Brain Behav. Immun.*, 23(8):1089-95.

Kahari, VM; Saarialho-Kere, U. (1997). Matrix metalloproteinases in skin. *Exp Dermatol.*,6, 199–213.

Kang, S; Chung, JH; Lee, JH; Fisher, GJ; Wan, YS; Duell, EA; Voorhees, JJ. (2003). Topical N-acetyl cysteine and genistein prevent ultraviolet-light-induced signaling that leads to photoaging in human skin in vivo. *J. Invest. Dermatol.*, 120(5), 835-41.

Kang, S; Fisher, GJ; Voorhees JJ. (1997). Photoaging and topical tretinoin: therapy, pathogenesis, and prevention. *Arch. Dermatol.*, 133(10), 1280-4.

Kang, S; Fisher, GJ; Voorhees, JJ. (2001). Photoaging: pathogenesis, prevention, and treatment. *Clin. Geriatr. Med.*, 17(4), 643-59, v-vi.

Kao, JS; Garg, A; Mao-Qiang, M; Crumrine, D; Ghadially, R; Feingold, KR; Elias, PM. (2001). Testosterone perturbs epidermal permeability barrier homeostasis.*J. Invest. Dermatol.*, 116(3), 443-51.

Kasper, M; Funk, RH. (2001). Age-related changes in cells and tissues due to advanced glycation end products (AGEs). *Arch. Gerontol. Geriatr*, 32, 233-243.

Kasprzak, KS. (1995). Possible role of oxidative damage in metal-induced carcinogenesis. *Cancer Invest.*, 13, 411–430.

Kasprzak, KS. (1991). The role of oxidative damage in metal carcinogenicity. *Chem. Res. Toxicol.*, 4, 604–615.

Kathryn, J; Martires, BA; Pingfu Fu; Amy M. Polster; Kevin D. Cooper; Elma D. Baron. (2009). Factors That Affect Skin Aging. A Cohort-Based Survey on Twins.*Arch. Dermatol.*, 145(12), 1375-1379.

Katiyar, SK; Ahmad, N; Mukhtar, H. (2000). Green tea and skin. *Arch. Dermatol*, 136, 989–94.

Katiyar, SK; Matsui, MS; Elmets, CA; Mukhtar, H. (1999). Polyphenolic antioxidant (-)-epigallocatechin-3-gallate from green tea reduces UVB-induced inflammatory responses and infiltration of leukocytes in human skin. *Photochem Photobiol.*, 69(2), 148-53.

Katiyar, SK; Vaid, M; van Steeg, H; Meeran, SM. (2010). Green tea polyphenols prevent UV-induced immunosuppression by rapid repair of DNA damage and enhancement of nucleotide excision repair genes. *Cancer Prev Res* (Phila Pa)., 3(2), 179-89.

Katiyar, SK. (2003). Skin photoprotection by green tea: antioxidant and immunomodulatory effects. *Curr Drug Targets Immune Endocr Metabol Disord.*, 3(3), 234-42.

Katiyar, S; Elmets, CA; Katiyar, SK. (2007). Green tea and skin cancer: photoimmunology, angiogenesis and DNA repair. *J. Nutr. Biochem.*, 18(5), 287-96.

Katiyar, SK. (2010). Green tea prevents non-melanoma skin cancer by enhancing DNA repair. *Arch. Biochem. Biophys.* [Epub ahead of print.

Katiyar, SK; Vaid, M; van Steeg, H; Meeran, SM. (2010). Green tea polyphenols prevent UV-induced immunosuppression by rapid repair of DNA damage and enhancement of nucleotide excision repair genes. *Cancer Prev Res* (Phila)., 3(2), 179-89.

Katiyar, SK; Mukhtar, H. (2001). Green tea polyphenol (-)-epigallocatechin-3-gallate treatment to mouse skin prevents UVB-induced infiltration of leukocytes, depletion of antigen-presenting cells, and oxidative stress. *J. Leukoc. Biol.*, 69(5), 719-26.

Katz, MS. (2000). Geriatrics grand rounds: Eve's rib, or a revisionist view of osteoporosis in men. *J. Gerontol. A. Biol. Sci. Med. Sci.*, 55(10), M560-9.

Kaul, N; Forman, HJ. Reactive oxygen species in physiology and toxicology: from lipid peroxidation to transcriptional activation. In: Rhodes Cr (ed): *Toxicology of the Human Environment: The Critical Role of Free Radicals*. New York: Taylor and Francis, 2000, pp. 310-335.

Kavouras, SA; Panagiotakos, DB; Pitsavos, C; Chrysohoou, C; Arnaoutis, G; Skoumas, Y; Stefanadis, C. (2010). Physical Activity and Adherence to Mediterranean Diet Increase Total Antioxidant Capacity: The ATTICA Study. *Cardiol. Res. Pract.*, 2011. 248626.

Kawano, Y; Matsuoka, H; Takishita, S; Omae, T. (1998). Effects of magnesium supplementation in hypertensive patients: assessment by office, home, and ambulatory blood pressures. *Hypertension.*, 32(2), 260-5.

Kawada S, Ohtani M, Ishii N.Increased oxygen tension attenuates acute ultraviolet-B-induced skin angiogenesis and wrinkle formation. *Am. J. Physiol. Regul. Integr. Comp. Physiol.* (May 26, 2010). doi:10.1152/ajpregu.00199.2010.

Kell, BD. Iron behaving badly: inappropriate iron chelation as a major contributor to the aetiology of vascular and other progressive inflammatory and degenerative diseases http://arxiv.org/ftp/arxiv/papers/0808/0808.1371.pdf. Accessed: 14.3.2010.

Kelley, R; Ideker, T. (2009). "Genome-Wide Fitness and Expression Profiling Implicate Mga2 in Adaptation to Hydrogen Peroxide." *PLoS Genet.*, 5(5):e1000488.

Kelly, FJ. (2004). Dietary antioxidants and environemtal stress. *Proceedings of the Nutrition Society*, 63,579-585.

Kemnitz, JW; Roecker, EB; Weindruch, R; Elson, DF; Baum, ST; Bergman, RN. (1994). Dietary restriction increases insulin sensitivity and lowers blood glucose in rhesus monkeys. *Am. J. Physiol.*, 266(4 Pt 1), E540-7.

Kensler, T; Guyton, K; Egner, P; McCarthy, T; Lesko, S; Akman, S. (1995). Role of reactive intermediates in tumor promotion and progression. *Prog. Clin. Biol. Res.*, 391, 103–116.

Kensler, TW; Taffe, BG. (19869. Free radicals and tumor promotion. *Adv. Free Rad. Biol.Med.,*2, 347–387.

Kenyon, C. (2001). A conserved regulatory mechanism of aging. *Cell*, 105, 165-168.

Ketterer, B; Meyer, DJ. (1989). Glutathione transferases: a possible role in the detoxication and repair of DNA and lipid hydroperoxides. *Mut. Res.*,214, 33–40.

Keyer, K; Imlay, JA. (1996). Superoxide accelerates DNA damage by elevating free-iron levels. *Proc. Natl. Acad. Sci. USA*, 93, 13635-13640.

Keylock, KT; Vieira, VJ; Wallig, MA; DiPietro, LA; Schrementi, M; Woods, JA. (2007). Exercise accelerates cutaneous wound healing and decreases wound inflammation in aged mice. *Am. J. Physiol. Regul. Integr. Comp. Physiol.* 294(1):R179-84.

Keyse, SM; Tyrrell, RM. (1989). Heme oxygenase is the major 32-kDa stress protein induced in human skin fibroblasts by UVA radiation, hydrogen peroxide and sodium arsenite. *Proc. Natl. Acad. Sci.* (USA), 86: 99-103.

Khamaisi, M; Rudich, A; Potashnik, R; Tritschler, HJ; Gutman, A; Bashan, N. (1999). Lipoic acid acutely induces hypoglycemia in fasting nondiabetic and diabetic rats. *Metabolism.*, 48(4), 504-10.

Khlat, M; Vail, A; Parkin, M; Green, A. (1992). Mortality from melanoma in migrants to Australia: variation by age at arrival and duration of stay. *Am. J. Epidemiol.*, 135 (10), 1103-13.

Kim, DW; Hwang, IK; Kim, DW; Yoo, KY; Won, CK; Moon, WK; Won, MH. (2007). Coenzyme Q_{10} effects on manganese superoxide dismutase and glutathione peroxidase in the hairless mouse skin induced by ultraviolet B irradiation. *Biofactors.*, 30(3), 139-47.

Kim, EJ; Jin, XJ; Kim, YK; Oh, IK; Kim, JE; Park, CH; Chung, JH. (2010). UV decreases the synthesis of free fatty acids and triglycerides in the epidermis of human skin in vivo, contributing to development of skin photoaging. *J. Dermatol. Sci.*, 57(1), 19-26.

Kimata, H; Hirata, H. (1999). Redox regulation and cellular signaling. *Cell signal*, 11, 1-14.

Kipp, C; Young, AR. (1999). The soluble eumelanin precursor 5,6 hydroxyindole-2-carboxylic acid enhances oxidative damage in human keratinocyte DNA after UVA irradiation. *Photochem. Photobiol.*, 70, 191-198.

Kirkwood, B; Mathers, JC. (2009). The basic biology of aging. In: Stanner, S; Thompson, R; Buttriss, J. *Healthy aging—The role of nutrition and lifestyle*. Wiley-Blackwell, 2009.

Kirkwood, TBL. (1977). Evolution of aging. *Nature*, 270, 301-304.

Kirkwood, B; Mathers, JC. The basic biology of aging. In: Stanner S, Thompson R, Buttriss J (eds.): *Healthy aging—The role of nutrition and lifestyle*. Wiley-Blackwell, 2009.

Kitazawa, M; Ishitsuka, Y; Kobayashi, M; Nakano, T; Iwasaki, K; Sakamoto, K; Arakane, K; Suzuki, T; Kligman, LH. (2005). Protective effects of an antioxidant derived from serine and vitamin B6 on skin photoaging in hairless mice. *Photochem Photobiol.*, 81(4), 970-4.

Kitazawa, M; Iwasaki, K; Sakamoto, K. (2006). Iron chelators may help prevent photoaging. *J. Cosmet. Dermatol.*, 5(3), 210-7.

Kitazawa, M; Ishitsuka, Y; Kobayashi, M; Nakano, T; Iwasaki, K; Sakamoto, K; Arakane, K; Suzuki, T; Kligman, LH. (2005). Protective effects of an antioxidant derived from serine and vitamin B6 on skin photoaging in hairless mice. *Photochem. Photobiol.*, 81(4), 970-4.

Kitazawa, M; Iwasaki, K; Sakamoto, K. (2006). Iron chelators may help prevent photoaging. *J. Cosmet. Dermatol.*, 5(3), 210-7.

Klapper, W; Parwaresch, R; Krupp, G. (2001). Telomere biology in human aging and aging syndromes. *Mech. Aging. Dev.*, 122, 695-712.

Klein, CB; Frenkel, K; Costa, M. (1991). The role of oxidative processes in metal carcinogenesis. *Chem. Res. Toxicol.*, 4, 592–604.

Kligman, LH; Kligman, AM. (1984). Reflections on heat. *Br. J. Dermatol.*, 110, 369-75.

Kligman, AM; Zheng, P; Lavker, RM. (1985). The anatomy and pathogenesis of wrinkles. *Br. J. Dermatol.*, 113(1), 37-42.

Kligman, AM; Grove GL; Hirose R; Leyden, JJ. (1986). Topical tretinoin for photoaged skin. *Journal of the AmericanAcademy of Dermatology*, 15, 836-859.

Kligman, LH; Kligman, AM. (1986). The nature of photoaging: Its prevention and repair. *Photodermatology*, 3, 215-227.

Kochevar, IE; Pathak, MA; Parrish, JA. Photophysics, photochemistry, and pathobiology. In: Freedberg, IM; Eisen, AZ; Wolff, K; et al. (eds). *Fitzpatrick's dermatology in general medicine*. McGraw-Hill, New York, 1999.

Kochevar, IE; Taylor, CR; Krutman, J. Fundamentals of cutaneousphotobiology and photoimmunology. In: Wolff, K; Austen, KF; Goldshmith, LA; et al. (Eds)*Fitzpatrick's dermatology in general medicine*. New York: McGraw-Hill, 2007.

Koizumi, A; Weindruch, R; Walford, RL. (1987). Influences of dietary restriction and age on liver enzyme activities and lipid peroxidation in mice. *J. Nutr.*, 117(2), 361-7.

Koh, HK; Kligler, BE; Lew, RA. (1990). Sunlight and cutaneous malignant melanoma: evidence for and against causationPhotochem. *Photobiol.*, 51, 765-79.

Koh, JS; Kang, H; Choi, SW; Kim, HO. (2002). Cigarette smoking associated with premature facial wrinkling: image analysis of facial skin replicas. *International Journal of Dermatology*, 41(1), 21-27.

Koizumi, A; Tsukada, M; Weindruch,W. (1992). Mitotic activity in mice suppressed by energy restriction-induced torpor. *J. Nutr.*, 122, 1446-1455.

Kollias, N; Sayre, RM; Zeise, L; Chedekel, MR. (1991). Photoprotection by melanin. *J. Photochem. Photobiol. B.*, 9(2), 135-160.

Kohen, R; Oron, M; Zelkowicz, A; Kanevsky, E; Farfouri, S; Wormser, U. (2004). Low molecular weight antioxidants released from the skin's epidermal layers: an age dependent phenomenon in the rat. *Exp Gerontol.*, 39(1), 67-72.

Kokkinos, A; W. le Roux, C; Alexiadou, K; Tentolouris, N; Royce P; Despoina, D; Kyriaki, DP, Ghatei, MA; Bloom, R.S; Katsilambros, N. (2010). Eating Slowly Increases the Postprandial Response of the Anorexigenic Gut Hormones, Peptide YY and Glucagon-Like Peptide-1. *J. Clin. Endocrinol. Metab.*, 95(1), 333-7.

Konrad, T; Vicini, P; Kusterer, K; Höflich, A; Assadkhani, A; Böhles, HJ; Sewell, A; Tritschler, HJ; Cobelli, C; Usadel, KH. (1999). alpha-Lipoic acid treatment decreases serum lactate and pyruvate concentrations and improves glucose effectiveness in lean and obese patients with type 2 diabetes. *Diabetes Care.*, 22(2), 280-7.

Kontush, K; Schekatolina, S. (2004). Vitamin E in neurodegenerative disorders: Alzheimer's disease. *Ann. N. Y. Acad. Sci.*, 1031, 249–62.

Korshunov, SS; Skulachev, VP; Starkov, AA. (1997). High protonic potential actuates a mechanism of production of reactive oxygen species in mitochondria. *Febs. Lett.*, 416, 15–18.

Kosmadaki, MG; Gilchrest, BA. (2004). *The role of telomeres in skin aging/photoaging. Micron.*, 35, 155-159.

Koster, JF; Sluiter, W. (1995). Is increased tissue ferritin a risk factor for atherosclerosis and ischaemic heart disease? *Br. Heart J,* 73, 208-9.

Kotova, N; Hemminki, K; Segerback D. (2005). Urinary thymidine dimer as a marker of total body burden of UV-inflicted DNA damage in humans. *Cancer Epidemiol Biomarkers Prev.*, (12), 2868-72.

Kovac, V; Alonso, B; Bourzeiix, M; Revilla, E. (1992). Effect of several ecological practices on the content of catechins and proanthocyanidins of red wine. *J. Agic. Food Chem.*, 40, 1953-1957.

Kowald, A; Kirkwood, TB. (1994). Towards a network theory of aging: A model combining the free radical theory and the protein error theory. *J. Theoret. Biol*, 168, 75-94.

Kowald, A; Kirkwood, TB. (1996). A network theory of aging: The interactions of defective mitochondria, aberrant proteins, free radicals and scavengers in the aging process. *Mutat Res*, 316, 209-236.

Kozarev, J. (1998). Use of photoprotective measures in relation to actual exposure to solar rays.*Med. Pregl.*, 51(11-12), 555-8.

Krauss, S; Zhang, CY; Lowell, BB. (2005). The mitochondrial uncoupling protein homologues. *Nat. Rev. Mol. Cell Biol*, 6, 248-261.

Krebs, HA. (1972). Some aspects of the regulation of fuel supply in omnivorous animals. *Adv Enzyme Regul.*, 10, 397-420.

Kregel, KC; Zhang, HJ. (2007). An integrated view of oxidative stress in aging: Basic mechanisms, functional effects and pathological considerations. *Am. J. Physiol. Regul. Integr. Physiol*, 292, 18-36.

Kripke, M. (1984). Immunologic unresponsiveness induced by UV radiation. *Immunol Rev.*, 80, 87-102.

Krol, ES; Kramer-Stickland, KA; Liebler, DC. (2000). Photoprotective actions of topically applied vitamin E. *Drug Metab Rev.*, 32(3-4), 413-20.

Krutman, J; Gilchrest, BA. Photoaging of skin. In: *Skin aging*, Gilchrest, B; Krutmann, J. (Eds.). Springer-Verlag, Berlin 2006.

Krutmann, J; Yarosh, D. Modern photoprotection of human skin. In: *Skin aging*, Gilchrest, B; Krutmann, J. (Eds.). Springer-Verlag, Berlin 2006.

Krutmann, J. Pathomechanisms of photoaged skin. In: *Farage*, MA; Miller, KW; Maivach, HI. (Eds). Springer-Verlag, Berlin, 2010

Kurapati, R; Passananti, HB; Rose, MR; Tower, J. (2000). Increased hsp22 RNA levels in Drosophila lines genetically selected for increased longevity. *J. Gerontol. Biol. Sci. Med. Sci.*, 55, B552-B559.

Kurfürst, R; Joly, R; Notarnicola, C; Crabbé, I; André, P; Bonté, F; Perrier, P. (2000). Epidermal prevention of premature cellular senescence by telomerase and DNA protection, *J. Invest Dermatol*, 115 (3), 546.

Kuriyama, S; Shimazu, T; Ohmori, K; Kikuchi, N; Nakaya, N; Nishino, Y; Tsubono, Y; Tsuji, I. (2006). Green tea consumption and mortality due to cardiovascular disease, cancer, and all causes in Japan: the Ohsaki study. *JAMA*, 13, 296(10),1255-65.

Kurz, DJ; Decary, S; Hong, Y; Trivier, E; Akhmedov, A; Erusalimsky, JD. (2004). Chronic oxidative stress compromises telomere integrity and accelerates the onset of senescence in human endothelial cells. *J. Cell Sci*, 117, 2417 - 2426.

Kushelevsky, AP; Slifkin, MA. (1975). Ultraviolet measurements at the Dead Sea and Beersheba Isr. *J. Med. Sci.*, 11, 488-90.

Kvam, E; Tyrell, RM. (1887). Induction of oxidative DNA base damage in human skin cells by UV and near visible radiation. *Carcinogenesis.*, 18, 2379-2384.

Kyo, S; Takakura, M; Kanaya, T; Zhuo, W; Fujimoto, K; Nishio, Y; Orimo, A; Inoue M. (1999). Estrogen activates telomerase. *Cancer Res*, 59, 5917-21.

La Ruche, G; Cesarini, JP. (1991). Protective effects of oral selenium plus copper associated with vitamin complex on sunburn cell formation in human skin. *Photodermatol. Photoimmunol. Photomed.*, 8, 232–5.

Lahmann, C; Bergemann, J, Harrison, G; Young, AR. (2001). Matrix metalloproteinase-1 and skin ageing in smokers. *Lancet.*, 357(9260), 935-6.

Lakshmi, AV. (1998). Riboflavin metabolism—relevance to human nutrition. *Indian J. Med Res.* 108, 182-90.

Lal, A; Atamna, W; Killilea, DW; Suh, JH; Ames, BN. (2008). Lipoic acid and acetyl-carnitine reverse iron-induced oxidative stress in human fibroblasts. *Redox Rep.*, 13(1), 2-10.

Laloeuf, A; Byrne, AJ. The molecular aspects of dry, flaky skin conditions. In: *Skin moisturization.* (Eds.: Rawlings, AV; Leyden, JJ.). Infotma Healthcare, New York, 2009.

Lamming, DW; Wood, JG; Sinclair, DA. (2004). Small molecules that regulate lifespan: evidence for xenohormesis. *Molecular Microbiology*, 2004, 53, 1003-1009.

Lands, WEM. (1992). Biochemistry and physiology of n-3 fatty acids. *FASEB J.*, 6(8), 2530-6.

Lane, MA; Tilmont, EM; De Angelis, H; Ingram, DK; Kemmnitz, JW; Roth, GS. (2000). Short-term Calorie Restriction Improves Disease-related Markers in Older male Rhesus Monkey (Maccaca mulatta). *Mexh. Ageing Dev.*, 112, 185-196.

Lane, MA; Baer, DJ; Rumpler, WV; Weindruch, R; Ingram, DK; Tilmont, EM; Cutler, RG; Roth, GS. (1996). Calorie restriction lowers body temperature in rhesus monkeys, consistent with a postulated anti-aging mechanism in rodents. *Proc. Natl. Acad. Sci. USA*, 93, 59-64.

Lane, N. Power, Sex, Suicide: *Mitochondria and the Meaning of Life.* Oxford University Press, 2006.

Larsen, P. (1993). Aging and resistance to oxidative damage in Caenorhabditis elegans. *Proc. Natl. Acad. Sci. USA*, 90, 19, 8905–9.

Lasch, J; Schonfelder, U; Walke, M; Zellmer, S; Beckert, D. (1997). Oxidative damage of human skin lipids. Dependence of lipid peroxidation on sterol concentration. *Biochim Biophys Acta.*, 1349, 171-181.

Latonen, L; Laiho, M. (2005). Cellular UV damage responses—functions of tumor suppressor p53. *Biochim. Biophys. Acta*, 1755, 71-89.

Laurent-Applegate, LE; Schwarzkopf, S. Photooxidative Stress in Skin and Regulation of Gene Expression. In: *Environmental stressors in health and disease* (Ed. Fuchs, J; Packer, L.). Marcel Dekker, Inc.,2001.

Laval, F. (1988). Pretreatment with oxygen species increases the resistance of mammalian cells to hydrogen peroxide and gamma-rays. *Mutat Res.*, 201(1), 73-9.

Lavker, RM; Kligman, A. (1988). Chronic heliodermatitis: amorphologic evaluation of chronic actinic dermal damage with emphasis on the role of mast cells. *J. Invest. Dermatol.*, 90, 325-330.

Lavker, RM. Cutaneous aging: Chronologic versus photoaging. In B. Gilchrest (Ed.), *Photodamage*(Vol. 1, pp. 123-135). Cambridge: Blackwell, 1995.

Lawrence, N. (2000). History of dermabrasion. *Dermatol Surg*, 26, 95-101.

Le Bourg, E. (2005). Is caloric restriction a means of delaying ageing and increasing longevity? *Presse Med.*, 34,121–127.

Le Bourg, E; Rattan, S. (eds.). *Mild Stress and Healthy Aging: Applying hormesis in aging research and interventions.*Springer Science, 2008, 187 pp.

Le Curieux, F; Hemminki K. (2001). Cyclobutane thymidine dimers are present in human urine following sun exposure: quantitation using 32P-postlabeling and high-performance liquid chromatography. *J. Invest. Dermatol.*, 117(2), 263-8.

Le Varlet, B; Dumay, C; Barré, P; Bonté, F. (1999). Influence of advanced glycation end products on the adhesion of normal human keratinocytes, *J. Invest. Dermatol*, 113.

Lea, CS; Scotto, JA; Buffler, PA; Fine, J; Barnhill, RL; Berwick, M. (2007). Ambient UVB and melanoma risk in the United States: a case-control analysis. *Ann. Epidemiol*, 17(6), 447-53.

Lee, DW; Yu, BP. (1991). Food restriction as an effective modulator of free radical metabolism in rats. *Korean Biochem. J.*, 1991, 24, 148-154.

Lee, IM; Hsieh, CC; Paffenbarger, RS Jr. (1995). Exercise intensity and longevity in men. The Harvard Alumni Health Study. *JAMA.*, 273(15), 1179-84.

Lee, J; Jiang, SG; Levine, N; Watson, RR. (2000). Carotenoid supplementation reduces erythema in human skin after simulated solar radiation exposure. *Proc. Soc. Exp. Biol. Med.*, 223, 170–4.

Lee, KS; Oh, KY; Kim, BC. (2000). Effects of dehydroepiandrosterone on collagen and collagenase gene expression by skin fibroblasts in culture.*J. Dermatol. Sci.*, 23(2), 103-10.

Lee, KW; Kim, YJ; Lee, HJ; Lee, CY. (2003). Cocoa has more phenolic phytochemicals and a higher antioxidant capacity than teas and red wine. *J. Agric. Food Chem.*,51(25), 7292–5.

Lee, KW; Kundu, JK; Kim, SO; Chun, KS; Lee, HJ; Surh, YJ. (2006). Cocoa polyphenols inhibit phorbol ester-induced superoxide anion formation in cultured HL-60 cells and expression of cyclooxygenase-2 and activation of NF-kappaB and MAPKs in mouse skin in vivo. *J. Nutr.*, 136(5), 1150-5.

Lee, MS; Lee, KH; Sin, HS; Um, SJ; Kim, JW; Koh, BK. (2006). A newly synthesized photostable retinol derivative (retinyl N-formyl aspartamate) for photodamaged skin: profilometric evaluation of 24-week study. *J. Am. Acad. Dermatol.*, 55(2), 220-4.

Leeuwenburgh, C; Fiebig, R; Chandwaney, R; Ji, L. (1994). Aging and exercise training in skeletal muscle: responses of glutathione and antioxidant enzyme systems. *Am. J. Physiol,* 267, 439–45.

Legrain, S; Massien, C; Lahlou, N; Roger, M; Debuire, B; Diquet, B; Chatellier, G; Azizi, M; Faucounau, V; Porchet, H; Forette, F; Baulieu, EE. (2000). Dehydroepiandrosterone replacement administration: Pharmacokinetic and pharmacodynamic studies in healthy elderly subjects. *Journal of Clinical Endocrinology and Metabolism*, 85(9), 3208-3217.

Yin, L; Morita, A; Tsuji, T. (2001). Skin premature aging induced by tobacco smoking: the objective evidence of skin replica analysis. *J. Dermatol. Sci.*, 27(1), S26-31.

Lenz, H; Schmidt, M; Welge, V; Schlattner, U; Wallimann, T; Elsässer, HP; Wittern, KP; Wenck, H; Stäb, F; Blatt, T. (2005). The creatine kinase system in human skin: protective effects of creatine against oxidative and UV damage in vitro and in vivo. *J. Invest. Dermatol.* 124(2), 443-52.

Letavayová, L; Vlcková, V; Brozmanová, J. (2006). Selenium: from cancer prevention to DNA damage. *Toxicology*, 227(1-2), 1-14.

Leung, W; Harvey, I. (2002). Is skin aging in the elderly caused by sun exposure or smoking? *Br. J. Dermatol*, 147(6), 1187-1191.

Lever, L; Kumar, P; Marks, R. (1990). Topical retinoic acid for treatment of solar damage. *Br. J. Dermatol.*, 122(1), 91-8.

Levi, B; Werman, MJ. (1998). Long-term fructose consumption accelerates glycation and several age-related variables in male rats. *J. Nutr.*, 128(9), 1442-9.

Levin, J; Momin, SB. (2010). How much do we really know about our favorite cosmeceutical ingredients? *J. Clin. Aesthet. Dermatol.*, 3(2), 22-41.

Levine, B; Kroemer, G. (2008). Autophagy in the pathogenesis of disease, *Cell*, 132 27–42.

Leyden, JJ; Grove, GL; Grove, MJ; Thorne, EG; Lufrano, L. (1989). Treatment of photodamaged facial skin with topical tretinoin. *J. Am. Acad. Dermatol.*, 21(3 Pt 2), 638-44.

Leyden, JJ; Parr, L. (2010). Treating photodamage of the décolletage area with a novel copper zinc malonate complex plus hydroquinone and tretinoin. *J. Drugs Dermatol.*, 9(3), 220-6.

Leyden, JJ. (1998). Treatment of photodamaged skin with topical tretinoin: an update. *Plast Reconstr. Surg.*, 102(5), 1667-71; discussion 1672-5.

Li, G; Mitchell, DL; Ho, VC; Reed, JC; Tron, VA. (1996). Decreased DNA repair but normal apoptosis in ultraviolet-irradiated skin of p53-transgenic mice. *Am. J. Pathol.*, 148, 1113–1123.

Li, JJ; Yu, BP. (1994). Alterations in mitochondrial membrane fluidity by lipid peroxidation products. *Free Radic. Biol. Med*, 17, 411-418.

Li, WQ; Kuriyama, S; Li, Q; Nagai, M; Hozawa, A; Nishino, Y; Tsuji, I. (2010). Citrus consumption and cancer incidence: The Ohsaki Cohort Study. *Int. J. Cancer*, [Epub ahead of print].

Li, YF; Kim, ST; Sancer, A. (1993). Evidence for lack of DNA photoreactivity enzyme in humans. *Proc. Natl. Acad. Sci. (USA)*, 90, 4389-4393.

Lin, JY; Selim, MA; Shea, CR ;Grichnik, JM; Omar, MM; Monteiro-Riviere, NA; Pinnell, SR. (2003). UV photoprotection by combination topical antioxidants vitamin C and vitamin E. *J. Am. Acad. Dermatol.*, 48(6), 866-74.

Lin, YJ; Seroude, L; Benzer, S. (1998). Extended lifespan and stress resistance in the Drosophila mutant methuselah. *Science*, 282, 943-946.

Lingelbach, LB; Mitchell, AE; Rucker, RB; McDonald, RB. (2000). Accumulation of advanced glycation end products in aging male Fischer 344 rats during long-term feeding of various dietary carbohydrates. *J. Nutr.*, 130(5), 1247-55.

Lima, CF; Pereira-Wilson, C; Rattan, SI. (2010). Curcumin induces heme oxygenase-1 in normal human skin fibroblasts through redox signaling: Relevance for anti-aging intervention. *Mol. Nutr. Food Res.*, [Epub ahead of print].

Lithgow, GJ; White, TM; Melov, S; Johnson, TE. (1995). Thermotolerance and extended lifespan conferred by single-gene mutations and induced by thermal stress. *Proc. Natl. Acad. Sci.* USA,92(16), 7540-4.

Littarru, GP; Tiano, L. (2007). Bioenergetic and antioxidant properties of coenzyme Q10: recent developments. *Mol. Biotechnol.*, 37(1), 31-7.

Liu, J. (1996). Immobilization stress causes oxidative damage to lipid, protein, and DNA in the brain of rats. *Faseb J.*, 10, 1532—1538.

Liu, JP. (1999). Studies of the molecular mechanisms in the regulation of telomerase activity, *FASEB J.*, 13, 2091-104.

Liu, RK; Walford, LR. (1970). Observations on the lifespans of several species of annual fish and of world' s smallest fish. *Exp. Gerontol.*, 5, 241-246.

Liu, RK; Walford, RL. (1972). The effect of lowered body temperature on lifespan and immune and non-immune processes. *Gerontologia*, 18, 363-388.

Liu, Y; Hong, L; Kempf, VR; Wakamatsu, K, Ito, S; Simon, JD. (2004). Ion-exchange and adsorption of Fe(III) by Sepia melanin. *Pigment Cell Research*,17(3), 262–9.

Loggie, BW; Eddy, JA. (1988).Solar considerations in the development of cutaneous melanomaSemin. *Oncol.*, 15, 494-9.

López-Torres, M; Barja, G. (2008). Lowered methionine ingestion as responsible for the decrease in rodent mitochondrial oxidative stress in protein and dietary restriction: Possible implications for humans. *Biochemica et BiophysicaActa*, 1780, 1337-1347.

Lopez-Torres, M; Gredilla, R; Sanz, A; Barja, G. (2002). Influence of aging and long-term caloric restriction on oxygen radical generation and oxidative DNA damage in rat liver mitochondria. *Free Radic. Biol. Med*, 32, 882–889.

Lorenz, M; Saretzki, G; Sitte, N; Metzkow, S; von Zglinicki, T. (2001). BJ fibroblasts display high antioxidant capacity and slow telomere shortening independent of hTERT transfection. *Free Rad. Biol. Med*, 31, 824-31.

Lotito, SB; Frei, B. (2006). Consumption of flavonoid-rich foods and increased plasma antioxidant capacity in humans: cause, consequence, or epiphenomenon? *Free Radic. Biol. Med.*, 41, 1727–46.

Lowe, NJ; Shauth, NA; Patahk, MA. (1997). *Sunscreens—development, evaluation and regulatory aspects*. Marcel Dekker, New York, 1997.

Lu J, Xie L, Sylvester J, et al. (2007). Different gene expression of skin tissues between mice with weight controlled by either CR or physical exercise. *Exp. Biol. Med.*, 232, 473-480.

Lu, YP; Lou, YR; Peng, QY; Xie, JG; Nghiem, P; Conney, AH. (2008). Effect of caffeine on the ATR/Chk1 pathway in the epidermis of UVB-irradiated mice. *Cancer Res.*, 68(7), 2523-9.

Lu, YP; Lou, YR; Peng, QY; Xie, JG; Nghiem, P; Conney, AH. (2008). Effect of caffeineon the ATR/Chk1 pathway in theepidermis of UVB-irradiated mice. *Cancer Res.*, 68, 2523-2529.

Lui, J; Killilea, DW; Ames, BN. (2002). Age-associated mitochondrial oxidative decay: Improvement of carnitine acetyltransferase substrate-binding affinity and activity in brain by feeding old rats acetyl-L-carnitine and/or R-a-lipoic acid. *Proceedings of the National Academy of Sciences.*, 99, 1876-1881.

Lunec, J; Griffits, HR. *Measuring in vivo oxidative damage*. New York: John Willey and Sons, Ltd., 2000.

Lushchak, VI. (2001). Oxidative stress and mechanisms of protection against it in bacteria. *Biochemistry* (Moscow), 66, 476-489.

Lutz, PL; Prentice, HM; Milton, SL. (2003). Is turtle longevity linked to enhanced mechanisms for surviving brain anoxia and reoxygenation? *Exp Gerontol*, 38, 797–800.

Mac Cawley, LJ; Matrisian, LM. (2000). Matrix metalloproteinase: Multifunctional contributors to tumor progression. *Mol Med Today*, 6, 149-56.

Mac Cawley, LJ; Matrisian, LM. (20019. Matrix metalloproteinase: they're not just for matrix anymore! *Curr. Opinion in Cell Biol*, 2001, 13, 534-40.

MacKie, RM; Freudenberger, T; Aitchison, TC. (1989). Personal risk-factor chart for cutaneous melanoma, *Lancet*, 2(8661), 487-90.

Maes, D; Collins,D; Declercq,L; Foyouzi-Yousseffi, R; Gan, D; Mammone, T; Pelle, E; Marenus, K; Gedeon, H. (2004). Improving cellular function through modulation of energy metabolism. *International Journal of Cosmetic Science*, 26(5), 268–269.

Mager, WH; Hohmann, S. (1997). Stress response mechanisms in the yeast Saccharomyces cerevisiae. In: *Yeast stress responses* (Hohmann, S; Mager HRG, Eds..). Austin: Landes Company, 1-5.

Mahoney, MG; Brennan, D; Starcher, B; Faryniarz, J; Ramirez, J; Parr, L; Uitto, J. (2009). Extracellular matrix in cutaneous ageing: the effects of 0.1% copper-zinc malonate-containing cream on elastin biosynthesis. *Exp. Dermatol.*, 18(3), 205-11.

Maiani, G; Periago Castón, MJ; Catasta, G. (2008). Carotenoids: Actual knowledge on food sources, intakes, stability and bioavailability and their protective role in humans. *Mol. Nutr. Food Res*, 53, 194-218.

Maier, T; Korting, HC. (2005). Sunscreens—which and what for? *Skin Pharmacol. Physiol.*, 18(6), 253-62.

Maillard, JL; Favreau, C; Reboud-Ravaux, M. (1995). Role of monocyte/macrophage derived matrix metalloproteinases(gelatinases) in prolonged skin inflammation. *Clin. Chim. Acta.*, 233, 61–74.

Makrantonaki, E; Adjaye, J; Herwig, R, et al. (2006). Age-specific hormonal decline is accompanied by transcriptional changes in human sebocytes in vitro. *Aging Cell*, 5, 331-344.

Makrantonaki, E; Schönknecht, P; Hossini, AM; Kaiser, E; Katsouli, MM; Adjaye, J; Schröder, J; Zouboulis, CC. (2010). Skin and brain age together: The role of hormones in the ageing process. *Exp. Gerontol.* 45(10):801-13.

Makrantonaki, E; Zouboulis, CC. *Pathomechanisms of endogenously aged skin.*In: Farage, MA; Miller, KW; Maivach, HI. (Eds). Springer-Verlag, Berlin, 2010.

Mammone, T; Gan, D; Foyouzi-Youssefi, R. Apoptotic cell death increases with senescence in normal human dermal fibroblast cultures. *Cell Biol. Int.*, 30(11), 903-9.

Manaka, I; Kadono, S; Kawashima, M; Kobayashi, T; Imokawa, G. (2001). The mechanisms of hyperpigmentation in seborrhoeic keratosis involve the high expression of endothelin-converting enzyme-1? and TNF-?, which stimulate secretion of endothelin 1, *Brit. J. Dermatol*, 145, 895-903.vv.

Mandel, S; Amit, T; Bar-Am, O; Youdim, MB. (2007). Iron dysregulation in Alzheimer's disease: multimodal brain permeable iron chelating drugs, possessing neuroprotective-neurorescue and amyloid precursor protein-processing regulatory activities as therapeutic agents. *Prog. Neurobiol.*, 82, 348-60.

Mandic, S; Myers, JN; Oliveira, RB; Abella, JP; Froelicher, VF. (2009). Characterizing differences in mortality at the low end of the fitness spectrum. *Med. Sci. Sports Exerc.*, 41(8), 1573-9.

Mangelsdorf, DJ. (1994).Vitamin A receptors. *Nutr. Rev.* 52(2 Pt 2), S32-44.

Mao-Qiang, M; Feingold, KR; Thornfeldt, CR; Elias, PM. (19969. Optimization of physiological lipid mixtures for barrier repair. *J. Invest. Dermatol*, 106, 1096–1101.

Marks, F; Fürstenberger, G. Tumor promotion in skin: Are active oxygen species involved? In: Sies H, ed. *Oxidative Stress.* London: Academic Press, Inc, 1985, 437–475.

Marnett, LJ. (2000). Oxyradicals and DNA damage. *Carcinogenesis*, 21, 361-370.

Marquardt, H; Schafer, SG; McClellan, RO; Welsch, F. (1999). *Toxicology.* San Diego: Academic Press.

Martin, GM. (1987). Interaction of aging and environmental agents: The gerontological perspective. *Prog. Clin. Bio. Res*, 228, 25-80.

Martin, GM; Austad, SN; Johnson, TE. (1996). Genetic analysis of ageing: Role of oxidative damage and environmental stress. *Nat. Genet*, 13, 25-34.

Martin-Du Pan RC. (1999). Are the hormones of youth carcinogenic? *Ann Endocrinol* (Paris), 60(5), 392-7.

Martires, KJ; Fu, P; Polster, AM; Cooper, KD; Baron, ED. (2009). Factors that affect skin aging: a cohort-based survey on twins. *Arch. Dermatol.* 145(12), 1375-9.

Martínez-González, MA; de la Fuente-Arrillaga, C; Nunez-Cordoba, JM; et al. (2008). Adherence to Mediterranean diet and risk of developing diabetes: prospective cohort study. *BMJ*, 336(7657), 1348–51.

Martindale, JL; Holbrook, NJ. (2002). Cellular response to oxidative stress: signaling for suicide and survival. *J. Cell Physiol.*, 192, 1–15.

Masaki, H. (2010). Role of antioxidants in the skin: anti-aging effects. *J. Dermatol. Sci.*, 58(2), 85-90.

Masoro, EJ. (1993). Dietary restriction and aging. *J. Am. Geriatr. Soc.*, 41, 994-9.

Massagué, J. (1998). TGF-beta signal transduction. *Annu. Rev. Biochem.*, 67, 753-91.

Mathews-Roth, MM; Krinsky, NI. (1987). Carotenoids affect development of UVB-induced skin cancer. *Photochem. Photobiol*, 46, 507-509.

Mattson MP. (2003). Energy Metabolism and Lifespan Determination, *Adv. Cell Aging Geronto*, 14, 105-122.

Matsuda, M; Hoshino, T; Yamashita, Y; Tanaka, K; Maji, D; Sato, K; Adachi, H; Sobue, G; Ihn, H; Funasaka, Y; Mizushima, T. (2010). Prevention of UVB radiation-induced epidermal damage by expression of heat shock protein 70. *J. Biol. Chem.*, 285(8), 5848-58.

Matsui, M; Miyasaka, J; Hamada, K; Ogawa, Y; Hiramoto, M; Fujimori, R; Aioi, A. (2000). Influence of aging and cell senescence on telomerase activity in keratinocytes. *J. Dermatol. Sci*, 22, 80-7.

Mattson, MP; Chan, SL; Duan, W. (2002). Modification of brain aging and neurodegenerative disorders by genes, diet, and behavior. *Physiological Reviews*, 82, 637-672.

Mattson, MP; Duan, Wenzhen; Wan, Ruiqian; Guo, Zhihong. (2003). Cellular and molecular mechanisms whereby dietary restriction extends healthspan: a beneficial type of stress; in Mattson, Mark P. (editor). Energy metabolism and Lifespan Determination; *Advances in cell aging and gerontology*, Vol. 14, 87-103.

Mattson, MP. (2003). The search for energy: a driving force in evolution and aging; in Mattson, Mark P. (editor). Energy metabolism and Lifespan Determination; *Advances in cell aging and gerontology*. Vol. 14, 1-11.

Mattson, MP; Chan, SI; Duan, W. (2000). Modification of Brain Aging and Neurodegenerative Disorders by Genes, Diet and Behavior. *Physiol. Rev.*, 82, 637-672.

Mauviel, A. (1993). Cytokine regulation of metalloproteinase gene expression. *J. Cell Biochem,* 53, 288-95.

Mazat, JP; Rossignol, R; Malgat, M; Rocher, C; Faustin, B; Letelliner, T. (2001). What do mitochondrial diseases teach us about normal mitochondrial functions... that we already knew: threshold expression of mitochondrial defects. *Biochimica et Biophysica Acta*, 1504, 20.

May, JM; Cobb, CE; Mendiratta, S; Hill, KE; Burk, RF. (1998). Reduction of the ascorbyl free radical to ascorbate by thioredoxin reductase. *J. Biol. Chem*, 273, 23039–23045.

McArdle, F; Rhodes, LE; Parslew, R; Jack, CI; Friedmann, PS; Jackson, MJ. (2002). UVR-induced oxidative stress in human skin in vivo: effects of oral vitamin C supplementation. *Free Radic. Biol. Med.*, 33(10), 1355-62.

McArdle, F; Rhodes, LE; Parslew, RA; Close, GL; Jack, CI; Friedmann, PS; Jackson, MJ. (20049. Effects of oral vitamin E and beta-carotene supplementation on ultraviolet radiation-induced oxidative stress in human skin. *Am. J. Clin. Nutr.*, 80(5), 1270-5.

McCall, MR; Frei, B. (1999). Can antioxidant vitamins materially reduce oxidative damage in humans?, *Free Radic. Biol. Med.*, 26, 1034–1053.

McCormick, JP; Fisher, JR; Pachlatko, JP; Eisenstark, A. (1976). Characterization of a cell lethal product from the photooxidation of tryptophan: hydrogen peroxide. *Science*, 198, 468-469.

McCullough, EC. (1970). Qualitative and quantitative features of the clear day terrestrial solar ultraviolet radiation environmentPhys. *Med. Biol.*, 15, 723-34.

McDaniel, DH; Neudecker, BA; DiNardo, JC; Lewis, JA; Maibach, HI. (2005). Clinical efficacy assessment in photodamaged skin of 0.5% and 1.0% idebenone. *Journal of Cosmetic Dermatology*, 4, 167-173.

McCay, CM; Crowell, MF; Maynard, LA. (1935). *The Effect of Retarded Growth upon the Length of the Lifespan and Upon the Ultimate Body Size*, 10, 63-79.

McKersie, BD. Oxidative stress. Dept of Crop science, University of Guelph. http://www.agronomy.psu.edu/Courses/AGRO518/Oxygen.htm#activation (8.2.2004).

McMichael, AJ; Giles, GG. (1988). Cancer in migrants to Australia: extending the descriptive epidemiological data. *Cancer Res.*, 48(3), 751-6.

McVean, M; Liebler, DC. (1999). Prevention of DNA photodamage by vitamin E compounds and sunscreens: roles of ultraviolet absorbance and cellular uptake. *Mol. Carcinog.*, 24(3), 169-76.

Medrano, E. (1998). Aging, replicative senescence, and the differentiated function of the melanocyte. *The pigmenary system*, Oxford University Press, 151-8.

Medvedev, ZA. (1990). An attempt at a rational classification of theories of ageing. *Biol. Rev. Camb. Philos. Soc.*, 65(3), 375–398.

Melov, S; Ravenscroft, J; Malik, S; et al. (2000). Extension of lifespan with superoxide dismutase/catalase mimetics. *Science*, 289, 1567–1569.

Mendiratta, S; Qu, Z; May, J. (1998). Erythrocyte ascorbate recycling: antioxidant effects in blood. *Free Radic. Biol. Med*, 24, 789-797.

Mendiratta, S; Qu, Z; May, JM. (1998). Erythrocyte defenses against hydrogen peroxide: The role of ascorbic acid. *Biochim. Biophys. Acta*, 1380(3), 389-95.

Menon, EL; Morrison, H. (2002). Formation of singlet oxygen by UVA irradiation and some consequences thereof. *Photochem. Photobiol*, 75, 565-569.

Merker, K; Sitte, N; Grune, T. (2000). Hydrogen peroxide-mediated protein oxidation in young and old human MRC-5 fibroblasts. *Arch. Biochem. Biophys.*, 375(1), 50-4.

Merry, BJ. (2004). Oxidative stress and mitochondrial function with aging—the effects of calorie restriction. *Aging Cell*, 3, 7–12.

Meydani, M. (2001). Nutrition interventions in aging and age-associated disease. *Ann. N Y Acad. Sci.*, 928, 226-35.

Meyers, DG; Maloley, PA; Weeks, D. (1996). Safety of antioxidant vitamins. *Arch. Intern. Med.*, 156, 925–35.

Middleton Fillmore, K; Kerr, WC; Stockwell, T; Chikritzhs, T; Bostrom, M. (2006). Moderate alcohol use and reduced mortality risk: Systematic error in prospective studies. *Addiction Research & Theory*, 101–132.

Miescher, G. (1930). Das problem des Lichtschutzes und der Lichtgewohnung. *Strahlentherapie*, 35, 403-43.

Milbury, PE; Richer, AC. (2008). *Understanding the Antioxidant Controversy: Scrutinizing the "fountain of Youth,"* Greenwood Publishing Group, p. 99.

Miller, DL; Weinstock, MA. (1994). Nonmelanoma skin cancer in the United States: incidence. *J. Am. Acad. Dermatol.*, 30(5 Pt 1), 774-8.

Miller, ER; Pastor-Barriuso, R; Dalal, D; Riemersma, R; Appel, LJ; Guallar, E. (2005).Meta-Analysis: High-Dosage Vitamin E Supplementation May Increase All-Cause Mortality. *Annals of Internal Medicine*, 142, 37-46.

Miller, R; Austad, SN. Growth and aging: why do big dogs die young? In: *Handbook of the biology of aging.* Sixthedition. Ed: Masoro, EJ; Austad, S. Elsevier, 2006.

Mills, SJ; Ashworth, JJ; Gilliver, SC; Hardman, MJ; Ashcroft, GS. (2005). The sex steroid precursor DHEA accelerates cutaneous wound healing via the estrogen receptors. *J. Invest Dermatol.*, 125(5), 1053-62.

Milton, NGN. (2004). Role of hydrogen peroxide in the aetiology of Alzheimer's disease—Implications for treatment. *Drugs & Aging*, 21, 81-100.

Mineharu, Y; Koizumi, A; Wada, Y; Iso, H; Watanabe, Y; Date, C; Yamamoto, A; Kikuchi, S; Inaba, Y; Toyoshima, H; Kondo, T; Tamakoshi, A. (2009/2010). Coffee, green tea, black tea and oolong tea consumption and risk of mortality from cardiovascular disease in Japanese men and women. *J. Epidemiol. Community Health*, [Epub ahead of print].

Miquel, J; Fleming, J; Economos, AC. (19829. Antioxidants, metabolic rate and aging in Drosophila. *Arch. Gerontol. Geriatr.*,1, 159-165.

Miquel, J; Johnson, JR. (1975). Effects of various antioxidants and radiation protectants on the lifespan and lipofuscin of Drosophila and C57BL/6J mice. *Gerontologist*, 15- 25.

Mirzoeva, OK; Calder, PC. (1996). The effect of propolis and its components on eicosanoid production during the inflammatory response. *Prostaglandins Leukot Essent Fatty Acids*, 55, 441–449.

Missirlis, F. (2003). Understanding the Aging Fly through Physiological Genetics. In: Mattson MP. (editor): Energy Metabolism and Lifespan Determination, *Adv. Cell Aging Gerontol.* 2003; 14: 123-141.

Miyachi, Y; Uchida, K; Komura, J; Asada, Y; Niwa, Y. (1985). Auto oxidative damage in cement dermatitis. *Arch. Dermatol. Res.*, 277, 288–292.

Miyamoto, K; Hillebrand, GG. (2002). The Beauty Imaging System: for the objective evaluation of skin condition. *J. Cosmetic. Sci.*, 53, 62–5.

Mlekusch, W; Tillian, H; Lamprecht, M; Trutnovsky, H; Reibnegger, G. (1996). The effect of reduced physical activity on longevity of mice. *Mech. Ageing Dev*, 88, 159-168.

Moan, J; Dahlback, A; Setlow, RB. (1999). Epidemiological support for a hypothesis for melanoma induction indicating a role for UVA radiation. *Photochem. Photobiol.*, 70(2), 243-7.

Moan, J; Porojnicu, AC; Dahlback, A. (2008). Ultraviolet radiation and malignant melanoma. *Adv. Exp. Med. Biol.*, 624, 104-16.

Molina, MJ; Rowland, FS. (1974).Stratospheric sink for chlorofluoromethanes: chlorine atom-catalyzed destruction of ozone. *Nature*, 249, 810-2.

Moloney, FJ; Collins, S; Murphy, GM. (2002). Sunscreens: safety, efficacy and appropriate use. *Am. J. Clin. Dermatol.*, 3(3), 185-91.

Monnier, VM; Sell, DR; Saxena, A; et al. Glycoxidatative and carbonyl stress in aging and age-related diseases. In: *Critical reviews of oxidative stress and aging* (Eds: Cutler, RG; Rodriguez, H). World Scientific, New Jersey, 2003.

Mooijaart, SP; van Heemst, D; Schreuder, J; van Gerwen, S; Beekman, M; Brandt, BW. (2004). Variation in the SHC1 gene and longevity in humans. *Exp. Gerontol*, 39, 263-8.

Moran, J. F; Klucas, R. V; Grayer, R. J; Abian, J; Becana, M. (1997). Complexes of iron with phenolic compounds from soybean nodules and other legume tissues: pro-oxidant and antioxidant properties. *Free Radic. Biol. Med.*, 22, 861-70.

Morano, KA. (2007). New tricks for an old dog: the evolving world of Hsp70. *Ann. N.Y. Acad. Sci.*,1113, 1–14.

Morita, A. (2007). Tobacco smoke causes premature skin aging. *J. Dermatol. Sci.*, 48(3), 169-75.

Morrow, GS; Battistini, S; Zhang, P; Tanguay, RM. (2004). Decreased lifespan in the absence of expression of the mitochondrial small heat shock protein hsp22 in Drosophila. *J. Biol. Chem.*, 279, 43382-43385.

Moschella, S; Hurley, H. (1992). *Aging and Its Effects on the Skin. Dermatology: Third Edition*. Philadelphia: W.B. Saunders Company, 1992.

Moskaug, JØ; Carlsen, H; Myhrstad, MC; Blomhoff, R. (2005). Polyphenols and glutathione synthesis regulation. *Am. J. Clin. Nutr.*, 81(1), 277S-283S.

Moyal, DD; Fourtanier, AM. (2008). Broad-spectrum sunscreens provide better protection from solar ultraviolet-simulated radiation and natural sunlight-induced immunosuppression in human beings. *J. Am. Acad. Dermatol.*, 58(5 Suppl 2), S149-54.

Moysan, A; Cle´ment-Lacroix, P; Michel, L; Dubertret, L; Morliere, P. (1995). Effects of ultraviolet A and antioxidant defense in cultured fibroblasts and keratinocytes. *Photodermatol. Photoimmunol. Photomed.*, 1995, 11, 192–197.

Moysan, A; Marquis, I; Gaboriau, F; Santus, R; Dubertret, L; Morliere P. (1993). Ultraviolet A-induced lipid peroxidation and antioxidant defense systems in cultured human skin fibroblasts. *J. Invest. Dermatol.*, 1993, 100, 692–698.

Muizzuddin, N; Maes, D; Giacomoni, P. Psychological stress and the skin. In: *Skin Moisturization*, Informa Healthcare, New York, 2009.

Murakami, K; Inagaki, J; Saito, M; Ikeda, Y; Tsuda, C; Noda, Y; Kawakami, S; Shirasawa, T; Shimizu, T.(2009). Skin atrophy in cytoplasmic SOD-deficient mice and its complete recovery using a vitamin C derivative. *Biochem. Biophys. Res. Commun.*, 382(2), 457-61.

Mustafa, MG. (1990). Biochemical basis of ozone toxicity. *Free Radic. Biol. Med.*, 9, 245–265.

Muldoon, MF; Kritchevsky, SB. (1996). Flavonoids and heart disease. *BMJ.*, 312(7029), 458-9.

Muta-Takada, K; Terada, T; Yamanishi, H; Ashida, Y; Inomata, S; Nishiyama, T; Amano, S. (2009). Coenzyme Q10 protects against oxidative stress-induced cell death and enhances the synthesis of basement membrane components in dermal and epidermal cells. *Biofactors.*, 35(5), 435-41.

Nandhini, AT; Thirunavukkarasu, V; Anuradha, CV. (2005). Taurine prevents collagen abnormalities in high fructose-fed rats. *Indian J. Med. Res.*,122 (2), 171–7.

Narayanan, BA. (2006). Chemopreventive agents alters global gene expression pattern: predicting their mode of action and targets. *Curr. Cancer Drug Targets*, 6, 711–727.

National Institutes of Health. (2006). NIH State-of-the-Science Conference Statement on Multivitamin/Mineral Supplements and Chronic Disease Prevention. *NIH Consens State Sci Statements.*, 23(2), 1-30.

Nedergaard, J; Ricquier, D; Kozak, LP. (2005). Uncoupling proteins: current status and therapeutic prospects. *EMBO Rep.*, 6 (10), 917–21.

Neer, RM. (1975). The evolutionary significance of vitamin D, skin pigment, and ultraviolet light. *Am. J. Phys. Anthropol.*, 43(3), 409-16.

Nemoto, S; Otsuka, M; Arakawa, N. (1997). Effect of high concentration of ascorbate on catalase activity in cultured cells and tissues of guinea pigs. *J. Nutr. Sci. Vitaminol.*, 43, 297-203.

Neukam, K; Stahl, W; Tronnier, H; Sies, H; Heinrich, U. (2007). Consumption of flavanol-rich cocoa acutely increases microcirculation in human skin. *European Journal of Nutrition*, 46(1),53-56.

Nicholls, D. (2002). Mitochondrial bioenergetics, aging, and aging-related diseases. *Sci. Aging Knowl. Environ.*, 2002(31), 12.

Nicholls, DG; Locke, RM.(1984). Thermogenic mechanisms in brown fat. *Physiol Rev.*, 64(1), 1-64.

Nishikawa, T; Edelstein, D; Du, XL; Yamagishi, S; Matsumura, T; Kaneda, Y; Yorek, MA; Beebe, D; Oates, PJ; Hammes, HP; Giardino, I; Brownlee, M. (2000). Normalizing mitochondrial superoxide production blocks three pathways of hyperglycaemic damage. *Nature.*, 404(6779), 787-90.

Nofsinger, JB; Liu, Y; Simon, JD. (2002). Aggregation of eumelanin mitigates photogeneration of reactive oxygen species. *Free Rad. Biol. Med,* 32, 720-30.

Nohynek, GJ; Antignac, E; Re, T; Toutain, H. (2010). Safety assessment of personal care products/cosmetics and their ingredients. *Toxicol. Appl. Pharmacol.*, 243(2), 239-59.

Nohynek, GJ; Schaefer, H. (2001). Benefit and risk of organic ultraviolet filters. *Regul. Toxicol. Pharmacol.*, 33(3), 285-99.

Nohynek, GJ; Lademann, J; Ribaud, C; Roberts, MS. (2007). Gray Goo on the skin? Nanotechnology, cosmetic and sunscreen safety. *Crit. Rew. Toxicol.*, 37, 251-277.

Norbury, CJ; Hickson, ID. (2001). Cellular responses to DNA damage. *Annu. Rev. Pharmacol. Toxicol.*, 41, 367-401.

Nordberg, J; Arner, ESJ. (2001). Reactive oxygen species, antioxidants, and the mammalian thioredoxin system. *Free Radic. Biol. Med.*, 31, 1287-1312.

Nordmann, R. (1994). Alcohol and antioxidant systems. *Alcohol.* 29(5), 513-22.

Norman, KG; Eshaghian, A; Sligh, J. DNA biomarkers in aging skin. In: *Textbook of aging skin* (Farage, MA; Miller, KW; Maibach HI (Eds). Springer-Verlag, Berlin, 2010

Norlen L. Untangling the role of keratin in stratum corneum. In: *Skin moisturization*. (Eds.: Rawlings, AV; Leyden, JJ). Infotma Healthcare, New York, 2009.

Nouveau, S; Bastien, P; Baldo, F; de Lacharriere, O. (2008). Effects of topical DHEA on aging skin: a pilot study. *Maturitas.*,59(2) 174-81.

Nusgens, BV; Humbert, P; Rougier, A; Richard, A; Lapière, CM. (2002). Stimulation of collagen biosynthesis by topically applied vitamin C. *EuropeanJournal of Dermatology*, 12(4):XXXII-XXXIV.

Offord, EA; Gautier, JC; Avanti, O; Scaletta, C; Runge, F; Krämer, K; Applegate, LA. (2002). Photoprotective potential of lycopene, beta-carotene, vitamin E, vitamin C and carnosic acid in UVA-irradiated human skin fibroblasts. *Free Radic. Biol. Med.*, 32(12), 1293-303.

Ohman, H; Vahlquist, A. (1994). In vivo studies concerning a pH gradient in human stratum corneum and upper epidermis. *Acta Derm. Venereol*, 74, 375–379.

Oikarinen A. (1994). Aging of the skin connective tissue: how to measure the biochemical and mechanical properties of aging dermis. *Photodermatology, Photoimmunology and Photomedicine*, 10(2), 47-52.

Oishi, K; Yokoi, M; Maekawa, S; Sodeyama, C; Shiraishi, T; Kondo, R; Kuriyama, T; Machida, K. (1999). Oxidative stress and haematological changes in immobilized rats. *Acta Physiol. Scand.*, 165(1), 65-9.

Okazaki, M. Aging and Melanocytes Stimulating Cytokine Expressed by Keratinocyte and Fibroblast. *Textbook of aging skin*. Berlin: Springer-Verlag, 2010.

Oleinck, NL; Chiu, S; Ramakrishman, N; Xue, L. (1986). The formation, identification, and significance of DNA- protein cross-links in mammalian cells. *Brit. J. Cancer*, 55, 135-140.

Olivenza, R; Moro, MA; Lizasoain, I; Lorenzo, P; Fernández, AP; Rodrigo, J; Boscá, L; Leza, JC. (2000). Chronic stress induces the expression of inducible nitric oxide synthase in rat brain cortex. *J. Neurochem.*, 74(2), 785-91.

Oliver, CN; Ahn, BW; Moerman, EJ; Goldstein, S; Stadtman, ER. (1987). Age-related changes in oxidized proteins. *J. Biol. Chem.*, 262(12), 5488-91.

Olsen, EA; Katz, HI; Levine, N; Shupack, J; Billys, MM; Prawer, S; Gold, J; Stiller, M; Lufrano, L; Thorne, EG. (1992). Tretinoin emollient cream: a new therapy for photodamaged skin. *J. Am. Acad. Dermatol.*, 26(2 Pt 1), 215-24.

Olshansky, SJ; Carnes, BA. *Science at the frontiers of aging. The quest for immortality.* W.W. Norton & Company, New York, 2001.

Olson, RL; Sayre, RM; Everett, MA. (1966). Effect of anatomic location and time on ultraviolet erythema. *Arch. Dermatol.*, 93, 211-5.

Omenn, GS; Goodman, GE; Thornquist, MD; Balmes, J; Cullen, MR; Glass, A; Keogh, JP; Meyskens, FL; Valanis, B; Williams, JH; Barnhart, S; Hammar, S. (1996). Effects of a combination of beta-carotene and vitamin A on lung cancer and cardiovascular disease. *The New England journal of Medicine*, 334, 1150-5.

Onorato, JM; Jenkins, AJ; Thorpe, SR; Baynes, JW. (2000). Pyridoxamine, an inhibitor of advanced glycation reactions, also inhibits advanced lipoxidation reactions. Mechanism of action of pyridoxamine. *J. Biol. Chem.*, 275(28), 21177-84.

Orengo, IF; Black, HS; Wolf, JE. (1992). Influence of fish oil supplementation on the minimal erythema dose in humans. *Arch Dermatol Res.*, 284, 219–21.

Orengo, IF; Black, HS; Kettler, AH; Wolf, JE Jr. (1989). Influence of dietary menhaden oil upon carcinogenesis and various cutaneous responses to ultraviolet radiation. *Photochem. Photobiol.*, 49(1), 71-7.

Orentreich, N; Matias, JR; DeFelice, A; Zimmerman, JA. (1993). Low methionine ingestion by rats extends lifespan. *Journal of Nutrition*, 123, 269-274.

Oresajo, C; Stephens, T; Hino, PD; Law; RM; Yatskayer, M; Foltis, P; Pillai, S; Pinnell, SR. (2008). Protective effects of a topical antioxidant mixture containing vitamin C, ferulic acid, and phloretin against ultraviolet-induced photodamage in human skin.*J. Cosmet. Dermatol.*, 7(4), 290-7.

Oresajo, C; Yatskayer, M; Galdi, A; Foltis, P; Pillai S. (2010). Complementary effects of antioxidants and sunscreens in reducing UV-induced skin damage as demonstrated by skin biomarker expression.*J. Cosmet. Laser Ther.* [Epub ahead of print].

Ornish, D; Lin, J; Daubenmier, J; Weidner, G; Epel, E; Kemp, C; Magbanua, MJ; Marlin, R; Yglecias, L; Carroll, PR; Blackburn, EH. (2008). Increased telomerase activity and comprehensive lifestyle changes: a pilot study. *Lancet Oncol.*. 9(11), 1048-57.

Orr, WC; Radyuk, SN; Prabhudesai, L; Toroser, D; Benes, JJ; Luchak, JM; Mockett, RJ; Rebrin, I; Hubbard, JG; Sohal, RS. (2005). Overexpression of glutamate-cysteine ligase extends lifespan in Drosophila melanogaster. *The Journal of Biological Chemistry*, 280, 37331–37338.

Ortega, RM. (2006). Importance of functional foods in the Mediterranean diet. *Public Health Nutr.*, 9(8A), 1136-40.

Osborne, R; Mullins, LA; Jarrold, BB. (2009). Understanding metabolic pathways for skin anti-aging. J. *Drugs Dermatol.*, 8(7 Suppl), s4-7.

Osler, M; McGue, M; Lund, R; Christensen, K. (2008). Marital status and twins' health and behavior: an analysis of middle-aged Danish twins. *Psychosom. Med.*, 70(4), 482-7.

Ostan, I; Poljšak, B; Simčič, M; Tijskens, L.M.M. Nutrition for the Selfish Gene. *Trends in food science& technology,*20(8,), 313-374.

Oudart, H; Groscolas, R; Calgari, C; Nibbelink, M; Leray, C; Le Maho, Y; Malan, A. (1997). Brown fat thermogenesis in rats fed high-fat diets enriched with n-3 polyunsaturated fatty acids. *Int. J. Obes. Relat. Metab. Disord.*, 21(11), 955-62.

Ouwehand, AC; Tiihonen, K; Lahtinen, S. The potential of probiotics and prebiotics for skin health. In: Farage, MA; Miller, KW; Maibach, HI. *Textbook of aging skin.* Berlin: Springer-Verlag, 2010.

Ouwor, ED; Kong AN. (2002). Antioxidants and oxidants regulate signal transduction pathways. *Pharmacol.*, 64, 765-770.

Ozturk, F; Kurt, E; Cerci, M; Emiroglu, L; Inan, U; Turker, M; Ilker, S. (2000). The effect of propolis extract in experimental chemical corneal injury. *Ophthalmic Res*, 32, 13–18.

Packer, JE; Slater, TF; Willson, RL. (1979). Direct observation of a free radical interaction between vitamin E and vitamin C. *Nature*, 278, 737–738.

Packer, L; Valacchi, G. (2002). Antioxidants and the response of skin to oxidative stress: vitamin E as a key indicator. *Skin Pharmacol. Appl. Skin. Physiol.*, 15(5), 282-90.

Packer, L; Weber, SU; Rimbach, G. (2001). Molecular aspects of alpha-tocotrienol antioxidant action in cell signaling. *J. Nutr.*, 131, 369S-373S.

Pajk Žontar, T; Rezar, V; Levant, A; Salobir, J. Efficiency of various nutrients on reduction for oxidative stress in pigs as model for humans; In: Gašperlin, L; Žlender, B.: Carcinogenic and anticarcinogenic food components: 24th Food Technology days. 2006 dedicated to Prof. F. Bitenc.—Ljubljana: University of Ljubljana, Biotechnical faculty, 199-206.

Pak, JW; Herbst, A; Bua, E; Gokey, N; McKenzie, D; Aiken, JM. (2003). Rebuttal to Jacobs: the mitochondrial theory of aging: alive or dead. *Aging Cell*, 2, 9.

Pallàs, M; Verdaguer, E; Tajes, M; Gutierrez-Cuesta, J; Camins, A. (2008). Modulation of sirtuins: new targets for anti-aging. *Recent Pat CNS Drug Discov.* 3(1), 61-9.

Palmer, RM; Ferrige, A; Moncada, S. (1987). Nitric oxide release accounts for the biological activity of endothelium-derived relaxing factor. *Nature*, 327, 524-526.

Palmer, DM; Kitchin, JS. (2010). Oxidative damage, skin aging, antioxidants and a novel antioxidant rating system. *J. Drugs Dermatol.*, 9(1), 11-5.

Palozza, P. (1998). Pro-oxidant action of carotenoid in biologic systems. *Nutr. Rev.*, 56, 257–265.

Palozza, P; Serini, S; Di Nicuolo, F; Piccioni, E; Calviello, G. (2003). Pro-oxidant effects of beta-carotene in cultured cells. *Mol. Aspects Med.*, 24(6), 353-62.

Paltridge, GW; Barton, IJ. (1978). Erythemal ultraviolet radiation distribution over Australia—the calculations, detailed results and input data Division of Atmospheric Physics Technical Paper 33 (Australia: Commonwealth Scientific and Industrial Research Organization).

Pandey, R; Muller, A; Napoli, CA; Selinger, DA; Pikaard, CS; Richards, EJ; Bander, J; Mount, DW; Jorgensen, RA. (2002). Analysis of histone acetyltransferase and histone deacetylase families of Arabidopsis thaliana suggests functional diversification of chromatin modification among multicellular eukaryotes, *Nucleic acid research*, 30, 5036-5055.

Paolini, M; Pozzetti, L; Pedulli, GF; Marchesi, E; Cantelli-Forti, G. (1999). The nature of pro-oxidant activity of vitamin C. *Life Sci,* 23(64), 273-278.

Palmer, RM; Ferrige, A; Moncada, S.(1987).Nitric oxide release accounts for the biological activity of endothelium-derived relaxing factor. *Nature*, 327, 524-526.

Pamplona, R; Barja, G; Portero-Otín, M. (2002). Membrane fatty acid unsaturation, protection against oxidative stress, and maximum lifespan: a homeoviscous-longevity adaptation? *Ann. N Y Acad. Sci.*, 959, 475-90.

Pardini, RS; Heidker, JC; Fletcher, DC. (1970). Inhibition of mitochondrial electron transport by nordihydroguaiaretic acid. *Biochem. Pharmacol.*, 19, 2695-2699.

Parhani, F. (2003). Possible role of oxidized lipids in osteoporosis: could hyperlipidemia be a risk factor? *Prostagland. Leuk. Essent. Fatty. Acids*, 68, 373.

Park, SK; Prolla, TA. (2005). Gene expression profiling studies of aging in cardiac and skeletal muscles. *Cardiovasc. Res.,* 66, 205-212.

Park, JB; Levine, M. (1996). Purification, cloning and expression of dehydroascorbic acid-reducing activity from human neutrophils: Identification as glutaredoxin. *Biochem J*, 315, 931–938.

Park, HY; Gilchrest, BA. (1999). Signaling pathways mediating melanogenesis. *Cell Mol Biol* (Noisy-le-grand), 45(7), 919-30.

Park, J; Halliday, GM; Surjana, D; Damian, DL. (2010). Nicotinamide prevents ultraviolet radiation-induced cellular energy loss. *Photochem. Photobiol.*, 86(4), 942-8.

Parker, J; Klein, SL; McClintock, MK; Morison, WL; Ye, X; Conti, CJ; Peterson, N; Nousari, CH; Tausk, FA. (2004). Chronic stress accelerates ultraviolet-induced cutaneous carcinogenesis. *J. Am. Acad. Dermatol.*, 51(6), 919-22.

Patrick, H; Rahn, RO. (1976). *Photochemistry of DNA and polynucleotides: photoproducts Photochemistry and Photobiology of Nucleic Acids vol. II.* (Ed. Wang, SY). New York: Academic, pp 35-95.

Patronek, GJ; Waters, DJ; Glickman, LT. (1997). Comparative longevity of pet dogs and humans: implications for gerontology research. *Journals of gerontology series A: Biological sciences and medical sciences*, 52, B171.

Pattison, DI; Davies, MJ. (2006). Actions of ultraviolet light on cellular structures. *EXS.*, (96), 131-57.

Pavicic, T; Steckmeier, S; Kerscher, M; Korting, HC. (2009). Evidence-based cosmetics: concepts and applications in photoaging of the skin and xerosis. *Wien Klin Wochenschr.*, 121(13-14), 431-9.

Peak, JG; Peak, MJ; Sikorski, RA; Jones, RA. (1988). Induction of DNA-protein cross-links in human cells by ultraviolet and visible radiations: action spectrum. *Photochem. Photobiol*, 41(3), 295-302.

Peak, MJ; Ito, A; Foote, CS; Peak JG. (1988). Photosensitized inactivation of DNA by monochromatic 334-nm radiation in the presence of 2-thiouracil: genetic activity and backbone breaks. *Photochem. Photobiol*, 47, 809–813.

Peak, MJ; Peak, JG; Carnes, BA. (1987). Induction of direct and indirect single-strand breaks in human cell DNA by far- and near-ultraviolet radiations: action spectrum and mechanisms. *Photochem. Photobiol*, 45, 381–387.

Peak, MJ; Peak, JG; Jones, CA. (1985). Different (direct and indirect) mechanisms for the induction of DNA-protein cross-links in human cells by far- and near ultraviolet radiations (290 and 405 nm). *Photochem. Photobiol.*, 42, 141–146.

Peak, MJ; Peak, JG. (1986). Molecular photobiology of UVA. In: *The Biological Effects of UVA Radiation*. (Edited by Urbach, F; Gange, RW.), pp. 42-52, Praeger Publishers, New York.

Peak, MJ; Peak, JG. (1989). Solar-ultraviolet-induced damage to DNA. *Photodermatology*, 6, 1–15.

Pehowich, DJ. (1999).Thyroid hormone status and membrane n-3 fatty acid content influence mitochondrial proton leak. *Biochim. Biophys. Acta.*, 1411(1), 192-200.

Pelletier, G; Ren, L. (2004). Localization of sex steroid receptors in human skin. *Histol. Histopathol.*, 19(2), 629-36.

Peppa, M; Uribarri, J; Vlassara, H. (2003). Glucose, Advanced Glycation End Products, and Diabetes Complications: What Is New and What Works. *Clinical Diabetes*, 21(4), 186-187.

Percheron, G; Hogrel, JY; Denot-Ledunois, S; Fayet, G; Forette, F; Baulieu, EE; Fardeau, M; Marini, JF. (2003). Double-blind placebo-controlled trial. Effect of one-year oral administration of dehydroepiandrosterone to 60- to 80-year-old individuals on muscle function and cross-sectional area: a double-blind placebo-controlled trial. *Arch. Intern. Med.*, 163(6), 720-7.

Pérez-López, FR; Chedraui, P; Haya, J; Cuadros, JL. (2009). Effects of the Mediterranean diet on longevity and age-related morbid conditions. *Maturitas*, 64(2), 67-79.

Persky, AM; Green, PS; Stubley, L; Howell, CO; Zaulyanov, L; Brazeau, GA; Simpkins, JW. (2000). Protective effect of estrogens against oxidative damage to heart and skeletal muscle in vivo and in vitro. *Proc. Soc. Exp. Biol. Med.*, 223(1), 59-66.

Peters, A. (2002). Structural changes that occur during normal aging of primate cerebral hemispheres. *Neurosci. Biobehav. Rev.*,26, 733-741.

Petersen, KF; Shulman, GI. (2002). Pathogenesis of skeletal muscle insulin resistance in type 2 diabetes mellitus. *Am. J. Cardiol.*, 90(5A), 11G-18G.

Petropoulos, I; Conconi, M; Wang, X; Hoenel, B; Brégégère, F; Milner, Y; Friguet, B. (2000). Increase of oxidatively modified protein is associated with a decrease of proteasome activity and content in aging epidermal cells. *J. Gerontol. A. Biol. Sci. Med. Sci.*, 55(5), B220-7.

Phelan, JP; Rose, MR. (2006). Caloric restriction increases longevity substantially only when the reaction norm is steep. *Biogerontology*, 7(3), 161-164.

Phelan, JP; Rose, MR. (2005). Why dietary restriction substantially increases longevity in animal models but won't in humans. *Ageing Res. Rev.*, 4, 339–350.

Phelan, JP; Austad, SN. (1989).Natural-selection, dietary restriction, and extended longevity. *Growth Dev. Aging*, 53, 4–5.

Philpott, MP; Kealey, T. (1991). Metabolic studies on isolated hair follicles: hair follicles engage in aerobic glycolysis and do not demonstrate the glucose fatty acid cycle. *J. Invest. Dermatol.*, 96(6), 875-9.

Philips, N; Hwang, H; Chauhan, S; Leonardi, D; Gonzalez, S. (2010). Stimulation of cell proliferation and expression of matrixmetalloproteinase-1 and interluekin-8 genes in dermal fibroblasts by copper. *Connect Tissue Res.*, 51(3), 224-9.

Phillips, TJ; Demircay, Z; Sahu, M. (2001). Hormonal effects on skin aging. *Clin. Geriatr. Med.*, 17, 661–72.

Pierard, GE; Letawe, C; Dowlati, A; Pierard-Franchimont, C. (1995). Effect of hormone replacement therapy for menopause on the mechanical properties of the skin. *J. Am. Geriat. Soc.*,42, 662-665.

Pierard, GE; Paquet, P; Uhoda, E; Quatresooz, P. Physiological variations during aging. In: Farage, MA; Miller, KW; Maivach, HI (Eds). Springer-Verlag, Berlin, 2010.

Pierard, GE; Uhoda, I; Pierard-Franchimont, C. (2003). From skin microrelief to wrinkles. An area ripe for investigation. *J. Cosmet. Dermatol.*, 2, 21–8.

Pierard-Franchimont, C; Quatresooz, P; Pierard GE. Sebum production. In: *Textbook of aging skin*. (Farage, MA; Miller, KW; Maibach, HI (Eds). Springer-Verlag, Berlin, 2010.

Pillai, S; Oresajo, C; Hayward, J. (2005). Ultraviolet radiation and skin aging: roles of reactive oxygen species, inflammation and protease activation, and strategies for prevention of inflammation-induced matrix degradation—a review. *Int. J. Cosmet. Sci.*, 27(1), 17-34.

Pitsavos, C; Panagiotakos, DB; Tzima, N; Chrysohoou, C; Economou, M; Zampelas, A; Stefanadis, C. (2005). Adherence to the Mediterranean diet is associated with total antioxidant capacity in healthy adults: the ATTICA study. *Am. J. Clin. Nutr.*, 82(3), 694-9.

Pitti-Ferrandi, H. DHEA and aging. *Psychol Neuropsychiatr Vieil.*, 1(2), 111-9.

Podda, M; Traber, MG; Weber, C; Yan, LJ; Packer, L. (1998). UV-irradiation depletes antioxidants and causes oxidative damage in a model of human skin. *Free Radic. Biol. Med.*,24(1), 55-65.

Podmore, ID; Griffiths, HR; Herbert, KE; Mistry, N; Mistry, P; Lunec, J. (1998). Vitamin C exhibits pro-oxidant properties. *Nature*, 392, 559–559.

Poeggeler, B; Saarela, S; Reiter, RJ. (1994). Melatonin—a highly potent endogenous radical scavenger and electron donor: new aspects of the oxidation chemistry of this indole accessed in vitro. *Ann. N. Y. Acad. Sci.*, 738, 419–20.

Poljsak, B; Gazdag, Z; Jenko-Brinovec, Š; Fujs, Š; Pesti, M; Belagyi, J; Plesnicar, S; Raspor, P. (2005). Pro-oxidative vs. antioxidative properties of ascorbic acid in chromium(VI)-induced damage : an in vivo and in vitro approach. *J. Appl.Ttoxicol.*, 25, 535-548.

Poljsak, B; Gazdag, Z; Pesti, M; Jenko-Brinovec, Š; Belagyi, J; Plesnicar, S; Raspor, P. (2006). Pro-oxidative versus antioxidative reactions between trolox and Cr(VI) : the role of H2O2. *Environ. Toxicol. Pharmacol.* 22, 15-19.

Poljsak, B; Pesti, M; Jamnik, P; Raspor P. (2011). Impact of environmental pollutants on oxidation-reduction processes in the cell environment. In: Dr. Jerome Nriagu (Ed.).*Encyclopedia of Environmental Health*.Elsevier.

Poljsak, B. *Decreasing Oxidative Stress and Retarding the Aging Process*, Nova SciencePublishers, 2010.

Ponticos, M; Lu, QL; Morgan, JE; et al. (1998). Dual regulation of AMP-activated protein kinase provides a novel mechanism for the controlof creatine kinase in skeletal muscle. *EMBOJ*, 17,1688-1699.

Poljsak, B; Jamnik, P. Methodology for Oxidative State Detection in Biological Systems. In: *Handbook of Free Radicals: Formation, Types and Effects*. New York: Nova Science Publishers, 2010.

Pons-Guiraud, A. (2007). Dry skin in dermatology: A complex physiopathology. *J. Eur. Acad. Dermatol. and Venereol.*,21(2), 1-4.

Postaire, E; Jungmann, H; Bejot, M; Heinrich, U; Tronnier, H. (1997). Evidence for antioxidant nutrients-induced pigmentation in skin: results of a clinical trial. *Biochem. Mol. Biol. Int.*, 42, 1023–33.

Poswig, A; Wenk, J; Brenneisen, P; Wlaschek, M; Hommel, C; Quel, G; Faisst, K; Dissemond, J; Briviba, K; Krieg, T; Scharffetter-Kochanek, K. (1999). Adaptive antioxidant response of manganese-superoxide dismutase following repetitive UVA irradiation. *J. Invest. Dermatol.* 112(1), 13-8.

Poulsen, HE; Loft, S; Vistisen, K. (1996). Extreme exercise and oxidative DNA modification. *J. Sports. Sci.*, 14, 343-346.

Powers, SK; Ji, LI; Leeuwenburgh, C. (1999). Exercise training-induced alterations in skeletal muscle antioxidant capacity: a brief review. *Medicine & Science in Sports & Exercise*, 31(7), 987.

Prahl S; Kueper T; Biernoth T; Wöhrmann Y; Münster A; Fürstenau M; Schmidt M; Schulze C; Wittern KP; Wenck H; Muhr GM; Blatt T.(2008) Aging skin is functionally anaerobic: importance of coenzyme Q10 for anti-aging skin care. *Biofactors*; 32(1-4):245-55.

Price, A; Lucas, PW; Lea, PJ. (1990) Age-dependent damage and glutathione metabolism in ozone fumigated barley: a leaf section approach. *J. Exptl. Bot.*,41, 1309-1317.

Proksch E; Holleran WM; Menon GK et al. (1993). Barrier function regulates epidermal lipid and DNA synthesis. *Br. J. Dermatol.*, 128(5), 473-482.

Proksch, E. (2008). The role of emollients in the management of diseases with chronic dry skin. *Skin Pharmacol. Physiol*, 21, 75-80.

Promislow, DE. (1994). DNA repair and the evolution of longevity: a critical analysis, *J. Theor. Biol.*,170, 291–300.

Pryor, WA. (1997). Cigarette smoke radicals and the role of free radicals in chemical carcinogenicity. *Environ. Health Perspect.*, 105(4), 875–882.

Pryor, WA. (2000).Vitamin E and heart disease: basic science to clinical intervention trials. *Free Radic. Biol. Med.*, 28, 141–64.

Puizina-Ivic, N. (2008). *Skin aging. Acta Dermatoven APA*, 17, 47-52.

Punnonen, K; Jansen, CT; Puntala, A; Ahotupa, M. (1991). Effects of in vitro UVA irradiation and PUVA treatment on membrane fatty acids and activities of antioxidant enzymes in human keratinocytes. *J. Invest. Dermatol.*, 96, 255–259.

Purba, MB; Kouris-Blazos, A; Wattanapenpaiboon, N; Lukito, W; Rothenberg, E; Steen, B; Wahlqvist, ML. (2001). Can skin wrinkling in a site that has received limited sun exposure be used as a marker of health status and biological age? *Age Ageing.*, 30(3), 227-34.

Purba, MB; Kouris-Blazos, A; Wattanapenpaiboon, N; Lukito, W; Rothenberg, EM; Steen, BC; Wahlqvist, ML. (2001). Skin wrinkling: can food make a difference?*J. Am. Coll. Nutr.*, 20(1), 71-80.

Quan, T; Qin, Z; Xu, Y; He, T; Kang, S; Voorhees, JJ; Fisher, GJ. (2010). Ultraviolet irradiation induces CYR61/CCN1, a mediator of collagen homeostasis, through activation of transcription factor AP-1 in human skin fibroblasts. *J. Invest. Dermatol.*, 130(6), 1697-706.

Quan, T; He, T; Kang, S; Voorhees, JJ; Fisher, GJ. (2002). Ultraviolet irradiation alters transforming growth factor beta/smad pathway in human skin in vivo. *Journal of Investigative Dermatology,*119(2), 499-506.

Quatresooz, P; Pierard Franchimont, C; Pierard, GE. Climacteric aging and oral hormone replacement therapy. In: *Textbook of aging skin* (Farage, MA; Miller, KW; Maibach, HI (Eds). Springer-Verlag, Berlin, 2010.

Quinton, ND; Laird, SM; Okon, MA; Smith, RF; Ross, RJ; Blakemore, AI. (1999). Serum leptin levels during the menstrual cycle of healthy women. *Br. J. Biomed. Sci*, 56, 16-9.

Quinton, ND; Smith, RF; Clayton, PE; Gills, MS; Shalet, S; Justice, SK; Walters, S; Postel-Vinay-MC; Blakemore, AI; Ross, RJ. (1999). Leptin binding activity changes with age: the link between leptin and puberty. *J. Clin. Endocrinol. Metab*, 84, 2336-41.

Wayne RP. *Chemistry of the Atmospheres,*Seconded. Oxford, 1991.

Radak, Z; Naito, H; Kaneko T; Nakamoto, H; Ohno, H; Ookawara, T; Goto S. (2002). Exercise training decreases DNA damage and increases DNA repair and resistance against oxidative stress of proteins in aged rat skeletal muscle. *Pflugers Archiv: Eur. J. Physiol.*, 445, 273-278.

Radak, Z; Nakamura, A; Nakamoto, H et al. (1998). A period of exercise increases the accumulation of reactive carbonyl derivatives in the lungs of rats. *Pfluger Arch: Eur. J. Physiol.* 435, 439-441.

Radák Z; Pucsuk J; Boros S; Josfai L; Taylor AW.(2000). Changes in urine 8-hydroxydeoxyguanosine levels of super-marathon runners during a four-day race period. *Life Sci.* 66(18), 1763-7.

Radák, Z; Young Chung, H; Naito, H; Takahashi, R; Jin Jung, K; Hyon-Jeen, K; Goto, S. (2004). Age-associated increases in oxidative stress and nuclear transcription factor κB activation are attenuated in rat liver by regular exercise. *The Faseb Journal express article*, 749-750.

Raine-Fenning NJ; Brincat MP; Muscat-Baron Y. (2003). Skin aging and menopause : implications for treatment. *Am. J. Clin. Dermatol.*, 4(6), 371-8.

Rajar, A; Gašperlin, L; Žlender, B.(2006). Karcinogene komponente v predelanih in toplotno obdelanih živilih/ Carcinogenic Components in Heat-treated and Processed Foods; v Gašperlin, L; Žlender, B (ured.): Karcinogene in antikarcinogene komponente živil; 24. Bitenčevi živilski dnevi 2006.—Ljubljana: Univerza v Ljubljani, Biotehniška fakulteta, 89-102.

Ramsey, JJ; Colman, RJ; Binkley, NC; Christensen, JD; Gresl, TA; Kemnitz, JW; Weindruch, R. (2000). Dietary Restriction and Aging in Rhesus Monkeys: The University of Wisconsin Study. *Exp. Gerontiol.*, 35, 1131-1149.

Rangarajan, V; Dreher, F. Topical growth factors for skin rejuvenation In: Farage, MA; Miller, KW; Maibach, HI. *Textbook of aging skin*. Berlin: Springer-Verlag, 2010.

Rasche, C; Elsner, P. Skin aging: A brief summary of characteristic changes. In: *Textbook of aging skin*. Ferage, MA; Miller, KW; Maibach, HI (Eds). Springer-Verlag, Berlin, 2010.

Rasmussen, UF; Vielwerth, SE; Rasmussen, HN. (2004). Skeletal muscle bioenergetics: a comparative study of mitochondria isolated from pigeon pectoralis, rat soleus, rat biceps brachii, pig biceps femoris and human quadriceps. *Comp. Biochem. Physiol. A. Mol. Integr. Physiol.* 137(2), 435-46.

Rattan, S. (2006). Theories of biological aging: genes, proteins, and free radicals. *Free Radic. Res*, 40, 1230–8.

Rattan, SI. (2008). Hormesis in aging. *Ageing Res. Rev.*, 1, 63-78.

Rattan, SI; Fernandes, RA; Demirovic, D; Dymek, B; Lima, CF. (2009). Heat stress and hormetin-induced hormesis in human cells: effects on aging, wound healing, angiogenesis, and differentiation. *Dose Response.* 7(1), 90-103.

Rattan, SI; Gonzalez-Dosal, R; Nielsen, ER; Kraft, DC; Weibel, J; Kahns, S. (2004). Slowing down aging from within: mechanistic aspects of anti-aging hormetic effects of mild heat stress on human cells. *Acta Biochim. Pol.*, 51(2), 481-92.

Rattan, SI. (2004).Hormetic mechanisms of anti-aging and rejuvenating effects of repeated mild heat stress on human fibroblasts in vitro. *Rejuvenation Res.* 7(1), 40-8.

Rattan, SI. (2008). Hormesis in aging. *Ageing Res. Rev.*, 1, 63-78.

Rattan, SI. (1998). Repeated mild heat shock delays ageing in cultured human skin fibroblasts.*Biochem Mol. Biol. Int.*, 45(4), 753-9.

Rawlings, A; Canestrari, D; Dobkowski, B. (2004). Moisturizer technology versus clinical performance. *Dermatologic. Therapy*, 17, 49-56.

Rawlings, AV; Harding, CR. (2004). Moisturization and skin barrier function. *Dermatol. Ther,* 17, 43-48.

Rawlings, AV; Matts, J. (2005). Stratum corneum moisturization at the molecular level: An update in relation to the dry skin cycle. *J. Invest. Dermatol*, 124, 1099-1110.

Reddy, BS; Rao, CV. (2002). Novel approaches for colon cancer prevention by cyclooxygenase-2 inhibitors. *J. Environ. Pathol. Toxicol. Oncol.*, 21, 155-64.

Rhee, SG. (1999).Redox signaling: hydrogen peroxide as intracellular messenger. *Exp. Mol. Med*, 31, 53-59.

Reenstra, WR; Yaar, M; Gilchrest, BA. (1993). Effect of donor age on epidermal growth factor processing in man, *Exp. Cell Res*, 209, 118-122.

Rehman, A; Collis, CS; Yang, M; Kelly, M; Diplock, AT; Halliwell, B; Fuce-Evans, C. (1998). The effects of iron and vitamin C co-supplementation on oxidative damage to DNA in healthy volunteers. *Biochem. Biophys. Res. Commun*, 246, 293-298.

Reiter, RJ. (1995). Oxygen radical detoxification processes during aging: The functional importance of melatonin. *Aging* (Milano), 7, 340-51.

Reverter-Branchat, G; Cabiscol, E; Tamarit, J; Ros, J. (2004). Oxidative damage to specific proteins in replicative and chronological-aged Saccharomyces cerevisiae—Common targets and prevention by calorie restriction. *J. Biol. Chem.*, 279, 31983-31989.

Rexbye, H; Petersen, I; Johansens, M; Klitkou, L; Jeune, B; Christensen, K. (2006). Influence of environmental factors on facial ageing. *Age Ageing.* 35(2),110-5.

Kafi, R; Kwak, HS; Schumacher, WE; Cho, S; Hanft, VN; Hamilton, TA; King, AL; Neal, JD; Varani, J; Fisher, GJ; Voorhees, JJ; Kang, S. (2007). Improvement of naturally aged skin with vitamin A (retinol). *Arch. Dermatol.*, 143(5), 606-12.

Reznick, AZ; Kegan, VE; Ramasey, R; Tsuchiya, M; et al. (1992). Antiradical effects in L-propionyl carnitine protection of the heart against ishemia-reperfusion injury: the possible role of iron chelation. *Arch. Biochem. Biophys*, 394-401.

Rhie, G; Shin, MH; Seo, JY; Choi, WW; Cho, KH; Kim, KH; Park, KC; Eun, HC; Chung, JH. (2001). Aging- and photoaging-dependent changes of enzymic and nonenzymic antioxidants in the epidermis and dermis of human skin in vivo.*J. Invest. Dermatol.*, 117(5), 1212-7.

Rhodes, LE; Azurdia, RM; Dean, M, et al. (2000). Systemic eicosapentaenoic acid reduces UVB-induced erythema and p53 induction in skin, while increasing oxidative stress, in a double-blind randomized study. *Br. J. Dermatol.*, 142(3), 601-602.

Rhodes, LE; Webb, AR; Fraser, HI; Kift, R; Durkin, MT; Allan, D; O'Brien, SJ; Vail, A; Berry, JL. (2010). Recommended summer sunlight exposure levels can produce sufficient (> or =20 ng ml(-1)) but not the proposed optimal (> or =32 ng ml(-1)) 25(OH)D levels at UK latitudes. *J. Invest. Dermatol.*, 130(5), 1411-8.

Rhodes, LE; Durham, BH; Fraser, WD; Friedmann, PS. (1995). Dietary fish oil reduces basal and ultraviolet B-generated PGE_2 levels in skin and increases the threshold to provocation of polymorphic light eruption. *J. Invest. Dermatol*, 105, 532–5.

Rhodes, LE; O'Farrell, S; Jackson, MJ; Friedmann, PS. (1994). Dietary fish oil supplementation in humans reduces UVB-erythemal sensitivity but increases epidermal lipid peroxidation. *J. Invest. Dermatol*, 103, 151–4.

Rhodes, C. *Toxicology of the human environment. The critical role of free radicals.* New York: Taylor & Francis, 2000.

Rial, E; Zardoya, R. (2009). Oxidative stress, thermogenesis and evolution of uncoupling proteins. *Journal of Biology*, 8, 1-5.

Ribaya-Mercado, JD; Gramyn, M; Gilchrest, BA; Russell, RM. (1995). Skin lycopene is destroyed preferentially over ß-carotene during ultraviolet irradiation in humans. *J. Nutr.* 125, 1854–9.

Rice-Evans, C. (2001). Flavonoid antioxidants. *Curr. Med. Chem*, 8, 797-807.

Ricquier, D. (2002). To burn or to store.*Ann. Endocrinol.* (Paris), 63(6 Pt 2), S7-14.

Richard, MJ, Guiraud, P, Leccia, MT, Beani, JC, Favier, A. (1993). Effect of zinc supplementation on resistance of cultured human skin fibroblasts toward oxidant stress. *Biol. Trace Elem. Res.*, 37(2-3), 187-99.

Richie, JP; Leutzinger, Y; Parthasarathy, S; Malloy, V; Orentreich, N; Zimmerman, JR. (1994). Methionine restriction increases blood glutathione and longevity in F344 rats. *FASEB Journal*, 8, 1302.

Ridley, M. Genome: The Autobiography of a Species in 23 Chapters/ Genom: Biografija človeške vrste.—Tržič: Učila International,1999/2002.

Rietjens, I; Boersma, M; de Haan, L. (2001). The pro-oxidant chemistry of the natural antioxidants vitamin C, vitamin E, carotenoids and flavonoids. *Environ Toxicol. Pharmacol*, 11, 321-333.

Rikke, BA; Johnson, TE. (2004). Lower body temperature as a potential mechanism of life extension in homeotherms. *Exp. Gerontol.*, 39, 6, 927-30.

Rimm, EB; Stampfer, MJ; Ascherio, A; Giovannucci, E; Colditz, GA; Willett, WC. (1993). Vitamin E consumption and the risk of coronary disease in men. *The New EnglandJournal of Medicine*, 328, 1450-56.

Rittie, L; Fisher, GJ; Voorhees; J. Retinoid therapy for photoaging. In: *Skin aging, Gilchrest*, B; Krutmann, J (Eds.). Springer-Verlag, Berlin, 2006.

Ritter, EF; Axelrod, M; Minn, KW; Eades, E; Rudner, AM; Serafin, D; Klitzman, B. (1997). Modulation of ultraviolet light-induced epidermal damage: beneficial effects of tocopherol. *Plast. Reconstr. Surg.* 100(4), 973-80.

Rockenfeller, P; Madeo, F. (2010). Ageing and eating, *Biochim. Biophys. Acta*, doi:10.1016/j.bbamcr.2010.01.001.

Rocquet, C; Bonté, F. (2002). Molecular aspects of skin ageing—recent data. Acta dermatologica Alpina, Pannonica ed. *Adriatica*, 11(3), 71–94.

Roe, D.(1986). Current etiologies and cutaneous signs of vitamin deficiencies. In: Roe, D. ed. *Nutrition and the skin. Contemporary issues in clinical nutrition*. New York: Alan R Liss Inc, 81–98.

Roe, FJC. (1981). Are Nutritionists Worried about the Epidemic of Tumors in Laboratory Animals? *Proc. Nutr. Soc*, 40, 57-65.

Rogiers, V; Derde, MP; Verleye, G: et al. (1990). Standardized conditions needed for skin surface hydration measurements. *Cosmet Toiletries*, 105, 73-82.

Roman, B; Carta, L; Martínez-González, MA; Serra-Majem, L. (2008). Effectiveness of the Mediterranean diet in the elderly. *Clin. Interv. Aging*, 3(1), 97-109.

Rona, C: Berardesca, E. (2008). Aging skin and food supplements: the myth and the truth. *Clinics in Dermatology*, 26(6), 641-647.

Rosenstein, BS; Ducore, JM. (1983). Induction of DNA strand breaks in normal human fibroblasts exposed to monochromatic ultraviolet and visible wavelengths in the 240–546 nm range. *Photochem. Photobiol*, 38, 51–55.

Rossi, A; Longo, R; Russo, A; Borrelli, F; Sautebinm, L. (2002). The role of the phenethyl ester of caffeic acid (CAPE) in the inhibition of rat lung cyclooxygenase activity by propolis. *Fitoterapia*, 73, 30–37.

Roos, TC; Jugert, FK; Merk, HF; Bickers, DR. (1998). Retinoid metabolism in the skin. *Pharmacol. Rev*, 50(2),315-33.

Rottkamp, CA; Raina, AK; Zhu, X; Gaier, E; Bush, AI; Atwood, CS. (2001). Redox-active iron mediates amyloid-beta toxicity.*Free Radic. Biol. Med.*, 30, 447-50.

Ruffien-Ciszak, A; Gros, P; Comtat, M; Schmitt, AM; Questel, E; Casas, C; Redoules, D. (2006). Exploration of the global antioxidant capacity of the stratum corneum by cyclic voltammetry. *Journal of Pharmaceutical and Biomedical Analysis*, 40(1), 162-7.

Rousset, S; Alves-Guerra, MC; Mozo, J; Miroux, B; Cassard-Doulcier, A.M; Bouillaud, F; Ricquie, D. (2004). The Biology of Mitochondrial Uncoupling Proteins. *Diabetes*, 53, 130-135.

Rowe, DJ; Guyuron, B.Environmental and genetic factors in facial aging in twins. In: *Textbook of aging skin* (Farage, MA; Miller, KW; Maibach, HI, Eds.). Springer-Verlag, Berlin, 2010.

Ruano-Ravina, A; Figueiras, A; Freire-Garabal, M; Barros-Dios, JM. (2006). Antioxidant vitamins and risk of lung cancer. *Curr. Pharm. Des.*, 12, 599–613.

Rubenowitz, E; Molin, I; Axelsson, G; Rylander, R. (2000). Magnesium in drinking water in relation to morbidity and mortality from acute myocardial infarction. *Epidemiology*, 11(4), 416-21.

Rudich, A; Tirosh, A; Potashnik, R; Khamaisi, M; Bashan, N. (1999). Lipoic acid protects against oxidative stress-induced impairment in insulin stimulation of protein kinase B and glucose transport in 3T3-L1 adipocytes. *Diabetologia*, 42(8),949-57.

Rudman, D; Feller, AG; Nagraj, HS; Gergans, GA; Lalitha, PY; Goldberg, AF; Schlenker, RA; Cohn, L; Rudman, IW; Mattson, DE. (1990). Effects of human growth hormone in men over 60 years old. *The New EnglandJournal of Medicine*, 323(1), 1-6.

Rumsey, SC; Levine, M. (1998). Absorption, transport and disposition of ascorbic acid in humans. *Nutr. Biochem.*, 9, 113–130.

Sacher, R; McPherson, RA. (2000). *Wildmann's Clinical Interpretation of Laboratory Tests*, 11th ed. F.A. Davis Company. ISBN 0-8036-0270-7.

Sahyoun, NR; Jacques, PF; Russell, RM. (1996).Carotenoids, vitamins C and E, and mortality in an elderly population, *Am. J. Epidemiol.*, 144, 501–511.

Saliou, C; Rimbach, G; Moini, H; McLaughlin, L; Hosseini, S; Lee, J; Watson, RR; Packer, L.(2001). Solar ultraviolet-induced erythema in human skin and nuclear factor-kappa-B-dependent gene expression in keratinocytes are modulated by a French maritime pine bark extract. *Free Radic. Biol. Med.*, 30(2), 154-60.

Samuel, M; Brooke, RC; Hollis, S; Griffiths, CE. (2005). Interventions for photodamaged skin. *Cochrane Database Syst Rev.* 25(1), CD001782.

Sander, CS; Chang, H; Salzmann, S; Müller, CS; Ekanayake-Mudiyanselage, S; Elsner, P; Thiele, JJ. (2002). Photoaging is associated with protein oxidation in human skin in vivo. *J. Invest. Dermatol*, 118(4), 618-25.

Santoro, N; Thiele, DJ. (1997). Oxidative stress responses in the yeast Saccharomyces cerevisiae. In: Yeast stress responses In.: Hohmann, S; Mager, HRG. *Landes Company*, 171-204.

Santosh, K; Mukhtar, K; Mukhtar, H. (2001).Immunotoxicity of Environmental Agents in the Skin. In: *Environmental stressors in health and disease* (Ed. Fuchs, J; Packer, L.). Marcel Dekker.

Sapolsky, RM. (2004). Organismal stress and telomeric aging: an unexpected connection. *Proc. Natl. Acad. Sci. USA*, 101, 17323-17324.

Sarnstrand, B; Jansson, AH; Matuseviciene, G; Scheynius, A; Pierrou, S; Bergstrand, H. (1999). N,N'- Diacetyl-L-cystine—the disulfide dimer of N-acetylcysteine—is a potent modulator of contact sensitivity/delayed type hypersensitivity reactions in rodents. *J. Pharmacol. Exp. Ther*, 288, 1174–1184;

Sato, K; Taguchi, H; Maeda, T. (et al). (1995). The primary cytotoxicity in UVA-irradiated riboflavin solution is derived from hydrogen peroxide. *J. Invest. Dermatol*, 105, 608-612.

Saul, AN; Oberyszyn, TM; Daugherty, C; Kusewitt, D; Jones, S; Jewell, S; Malarkey, WB; Lehman, A; Lemeshow, S; Dhabhar, FS. (2005). Chronic stress and susceptibility to skin cancer. *J. Natl. Cancer Inst.*, 97(23), 1760-7.

Scarborough, D; Eickhorst, KM; Bisaccia, W. Cosmetic surgery in the elderly. In: Farage, MA; Miller, KW; Maibach, HI. *Textbook of aging skin*. Berlin: Springer-Verlag, 2010.

Schafer, ZT.(2009). Antioxidant and oncogene rescue of metabolic defects caused by loss of matrix attachment. *Nature*, 461, 109-113.

Schaefer, T; Dirschedl, P; Kunz, B; Ring, J; Ueberla, K. (1997). Maternal smoking during pregnancy and lactation increases the risk for atopic eczema in the offspring. *J. Am. Acad. Dermatol*, 36, 550–556.

Schallreuter, KU. (2007). Advances in melanocyte basic science research. *Dermatol. Clin.*,25, 283-291.

Scharffetter-Kochanek, K; Brenneisen, P; Wenk, J; Herrmann, G; Ma, W; Kuhr, L; Meewes, C; Wlaschek, M. (2000). Photoaging of the skin from phenotype to mechanisms. *Exp. Gerontol.*, 35(3), 307-16.

Scharffetter-Kochanek, K; Wlaschek, M; Brenneisen, P; Schauen, M; Blaudschun, R; Wenk, J. (1997). UV-induced reactive oxygen species in photocarcinogenesis and photoaging. *Biol. Chem.*, 378(11), 1247-57.

Schenk, H; Klein, M; Erdbrügger, W; Dröge, W; Schulze-Osthoff, K. (1994). Distinct effects of thioredoxin and antioxidants on the activation of transcription factors NF-kappa B and AP-1. *Proc. Natl. Acad. Sci. USA*, 91(5), 1672-6.

Schmid, D; Muggli, R; Zülli, F. (2002). Collagen glycation and skin aging. *Cosm. Toil.*, 118-24.

Schneider, RH; Nidich, SI; Salerno, JW; Sharma, HM; Robinson, CE; Nidich, RJ; Alexander, CN. (1998). Lower lipid peroxide levels in practitioners of the Transcendental Meditation program. *Psychosom. Med.*, 60(1), 38-41.

Schriner, SE; Linford, NJ; Martin, GM; Treuting, P; Ogburn, CE; Emond, M; Coskun, PE; Ladiges, W; Wolf, N; Van Remmen, H; Wallace, DC; Rabinovitch, PS. (2005). Extension of murine lifespan by overexpression of catalase targeted to mitochondria. *Science*, 308, 1909–1911.

Schröder, P; Krutmann, J.Environmental Oxidative Stress –Environmental Sources of ROS. In Hutzinger O. (eds.).*The Handbook of Environmental Chemistry*, pp 19-31. Berlin: Springer-Verlag, 2004.

Schroder, P; Schieke, SM; Morita, A. (2006). Premature skin aging by infrared radiation, tobacco smoke and ozone. In: Gilchrest, BA; Krutmann, J. (eds). *Skin Aging*. Springer: New York, 45–55.

Schroeder, P; Krutmann, J. Infrared A-induced skin aging. In: *Textbook of aging skin* (Farage, MA; Miller, KW; Maibach, HI (Eds). Springer-Verlag, Berlin, 2010.

Schroeder, P; Wild, S; Schieke, SM; Krutmann, J. (2004). Further analysis of infrared a radiation-induced MMP-1 expression, *J. Invest. Dermatol*, 122(3), 140.

Schrauwen, P; Hesselink, M. (2003). Uncoupling protein 3 and physical activity: the role of uncoupling protein 3 in energy metabolism revisited. *Proc. Nutr. Soc.*, 62, 635-43.

Schulz, TJ; Zarse, K; Voigt, A; Urban, N; Birringer, M; Ristow, M. (2007). Glucose Restriction Extends Caenorhabditis elegans Lifespan by Inducing Mitochondrial Respiration and Increasing Oxidative Stress. *Cell Metabolism*, 6, 280-293.

Schuppe, HC; Ro¨nnau, AC; von Schmiedeberg, S; Ruzicka, T; Gleichmann, E; Griem, P. (1998). Immunomodulation by heavy metal compounds. *Clin. Dermatol*, 16, 149–157.

Schutzer, WE; Mader, SL. (2003). Age-related changes in vascular andrenergic signaling: clinical and mechanistic implications.*Ageing Res. Rev*, 2, 169-190.

Schwarz, T; Urbanski, A; Luger, TA. (1994). Ultraviolet light- and epidermal cell-derived cytokines. In: *Epidermal Growth Factors and Cytokines*. Ed. Luger, TA; Schwarz, T., Marcel Dekker, New York, 303-363.

Schwedhelm, E; Maas, R; Troost, R; Böger, RH. (2003). Clinical pharmacokinetics of antioxidants and their impact on systemic oxidative stress. *Clinical Pharmacokinetics*, 42, 437-59.

Scientific Committee on Consumer Products (SCCP), 18 December 2007. *Safety of nanomaterial in cosmetic products.* SCCP/1147/07, 1-63.

Seiberg, M. (2001). Keratinoyte-melanocyte Interactions during melanosome transfer. *Pigment Cell Res*, 14, 236-42.

Sejersen, H; Rattan, SI. (2007). Glyoxal-induced premature senescence in human fibroblasts. *Ann. N Y Acad. Sci.*, 1100, 518-23.

Sell, DR; Kleinman, NR; Monnier, VM. (2000).Longitudinal determination of skin collagen glycation and glycoxidation rates predicts early death in C57BL/6NNIA mice. *FASEB J.*, 14(1), 145-56.

Sell, DR; Lane, MA; Johnson, WA; Masoro, EJ; Mock, OB; Reiser, KM; Fogarty, JF; Cutler, RG; Ingram, DK; Roth, GS; Monnier, VM. (1996). Longevity and the genetic determination of collagen glycoxidation kinetics in mammalian senescence. *Proc. Natl. Acad. Sci.*USA, 93(1), 485-90.

Sell, DR; Monnier, VM. *Aging of Long-lived Proteins: Extracellular Matrix* (Collagens, Elastins, Proteoglycans) and Lens Crystallins, Oxford University Press, New York, 1995.

Selman, C; McLaren, J; Meyer, C; Duncan, J; Redman, P. (2006). Life-long vitamin C supplementation in combination with cold exposure does not affect oxidative damage or lifespan in mice, but decreases expression of antioxidant protection genes. In: *Mechanisms of ageing and development*, 127, 897-904.

Selman, C; McLaren, JS; Himanka, MJ; Speakman, JR. (2000). Effect of long-term cold exposure on antioxidant enzyme activities in a small mammal. *Free Radic. Biol. Med.*, 28(8), 1279-85.

Sen, CK; Khanna, S; Roy, S. (2003). α-lipoic acid. In: *Criticalm reviews of oxidative stress and aging*. Edited by Cutler, RG. and Rodriguez, H. World Scientific Publishing. 759-778.

Sen,CK; Packer, L; Hanninen, O.Editors, *Handbook of oxidants and antioxidants in exercise*, Elsevier Science, The Netherlands, 2000.

Seo, JY; Lee, SH; Youn, CS; Choi, HR; Rhie, G; Cho, K; Kim, KH; Park, C; Eun, HC; Chung, JH. (2001). Ultraviolet radiation increases tropoelastin mRNA expression in the epidermis of human skin in vivo. *J. Invest. Dermatol*, 116, 915-9.

Seo, YR; Kelley, MR; Smith, ML. (2002).Selenomethionine regulation of p53 by a refl-dependent redox mechanism. *Proc. Natl. Acad. Sci.* USA,99(22), 14548-53.

Serafini, M.Role of the Antioxidant Network in the Prevention of Age-Related Diseases. In: Miwa, S; Beckman, KB; Muller, FL. *Oxidative Stress in Aging. From Model Systems to Human Diseases*.Totowa: Humana Press, 2008.

Serpone, N; Salinaro, E; Emeline,A. (2001). Deleterious effects of sunscreen titanium dioxide nanoparticles on DNA: efforts to limit DNA damage by particle surface modification. *Proc. SPIE.*, 4258, 86-98.

Serri, R; Iorizzo, M. (2008). Cosmeceuticals: focus on topical retinoids in photoaging. *Clin. Dermatol.*, 26(6), 633-5.

Shackelford, RE; Kaufman, W; Paules, RS. (1999). Cell cycle control, checkpoint mechanisms and genotoxic stress. *Environ Health Perspect*, 107(1), 5-24.

Sharkey, P; Eedy, DJ; Burrows, D; McCaigue, MD; Bell, AL. (1991). A possible role for superoxide production in the pathogenesis of contact dermatitis. *Acta Dermato-Venereol*, 71, 156–159.

Sharma, H; Sen, S; Singh, A; Bhardwaj, NK; Kochupillai, V; Singh, N. (2003). Sudarshan Kriya practitioners exhibit better antioxidant status and lower blood lactate levels. *Biol. Psychol.*, 63(3), 281-91.

Shapira, N. (2010). Nutritional approach to sun protection: a suggested complement to external strategies. *Nutr. Rev.*, 68(2), 75-86.

Shao, L; Li, QH; Tan, Z. (2004). L-carnosine reduces telomere damage and shortening rate in cultured normal fibroblasts. *Biochem. Biophys. Res. Commun.*, 324(2), 931-6.

Sheehy, MRJ; Greenwood, JG; Fielder, DR. (1995). Lipofuscin as a record of "rate of living" in an aquatic poikilotherm. *J. Gerontol. Biol. Sci.*, 50, 322- 326.

Shen, CL; Song, W; Pence, BC. (2001). Interactions of selenium compounds with other antioxidants in DNA damage and apoptosis in human normal keratinocytes. *Cancer Epidemiol. Biomarkers Prev.*, 10(4), 385-90.

Shenkin, A. (2006). The key role of micronutrients. *Clin. Nutr.*, 25, 1–13.

Sherrington, R; Rogaev, EI; Liang, Y; Rogaeva, EA; Levesque, G; Ikeda, M. (1995).Cloning of a gene bearing missense mutations in early-onset familial Alzheimer's disease. *Nature*, 375, 754-60.

Shi. J; Le Maguer, M. (2000). Lycopene in tomatoes: chemical and physical properties affected by food processing. *Crit. Rev. Biotechnol.*, 20(4), 293-334.

Shigenaga. MK; Hagen, TM; Ames, BN. (1994). Oxidative damage and mitochondrial decay in aging. *Proc. Natl. Acad. Sci.* USA, 91(23), 10771-8.

Shin, MH; Rhie, GE; Park, CH; Kim, KH; Cho, KH; Eun, HC; Chung, JH. (2005). Modulation of collagen metabolism by the topical application of dehydroepiandrosterone to human skin. *J. Invest. Dermatol.*, 124(2),315-23.

Shindo, Y; Witt, E; Han, D; Epstein, W; Packer, L. (1994). Enzymic and non-enzymic antioxidants in epidermis and dermis of human skin. *J. Invest. Dermatol*, 102, 122–124.

Shindo, Y; Witt, E; Han, D; Tzeng, B; Aziz, T; Nguyen, L; Packer, L. (1994). Recovery of antioxidants and reduction in lipid hydroperoxides in murine epidermis and dermis after acute ultraviolet radiation exposure. *Photodermatol. Photoimmunol. Photomed*, 10, 183–191.

Shindo, Y; Witt, E; Packer, L. (1993). Antioxidant defense mechanisms in murine epidermis and dermis and their responses to ultraviolet light. *J. Invest. Dermatol*, 100, 260–265.

Shindo, Y; Witt, E; Han, D; Tzeng, B; Aziz, T; Nguyen, L; Packer, L. (1994). Recovery of antioxidants and reduction in lipid hydroperoxides in murine epidermis and dermis after acute ultraviolet radiation exposure. *Photodermatol. Photoimmunol. Photomed*, 10(5), 183-91.

Shpall, R; Beddingfield, FC 3rd; Watson, D; Lask, GP. (2004). Microdermabrasion: a review. *Facial. Plast. Surg.*, 20(1), 47-50.

Shringarpure, R; Davies, KJ. (2002). Protein turnover by the proteasome in aging and disease. *Free Radic. Biol. Med.*, 32, 1084-9.

Siemieniuk, E; Skrzydlewska, E. (2005). Coenzyme Q10: its biosynthesis and biological significance in animal organisms and in humans.*Postepy Hig Med. Dosw,* 59,150-9.

Siems, W; Wiswedel, I; Salerno, C; Crifò, C; Augustin,W; Schild,L; Langhans, CD; Sommerburg O. (2005). Beta-carotene breakdown products may impair mitochondrial functions—potential side effects of high-dose beta-carotene supplementation. *J. Nutr. Biochem.*, 16(7), 385-97.

Sies, H; Stahl, W; Sundquist. AR. (1992). Antioxidant functions of vitamins. Vitamins E and C, beta-carotene, and other carotenoids. *Ann. N Y Acad. Sci.*, 30(669), 7-20.

Sies, H; Stahl, W; (1998). Lycopene: antioxidant and biological effects and its bioavailability in the human. *Proc. Soc. Exp. Biol. Med.*, 218(2), 121-4.

Sies, H; Stahl, W. (2004). Carotenoids and UV protection. *Photochem. Photobiol. Sci.*, 3(8), 749-52.

Sigler, K; Chaloupka, J; Brozmanova, J; Stadler, N; Hofer, M. (1999). Oxidative stress in microorganisms. *Folia Microbiol.* (Praha), 44, 587-624.

Sil, H; Sen, T; Moulik, S; Chatterjee, A. (2010). Black tea polyphenol (theaflavin) downregulates MMP-2 in human melanoma cell line A375 by involving multiple regulatory molecules. *J. Environ. Pathol. Toxicol. Oncol.*, 29(1), 55-68.

Silva, RH; Chehin, AB; Kameda, SR; Takatsu-Coleman, AL; Abílio, VC; Tufik, S; Frussa-Filho, R. (2004). Effects of pre- or post-training paradoxical sleep deprivation on two animal models of learning and memory in mice. *Neurobiol. Learn. Mem.*, 82(2), 90-8.

Silva, RH; Kameda, SR; Carvalho, RC; Takatsu-Coleman, AL; Niigaki, ST; Abílio, VC; Tufik, S; Frussa-Filho, R. (2004).Anxiogenic effect of sleep deprivation in the elevated plus-maze test in mice. *Psychopharmacology* (Berl), 176(2), 115-22.

Sime, S; Reeve, VE. (2004). Protection from inflammation, immunosuppression and carcinogenesis induced by UV radiation in mice by topical Pycnogenol. *Photochem. Photobiol.*, 79(2), 193-8.

Sinclair, DA; Howitz, TK. Dietary restriction, hormesis, and small molecule mimetics. In: Handbook of the biology of aging, Sixth edition. Academic Press, 2006.

Singh, D. (1995). Electron spin resonance spectroscopic demonstration of the generation of reactive oxygen species by diseased human synovial tissue following ex vivo hypoxia-reoxygenation. *Ann. Rheum. Dis.*, 54, 94-99.

Singh, RP; Agarwal, R. (2002). Flavonoid antioxidant silymarin and skin cancer. *Antioxid. Redox Signal.*, 4(4), 655-63.

Sivapirabu, G; Yiasemides, E; Halliday, GM; Park, J; Damian, DL. (2009). Topical nicotinamide modulates cellular energy metabolism and provides broad-spectrum protection against ultraviolet radiation-induced immunosuppression in humans. *Br. J. Dermatol.*, 161(6), 1357-64.

Sivonova, M; Tatarkova, Z; Durackova, Z; et al. (2007). Relation between antioxidant potential and oxidative damage to lipids, proteins and DNA in aged rats. *Physiol. Res,* 56:, 757-764;

Sjerobabski, MI; Poduje, S. (2008). *Photoaging. Coll. Antropol.*, 32(2), 177-80.

Skulacev, VP. (1998). Uncoupling: new approaches to an old problem of bioenergetics. *Rev. Biochim. Biophys. Acta,* 1363, 100-124.

Skulachev, VP. (1996). Role of uncoupled and non-coupled oxidations in maintenance of safely low levels of oxygen and its one-electron reductants. *Q Rev. Biophys.*, 29(2), 169-202.

Slaga, TJ. (1998). Tumor promotion and-or enhancement models. *Int. J. Toxicol*, 17(3),109–127.

Slagboom, PE;Heijmans, BT; Beekman, M; Westendorp, RG; Meulenbelt, I. (2000). Genetics on human aging. The search for genes contributing to human longevity and diseases of the old. *Ann. NY Acad. Sci.*, 908, 50-63.

Sliney, DH. (1983). Eye protective techniques for bright light. *Ophthalmology*, 90(8), 937-944.

Sliney, D. (1986). Physical factors in cataractogenesis: ambient ultraviolet radiation and temperature. *Invest. Ophthalmol. Vis. Sci.*, 27(5), 781-790.

Smelick, C. (2003).http://www.biologicalgerontology.com/ accessed March 2010.

Smith, JB; Fenske, NA. (1996). Cutaneous manifestations and consequence of smoking. *J. Am. Acad. Dermatol.* 34, 717–32.

Smith, MAL; Marley, KA;. Seigler, D; Singletary, KW; Meline, B. (2000). Bioactive Properties of Wild Blueberry Fruits. *Journal of Food Science*, 65, 352-356.

Smutzer, G. (2002). Molecular demolition. *The Scientist*, 34-6.

Sober; AJ. (1987). Solar exposure in the etiology of cutaneous melanoma.*Photodermatology*, 4, 23-31.

Sofi, F; Cesari, F; Abbate, R; Gensini, GF; Casini, A. (2008). Adherence to Mediterranean diet and health status: meta-analysis. *BMJ*, 11, 337- 1344.

Sohal, R. (2002). Role of oxidative stress and protein oxidation in the aging process. *Free Radic Biol. Med.*, 33, 37–44.

Sohal, R; Mockett, R; Orr, W. (2002). Mechanisms of aging: an appraisal of the oxidative stress hypothesis. *Free Radic. Biol. Med.*, 33, 575–86.

Sohal, R; Weindruch, R. (1996). Oxidative stress, caloric restriction, and aging. *Science*, 273, 59-63.

Sohal, RS. (1976). Metabolic rate and lifespan. In: Witler, R. *Cellular aging: Concepts and metabolism*. Basel: Karger, 25-40.

Sohal, RS; Hu, H; Agarwal, S; Forster, MJ; Lal, H. (1994). Oxidative damage, mitochondrial oxidant generation and antioxidant defenses during aging and in response to food restriction in the mouse. *Mech. Ageing Dev.*, 74, 121-133.

SORG (1990). United Kingdom Stratospheric Ozone Review Group. Third Report. London: HMSO.

Sorg, O; Tran, C; Carraux, P; Didierjean, L; Falson, F; Saurat, JH. (2002). Oxidative stress-independent depletion of epidermal vitamin A by UVA. *J. Invest. Dermatol*, 118, 513-8.

Sorlie, T. (2001). Gene expression patterns of breast carcinomas distinguish tumor subclasses with clinical implications. *Proc. Natl. Acad. Sci.*, 98, 10869–10874.

Speakman, JR; Talbot, DA; Selman, C; Snart, S; McLaren, JS; Redman, P; Krol, E; Jackson, DM; Johnson, MS; Brand, MD. (2004). Uncoupled and surviving: individual mice with high metabolism have greater mitochondrial uncoupling and live longer. *Aging Cell*, 3, 87.

Speakman, JR; Krol, E. (2005). Limits to sustained energy intake IX: A review of hypotheses. *J. Comp. Physiol.*, 175, 375-394.

Speakman, JR; van Acker, A; Herper, EJ. (2003). Age-related changes in the metabolism and body composition of three dog breeds and their relationship to life expectancy. *Aging cell*, 2, 265-275.

Sreekumar, R; Unnikrishnan, J; Fu, A. (2002). Effects of caloric restriction on mitochondrial function and gene transcripts in rat muscle. *Am. J. Physiol. Endocrinol. Metab.*, 283, 38-43.

Staal, FJT; Roederer, M; Herzenberg, LA; Herzenberg, LA. (1990). Intracellular thiols regulate activation of nuclear factor κB and transcription of human immunodeficiency virus. *Proc. Natl. Acad. Sci. USA*, 87,9943–9947.

Stadtman, ER. (1992). Protein oxidation and aging. *Science*, 257, 1220-4.

Stadtman, ER; Berlett, BS. (1997). Reactive oxygen mediated protein oxidation in aging and disease. *Chem. Res. Tox,* 10, 485-94.

Stadtman, ER; Berlett, BS. (1998). Reactive oxygen-mediated protein oxidation in ageing and disease. *Drug Metab. Rev.*, 30, 225-243.

Stadtman, ER; Starke-Reed, PE; Oliver, CN, et al. Protein modification in aging. In: Emerit I, Chance B, Eds., *Free radicals in aging*. Basel: Birkhauser Verlag, 1992.

Stahl, W; Heinrich, U; Jungmann, H; Sies, H; Tronnier, H; (2000). Carotenoids and carotenoids plus vitamin E protect against ultraviolet light-induced erythema in humans. *Am. J. Clin. Nutr.*, 71(3), 795-8.

Stahl, W; Junghans, A; de Boer, B; Driomina, ES; Briviba, K; Sies, H. (1998). Carotenoid mixtures protect multilamellar liposomes against oxidative damage: synergistic effects of lycopene and lutein. *FEB S Lett.*, 427(2), 305-8.

Stahl, W; Mukhtar, H; Afaq, F; Sies, H. Vitamins and polyphenols in systemic photoprotection. In: *Skin aging*, Gilchrest B, Krutmann J (Eds.). Springer-Verlag, Berlin, 2006.

Stahl, W; Krutmann, J.(2006). Systemic photoprotection through carotenoids. *Hautarzt.*, 57(4), 281-5.

Stahl, W; Sies, H. (2005). Bioactivity and protective effects of natural carotenoids. *Biochim. Biophys. Acta.*, 1740(2), 101-7.

Stampfer, MJ; Hennekens, CH; Manson, JE; Colditz, GA; Rosner, B; Willett, WC. (1993). Vitamin E consumption and risk of coronary disease in women. *The New England Journal of Medicine,* 328, 1444-49.

Standeven, AM; Wetterhahn, KE. (1991). Is there a role for reactive oxygen species in the mechanism of chromium (VI) carcinogenesis? *Chem. Res. Toxicol*, 4, 616–625.

Staniek, K; Nohl, H. (1999). H2O2 detection from intact mitochondria as a measure for one-electron reduction of dioxygen requires a non-invasive assay system. *Biochim. Biophys. Acta.*,1413, 70–80.

Staniek, K; Nohl, H. (2000). Are mitochondria a permanent source of reactive oxygen species? *Biochim. Biophys. Acta.*, 1460, 268–75.

Stanner, SA; Hughes, J; Kelly, CN; Buttriss, J. (2004). A review of the epidemiological evidence for the "antioxidant hypothesis."*Public Health Nutr.*, 7, 407–22.

Starkov, AA. (1997). "Mild" uncoupling of mitochondria. *Biosci. Rep.*, 17, 273–279.

Stephens, NG; Parsons, A; Schofield, PM; Kelly, F; Cheeseman, K; Mitchinson, MJ. (1996). Randomized controlled trial of vitamin E in patients with coronary disease: Cambridge Heart Antioxidant Study (CHAOS), 347, 781-86.

Stipanuk, MH. (2006). *Biochemical, physiological, molecular aspects of human nutrition* (2nd ed.). St Louis: Saunders Elsevier, p. 667.

Stocker, R. (1999). The ambivalence of vitamin E in atherogenesis. *TIBS*, 24, 219.

Stocker, R; Frei, B. (1991). Endogenous antioxidant defenses in human blood plasma. In: *Oxidative stress: oxidants and antioxidants*. London: Academic press, 213-42.

Stocker, R; Weidemann, MJ; Hunt, NH. (1986). Possible mechanisms responsible for the increased ascorbic acid content of Plasmodium vinckei-infected mouse erythrocytes. *Biochim. Biophys. Acta*, 881, 391–397.

Stöckl, P; Hütter, E; Zwerschke, W; Jansen-Dürr, P. (2006). Sustained inhibition of oxidative phosphorylation impairs cell proliferation and induces premature senescence in human fibroblasts. *Exp. Gerontol.*, 47(7), 674-82.

Streilein, J. (1991). Immunogenic factors in skin cancer. *N. Engl. J. Med.*, 325, 884-887.

Streppel, MT; Ocké, MC; Boshuizen, HC; Kok, FJ; Kromhout, D. (2009). Long-term wine consumption is related to cardiovascular mortality and life expectancy independently of moderate alcohol intake: the Zutphen Study. *J. Epidemiol. Community Health.*, 63(7), 534-40.

Strickland, M. (2009). Basic Immunology, http://www.photobiology.info/Strickland.html.

Strom, A; Jensen, RA. (1951). Mortality from circulatory diseases in Norway 1940-1945. *Lancet*, 258, 126- 129.

Stücker, M; Struk, PA; Hoffmann, K; Schulze, L; Röchling, A; Lübbers, DW. (2000). The transepidermal oxygen flux from the environment is in balance with the capillary oxygen supply. *J. Invest. Dermatol.*, 114(3),533-40.

Sun, Y. (1990).Free radicals, antioxidant enzymes and carcinogenesis. *Free Rad. Biol. Med.*, 8, 583–597.

Sullivan, MF; Ruemmler, PS. (1987). Effect of excess Fe on Cd or Pb absorption by rats. *J. Toxicol. Environ Health.*, 22(2), 131-9.

Sugimura, T; Wakabayashi, K; Nakagama, H; Nagao, M. (2004). Heterocyclic amines: Mutagens/carcinogens produced during cooking of meat and fish. *Cancer Sci.*, 95(4), 290-9.

Swift, ME; Burns, AL; Gray, KL; DiPietro, LA. (2001). Age-relatedalterations in inflammatory response to dermal injury. *J. Invest. Dermatol.*, 117, 1027–35.

Tagami, H. (2008). Functional characteristics of the stratum corneum in photoaged skin in comparison with those found in intrinsic aging. *Arch. Dermatol. Res.*, 300, S1-S6.

Tagami, H. (1994). Quantitative measurements of water concentration of the stratum corneum in vivo by high-frequency current. *Acta Derm. Venerol. Suppl.* (Stockh), 185, 29-33.

Tahara, S; Matsuo, M; Kaneko, T. (2001). Age-related changes in oxidative damage to lipids and DNA in rat skin. *Mech. Ageing Dev*, 122,415-426.

Tajima, S; Manaka, I; Kawashima, M; Kobayashi, T; Imokawa, G. (1998). Role of endothelin cascade between keratinocytes and melanocytes in hyperpigmentation in senile freckles, *J. Invest. Dermatol*, 110 (4).

Talwar, HS; Griffiths, CE; Fisher, GJ; Hamilton, TA; Voorhees, JJ. (1995). Reduced type I and type III procollagens in photodamaged adult human skin. *J. Invest. Dermatol.*, 105(2), 285-90.

Tamagno, E; Aragno, M; Boccuzzi, G; Gallo, M; Parola, S; Fubini, B; Poli, G; Danni, O. (1998). Oxygen free radical scavenger properties of dehydroepiandrosterone. *Cell Biochem. Funct.*, 16(1), 57-63.

Tan, DX; Chen, LD; Poeggeler, B; Manchester, LC; Reiter, RJ. (1993).Melatonin: a potent, endogenous hydroxyl radical scavenger. *Endocr. J.*, 1, 57-60.

Tapia, PC. (2006). Sublethal mitochondrial stress with an attendant stoichiometric augmentation of reactive oxygen species may precipitate many of the beneficial alterations in cellular physiology produced by caloric restriction, intermittent fasting, exercise and dietary phytonutrients: "Mitohormesis for health and vitality." *Med. Hypotheses*, 66, 832-43.

Tapiero, H; Townsend, DM; Tew, KD. (2003) The antioxidant role of selenium and selenocompounds. *Biomed. Pharmacother.*, 57(3-4), 134-44.

Tate, DJ Jr; Miceli, MV; Newsome, DA. (1999).Zinc protects against oxidative damage in cultured human retinal pigment epithelial cells. *Free Radic. Biol. Med.*, 26(5-6), 704-13.

Tavaria, M; Gabriele, T; Kola, I; Anderson, RL. (1996). A hitchhiker's guide to the human Hsp70 family. *Cell Stress Chaperones*, 1(1), 23–8

Terman, A. (2001). Garbage catastrophe theory of aging: Imperfect removal of oxidative damage? *Redox. Rep.*, 6, 15-26.

Terman, A; Brunk, UT. (2006). Oxidative stress, accumulation of biological "garbage," and aging. *Antioxid. Redox Signal*, 8, 197-204.

Thibodeau, A. (2000). Metalloproteinase inhibitors. *Cosmetics & Toiletries*, 115, 75-80.

Thiboutot, DM. (1995). Dermatological manifestations of endocrine disorders. *J. Clin. Endocrinol. Metab*, 80, 3082-3087.

Thiele, J; Barland, CO; Ghadially, R; Elias, P. Permeability and antioxidant barriers in aged skin. In: *Skin aging*, Gilchrest, B; Krutmann, J. (Eds.). Springer-Verlag, Berlin, 2006.

Thiele, J; Schroeter, C; Hsieh, SN; Podda, M; Packer, L. (2001). The antioxidant network of the stratum corneum. *Curr. Probl. Dermatol*, 29, 26-42.

Thiele, J; Traber, MG; Packer, L. (1998). Depletion of human stratum corneum vitamin E: an early and sensitive in vivo marker of UV-inducedphotooxidation. *J. Invest. Dermatol*, 110, 756–761.

Thiele, J. (2001). Oxidative targets in the stratum corneum. A new basis for antioxidative strategies. *Skin Pharmacol. Appl. Skin Physiol*, 1, 87-91.

Thirunavukkarasu, V; Nandhini, AT; Anuradha, CV. (2004).Fructose diet-induced skin collagen abnormalities are prevented by lipoic acid. *Exp. Diabesity Res.*, 5(4), 237-44.

Thomas, JH; Inoue, T. (1998). Methuselah meets diabetes. *Bioessays*, 20, 113.

Thomas, JP; Maiorino, M; Ursini; Girotti, AW. (1990). Protective action of phospholipid hydroperoxide glutathione peroxidase against membrane-damaging lipid peroxidation. *J. Biol. Chem*, 265, 454–461.

Thomas, JR. (2005). Effects of age and diet on rat skin histology. *Laryngoscope*, 115, 405-411.

Thomas, D. (2004). Vitamins in health and aging. *Clin. Geriatr. Med.*,20(2), 259–74.

Thornton, MJ. (2002). The biological actions of estrogens on skin. *Exp. Dermatol.*, 11(6), 487-502.

Tian, WD; Gillies, R; Brancaleon, L; Kollias, N. (2001). Aging and effects of ultraviolet A exposure may be quantified by fluorescence excitation spectroscopy in vivo. *J. Invest. Dermatol*, 116, 840-5.

Tijskens, P. *Discovering the Future: Modeling Quality Matters*. Wageningen University, 2004.

Tindle, HA; Chang, YF; Kuller, LH; Manson, JE; Robinson, JG; Rosal, MC; Siegle, GJ; Matthews, KA. (2009). Optimism, cynical hostility, and incident coronary heart disease and mortality in the Women's Health Initiative. *Circulation*, 120(8), 656-62.

Tindle, H; Davis, E; Kuller, L. (2010). Attitudes and cardiovascular disease. *Maturitas.*, 67(2), 108-13.

Tissenbaum, HA; Ruvkun, G.(1998). An insulin-like signaling pathway affects both longevity and reproduction in Caenorhabditis elegans. *Genetics.*, 148(2), 703-17.

Tixier, JM; Godeau, G; Robert, AM; Hornebeck, W. (1984). Evidence by in vivo and in vitro studies that binding of pycnogenols to elastin affects its rate of degradation by elastases. *Biochem. Pharmacol.*, 33(24), 3933-9.

Toba, Y; Kajita, Y; Masuyama, R; Takada, Y; Suzuki, K; Aoe, S. (2000). Dietary magnesium supplementation affects bone metabolism and dynamic strength of bone in ovariectomized rats. *J. Nutr.*, 130(2), 216-20.

Toews, GB; Bergstresser, PR; Streilein, JW. (1980). Epidermal Langerhans Cell Density Determines Whether Contact Hypersensitivity or Unresponsiveness Follows Skin Painting with DNFB," *J. Immunol.*, 124, 445-453.

Torres, CA;Perez, VI. (2008).Proteasome modulates mitochondrial function during cellular senescence. *Free Radic. Biol. Med.*, 44(3), 403-14.

Tourlouki, E; Polychronopoulos, E; Zeimbekis, A; Tsakountakis, N; Bountziouka, V; Lioliou, E; Papavenetiou, E; Polystipioti, A; Metallinos, G; Tyrovolas, S; Gotsis, E; Matalas, AL; Lionis, C; Panagiotakos, DB. (2010). The "secrets" of the long livers in Mediterranean islands: the MEDIS study. *Eur. J. Public Health*, 20(6), 659-64.

Touyz, RM; Milne, FJ. (1999). Magnesium supplementation attenuates, but does not prevent, development of hypertension in spontaneously hypertensive rats. *Am. J. Hypertens.*, 12(8-1), 757-65.

Toyokuni, S; Yasui, H; Date, A; Hakozaki, T; Akatsuka, S; Kohda, H; Yoshii, T; Sakurai, H. (2006).Novel screening method for ultraviolet protection: combination of a human skin-equivalent model and 8-hydroxy-2'-deoxyguanosine. *Pathol. Int.*, 56(12), 760-2.

Traber, MG; Packer, L. Vitamin E: beyond antioxidant function. *Am. J. Clin. Nutr.*, 62, 1501S–9S.

Trautinger, F; Kindås-Mügge, I; Knobler, RM; Hönigsmann, H. (1996).Stress proteins in the cellular response to ultraviolet radiation. *J. Photochem. Photobiol. B.*, 35(3), 141-8.

Treina, G; Scaletta, C; Fourtanier, A; Seite, S; Frenk, E; Applegate, LA. (1996).Expression of intracellular adhesion molecule-1 in UVA-irradiated human skin cells in vitro and in vivo. *J. Dermatol*, 135, 241–247.

Trichopoulou, A; Costacou, T; Bamia, C; Trichopoulos, D. (2003). Adherence to a Mediterranean diet and survival in a Greek population. *N. Engl. J. Med.*, 26, 2599-608.

Trifunovic, A; Wredenberg, A; Falkenberg, M. et al. (2004).Premature ageing in mice expressing defective mitochondrial DNa polymerase. *Nature*, 429, 417-423.

Troll, W; Wiesner, R. (1985). The role of oxygen radicals as a possible mechanism of tumor promotion.*Ann. Rev. Pharmacol. Toxicol*, 25, 509–528.

Trouba, KJ; Hamadeh, KH; Amin, RP; Germolec, DDR. (2002). Oxidative Stress and Its Role in Skin Disease. *Antioxidants & Redox Signaling*, 4(4), 665-673.

Trounce, I; Byrne, E; Marzuki, S. (1989). Decline in skeletal muscle mitochondrial respiratory chain function: possible factor in ageing. *Lancet.*, 1(8639), 637-9.

Trüeb, RM. (2003).Association between smoking and hair loss: another opportunity for health education against smoking? *Dermatology.*, 206(3), 189-91.

Trüeb, RM. (2009).Oxidative stress in ageing of hair. *Int. J. Trichology.*, 1(1), 6-14.

Trüeb, RM. (2005). Aging of skin and hair. *Ther. Umsch.*, 62(12), 837-46.

Trush, MA; Kensler, TW. (1991). An overview of the relationship between oxidative stress and chemical carcinogenesis. *Free Rad. Biol. Med.*, 10, 201–209;

Tsuchiya, T; Horii, IN. (1996).Epidermal cell proliferative activity assessed by proliferating cell nuclear antigen (PCNA) decreases following immobilization-induced stress in male Syrian hamsters. *Psychoneuroendocrinology*, 21(1), 111-117.

Tsuji, N; Moriwaki, S; Suzuki, S; Takema, Y; Imokawa, G. (2001). The role of elastases secreted by fibroblasts in wrinkle formation: implication through selective inhibition of elastase activity. *Photochem. Photobiol.*, 74, 283-90.

Tsukahara, K; Takema, Y; Moriwaki, S; Tsuji, N; Suzuki, Y; Fujimura, T; Imokawa, G. (2001). Selective inhibition of skin fibroblast elastase elicits a concentration-dependent prevention of ultraviolet B-induced wrinkle formation. *J. Invest. Dermatol*, 117, 671-7.

Tucker-Samaras, S; Zedayko, T; Cole, C; Miller, D; Wallo, W; Leyden, JJ. (2009). A stabilized 0.1% retinol facial moisturizer improves the appearance of photodamaged skin in an eight-week, double-blind, vehicle-controlled study. *J. Drugs Dermatol.*, 8(10), 932-6.

Turner, N; Mitchell, TW; Else, PL; Hulbert, AJ. (2010). The ω-3 and ω-6 fats in meals: A proposal for a simple new label.*Nutrition.* [Epub ahead of print].

Turrens, JF. (1997). Superoxide production by the mitochondrial respiratory chain. *Biosci. Rep.*, 17, 3–8.

Turturro, A; Hass, BS; Hart, RW. (2000).Does caloric restriction induce hormesis? *Human experimental toxicology*, 19, 320-329.

Tyrrell, RM. (1991). UVA (320–380 nm) radiation as an oxidative stress. Oxidative Stress: Oxidants and Antioxidants. In: Sies H, ed. New York: Academic Press, 57–78.

Tyrrell, RM; Pidoux, M. (1989). Singlet oxygen involvement in the inactivation of cultured human fibroblasts by UVA (334 nm, 365 nm) and near-visible radiations. *Photochem. Photobiol*, 49, 407-412.

Tyrrell, RM; Pidoux, M. (1986). Endogenous glutathione protects human skin fibroblasts against the cytotoxic action of UVB, UVA and near-visible radiations. *Photochem. Photobiol*, 44, 561-564.

Tyrrell, RM; Pidoux, M: (1988). Correlation between endogenous glutathione content and sensitivity of cultured human skin cells to radiation at defined wavelengths in the solar UV range. *Photochem. Photobiol*, 47, 405-412.

U.S. Department of Health and Human Services. Washington, DC: U.S. Government Printing Office; Healthy People. 2010, 2000.

U.S. Department of Health and Human Services. Physical activity and health: a report of the Surgeon General. Atlanta, GA: U.S. Department of Health and Human Services, Centers for Disease Control and Prevention, National Center for Chronic Disease Prevention and Health Promotion, 1996.

U.S. Department of Health and Human Services, Public Health Service, CDC, National Center for Chronic Disease Prevention and Health Promotion, 1996.

Udelsman, R; Blake, MJ; Stagg, CA; Holbrook, NJ. (1994).Endocrine control of stress-induced heat shock protein 70 expression in vivo. *Surgery.*, 115(5), 611-6.

Ueda, M; Ouhtit, A; Bito, T; Nakazawa, K; Lübbe, J; Ichihashi, M; Yamasaki, H; Nakazawa, H. (1997).Evidence for UV-associated activation of telomerase in human skin, *Cancer Res*, 57, 370-4.

Uitto, J; Fazio, MJ; Olsen, DR. (1998). Cutaneous aging: Molecular alterations in elastic fibers. *J. Cuta. Aging & Cos. Derm*, 1(1), 13-26.

Vaid, M; Katiyar, SK. (2010).Molecular mechanisms of inhibition of photocarcinogenesis by silymarin, a phytochemical from milk thistle (Silybum marianum L. Gaertn.) (Review). *Int. J. Oncol.*, 36(5), 1053-60.

Vayalil, PK; Elmets, CA; Katiyar, SK. (2003). Treatment of green tea polyphenols in hydrophilic cream prevents UVB-induced oxidation of lipids and proteins, depletion of antioxidant enzymes and phosphorylation of MAPK proteins in SKH-1 hairless mouse skin. *Carcinogenesis.*, 24(5), 927-36.

Valacchi, G. Effect of ozone on cutaneous tissues. In: *Textbook of aging skin* (Farage, MA; Miller, KW; Maibach, HI. (Eds). Springer-Verlag, Berlin, 2010.

Valko, M; Morris, H; Cronin, MT. (2005).Metals, toxicity and oxidative stress. *Curr. Med. Chem.*, 12(10), 1161-208.

Valko, M; Morris, H; Cronin, MT. (2005). Metals, toxicity and oxidative stress. *Curr. Med. Chem.*, 12(10), 1161-208.

Valko, M; Leibfritz, D; Moncol, J; Cronin, MTD; Mazur, M; Telser, J. (2007). Free radicals and antioxidants in normal physiological functions and human disease. *The International Journal of Biochemistry & Cell Biology,* 39, 44–84.

Van der Leun, JC; de Gruijl, FR. (1993). Influences of ozone depletion on human and animal health. Chapter 4 inUVB radiation and ozone depletion: Effects on humans, animals, plants, microorganisms, and materials, ed. M. Tevini. Ann Arbor: Lewis Publishers,95-123.

Van der Leun, JC; van Weelden, H. (1986). UVB Phototherapy: Principles, Radiation Sources, Regimens.*Curr. Probl. Dermatol.*, 15, 39-51.

Van Weelden, H; Baart de la Faille, H; Young, E; van der Leun, JC. (1988). A New Development in UVB Phototherapy of Psoriasis, *Brit. J. Dermatol.*, 119, 11-19.

Vanfleteren, JR; Braeckman, BP. (1999).Mechanism of lifespan determination in Caenorhabditis elegans. *Neurobiol. Aging*, 20, 487.

Varani, J; Warner, RL; Gharaee-Kermani, M; Phan, SH; Kang, S; Chung, JH; Wang, ZQ; Datta, SC; Fisher, GJ; Voorhees, JJ. (2000). Vitamin A antagonizes decreased cell growth and elevated collagen-degrading matrix metalloproteinases and stimulates collagen accumulation in naturally aged human skin. *J. Invest. Dermatol.*, 114(3), 480-6.

Varani, J; Fisher, GJ; Kang, S; Voorhees, JJ. (1998). Molecular mechanisms of intrinsic skin aging and retinoid-induced repair and reversal. *J. Investig. Dermatol. Symp. Proc.*, 3(1), 57-60.

Vasankari, TJ; Kujala, UM; Vasankari, TM; Vuorimaa, T; Ahotupa, M. (1997). Effects of acute prolonged exercise on-serum and LDL oxidation and antioxidantdefenses. *Free Radic. Biol. Med.*, 22(3), 509-13.

Venditti, P; Masullo, P; Di Meo, S. (1999). Effect of training on H(2)O(2) release by mitochondria from rat skeletal muscle. *Arch. Biochem. Biophys.*, 372(2), 315-20.

Verani, J. et al. (2000). Vitamin A antagonizes decreased cell growth and elevated collagen-degrading matrix metalloproteinases and stimulates collagen accumulation in naturally aged human skin. *J. Invest. Dermatol*, 114, 480-486.

Varani, J; Perone, P; Fligiel, SEG; Fisher, GJ; Voorhees, JJ. (2002).Inhibition of type I procollagen production in photodamage: Correlation between presence of high molecular weight collagen fragments and reduced procollagen synthesis. *J. Invest. Dermatol*,119, 122–129.

Verbeke, P; Clark, BF; Rattan, SI. (2001).Reduced levels of oxidized and glycoxidized proteins in human fibroblasts exposed to repeated mild heat shock during serial passaging in vitro. *Free Radic. Biol. Med.*, 31(12), 1593-602.

Vercellotti, GM.(1996). A balanced budget-evaluating the iron economy. *Clin. Chem.*, 42, 657.

Vielhaber, G; Grether-Beck, S; Koch, O; Johncock, W; Krutmann, J. (2006). Sunscreens with an absorption maximum of > or =360 nm provide optimal protection against UVA1-induced expression of matrix metalloproteinase-1, interleukin-1, and interleukin-6 in human dermal fibroblasts. *Photochem. Photobiol. Sci.*, 5(3), 275-82.

Vierkötter, A; Schikowski, T; Ranft, U; Sugiri, D; Matsui, M; Krämer, U; Krutmann, J. (2010). Airborne particle exposure and extrinsic skin aging. *J. Invest. Dermatol.*, 130(12), 2719-26.

Vile, GF; Basu-Moda, S; Waltner, C; Tyrrell, RM. (1994) Haem oxygenase 1 mediates an adaptive response to oxidative stress in human skin fibroblasts. *Proc. Natl. Acad. Sci. USA*, 91, 2607-2610.

Villeponteau, B. (2003).Nutritional approaches to reducing oxidative stress. In: *Critical reviews of oxidative stress and aging.* (Cutler RG and Rodriguez H. Eds.).

Vinson, JA; Howard, TB. (1996).Inhibition of protein glycation and advanced glycation end products by ascorbic acid and other vitamins and nutrients. *National Biochemistry*, 7, 659-63.

Viola P, Viola M. (2009).Virgin olive oil as a fundamental nutritional component and skin protector. *Clin. Dermatol.*, 27(2), 159-65.

Virador, VM; Muller, J; Wu, X; Abdel-Malek, ZA; Yu, ZX; Ferrans, V; Kobayashi, N; Wakamatsu, K; Ito, S; Hammer, JA; Hearing, VJ. (2002). Influence of alpha-melanocyte-stimulating hormone and ultraviolet radiation on the transfer of melanosomes to keratinocytes, *FASEB J*, 16, 105-7.

Virtamo, J. (1999). Vitamins and lung cancer. *Proc. Nutr. Soc,* 58, 329.

Vitetta, A; Anton, B. (2007). Lifestyle and nutrition, caloric restriction, mitochondrial health and hormones: Scientific interventions for anti-aging. *Clin. Interv. Aging*, 2, 537–543.

Vivekananthan, DP; Penn, MS; Sapp, SK; Hsu, A; Topol, EJ. (2003). Use of antioxidant vitamins for the prevention of cardiovascular disease: meta-analysis of randomized trials. *Lancet*, 361, 2017–23.

Von Schacky, C. (2010). Omega-3 fatty acids vs. cardiac disease—the contribution of the omega-3 index. *Cell Mol. Biol* (Noisy-le-grand*)*, 56(1), 93-101.

Von Zglinicki, T; Nilsson, E; Döcke, WD; Brunk, UT. (1995). Lipofuscin accumulation and ageing of fibroblasts. *Gerontol*, 41(2), 95-108.

Von Zglinicki, T. (2002).Oxidative stress shortens telomeres. *Trends Biochem. Sci.,* 27, 339–44.

Von Zglinicki, T; Bürkle, A; Kirkwood, TB. (2001). Stress, DNA damage and ageing—an integrative approach. *Exp. Gerontol.*, 36, 1049–1062.

Voorhees, JJ. (1990). Clinical effects of long-term therapy with topical tretinoin and cellular mode of action. *J. Int. Med. Res.*, 18()3, 26C-28C.

Walford, RL; Weindruch, R; Fligiel, S; Guthrie, D. (1986). The Retardation of Aging in Mice by Dietary Restriction: Longevity, Cancer, Immunity and Lifetime Energy Intake. *J. Nutr*, 116, 641-654.

Wallace, DC. (2005). A mitochondrial paradigm of metabolic and degenerative diseases, aging, and cancer: A dawn for evolutionary medicine. *Annu. Rev. Genet.*, 39, 359–407.

Wallace, S. (1988). AP endonucleases and DNA glycosylases that recognize oxidative DNA damage. *Environ. Molec. Mutagen*, 12, 431–477.

Walker, AF. (1990). The contribution of weaning foods to protein-energy malnutrition. *Nutr. Res. Rev.*, 3, 25-47.

Wan, R; Camandola, S; Mattson, MP. (2004). Dietary supplementation with 2-deoxy-D-glucose improves cardiovascular and neuroendocrine stress adaptation in rats. *Am. J. Physiol. Heart Circ. Physiol.*, 287, 186-193.

Wang X, Liang J, Koike T, Sun H, Ichikawa T, Kitajima S, Morimoto M, Shikama H, Watanabe T, Sasaguri Y, Fan J. (2004). Overexpression of human MMP-12 enhances the development of inflammatory arthritis in transgenic rabbits. *Am. J. Pathol.*, 165, 1375.

Wani, G; Milo, GE; D'Ambrosio, SM. (1998). Enhanced expression of 8-OHdG triphosphatase gene in human breast tumor cells. *Cancer Lett*, 125, 123-130.

Ward, J. (1998). Should antioxidant vitamins be routinely recommended for older people? *Drugs Aging*, 12(3), 169–75.

Warner, D; Sheng, H; Batinić-Haberle, I. (2004).Oxidants, antioxidants and the ischemic brain. *J. Exp. Biol.*, 207, 3221–31.

Watson, JD; Berry, A. DNA: *The Secret of Life*. Ljubljana: Modrijan, 2007.

Watson, R; Griffiths, EM; Craven, NM; Shuttleworth, A; Kielty, CM. (1999). Fibrillin-rich microfibrils are reduced in photoaged skin. Distribution at the dermal-epidermal junction, *J. Invest. Dermatol*, 112, 782-7.

Webb, AR; Holick, MF. (1988). The role of sunlight in the cutaneous production of vitamin D3 *Ann. Rev. Nutr.*, 8, 375-99.

Webb, AR; DeCosta, BR; Holick, MF. (1989). Sunlight regulates the cutaneous production of vitamin D3 by causing its photodegradation, *J. Clin. Endocrinol. Metab.*, 68, 882-7.

Weber, SU; Packer, L. (2001). Ozone Stress in the Skin Barrier. In: *Environmental stressors in health and disease* (Ed. Fuchs J and Packer L.). Marcel Dekker, Inc.

Weber, SU; Thiele, JJ; Cross, CE; Packer, L. (1999). Vitamin C, uric acid, and glutathione gradients in murine stratum corneum and their susceptibility to ozone exposure. *J. Invest. Dermatol*, 113, 1128–1132.

Wei, H; Bowen, R; Cai, Q; Barnes, S; Wang, Y. (1995).Antioxidant and antipromotional effects of the soybean isoflavone genistein. *Proc. Soc. Exp. Biol. Med.*, 208(1), 124-30.

Weindruch, R; Kristie, JA; Cheney, K; Walford, RL. (1979). The influence of controlled dietary restriction on immunologic function and aging. *Fed. Proc.*, 38, 2007-2016.

Weindruch, RK; Walford, RL. *Retardation of aging and disease by dietary restriction*. Springfield: Charles C. Thomas, 1988.

Weinert, BT; Timiras, PS. (2003). Invited review: theories of aging. *J. Appl. Physiol.*, 95, 1706–1716.

Weinstein, GD; Nigra, TP; Pochi, PE; Savin, RC; Allan, A; Benik, K; Jeffes, E; Lufrano, L; Thorne, EG. (1991). Topical tretinoin for treatment of photodamaged skin. A multicenter study. *Arch Dermatol.*, 127(5), 659-65.

Weiss, JS; Ellis, CN; Headington, JT; Voorhees, JJ. (1988). Topical tretinoin in the treatment of aging skin. *J. Am. Acad. Dermatol.*, 19(1- 2), 169-75.

Weiss, JS; Ellis, CN; Headington, JT; Tincoff, T; Hamilton, TA; Voorhees, JJ. (1988). Topical tretinoin improves photoaged skin. A double-blind vehicle controlled study. *JAMA*, 259(4), 527-532.

Wenk, J; Brenneisen, P; Meewes, C; Wlaschek, M; Peters, T; Blaudschun, R; Ma, W; Kuhr, L; Schneider, L; Scharffetter-Kochanek, K. (2001). UV-induced oxidative stress and photoaging. *Curr. Probl. Dermatol.*, 29, 83-94.

Werninghaus, K; Meydani, M; Bhawan, J; Magolis, R; Blumberg, JB; Gilchrest, BA. (1994). Evaluation of the photoprotective effect of oral vitamin E supplementation. *Arch. Dermatol*, 130, 1257–61.

Wert, PW; van den Bergh, B. (1998). The physical, chemical and functional properties of lipids in the skin and other biological barriers. *Chem. Phys. Lipids*, 91, 85-96.

Wespes, E; Schulman, CC. (2002). Male andropause: myth, reality and treatment. *Int. J. Impot. Res.*, 14(1), 93–8.

Whiteman, M. et al. (2004). ONNO- mediates Ca-dependent mitochondrial dysfunction and cell death via activation of calpains. *FASEB J*, 18, 1395.

Whitney, Ellie; Rolfes, SR. *Understanding Nutrition 11th Ed*, California, Thomson Wadsworth, 2008, p.154.

WHO, Ultraviolet radiation, Environmental health criteria: 160.

Wiese, AG; Pacifici, RE; Davies, KJ. (1995). Transient adaptation of oxidative stress in mammalian cells. *Arch. Biochem. Biophys.*, 318(1), 231-40.

Wilhelm, KP; Cua, AB; Maibac, HI. (1991). Skin aging: Effect on transepidermal water loss, stratum corneum hydration, skin surface pH and casual sebum content. *Arch. Dermatol*, 127, 1806-1809.

Wilken, R. Healthy aging: Skeletal muscle. In: Stanner, S; Thompson, R; Buttriss, *J. Healthy aging—The role of nutrition and lifestyle*. Wiley-Blackwell, 2009.

Willcox, DC; Willcox, BJ; Todoriki, H; Curb, JD; Suzuki, M. (2006). Caloric restriction and human longevity: what can we learn from the Okinawans? *Biogerontology*, 7(3), 173.

Williams, IR; Kupper, TS. (1996). Immunity at the surface: Homeostatic mechanisms of the skin immune system. *Life Sci.*, 58, 1485–1507.

Williams, R; Philpott, MP; Kealey, T. (1993).Metabolism of freshly isolated human hair follicles capable of hair elongation: a glutaminolytic, aerobic glycolytic tissue. *J. Invest. Dermatol.*, 100(6), 834-40.

Williams, JD; Jacobson, MK. (2010). Photobiological implications of folate depletion and repletion in cultured human keratinocytes. *J. Photochem. Photobiol. B.*, 99(1), 49-61.

Wilson, J; Gelb, A. (2002). Free radicals, antioxidants, and neurologic injury: possible relationship to cerebral protection by anesthetics. *J. Neurosurg. Anesthesiol*, 14, 66–79.

Winyard, PG; Blake, DR. (1997). Antioxidants, redox-regulated transcription factors, and inflammation. In: Sies H, ed. *Advances in Pharmacology: Antioxidants in Disease Mechanism and Therapy*. San Diego: Academic Press, 403–421.

Wittgen, HG; van Kempen, LC. (2007). Reactive oxygen species in melanoma and its therapeutic implications. *Melanoma Res.*, 17(6),400-9.

Wolf, C; Steiner, A; Honigsmann, H. (1988). Do oral carotenoids protect human skin against ultraviolet erythema, psoralen phototoxicity, and ultraviolet-induced DNA-damage? *J. Invest. Dermatol*, 90, 55–7.

Wolf, FI; Fasanella, S; Tedesco, B; Cavallini, G; Donati, A; Bergamini, E; Cittadini, A. (2005). Peripheral lymphocyte 8-OHdG levels correlate with age-associated increase of tissue oxidative DNA damage in Sprague-Dawley rats. Protective effects of caloric restriction. *Exp. Gerontol.*, 40, 181-188.

Wondrak, GT; Roberts, MJ; Cervantes-Laurean, D; Jacobson, MK; Jacobson, EL. (2003). Proteins of the extracellular matrix are sensitizers of photooxidative stress in human skin cells. *J. Invest. Dermatol*, 121, 578-586.

Wondrak, GT; Roberts, MJ; Jacobson, MK; Jacobson, EL. (2004). 3-Hydroxypiridine chromophores are endogenous sensitizers of photooxidative stress in human skin cells. *J. Biol. Chem.*, 279, 30009-30020.

Wondrak, GT; Roberts, MJ; Jacobson, MK; Jacobson, EL. (2002). Photosensitized growth inhibition of cultured humans skin cells: mechanism and suppression of oxidative stress from solar irradiation of glycated proteins. *J. Invest. Dermatol*, 119, 489-498.

Wood, LC; Feingold, KR; Sequeira-Martin, SM; Elias, PM; Grunfeld, C. (1994).Barrier function coordinately regulates epidermal IL-1 and IL-1 receptor antagonist mRNA levels. *Exp. Dermatol*, 3, 56–60.

Wood, LC; Jackson, SM; Elias, PM; Grunfeld, C; Feingold, KR. (1992). Cutaneous barrier perturbation stimulates cytokine production in the epidermis of mice. *J. Clin. Invest*, 90, 482–487.

Wu, D; Cederbaum, AI. (2003). Alcohol, oxidative stress, and free radical damage. Alcohol Res. *Health*,27,277-284.

Wu, D.; Rea, SL; Yashin, AI; Johnson, TE. (2006). Visualizing hidden heterogeneity in isogenic populations of C. elegans. *Exp. Gerontol.*,41, 261–270.

www.spectracell.com.

www.nas.nasa.gov.

www.wikipedia.com.

http://www.iarc.fr/.

www.cancer.gov/.

www.merckmanuals.com/.

Xanthoudakis, S; Miao, G; Wang, F; Pan, YC; Curran, T. (1992). Redox activation of Fos-Jun DNA binding activity is mediated by a DNA repair enzyme. *EMBO J.,* 11(9), 3323-35.

Xianquan, S; Shi, J; Kakuda, Y; Yueming, J. (2005). Stability of lycopene during food processing and storage. *J. Med. Food*, 8, 413–22.

Yiasemides, E; Sivapirabu, G; Halliday, GM; Park, J; Damian, DL. (2009). Oral nicotinamide protects against ultraviolet radiation-induced immunosuppression in humans. *Carcinogenesis...*,30(1), 101-5.

Xu, X; Weisel, CP. (2005).Dermal uptake of chloroform and haloketones during bathing. *J. Expo. Anal. Environ. Epidemiol*, 15(4), 289-96.

Yaar, M; Gilchrest, BA.Aging of skin. In: Freedberg, IM; Eiser, AZ; Wolff, K; et al. (Eds). *Fitzpatrick's dermatology in general medicine*, vol. 2. McGraw-Hill, New York, 2003.

Yaar, M; Eller, MS; Gilchrest, BA. (2002). Fifty years of skin aging. *J. Invest. Symp. Proc*, 7, 51-58.

Yaar, M; Lee, MS; Rünger, TM; Eller, MS; Gilchrest, B. (2002). Telomere mimetic oligonucleotides protect skin cells from oxidative damage. *Ann. Dermatol. Venerol*, 129, 1-18.

Yaar, M. Clinical and histological features of intrinsic versus extrinsic skin aging. In: *Skin aging*, Gilchrest, B; Krutmann, J. (Eds.). Springer-Verlag, Berlin 2006.

Yamamoto, O; Bhawan, J; Solares, G; Tsay, AW; Gilchrest, BA. (1995). Ultrastructural effects of topical tretinoin on dermo-epidermal junction and papillary dermis in photodamaged skin. A controlled study. *Exp. Dermatol*, 4, 146-154.

Yamauchi, PS. (2010). Selection and preference for botulinum toxins in the management of photoaging and facial lines: patient and physician considerations. *Patient Prefer Adherence*, 4, 345-354.

Yang, JH; Lee, HC; Lin, KJ; Wei, YH. (1994). A specific 4977-bp deletion of mitochondrial DNA in human aging skin). *Arch. Dermatol. Res*, 286, 386-390.

Yang, CS; Wang, X. (2010). Green tea and cancer prevention. Nutr Cancer., 62(7), 931-7.

Yang, S. et al. (2004). Expression of Nox4 in osteoclasts. *J. Cell. Biochem*. 92, 238.

Yano, K; Ouira, H; Detmar, M. (2002). Targeted overexpression of the angiogenesis inhibitor thrombospondin-1 in the epidermis of transgenic mice prevents UVB-induced angiogenesis and cutaneous photodamage. *J. Invest. Dermatol*, 118, 800-805.

Yarosh, D; Bucana, C; Cox, P; Alas, L; Kibitel, J; Kripke, M. (1994). Localization of liposomes containing a DNA repair enzyme in murine skin. *J. Invest. Dermatol.*, 103(4), 461-8.

Yarosh, D. UV-DNA repair enzymes and liposomes. In: *Clinical reviews in oxidative stress and aging*. Cutler, RG and Rodriguez, H (Eds). World Scientific, 2003.

Yarosh, DB. DNA damage and repair in skin aging. In: *Textbook of aging skin*. Farage, MA; Miller, KW; Maibach, HI (Eds). Springer-Verlag, Berlin, 2010.

Yarosh, D; Dong, K; Smiles, K. (2008). UV-induced degradation of collagen I is mediated by soluble factors released from keratinocytes. *Photochem. Photobiol.*, 84(1), 67-8.

Yates, LB; Djoussé, L; Kurth, T; Buring, JE; Gaziano, JM. (2008). Exceptional longevity in men: modifiable factors associated with survival and function to age 90 years. *Arch. Intern.*, 168, 277-83.

Yeh, SL; Huang, CS; Hu, ML. (2005). Lycopene enhances UVA-induced DNA damage and expression of heme oxygenase-1 in cultured mouse embryo fibroblasts. *Eur. J. Nutr.*, 44(6), 365-70.

Yin, L; Morita, A; Tsuji, T. (2001). Skin aging induced by ultraviolet exposure and tobacco smoking: evidence from epidemiological and molecular studies. *Photodermatol. Photoimmunol. Photomed.*, 17(4), 178-83.

Yokoo, S; Furumoto, K; Hiyama, E; Miwa, N. (2004). Slow-down of age-dependent telomere shortening is executed in human skin keratinocytes by hormesis-like-effects of trace hydrogen peroxide or by antioxidative effects of pro-vitamin C in common concurrently with reduction of intracellular oxidative stress.*J. Cell Biochem.*, 93(3), 588-97.

Yoshino, M; Murakami, K. (1998). Interaction of iron with polyphenolic compounds: application to antioxidant characterization. *Anal. Biochem.*, 257, 40-4.

Yoshioka, MT; Tanaka, H; Shono, N; Snyder, E; Shindo, M; St-Amand, J. (2003). Serial analysis of gene expression in the skeletal muscle of endurance athletes compared to sedentary man. *FASEB J.,* 17, 1812-1819.

Yosipovitch G, Hu J. (2003). The importance of skin pH. *Skin & aging*, 11(3), 88-93.

Yu, BP; Masoro, EJ; McMahan, CA. (1985). Nutritional influences on aging of Fischer 344 rats: I- Physical, metabolic and longevity characteristics. *Journal of Gerontology*, 40, 657-670.

Yu, BP. (1995). Putative interventions. In: Masoro, E.J. Editor. *Handbook of Physiology* Oxford University Press, New York, 613–631.

Yu, BP. (1996). Aging and oxidative stress: modulation by dietary restriction. *Free Radic. Biol. Med.*, 21, 651–668.

Yu, ZF; Mattson, MP. (1999). Dietary restriction and 2-deoxyglucose administration reduce focal ischemic brain damage and improve behavioral outcome: evidence for a preconditioning mechanism. *J. Neurosci. Res.*, 57(6), 830-9.

Yue, Y; Zhou, H; Liu, G; Li, Y; Yan, Z; Duan, M. (2010). The advantages of a novel CoQ10 delivery system in skin photo-protection. *Int. J. Pharm.*, 392(1-2), 57-63.

Zhang, HJ; Doctrow, SR; Xu, L; Oberley, LW; Beecher, B; Morrison, J; Oberley, TD; Kregel, KC. (2004).Redox modulation of the liver with chronic antioxidant enzyme mimetic treatment prevents age-related oxidative damage associated with environmental stress. *Faseb J.*, 18, 1547–1549.

Zondlo, FM. (2002). Final report on the safety assessment of Tocopherol, Tocopheryl Acetate, Tocopheryl Linoleate, Tocopheryl Linoleate/Oleate, Tocopheryl Nicotinate, Tocopheryl Succinate, Dioleyl Tocopheryl Methylsilanol, Potassium Ascorbyl Tocopheryl Phosphate, and Tocophersolan. *Int. J. Toxicol.*, 3, 51-116.

Zouboulis, CC; Makrantonaki, E. The role of hormones in intrinsic aging. In: *Skin aging*, Gilchrest, B; Krutmann, J. (Eds.). Springer-Verlag, Berlin 2006.

Zouboulis, CC; Chen, WC; Thornton, MJ; Qin, K; Rosenfield, R. (2007). Sexual hormones in human skin. *Horm. Metab. Res.*, 39(2), 85-95.

Zouboulis, CC; Degitz, K. (2004). Androgen action on human skin— from basic research to clinical significance. *Exp. Dermatol.*, 13(4), 5-10.

Zouboulis, CC. (2000). Human skin: an independent peripheral endocrine organ. *Horn. Res.*, 54, 230-242.

Zouboulis, CC. (2003). Intrinsic skin aging. A critical appraisal of the role of hormones.*Hautarzt.*, 54(9), 825-32.

Zoubpulis, CC. (2004). The human skin as a hormone target and an endocrine gland. *Hormones*, 3, 9-26.

Zussman, J; Ahdout, J; Kim, J. (2010). Vitamins and photoaging: Do scientific data support their use?*J. Am. Acad. Dermatol.*, 63(3), 507-25.

Zwerschke, W; Mazurek, S; Stöckl, P; Hütter, E; Eigenbrodt, E; Jansen-Dürr, P. (2003). Metabolic analysis of senescent human fibroblasts reveals a role for AMP in cellular senescence. *Biochem J.*, 376(2), 403-11.

Index

A

Abraham, 322
accelerator, 55
access, 234, 236
accounting, 31, 68
acetaldehyde, 146
acidic, 27, 126, 140, 273, 281
acidity, 282
acne, 52, 136, 272, 292
acne vulgaris, 136
ACTH, 104
activation state, 263
active compound, 125
active oxygen, 88, 253, 286, 353
active site, 117, 235
activity level, 4, 239
acute stress, 218
adaptability, 120
adaptation, 105, 167, 187, 204, 205, 212, 225, 338, 340, 342, 361, 382, 383
adaptations, 213, 218, 219
additives, 6
adenine, 44, 88, 122, 126, 143, 151, 283
adenosine, 44, 46
adenosine triphosphate, 44
adhesion, 32, 232, 245, 332, 341, 350, 378
adipocyte, 224
adipose, 41, 139, 215, 225, 230, 321, 328
adipose tissue, 139, 215, 225, 230, 328
adiposity, 255
adjustment, 239
adolescents, 95, 178
ADP, 46, 79, 119, 147, 216, 224, 228, 320, 329, 336, 339
adrenal gland, 215, 263
adrenal glands, 215, 263

adsorption, 352
adulthood, 259, 260
adults, 93, 106, 135, 142, 178, 185, 213, 219, 238, 264, 273, 278, 287, 297, 363
adverse conditions, 203
adverse effects, 54, 109, 161, 180, 234
adverse event, 178
aerobic exercise, 4, 216, 218, 219, 340
aesthetic, 289, 290
aetiology, 345, 356
African Americans, 339
age spots, 41, 42, 57, 106, 107
age-related diseases, 8, 44, 185, 186, 209, 230, 236, 238, 244, 252, 260, 300, 357
aggregation, 20, 30, 107, 207, 334
aggression, 90, 144
agriculture, 186
AIDS, 194
air pollutants, 50, 191, 252, 253
alanine, 33
albumin, 193, 221
alcohol abuse, 23
alcohol consumption, 39, 50, 64, 183, 229, 240
alcohol use, 356
alcohols, 63, 117, 156, 191, 252
aldehydes, 61, 63, 83, 146, 201, 204, 235, 248
alkalinity, 282
alkoxyl radicals (LO$^\cdot$), 83
allele, 323
allergens, 40, 100, 279
allergic inflammation, 248
allergic reaction, 60
allergy, 101, 291
aloe, 323
alopecia, 35, 53, 85, 325
alpha-tocopherol, 122, 123, 124, 129, 130, 139, 141, 145, 238, 272, 275, 312, 315, 328, 332, 335
alters, 100, 232, 264, 316, 326, 358, 365

aluminium, 60
aluminum oxide, 292
ambivalence, 375
amines, 50, 63, 228, 329, 376
amino, 23, 30, 33, 36, 117, 144, 176, 212, 229, 230, 231, 298
amino acid, 23, 30, 33, 36, 117, 144, 176, 212, 229, 231, 298
amino acids, 23, 30, 33, 176, 229, 231, 298
amino groups, 230, 231
ammonium, 222
amphibians, 80
amyotrophic lateral sclerosis, 11
anaerobic bacteria, 43
anaphylactic shock, 248
anaphylaxis, 291
anatomy, 31, 37, 346
ancestors, 36, 250, 303, 307
anchoring, 138, 321
androgen, 35, 265, 266, 268
androgens, 265, 266, 268, 333
anemia, 144
anesthetics, 383
angiogenesis, 68, 238, 317, 344, 345, 366, 385
annual rate, 94
anoxia, 352
antagonism, 330
anthocyanin, 149
antibiotic, 248
anti-cancer, 149
antidepressants, 51, 65
antigen, 32, 99, 100, 101, 325, 345, 379
antigen-presenting cell, 101, 345
antihistamines, 109
antioxidant substances, 128, 136, 192, 236, 240, 297
antioxidative activity, 208
antioxidative potential, 170, 192, 272, 330
anxiety, 257
APA, 365
apoptosis, 9, 21, 29, 36, 53, 54, 66, 75, 79, 80, 97, 111, 137, 138, 143, 147, 148, 152, 179, 183, 184, 203, 214, 232, 234, 235, 238, 259, 270, 277, 296, 302, 305, 314, 318, 320, 324, 340, 351, 372
apoptosis pathways, 179, 184
appetite, 215
apples, 186, 249, 250
Arabidopsis thaliana, 361
arginine, 229, 231
aromatic rings, 149, 154
arrest, 183, 261
arsenic, 29, 60, 91, 220
arteries, 4, 231, 244
arteriosclerosis, 10

artery, 12
arthritis, 10
articular cartilage, 315
ascorbic acid, 26, 27, 118, 122, 123, 124, 125, 128, 140, 141, 168, 169, 170, 181, 182, 194, 197, 202, 205, 221, 229, 231, 272, 328, 332, 341, 355, 364, 369, 376, 381
assessment, 126, 146, 193, 197, 275, 286, 320, 323, 328, 334, 339, 345, 355, 358, 386
asthma, 244, 245, 246, 248
asymptomatic, 194, 333
atherogenesis, 331, 375
atherosclerosis, 10, 168, 230, 240, 244, 267, 321, 347
atherosclerotic plaque, 30
athletes, 218, 219, 331, 385
atmosphere, 49, 57, 58, 59, 70, 281, 303, 308
atoms, 56
atopic dermatitis, 52, 110, 256, 319
atopic eczema, 370
ATP, 5, 8, 9, 10, 42, 44, 46, 48, 49, 85, 143, 159, 180, 183, 204, 216, 217, 223, 224, 225, 226, 228, 251
atrophy, 41, 42, 53, 67, 83, 90, 158, 265, 268, 270, 357
attachment, 232, 370
authorities, 285
authority, 178
avoidance, 99, 111, 200, 249, 282, 287, 337
awareness, 326

B

baby boomers, 1
background radiation, 170
bacteria, 25, 34, 50, 116, 118, 248, 300, 352
bacterial infection, 186
bacteriostatic, 34
bacterium, 290
bad habits, 50, 65, 66
balanced budget, 381
barriers, 37, 377, 383
basal cell carcinoma, 80, 91, 93, 95, 97, 98, 282
basal lamina, 33
basal layer, 31, 32, 72, 107, 144, 259, 311
basal metabolic rate, 227
base, 10, 22, 29, 75, 76, 77, 79, 81, 106, 119, 208, 223, 230, 259, 271, 272, 312, 320, 339, 348
base pair, 10, 29, 77, 81, 259
basement membrane, 32, 145, 242, 276, 357
basic research, 386
baths, 236
beef, 149

beer, 150
behavioral dispositions, 255
behaviors, 64, 97, 106, 127, 143
beneficial effect, 66, 110, 136, 141, 142, 145, 161, 162, 170, 179, 184, 199, 206, 207, 208, 212, 213, 214, 227, 229, 236, 237, 239, 245, 276, 282, 313, 368
benefits, 4, 54, 110, 130, 136, 139, 151, 152, 171, 175, 176, 178, 191, 203, 213, 217, 218, 219, 223, 229, 235, 237, 238, 247, 248, 249, 285, 304, 317
benign, 39, 46, 67, 92, 94, 111
beryllium, 60
beta-carotene, 123, 124, 129, 131, 132, 133, 134, 135, 136, 139, 140, 141, 155, 168, 170, 176, 178, 181, 183, 245, 247, 311, 312, 317, 325, 332, 334, 335, 338, 339, 355, 359, 361, 373
beverages, 53, 150, 229, 240, 301
biceps brachii, 366
biceps femoris, 366
bilirubin, 122, 193
bioavailability, 19, 28, 60, 127, 130, 132, 139, 143, 150, 168, 179, 181, 221, 229, 353, 373
biochemistry, 41, 43, 146, 194, 321, 338
bioconversion, 132
biodegradables, 291
bioflavonoids, 150, 151, 154
biokinetics, 23
biological activity, 130, 361
biological consequences, 76, 286
biological processes, 43, 88, 138, 151, 305
biological samples, 5
biological systems, 21, 27, 28, 49, 77, 104, 175, 191, 244, 327
biomarkers, 3, 152, 194, 195, 212, 213, 239, 253, 274, 328, 338, 343, 358
biomolecules, 27, 29, 56, 115, 118, 121, 124, 169, 229, 231, 244, 283, 304
biopolymers, 229
biosphere, 303
biosynthesis, 48, 52, 265, 268, 272, 341, 353, 359, 372
biosynthetic pathways, 151
birds, 158, 307
birth control, 51, 106
black tea, 238, 356
black women, 255
blame, 231, 254
bleeding, 97, 291
blepharoplasty, 289
blood circulation, 40, 154
blood flow, 52, 153, 218, 219, 248, 270
blood plasma, 193, 331, 375
blood pressure, 4, 185, 215, 269, 345

blood stream, 235
blood supply, 37
blood vessels, 31, 37, 40, 57, 100, 102, 105, 268
blood-brain barrier, 179, 252
bloodstream, 49, 142, 179, 231, 232
BMI, 64, 65, 66, 212
body composition, 212, 374
body fat, 212, 250, 264, 270
body fluid, 124, 191
body mass index, 64, 65, 66, 212, 250
body shape, 301
body size, 227, 298
body weight, 31, 180, 226
bonding, 61, 139, 220, 231
bonds, 29, 92, 156
bone, 2, 42, 151, 178, 199, 238, 268, 378
bones, 42, 55, 142, 219, 268
botulism, 290
bowel, 179
brain, 183, 210, 211, 215, 218, 229, 248, 254, 267, 325, 327, 339, 351, 352, 353, 354, 359, 382, 386
brain damage, 386
brainstem, 254
breakdown, 33, 41, 55, 89, 264, 302, 373
breast augmentation, 290
breast cancer, 183, 270, 341, 342
breast carcinoma, 374
buccal mucosa, 140
burn, 73, 102, 152, 269, 367
by-products, 4, 7, 43, 46, 193, 236, 303

C

Ca^{2+}, 21, 29, 305
cadmium, 29, 60, 61, 220, 223
caffeine, 53, 152, 237, 352
calciferol, 142
calcium, 60, 123, 142, 178, 185, 210, 291
caloric intake, 23, 203, 209, 211, 213, 298, 300
caloric restriction, 177, 185, 201, 203, 209, 210, 211, 213, 234, 298, 299, 315, 326, 328, 335, 339, 349, 352, 374, 376, 379, 381, 384
calorie, 211, 212, 213, 214, 215, 223, 226, 227, 228, 229, 230, 233, 234, 239, 241, 256, 313, 316, 321, 328, 338, 340, 355, 367
campaigns, 287, 300
cancer cells, 21, 305
candidates, 153
CAP, 153
capillary, 52, 376
capsule, 140, 247
carbohydrate, 40, 48, 158, 230, 233, 234, 235, 329
carbohydrate metabolism, 48

carbohydrates, 50, 109, 111, 115, 127, 143, 158, 195, 228, 234, 235, 242, 247, 261, 351
carbon, 30, 150, 156
carbon atoms, 150, 156
carbonyl groups, 61, 339
carboxyl, 130, 156, 280
carboxylic acid, 36, 63, 156, 346
carboxylic acids, 63, 156
carcinogen, 92, 137, 152, 183, 274
carcinogenesis, 21, 54, 57, 60, 91, 92, 99, 135, 142, 143, 151, 154, 183, 237, 274, 305, 311, 315, 316, 336, 344, 346, 359, 361, 373, 375, 376, 378
carcinogenicity, 61, 73, 92, 98, 220, 254, 285, 329, 344, 364
carcinoma, 80, 93, 97, 135, 147
cardiac arrhythmia, 238
cardiovascular disease, 10, 19, 120, 129, 139, 176, 186, 212, 237, 238, 245, 339, 348, 356, 359, 377, 381
cardiovascular risk, 186, 239, 329
cardiovascular system, 235
carnivores, 131
carnivorous diet, 146, 340
carnosic acid, 141, 359
carnosine, 111, 146, 147, 235, 272, 312, 340, 372
carotene, 122, 126, 131, 132, 133, 134, 135, 136, 139, 140, 141, 168, 169, 179, 183, 184, 196, 245, 247, 296, 312, 335, 367, 373
carotenoids, 120, 121, 122, 123, 124, 131, 132, 133, 134, 136, 139, 140, 141, 142, 168, 170, 176, 179, 229, 245, 301, 321, 332, 335, 338, 368, 373, 375, 383
cartilage, 55
castration, 266
catabolism, 49, 61, 117
catalysis, 116
catalyst, 29, 61, 77, 169, 221
catalytic activity, 61
cataract, 10, 58, 115, 311
catecholamines, 217
category a, 160
cathepsin G, 242
Caucasians, 103, 339
causality, 181, 184, 199, 212
causation, 347
CDC, 219, 379
cell body, 276
cell culture, 90, 146, 169, 204
cell cycle, 12, 97, 147, 152, 183, 277, 296, 300, 311
cell death, 20, 61, 80, 113, 145, 147, 151, 153, 208, 243, 305, 334, 353, 357, 383
cell differentiation, 131
cell division, 12, 48, 80, 92, 105, 119, 235, 259, 261

cell invasion, 238
cell line, 300, 306, 373
cell lines, 300
cell membranes, 117, 129, 159, 179, 244, 247, 252, 304
cell metabolism, 60, 115, 118, 121, 143, 220, 264
cell organelles, 293
cell proliferation, 5, 20, 48, 79, 113, 138, 144, 183, 234, 238, 243, 256, 267, 363, 376
cell signaling, 107, 145, 152, 276, 305, 360
cell size, 207, 235
cell surface, 89
cellular maintenance, 211
Census, 1, 341
central nervous system, 232
cerebral cortex, 254
cerebral hemisphere, 362
ceruloplasmin, 169, 193, 221
chain propagation, 128
challenges, 179, 202, 204, 249
chaperones, 201, 206, 208, 210, 219
cheese, 149
cheilitis, 143
cheilosis, 143
chemical peel, 108, 289, 291, 322
chemical properties, 179
chemical reactions, 109, 226, 229
chemical structures, 126
chemicals, 19, 50, 75, 136, 151, 153, 235, 243, 279, 297, 305
chemiluminescence, 196
chemokines, 242, 264
chemoprevention, 153
chemopreventive agents, 237
chemotherapy, 23, 305
chicken, 149, 239
childhood, 95, 98, 254, 304
children, 3, 66, 93, 142, 178, 185, 287, 301
chimpanzee, 105
Chinese women, 237
chloasma, 106
chlorination, 170
chlorine, 50, 171, 236, 281, 321, 357
chloroform, 29, 384
cholecalciferol, 142
cholesterol, 4, 83, 150, 151, 170, 234, 239, 247, 279, 286
chromatid, 76
chromium, 28, 50, 60, 61, 169, 220, 223, 235, 301, 320, 336, 339, 364, 375
chromosome, 75, 76, 259, 260
chronic diseases, 178, 186, 238, 274, 305
chronic illness, 23

cigarette smoke, 19, 21, 23, 29, 53, 63, 64, 168, 242, 253, 296, 325
cigarette smoking, 52, 66, 168, 334
circadian rhythm, 251, 269, 328
circadian rhythms, 251, 328
circulation, 35, 99, 110, 131, 145, 153, 216, 230, 269
classes, 76, 210, 228, 279
classification, 84, 331, 343, 355
cleaning, 63, 271, 281
cleavage, 21, 29, 33, 77
clients, 106
climate, 54, 278, 291
climates, 67, 105, 281
clinical application, 157
clinical judgment, 110
clinical symptoms, 11
clinical trials, 137, 151, 160, 178, 187, 194, 249, 274, 300
cloning, 361
clothing, 70, 108, 143, 287
clusters, 149
CNS, 361
coal, 46, 51
coal tar, 51
cobalt, 60, 61, 220
cocoa, 149, 153, 154, 338, 358
coenzyme, 46, 121, 128, 143, 144, 182, 272, 275, 322, 351, 364
coffee, 53, 150, 152, 237, 246, 301
cognitive abilities, 4
cognitive deficit, 238
collaboration, 186
colon, 366
colon cancer, 366
color, 2, 31, 36, 40, 73, 84, 90, 97, 102, 105, 107, 131, 133, 134, 139, 247, 314
coma, 232
combustion, 253
commerce, 57
commercial, 237, 261
communication, 1, 139, 186, 254, 314
community, 135, 158
compaction, 137
compensation, 66, 187
competition, 146, 157
complement, 128, 141, 284, 372
complex carbohydrates, 235, 300
compliance, 312
complications, 11, 28, 147, 229, 230, 245, 290
composition, 31, 63, 139, 158, 159, 279, 318, 341
condensation, 230
conditioning, 54, 126, 129, 342
conduction, 37, 290

conference, 335
confounders, 239
confounding variables, 97
Congress, 328
conjugation, 118
connective tissue, 33, 34, 40, 52, 55, 89, 133, 359
consciousness, 232
consensus, 284
conservation, 207, 227
constant rate, 162
constituents, 8, 9, 14, 20, 27, 43, 117, 123, 154, 155
construction, 307
consumers, 105, 160, 175, 278
consumption, 47, 64, 139, 150, 152, 157, 159, 178, 179, 184, 185, 186, 214, 216, 217, 224, 229, 231, 234, 235, 237, 239, 274, 297, 300, 321, 348, 351, 356, 368, 375, 376
contact dermatitis, 60, 63, 372
contaminant, 71
contradiction, 14, 211, 291
control group, 133, 276
controlled studies, 266
controlled trials, 261, 271, 273
controversial, 10, 11, 93, 176, 183
COOH, 156
cooking, 185, 228, 229, 231, 376
coping strategies, 254
copper, 11, 60, 61, 146, 147, 148, 162, 169, 220, 221, 223, 274, 275, 301, 318, 348, 351, 353, 363
coronary artery disease, 244
coronary heart disease, 150, 212, 238, 239, 240, 333, 334, 339, 377
correlation, 15, 63, 79, 93, 146, 180, 233, 266
cortex, 267, 359
cortisol, 255, 264
cosmetic, 1, 2, 37, 54, 70, 105, 126, 129, 160, 271, 272, 274, 275, 280, 281, 285, 289, 290, 292, 293, 313, 317, 326, 358, 371
cosmetics, 51, 109, 126, 136, 272, 328, 358, 362
cost, 46, 171, 217, 223, 287, 292
counseling, 261
covalent bond, 21
covering, 36, 71
cracks, 84, 143
creatine, 10, 47, 159, 160, 228, 276, 350, 364
creatinine, 159
crises, 255
critical analysis, 364
cross links, 77
cross-linking reaction, 233
cross-sectional study, 232
CRP, 218, 245, 250
crystalline, 53

crystals, 292
CSF, 279
culture, 36, 136, 138, 141, 259, 261, 267, 316, 322, 350
culture medium, 322
curcumin, 208, 248, 284
cure, 1, 93, 176, 298, 309
CVD, 237, 238
cyanotic, 1
cycling, 60, 61, 152, 182, 220, 221, 252
cyclooxygenase, 154, 157, 248, 285, 350, 366, 368
cysteine, 146, 179, 231, 235, 277, 321, 344, 360
cystine, 53, 83, 325, 369
cytochrome, 19, 26, 29, 44, 46, 80, 229, 263, 293, 320
cytochromes, 267
cytokines, 9, 52, 53, 63, 66, 87, 89, 99, 100, 107, 111, 242, 243, 245, 250, 256, 264, 279, 293, 302, 371
cytoplasm, 88
cytosine, 75, 76, 77, 92
cytoskeleton, 231, 232
cytosolic, 11, 49, 116, 120, 203
cytotoxicity, 147, 148, 200, 285, 322, 369

D

daily living, 185
damages, 79, 99, 141, 147, 196
deaths, 51, 94, 233
decay, 8, 14, 352, 372
decomposition, 169
defects, 2, 48, 354, 370
defense mechanisms, 24, 43, 99, 101, 113, 204, 218, 372
deficiencies, 144, 249, 313, 368
deficiency, 23, 50, 125, 142, 144, 169, 178, 184, 185, 212, 223, 230, 265, 266, 275, 334, 340
deficit, 90, 279
deformation, 54
degradation, 33, 40, 52, 84, 90, 91, 136, 146, 154, 197, 203, 207, 233, 242, 257, 268, 273, 279, 302, 342, 363, 378, 385
dehydration, 236, 281, 282
dementia, 11, 12, 144, 218
demography, 12
denaturation, 63, 115, 203, 206
dendrites, 36
dendritic cell, 104, 242
Department of Agriculture, 241
Department of Health and Human Services, 212, 219, 379
Department of Transportation, 324

depolymerization, 42
deposition, 106, 292
deposits, 84
depression, 65, 66, 144, 255, 291
deprivation, 201, 246, 254, 303, 325, 373
depth, 73, 84, 145, 275, 276, 291, 292, 322
derivatives, 129, 136, 141, 150, 151, 170, 205, 231, 284, 365
dermabrasion, 289, 292, 349
dermatitis, 60, 63, 138, 143, 246, 356
dermatologist, 146, 333
dermatology, 93, 308, 315, 347, 364, 384
dermatoses, 272
dermis, 30, 31, 32, 33, 34, 35, 37, 40, 43, 49, 52, 54, 59, 67, 68, 70, 72, 73, 74, 84, 90, 91, 100, 102, 106, 111, 122, 123, 124, 127, 146, 155, 162, 231, 232, 242, 265, 276, 278, 280, 281, 291, 292, 316, 324, 359, 367, 372, 385
destruction, 8, 19, 90, 113, 136, 170, 202, 243, 244, 357
destructive process, 70
detectable, 124, 181, 222
detection, 5, 93, 196, 343, 375
detergents, 50, 278, 280
detoxification, 116, 117, 146, 201, 237, 337, 367
developed countries, 249, 297
developing countries, 160
diabetes, 215, 216, 229, 230, 232, 233, 244, 319, 329, 331, 339, 342, 354, 377
diabetic ketoacidosis, 234
dialysis, 23
diarrhea, 144
diastolic blood pressure, 238
dietary fat, 159
dietary habits, 237, 255
dietary intake, 156, 161, 185, 214, 231, 236, 249
dietary supplementation, 157
diffusion, 27, 49, 116, 182, 279, 286
digestion, 89
dimerization, 21
diodes, 293
diploid, 12, 13, 147, 334
disability, 2
disease progression, 327
disinfection, 236
disposition, 369
dissociation, 57
distortions, 77
distribution, 56, 94, 97, 104, 107, 169, 182, 264, 275, 280, 327, 335, 361
diversification, 361
dizygotic, 64
dizygotic twins, 64

DNA breakage, 92
DNA lesions, 26, 46, 79, 111, 119, 134, 206
DNA polymerase, 77, 259, 260
DNA repair, 9, 29, 42, 75, 77, 79, 80, 81, 82, 90, 97, 98, 99, 105, 111, 119, 123, 151, 177, 179, 187, 200, 202, 223, 237, 254, 270, 287, 298, 304, 307, 320, 323, 331, 334, 339, 344, 345, 351, 364, 365, 384, 385
DNA strand breaks, 76, 92, 111, 368
docosahexaenoic acid, 156, 157
doctors, 160
dogs, 227, 356, 362
donors, 9, 48, 145, 276
dopamine, 264
dopaminergic, 328
dosage, 134, 247
dose-response relationship, 207
dosing, 178
double bonds, 29, 156
drinking water, 53, 170, 236, 237, 281, 369
Drosophila, 177, 180, 206, 210, 215, 226, 314, 348, 351, 356, 357, 360
drought, 246
drug delivery, 276
drugs, 109, 136, 153, 160, 176, 285, 353
drying, 32, 50, 54, 236, 281
durability, 33
dyes, 131
dyslipidemia, 312

E

earnings, 309
East Asia, 339
ECM, 41
economic status, 261
ectoderm, 34
edema, 151
editors, 334
eicosapentaenoic acid, 157, 367
elastin, 33, 34, 40, 43, 55, 83, 84, 89, 151, 154, 231, 232, 270, 273, 275, 280, 293, 302, 353, 378
elderly population, 1, 239, 297, 369
electromagnetic, 23, 56, 57, 58, 59
electron microscopy, 334
electron paramagnetic resonance, 124, 191
electron transport chain (ETC), 44
electrons, 9, 10, 21, 25, 44, 45, 46, 116, 126, 128, 161, 162, 193, 210, 216, 220, 224, 251
elongation, 383
embryogenesis, 131
emission, 105, 145, 196, 234, 276
emotional state, 255

emphysema, 53
employment, 153
encephalopathy, 179
encoding, 81, 217, 297
endocrine, 14, 203, 215, 263, 267, 268, 269, 270, 377, 386
endocrine disorders, 377
endocrine system, 14, 203, 269, 270
endonuclease, 339, 343
endothelial cells, 15, 34, 52, 79, 120, 208, 233, 242, 348
endothelium, 361
endothermic, 225
endurance, 217, 218, 219, 329, 340, 385
energy efficiency, 199
energy expenditure, 185, 212, 217, 227
energy input, 21
energy supply, 159
energy transfer, 88
engineering, 197
England, 331
enlargement, 14, 81, 85
entropy, 212
environment, 19, 23, 26, 37, 39, 114, 128, 144, 167, 169, 181, 183, 184, 186, 200, 201, 203, 207, 227, 246, 263, 278, 304, 306, 307, 313, 335, 355, 364, 367, 376
environmental cigarette smoke, 53
environmental conditions, 206, 210, 295
environmental effects, 297
environmental factors, 2, 3, 5, 22, 39, 58, 66, 91, 282, 302, 367
environmental influences, 64, 305
environmental stress, 66, 128, 207, 246, 337, 354, 386
enzyme, 27, 43, 53, 79, 80, 89, 99, 104, 107, 116, 117, 118, 119, 120, 123, 124, 131, 140, 151, 162, 177, 180, 191, 218, 223, 227, 231, 245, 254, 259, 260, 299, 303, 304, 314, 343, 347, 350, 351, 353, 371, 384, 385, 386
eosinophils, 243, 244
EPA, 156, 157, 158
epidemic, 255
epidemiologic studies, 184, 212
epidemiology, 12, 102, 120, 176
epidermal cells, 35, 104, 145, 159, 276, 280, 324, 325, 357, 363
epithelial cells, 91, 244, 304, 343, 377
epithelium, 32, 92, 243
EPR, 124, 191, 343
equilibrium, 23, 59, 141, 184
equipment, 105
ergocalciferol, 142

erosion, 259
erythrocytes, 140, 376
ESR, 191, 192, 196
essential fatty acids, 156, 228
ester, 129, 131, 154, 264, 267, 277, 350, 368
estrogen, 23, 42, 106, 265, 266, 268, 269, 270, 301, 335, 356
ethanol, 29, 53, 170, 208, 229
ethers, 63
ethnic background, 250
ethnic groups, 36
etiology, 242, 374
EU, 54, 285
eukaryotic, 44, 75, 79, 104, 113, 116, 119, 144, 206, 207, 210, 221, 223, 224
eukaryotic cell, 75, 79, 113, 116, 119, 144, 206, 207, 223
Europe, 130, 285
European Union, 285
evaporation, 32, 34, 281
everyday life, 300
evolution, 43, 68, 97, 105, 159, 213, 303, 304, 306, 307, 343, 354, 364, 367
examinations, 97
excision, 22, 75, 77, 79, 119, 134, 223, 237, 238, 344, 345
excitation, 56, 109, 234, 377
excretion, 34, 159, 217, 343
exercise, 2, 4, 6, 23, 195, 200, 204, 216, 217, 218, 219, 228, 245, 246, 250, 261, 296, 308, 312, 321, 329, 333, 334, 337, 339, 340, 343, 350, 364, 365, 371, 377, 380
exocytosis, 107
expenditures, 217
exploitation, 185
external environment, 37
extinction, 283
extracellular matrix, 14, 33, 34, 40, 89, 138, 232, 268, 274, 285, 293, 384
extraction, 63, 261, 336
extracts, 161, 170, 186, 240, 247, 272, 274, 333

F

FAA, 324
facelift, 293
facial expression, 55, 83
facial muscles, 52, 54, 55
factories, 181
FAD, 44, 143
families, 63, 149, 323, 361
family history, 91
family members, 21

famine, 211, 303, 304
fantasy, 340
FAS, 158
fast food, 261
fasting, 203, 209, 211, 213, 215, 313, 346, 376
fat, 40, 42, 55, 56, 64, 85, 131, 156, 158, 161, 212, 224, 225, 229, 247, 250, 255, 261, 264, 289, 291, 293, 296, 298, 300, 358, 360
fat intake, 64
fatty acids, 32, 49, 115, 117, 121, 156, 157, 158, 161, 176, 185, 239, 243, 246, 250, 261, 279, 307, 317, 320, 346, 349, 365, 381
FDA, 160, 175, 176, 178, 215, 285, 290
FDA approval, 175, 290
feelings, 53, 281
ferritin, 61, 62, 169, 207, 208, 221, 347
fertility, 85, 211, 298, 307
fiber, 4, 43, 146, 155, 176, 186, 232, 235, 247, 261, 266, 300, 319, 340
fibers, 33, 34, 41, 52, 55, 83, 84, 138, 219, 231, 232, 274, 297, 379
fibrin, 240
fibroblast proliferation, 292
fibrosis, 53, 244, 304
fibrous tissue, 57
fidelity, 306
filament, 35
fillers, 289, 291, 319, 322
filters, 54, 59, 111, 284, 285, 287, 358
financial, 4, 253
fish, 4, 80, 156, 157, 185, 226, 228, 238, 239, 243, 245, 246, 249, 250, 261, 272, 351, 359, 367, 376
fish oil, 156, 157, 185, 245, 359, 367
fission, 21
fitness, 7, 218, 219, 298, 306, 328, 353
flavonoids, 120, 121, 149, 150, 151, 152, 153, 154, 155, 176, 178, 193, 238, 242, 246, 247, 248, 272, 278, 330, 337, 338, 339, 368
flavonol, 150, 153
flexibility, 219, 232
flight, 253
flour, 144
flowers, 247
fluctuations, 266
fluid, 34, 50, 157, 193
fluorescence, 196, 197, 232, 233, 234, 283, 377
folate, 105, 144, 383
folic acid, 144, 179, 184, 185, 228, 247, 319
follicle, 35, 265
follicles, 34, 35, 53, 265, 363
food additives, 23, 50
food habits, 105
food intake, 185, 186, 212, 213, 215, 217, 226, 250

Index

food products, 155, 297
force, 45, 46, 56, 223, 225, 354
formula, 182, 284, 324
fractures, 178
fragility, 67, 90
fragments, 217, 380
France, 333
free energy, 251
freedom, 176
fructose, 229, 231, 234, 351, 358
fruits, 4, 120, 121, 125, 139, 149, 150, 161, 176, 178, 181, 185, 186, 236, 238, 239, 240, 241, 243, 246, 261, 276, 296, 297, 298, 300, 321
functional changes, 212, 302, 329
functional food, 120, 155, 177, 250, 360
fungi, 50, 203, 248, 251
fusion, 76

G

gamma rays, 57
gamma-tocopherol, 130
garbage, 3, 7, 14, 118, 120, 377
gastritis, 14
gel, 136, 197, 277, 291
gelatinase A, 89
gene expression, 10, 20, 21, 40, 56, 79, 113, 123, 133, 147, 154, 187, 214, 215, 218, 228, 253, 260, 305, 325, 332, 335, 339, 340, 350, 352, 354, 358, 369, 385
gene regulation, 29, 99, 244
gene silencing, 151
gene therapy, 300
gene transfer, 306
genes, 2, 5, 7, 22, 36, 66, 76, 79, 80, 90, 92, 97, 107, 131, 143, 145, 158, 179, 186, 201, 206, 210, 213, 214, 215, 217, 218, 237, 238, 240, 243, 244, 251, 260, 263, 270, 276, 295, 297, 298, 299, 300, 304, 305, 314, 324, 344, 345, 354, 363, 366, 371, 374
genetic alteration, 76
genetic code, 13
genetic factors, 3, 91, 263, 369
genetic predisposition, 3, 66, 250, 280
genetic syndromes, 91
genetics, 2, 12, 184, 210, 249, 279, 301
genome, 8, 26, 81, 159, 260, 300, 306, 313
genomic instability, 144, 183
genomic stability, 337
genotype, 299, 328
genus, 105
Georgia, 219
germ cells, 260, 307
gerontology, 335, 340, 342, 354, 362

gestational age, 32
ginger, 235
ginseng, 155, 322
gland, 34, 35, 265, 267, 386
glasses, 55, 287, 301
glossitis, 143
glucose, 48, 49, 118, 122, 180, 195, 203, 210, 215, 227, 229, 230, 231, 232, 233, 234, 235, 245, 251, 256, 269, 298, 303, 313, 327, 328, 329, 332, 336, 345, 347, 363, 369, 382
glucose regulation, 195
glucose tolerance, 215, 233, 336
glucoside, 205
glutamate, 146, 251, 360
glutamine, 49
Glutathione (GSH), 117, 146
glycerol, 279, 281, 319
glycine, 33, 117, 146
glycogen, 230, 232
glycol, 120
glycolysis, 47, 48, 49, 85, 159, 215, 216, 219, 231, 363
glycoproteins, 40
glycosaminoglycans, 40, 280, 292
glycosylated hemoglobin, 195
glycosylation, 48, 195, 231, 319
gonads, 263
granules, 81, 104
gravitation, 56
gravitational force, 55, 56
gravity, 46, 50, 56, 264
Greece, 239, 249
green alga, 303
growth arrest, 80, 183, 201
growth factor, 40, 52, 89, 210, 217, 230, 260, 263, 264, 293, 298, 314, 316, 326, 366
growth hormone, 263, 264, 266, 269, 270, 298, 319, 369
growth rate, 207, 227
guanine, 29, 75, 229

H

hair, 2, 3, 31, 33, 34, 35, 36, 42, 52, 53, 72, 73, 102, 105, 109, 236, 265, 267, 271, 289, 293, 314, 363, 378, 383
hair follicle, 31, 33, 34, 35, 53, 72, 265, 314, 363, 383
hair loss, 35, 52, 53, 378
hairless, 54, 62, 68, 73, 89, 123, 124, 127, 151, 155, 156, 197, 205, 238, 321, 324, 329, 346, 380
half-life, 33, 127, 191, 228
halogen, 87

halogens, 63
happiness, 308
harbors, 311
harmful effects, 58, 104, 110, 142, 148, 207, 246, 253, 261, 277, 284, 317, 334
hazards, 50, 175, 239
HE, 331, 343, 364
healing, 40, 146, 148, 208, 244, 249, 266, 268, 274, 292, 322
Health and Human Services, 379
health care, 160, 186
health education, 378
health effects, 37, 56, 254, 317
health problems, 53, 281
health risks, 106
health status, 219, 238, 365, 374
heart attack, 10
heart disease, 115, 150, 176, 178, 187, 229, 255, 340, 357, 365
heart rate, 4, 215
heat shock protein, 175, 204, 206, 207, 208, 218, 264, 343, 354, 357, 379
heavy metals, 50, 206
heavy oil, 280
height, 3, 58, 247, 293
Helicobacter pylori, 243, 321
heme, 61, 109, 144, 207, 248, 313, 314, 351, 385
heme oxygenase, 61, 207, 248, 313, 314, 351, 385
hemisphere, 70
hemoglobin, 37, 195, 234
hemorrhagic stroke, 129
heterogeneity, 384
high blood pressure, 144, 185, 186, 255
hippocampus, 254, 331
histidine, 146, 235, 279, 283
histology, 377
histone, 215, 248, 361
histone deacetylase, 215, 361
histones, 81
history, 39, 64, 65, 68, 69, 90, 94, 95, 98, 106, 154, 291, 303, 304, 307, 316
HO-1, 62, 208, 248
HO-2, 62, 208
homeostasis, 60, 113, 121, 123, 144, 210, 215, 256, 265, 266, 280, 295, 326, 344, 365
hominids, 105
homocysteine, 144, 185, 319
homolytic, 21
honey bees, 159, 336
Hong Kong, 237
hormonal control, 260

hormone, 65, 107, 216, 226, 252, 264, 265, 267, 268, 269, 270, 279, 303, 320, 343, 362, 363, 365, 381, 386
hormone levels, 216, 226, 265
hormones, 12, 15, 65, 106, 120, 143, 156, 215, 255, 263, 264, 265, 267, 269, 353, 354, 381, 386
host, 101, 204, 218
hostility, 255, 377
housing, 343
hTERT, 352
human body, 1, 35, 118, 121, 142, 147, 161, 167, 179, 201, 241, 248, 271
human exposure, 56, 58
human genome, 46
human health, 54, 136, 184, 241
human immunodeficiency virus, 375
human lung fibroblasts, 320
human neutrophils, 361
human subjects, 127, 195
humidity, 54, 281
Hungary, 26, 49, 116
hybrid, 336
hydrocarbons, 228
hydroelectric power, 45
hydrogen, 11, 20, 25, 26, 27, 28, 29, 43, 46, 49, 60, 61, 88, 109, 116, 117, 126, 146, 156, 162, 180, 192, 193, 205, 208, 217, 220, 222, 223, 228, 244, 253, 264, 283, 286, 303, 304, 331, 341, 342, 346, 349, 355, 356, 366, 369, 385
hydrogen abstraction, 29, 88
hydrogen atoms, 126, 156, 193
hydrogen peroxide, 11, 20, 25, 26, 27, 28, 43, 46, 49, 60, 61, 88, 109, 116, 117, 146, 162, 180, 205, 208, 217, 220, 222, 223, 228, 244, 253, 264, 286, 303, 304, 331, 341, 342, 346, 349, 355, 356, 366, 369, 385
hydrogenation, 156
hydroperoxides, 50, 117, 193, 195, 345, 372
hydroquinone, 275, 351
hydroxyl, 11, 25, 27, 28, 29, 30, 43, 60, 61, 62, 77, 88, 109, 114, 117, 118, 126, 150, 154, 168, 182, 220, 221, 222, 244, 269, 280, 304, 376
hydroxyl groups, 62, 150, 154
hydroxylapatite, 291
hygiene, 307
hyperbaric chamber, 205
hyperglycemia, 230
hyperinsulinemia, 230
hyperlipidemia, 361
hyperplasia, 35, 103, 127, 205
hypersensitivity, 100, 101, 127, 369
hypertension, 12, 144, 230, 238, 378
hyperthermia, 206

hypertrophy, 62, 226
hypodermis, 35
hypoglycemia, 346
hypothalamus, 34
hypothesis, 11, 12, 35, 79, 95, 98, 158, 178, 183, 186, 187, 203, 205, 210, 212, 216, 217, 218, 225, 226, 227, 234, 295, 316, 319, 333, 334, 356, 374, 375
hypoxia, 373

I

ICAM, 341
ideal, 213, 280, 286, 293, 296, 297, 299, 300
identical twins, 65, 327, 336
identification, ix, 5, 124, 325, 359
IL-8, 100, 274
image, 55, 347
image analysis, 347
imbalances, 295
immobilization, 254, 379
immortality, 304, 306, 359
immune defense, 305
immune function, 2, 101, 143, 269, 314
immune response, 21, 66, 74, 99, 100, 101, 242
immune system, 32, 34, 37, 56, 58, 92, 99, 100, 142, 200, 242, 243, 244, 253, 257, 261, 383
immunity, 99, 100, 101, 131, 256, 344
immunohistochemistry, 196
immunomodulatory, 274, 284, 344
immunostimulatory, 155
immunosuppression, 91, 99, 100, 101, 102, 143, 151, 154, 237, 238, 274, 284, 344, 345, 357, 373, 384
immunosurveillance, 101
impairments, 208
improvements, 3, 137, 261, 275
in transition, 34
in utero, 2
incidence, 9, 37, 39, 93, 94, 97, 98, 99, 115, 129, 135, 137, 170, 178, 183, 187, 214, 218, 236, 237, 238, 267, 275, 278, 312, 339, 342, 351, 356
indirect effect, 260, 337
indirect measure, 161
individuals, 1, 3, 8, 9, 29, 30, 35, 36, 53, 64, 70, 77, 85, 93, 95, 102, 109, 135, 141, 155, 157, 171, 178, 194, 195, 200, 218, 219, 223, 250, 253, 255, 257, 268, 298, 304, 306, 338, 362
inducer, 215, 248
induction, 10, 15, 40, 48, 53, 59, 66, 79, 91, 95, 99, 100, 101, 102, 111, 136, 139, 147, 148, 152, 155, 157, 160, 162, 177, 201, 202, 204, 206, 209, 210, 227, 237, 248, 273, 314, 320, 329, 341, 356, 362, 367

industrialized countries, 69, 250
industries, 186
industry, 2, 57, 200, 271
inefficiency, 318
infants, 307
infarction, 194
infection, 50, 101, 243, 244, 275, 304
inflammation, 3, 9, 14, 22, 23, 28, 52, 53, 63, 87, 94, 102, 142, 143, 154, 155, 161, 186, 193, 200, 214, 217, 220, 229, 242, 243, 244, 245, 246, 248, 249, 250, 255, 266, 269, 274, 285, 290, 304, 332, 345, 353, 363, 373, 383
inflammatory arthritis, 382
inflammatory cells, 100, 266
inflammatory disease, 10
inflammatory mediators, 102
inflammatory responses, 15, 152, 238, 242, 243, 245, 249, 274, 344
infrared (IR) radiation, 57
ingest, 156, 170, 289, 300
ingestion, 49, 91, 135, 140, 148, 153, 154, 156, 167, 211, 236, 338, 352, 359
ingredients, 120, 126, 129, 139, 161, 177, 236, 250, 271, 272, 276, 281, 282, 285, 286, 324, 351, 358
inheritance, 295, 333
inhibition, 53, 84, 119, 127, 139, 147, 152, 155, 157, 206, 235, 237, 238, 248, 252, 274, 285, 290, 298, 332, 368, 376, 379, 380, 384
inhibitor, 215, 233, 234, 248, 359, 385
initiation, 22, 23, 30, 72, 77, 92, 99, 145, 244, 263, 305
initiation rates, 23
injections, 290
injuries, 12, 128, 176, 219
injury, 10, 22, 37, 41, 79, 102, 104, 105, 109, 119, 148, 170, 176, 182, 215, 222, 229, 244, 248, 269, 270, 273, 285, 292, 313, 321, 327, 360, 367, 376, 383
inositol, 235
insects, 226
insomnia, 144
instinct, 306
institutions, 142, 176
insulin, 3, 215, 217, 230, 235, 239, 243, 245, 246, 255, 256, 263, 264, 296, 298, 317, 327, 328, 329, 336, 341, 342, 345, 362, 369, 378
insulin resistance, 3, 317, 327, 362
insulin sensitivity, 217, 239, 296, 341, 342, 345
integration, 194
integrity, 13, 41, 52, 90, 105, 118, 231, 257, 261, 344, 348
integument, 105
interference, 269

interleukin-8, 274
internal influences, 39
internal processes, 302
internalization, 40, 264, 326
intervention, 4, 5, 12, 47, 129, 132, 135, 139, 154, 179, 182, 183, 186, 208, 213, 214, 233, 234, 243, 245, 248, 290, 299, 341, 351, 365
intervention strategies, 47
intestinal tract, 179
intestine, 131, 170
investment, 2, 211, 304, 306, 307
investments, 211, 300
ionization, 56
ionizing radiation, 23, 26, 40, 56, 75, 91, 170, 183, 191, 252, 315, 341
ions, 44, 46, 60, 62, 117, 182, 183, 220, 221, 279
iron, 11, 28, 44, 60, 61, 62, 88, 169, 170, 179, 184, 185, 193, 220, 221, 222, 223, 225, 230, 301, 316, 329, 330, 341, 345, 349, 353, 357, 366, 367, 368, 381, 385
irradiation, 59, 69, 84, 88, 90, 102, 103, 104, 107, 124, 133, 136, 140, 141, 145, 153, 155, 157, 162, 170, 201, 202, 204, 209, 232, 260, 269, 286, 290, 315, 322, 324, 346, 365, 384
ischaemic heart disease, 347
ischemia, 10
islands, 239, 378
isoflavone, 382
isoflavonoids, 150, 238
isolation, 183
isomerization, 139, 283
isomers, 109, 277
isoprene, 144
Israel, 72, 95, 342
issues, 178, 243, 309, 339, 368
Italy, 95

J

Japan, 54, 285, 325, 348
jaundice, 110
joints, 231

K

kaempferol, 151, 248
karyotype, 259
keratin, 31, 32, 35, 280, 283, 358
keratinocyte, 62, 90, 104, 107, 283, 293, 323, 346
keratosis, 84, 353
ketones, 61
kidney, 210, 211, 230, 241, 247, 254
kidneys, 142, 215
kill, 248, 281
kinetics, 14, 226, 233, 343, 371
Krebs cycle, 216

L

labeling, 176, 178
laboratory studies, 161
laboratory tests, 187, 193, 261
lack of control, 271
lactate level, 254, 372
lactation, 23, 52, 105, 370
lactic acid, 291
Langerhans cells, 31, 41, 83, 99, 100, 242, 269, 274
lasers, 289, 292
latency, 256
later life, 95
Latinos, 339
lattices, 340
LDL, 124, 218, 239, 319, 380
lead, 5, 7, 8, 28, 29, 35, 43, 54, 60, 61, 64, 70, 74, 75, 76, 81, 84, 90, 92, 93, 103, 110, 123, 144, 162, 170, 181, 201, 203, 209, 210, 213, 216, 217, 220, 221, 224, 228, 229, 230, 231, 242, 243, 253, 255, 263, 266, 273, 285, 296, 301, 302, 305
leakage, 9, 20, 22, 44, 46, 116, 200, 210, 297, 298
leaks, 251, 298
lean body mass, 227, 270
learning, 301, 373
legs, 94
legume, 357
leisure, 69, 95
leisure time, 95
lending, 9
lentigo, 106, 338, 344
leptin, 215, 264, 365
lesions, 49, 53, 57, 67, 74, 75, 76, 79, 85, 90, 91, 94, 97, 101, 111, 135, 168, 179, 184, 228, 282
liberation, 83, 89
libido, 268
life cycle, 195
life expectancy, 3, 180, 182, 212, 213, 214, 236, 303, 307, 374, 376
life experiences, 64
lifestyle changes, 261, 360
lifestyle decisions, 66
lifetime, 2, 31, 41, 65, 66, 69, 93, 94, 95, 97, 102, 191, 212, 298
ligand, 62
linoleic acid, 32, 127, 156, 158, 249, 279
lipases, 120
lipid oxidation, 156, 207

lipid peroxidation, 20, 42, 47, 48, 60, 83, 111, 118, 129, 131, 134, 145, 153, 157, 158, 159, 163, 168, 169, 223, 232, 234, 254, 274, 276, 307, 311, 312, 341, 345, 347, 349, 351, 357, 367, 377
lipid peroxides, 117, 280
lipids, 8, 9, 23, 30, 31, 32, 47, 62, 64, 66, 83, 109, 111, 115, 118, 120, 145, 158, 170, 175, 183, 218, 229, 230, 238, 242, 254, 274, 278, 279, 283, 318, 319, 349, 361, 373, 376, 380, 383
lipooxygenase, 157
lipoproteins, 156
liposomes, 139, 286, 375, 385
liposuction, 289, 293
liquid chromatography, 350
liver, 49, 92, 106, 110, 119, 130, 131, 142, 144, 156, 179, 182, 211, 215, 230, 232, 247, 253, 254, 311, 341, 347, 352, 365, 386
liver cells, 247
liver spots, 106
living conditions, 3
living environment, 66
locus, 191
longitudinal study, 233
loss of appetite, 297
low temperatures, 54
low-density lipoprotein, 124, 151
low-grade inflammation, 301
lubricants, 281
lung cancer, 53, 155, 168, 170, 176, 178, 312, 320, 359, 369, 381
lung function, 168
lupus, 10, 101
lutein, 122, 124, 132, 133, 134, 139, 140, 245, 375
lycopene, 122, 124, 132, 133, 134, 139, 140, 141, 229, 245, 314, 359, 367, 375, 384
lymph, 100
lymphocytes, 14, 100, 102, 120, 196
lysine, 23, 229, 231, 233, 321
lysosome, 9
lysosomes, 10, 11, 14, 120, 202, 230

M

machinery, 206, 227
macromolecules, 8, 9, 20, 25, 28, 41, 43, 47, 118, 183, 243, 283, 302
macrophages, 87, 100, 102, 142, 243, 244, 248
magnesium, 186, 221, 222, 223, 301, 324, 334, 345, 378
magnitude, 29, 70, 73, 77, 134, 136, 159, 168
Maillard reaction, 231, 232, 332
majority, 11, 44, 49, 60, 61, 63, 70, 79, 83, 94, 106, 111, 120, 217, 223, 259, 287, 288

malignancy, 97, 183
malignant growth, 91
malignant melanoma, 93, 94, 95, 96, 98, 158, 282, 314, 332, 347, 356
malnutrition, 185, 210, 212, 300, 382
mammal, 158, 182, 371
mammalian cells, 260, 313, 336, 349, 359, 383
mammalian tissues, 126, 204, 206
mammals, 8, 14, 80, 85, 120, 151, 158, 177, 182, 211, 213, 215, 217, 218, 224, 225, 226, 230, 252, 295, 298, 299, 304, 307, 314
man, 7, 79, 101, 125, 218, 252, 265, 268, 285, 328, 366, 385
management, 253, 272, 289, 292, 364, 385
manganese, 60, 162, 220, 234, 346, 364
manipulation, 183, 209, 227, 299
mannitol, 196
mantle, 282
marital status, 66
marketing, 54, 160, 176, 285
Maryland, 245, 281
mass, 33, 65, 195, 212, 239, 321
mast cells, 33, 41, 52, 242, 244, 349
materials, 50, 243, 291, 380
matrix, 9, 31, 32, 33, 34, 40, 52, 59, 81, 84, 89, 90, 91, 102, 111, 117, 133, 139, 183, 196, 197, 216, 224, 226, 232, 242, 265, 273, 279, 285, 302, 314, 328, 330, 335, 352, 353, 363, 370, 380, 381
matrix metalloproteinase, 33, 40, 52, 84, 89, 90, 111, 133, 273, 302, 314, 330, 335, 353, 380, 381
matrixes, 242
matter, 5, 19, 51, 56, 110, 187, 201, 218, 253, 268, 298, 301
Mauro Carratelli, 20, 193, 194
measurement, 97, 191, 192, 193, 194, 195, 196, 197, 240, 320
measurements, 70, 95, 136, 141, 197, 198, 241, 327, 336, 348, 368, 376
meat, 4, 144, 149, 228, 239, 250, 376
mechanical properties, 55, 278, 280, 343, 359, 363
mechanical stress, 54
media, 90
median, 70
mediation, 342
medical, 3, 12, 101, 110, 136, 149, 160, 185, 329, 338, 362
medical science, 362
medicine, 100, 131, 153, 289, 299, 313, 337, 347, 382, 384
Mediterranean, 238, 247, 248, 328, 331, 345, 354, 360, 362, 363, 368, 374, 378
melanin, 31, 35, 36, 37, 57, 62, 95, 104, 106, 107, 109, 111, 137, 141, 205, 283, 303, 330, 347, 352

Melanin particles, 104
melanoma, 32, 36, 51, 73, 91, 93, 94, 95, 97, 98, 105, 151, 158, 170, 205, 238, 239, 252, 274, 315, 325, 331, 335, 345, 346, 350, 352, 356, 373, 374, 383
melatonin, 61, 168, 170, 223, 252, 256, 264, 267, 269, 277, 325, 327, 330, 337, 342, 367
membrane permeability, 20, 109
membranes, 26, 27, 28, 32, 43, 61, 63, 85, 104, 115, 124, 156, 158, 159, 177, 200, 221, 235, 307, 336
memory, 373
menopause, 23, 35, 263, 265, 270, 317, 319, 363, 365
menstruation, 265
mercury, 29, 60, 61, 68, 220
mesoderm, 34
messages, 37
messengers, 21
meta-analysis, 181, 317, 374, 381
Metabolic, 22, 313, 363, 374, 386
metabolic changes, 203
metabolic pathways, 225, 231, 360
metabolic syndrome, 218
metabolites, 41, 75, 132, 152, 180, 203, 216, 268, 283, 305, 324
metabolized, 11, 49, 110, 116, 120, 159, 277
metabolizing, 36, 265
metal complexes, 168
metal ion, 11, 23, 26, 27, 34, 50, 60, 62, 127, 182, 183, 220, 221, 229, 283, 337
metal ions, 11, 26, 27, 34, 50, 60, 62, 127, 182, 183, 220, 221, 229, 283, 337
metal nanoparticles, 285
metal oxides, 285
metal salts, 50
metalloenzymes, 116
metalloproteinase, 41, 52, 89, 90, 133, 349, 352, 354
metals, 28, 60, 61, 89, 168, 191, 220, 231, 252
metastasis, 183, 238
meter, 59
metformin, 215
methodology, 240
microcirculation, 358
micronutrients, 123, 124, 160, 180, 185, 186, 236, 241, 245, 249, 296, 297, 313, 317, 372
microorganism, 304
microorganisms, 50, 105, 170, 206, 279, 304, 305, 307, 373, 380
microscopy, 316
microsomes, 44, 61
microwaves, 57
migrants, 94, 342, 346, 355
migration, 90, 101

misuse, 309
mitochondria, 8, 9, 10, 11, 14, 15, 28, 44, 45, 46, 48, 49, 61, 72, 80, 81, 113, 116, 144, 160, 177, 181, 199, 202, 207, 210, 216, 217, 223, 224, 225, 240, 246, 251, 267, 276, 295, 297, 298, 300, 303, 304, 307, 318, 319, 331, 334, 337, 338, 347, 348, 352, 366, 370, 375, 380
mitochondrial damage, 9, 48, 119, 301
mitochondrial DNA, 8, 9, 10, 20, 79, 81, 85, 187, 222, 252, 293, 296, 316, 333, 335, 385
mitochondrial proteases, 11, 120
mitogen, 107, 113, 237, 293
mitosis, 259
MMP, 10, 33, 40, 52, 89, 111, 141, 155, 238, 266, 274, 284, 285, 327, 329, 370, 373, 382
MMP-2, 41, 89, 238, 373
MMP-3, 89
MMP-9, 33, 155
MMPs, 33, 41, 52, 89, 136, 145, 276, 285, 314
model system, 140
models, 85, 100, 135, 146, 152, 160, 181, 185, 196, 211, 213, 227, 274, 300, 317, 328, 344, 363, 373
moderate activity, 219
modern society, 214, 253, 255
modifications, 28, 29, 30, 60, 75, 76, 79, 88, 109, 145, 162, 264, 295
modules, 54
moisture, 40, 52, 54, 266, 268, 280, 281
moisture content, 52, 280
mole, 97
molecular oxygen, 25, 26, 46, 57, 116, 117, 124, 162, 182, 224, 228
molecular structure, 72, 150
molecular weight, 197, 347, 380
monolayer, 138
monomers, 154
monounsaturated fatty acids, 158, 238, 239
Montenegro, 318
Moon, 346
morbidity, 51, 179, 184, 369
morphology, 119, 207, 234
mortality, 94, 97, 129, 179, 181, 183, 184, 212, 216, 218, 219, 237, 238, 245, 255, 306, 307, 333, 335, 336, 338, 339, 348, 353, 356, 369, 376, 377
mortality rate, 94, 219, 338
mortality risk, 356
Moscow, 352
mRNA, 52, 62, 84, 116, 123, 133, 141, 371, 384
mtDNA, 8, 9, 10, 81, 85, 111, 124, 160, 210, 302
mucosa, 54
mucous membrane, 271
mucous membranes, 271
mucus, 280

multiple factors, 184
multiplication, 12, 306
multipotent, 293
muscle mass, 2, 218
muscle strength, 219
muscles, 55, 148, 290, 312, 325
mutagenesis, 10, 91, 111, 316, 331
mutant, 93, 273, 327, 334, 351
mutation, 7, 9, 10, 23, 29, 75, 77, 81, 92, 119, 305
mutation rate, 9, 81
mutations, 7, 10, 42, 72, 76, 79, 80, 85, 92, 93, 97, 123, 160, 222, 243, 260, 283, 296, 302, 305, 307, 311, 315, 351, 372
mutilation, 119
myocardial infarction, 238, 333, 369
myocardial ischemia, 326

N

NAD, 44, 45, 124, 143, 151, 170, 180, 325, 341
NADH, 8, 44, 46, 88, 124, 126, 140, 180, 283, 324, 325
nanomaterials, 286
nanometer, 57
nanometers, 57
nanoparticles, 54, 285, 371
National Institutes of Health, 178, 212, 358
natural disaster, 3
natural disasters, 3
natural food, 246
natural killer cell, 101, 261
natural selection, 211
necrosis, 147, 179, 183, 184
negative consequences, 266
negative effects, 232
neonates, 35
neoplasm, 39
neovascularization, 302
nerve, 3, 32, 33, 37, 261, 290
nervous system, 156, 232
Netherlands, 150, 255, 371
network theory, 348
neural function, 238
neurodegeneration, 147
neurodegenerative diseases, 10, 20
neurodegenerative disorders, 347, 354
neuroendocrine system, 3, 102
neurological disease, 178
neurons, 3, 12, 118, 120, 210, 327, 328
neuroprotection, 335
neurotransmission, 21, 305
neurotransmitters, 248, 264
neutral, 21, 55, 129, 208, 243, 281

neutrophils, 25, 102, 242, 243, 244
New England, 359, 368, 369, 375
New Zealand, 95
niacin, 140, 143
niacinamide, 272
nickel, 60, 61, 220
nicotinamide, 44, 73, 88, 122, 126, 143, 151, 180, 283, 325, 373, 384
nicotinic acid, 180
nitric oxide, 19, 43, 44, 88, 234, 242, 359
nitric oxide synthase, 19, 44, 234, 359
nitrogen, 8, 21, 29, 61, 65, 102, 126, 220, 242, 253
nitrogen dioxide, 29
nitrosamines, 228
nitroxide, 126
nitroxide radicals, 126
NMR, 335
nodules, 357
non-enzymatic antioxidants, 24, 121, 122, 170, 192, 223
nonionic surfactants, 281
non-polar, 279
non-smokers, 52
normal aging, 5, 8, 229, 237, 329, 362
North America, 94, 130, 247
Norway, 95, 376
nuclear genome, 3
nuclear membrane, 169
nuclei, 105, 215, 265, 283
nucleic acid, 9, 23, 47, 77, 115, 170, 230, 235, 254, 283
nucleotides, 46, 259
nucleus, 81, 92, 119, 221, 276, 300
nutraceutical, 155
nutrient, 126, 127, 144, 155, 158, 181, 211, 212, 213, 228, 235, 240, 242, 246, 249, 274, 301, 303, 317, 323
nutrient concentrations, 317
nutrients, 15, 37, 41, 44, 141, 154, 161, 169, 176, 178, 181, 182, 185, 186, 211, 213, 216, 222, 223, 228, 235, 237, 240, 243, 245, 246, 247, 249, 287, 297, 300, 331, 332, 360, 364, 381
nutrition, 3, 23, 39, 50, 131, 136, 181, 184, 213, 228, 236, 241, 249, 261, 282, 289, 295, 296, 298, 300, 308, 320, 326, 329, 339, 343, 344, 346, 349, 368, 375, 381, 383
nutritional deficiencies, 228
nutritional status, 161, 185

O

obesity, 23, 212, 225, 238, 250, 261
obstacles, 278

occlusion, 279
OH, 25, 27, 29, 75, 78, 88, 143, 196, 222, 252, 254, 323, 367
oil, 33, 35, 51, 129, 132, 139, 144, 149, 155, 156, 157, 185, 238, 239, 245, 250, 282, 301, 321, 324, 359
old age, 180, 209, 250, 255, 296, 303
oleic acid, 157
olive oil, 139, 238, 249, 250, 381
omega-3, 121, 156, 157, 158, 261, 381
one dimension, 286
operations, 290
opportunities, 4
optimism, 255, 333
oral cavity, 54, 271
organ, 1, 10, 31, 36, 50, 91, 99, 101, 138, 215, 244, 263, 269, 315, 386
organelles, 14, 104, 233, 279
organic compounds, 128
organic peroxides, 123
organic solvents, 50, 63
organism, 12, 14, 37, 44, 50, 79, 80, 98, 171, 181, 186, 199, 201, 202, 203, 206, 211, 213, 216, 218, 220, 228, 229, 236, 262, 269, 275, 295, 300, 304, 306, 307, 308
organs, 3, 39, 76, 167, 179, 201, 211, 266, 271
osmotic stress, 202
osteoarthritis, 245
osteomalacia, 142
osteoporosis, 142, 185, 267, 316, 340, 345, 361
ovaries, 265
overlap, 15, 88, 201
overproduction, 74, 105
overweight, 23, 239, 250, 328, 338
ox, 37
oxidation products, 76, 78, 107, 126, 195
oxidative reaction, 61, 160, 202
oxygen consumption, 8, 10, 160, 210, 216, 224, 228, 312
ozone, 19, 29, 43, 50, 51, 57, 58, 59, 63, 68, 69, 70, 93, 94, 128, 167, 253, 290, 298, 301, 303, 329, 331, 333, 357, 364, 370, 380, 382

P

p53, 42, 61, 76, 80, 97, 152, 157, 223, 260, 318, 349, 351, 367, 371
pain, 102, 290
palladium, 60
palliative, 109
paradoxical sleep, 373
parallel, 69, 84, 128, 133, 141, 143, 157, 318
paralysis, 290

parasites, 248
parasitic diseases, 304
parents, 254, 309
participants, 64, 135, 239, 245, 287, 297
pathogenesis, 44, 124, 170, 175, 191, 212, 246, 316, 334, 344, 346, 351, 372
pathogens, 37, 305
pathology, 194, 227, 244
pathophysiological, 22, 305
pathophysiology, 63, 328, 339
pathways, 10, 25, 40, 48, 81, 89, 104, 113, 152, 159, 201, 204, 205, 206, 208, 219, 237, 263, 278, 286, 289, 296, 358, 360, 361
PBMC, 261
PCP, 50, 54
PDL, 206
pellagra, 144, 249
pepsin, 197
peptidase, 119
peptide, 30, 251, 267
peptide chain, 30
peptides, 104, 179, 235, 271, 274
periodicity, 32
peripheral blood, 255, 261, 342
peripheral blood mononuclear cell, 255, 261
permeability, 29, 41, 80, 102, 242, 257, 266, 286, 326, 328, 333, 344
permit, 34, 80, 105, 185
peroxidation, 30, 62, 83, 115, 145, 157, 158, 170, 223, 245, 312, 335, 336
peroxide, 21, 25, 88, 116, 117, 118, 162, 205, 221, 264, 303, 305, 355, 370
peroxynitrite, 123, 126
personal communication, 20, 25
personal history, 102
personal problems, 34
pessimists, 255
pests, 297
petroleum, 167
pH, 27, 126, 161, 233, 281, 282, 359, 383, 385
phagocytosis, 29, 244, 304
phalanges, 36
pharmaceutical, 155, 186, 200, 325
pharmaceuticals, 272
pharmacokinetics, 371
phenolic compounds, 149, 357
phenothiazines, 109
phenotype, 21, 24, 92, 102, 213, 230, 263, 287, 306, 370
phenotypes, 85, 103
phenoxyl radicals, 154
Philadelphia, 343, 357
phlebotomy, 329

phosphate, 46, 88, 118, 122, 126, 144, 183, 205, 231, 233
phosphatidylcholine, 47
phosphocreatine, 47, 159, 160
phospholipids, 61, 158, 279, 286
phosphorylation, 44, 46, 48, 113, 160, 208, 218, 224, 225, 228, 233, 238, 260, 305, 334, 376, 380
photochemical degradation, 88
photodegradation, 382
photographs, 309
photolysis, 57, 110
photons, 68, 76, 104, 253, 284
photooxidation, 83, 355, 377
photosensitivity, 109, 120, 176, 327
photosynthesis, 44, 142, 326
physical activity, 23, 217, 219, 239, 250, 301, 328, 341, 356, 370
physical and mechanical properties, 232
physical exercise, 352
physical properties, 372
physicians, 278, 291
Physiological, 41, 256, 298, 354, 356, 363
physiological factors, 43, 260
physiological mechanisms, 213
physiology, 10, 12, 31, 37, 213, 227, 251, 270, 330, 345, 349, 376
physiopathology, 364
phytosterols, 238
pigmentation, 16, 36, 39, 64, 67, 73, 74, 90, 94, 104, 105, 106, 107, 109, 114, 127, 141, 155, 197, 265, 267, 268, 272, 273, 320, 330, 334, 364
pigs, 186, 336, 358, 360
pilot study, 136, 358, 360
pineal gland, 252
pituitary gland, 267
placebo, 128, 133, 134, 135, 137, 140, 141, 157, 161, 268, 273, 311, 318, 322, 338, 341, 342, 362
plants, 80, 109, 126, 131, 147, 149, 150, 167, 203, 215, 246, 249, 251, 297, 318, 324, 337, 380
plasma levels, 153, 179, 195, 261
plasma proteins, 150
plastic surgeon, 291
plasticity, 305
platform, 327
platinum, 60, 197
playing, 21, 29, 33, 44, 192
pleiotropy, 7, 304
PM, 51, 168, 200, 282, 317, 326, 327, 328, 332, 333, 335, 339, 344, 353, 375, 384
point mutation, 85
polar, 279
policy, 300
pollen, 159

pollutants, 5, 19, 23, 50, 51, 63, 167, 171, 191, 194, 199, 242, 252, 253, 256, 298, 300, 308, 320, 364
pollution, 22, 23, 28, 40, 50, 51, 66, 168, 185, 200, 295, 301, 303
polycyclic aromatic hydrocarbon, 50
polymer, 36, 232
polymerase, 52, 79, 119, 147, 320, 329, 336, 378
polymerase chain reaction, 52
polymerase chain reactions, 52
polymethylmethacrylate, 291
polymorphisms, 7
polypeptide, 230
polyphenols, 120, 121, 123, 149, 151, 152, 153, 154, 155, 161, 169, 176, 181, 193, 237, 238, 246, 248, 274, 344, 345, 350, 375, 380
Polysaccharides, 323
polyunsaturated fat, 29, 60, 156, 157, 158, 159, 168, 229, 238, 239, 243, 245, 326, 333, 360
polyunsaturated fatty acids, 29, 156, 157, 158, 159, 168, 229, 238, 239, 243, 245, 333, 360
pools, 236
population, 1, 4, 31, 40, 69, 70, 94, 97, 127, 136, 143, 147, 155, 158, 160, 175, 178, 183, 196, 205, 207, 211, 212, 229, 236, 241, 260, 306, 378
population group, 143
porphyrins, 88, 109, 283
positive correlation, 119
positive feedback, 10, 87
positive relationship, 11, 97
potassium, 208
potato, 149, 241
potential benefits, 213
poultry, 246
power plants, 46
predation, 306
predators, 304, 306
pregnancy, 23, 52, 105, 106, 213, 301, 370
preparation, 134, 176, 215, 229, 271, 297
preservation, 4
preservative, 126, 247
President, 1
preventive approach, 91, 156, 236, 286, 289
primary function, 32, 33, 104, 225
primary products, 72, 77
primate, 362
priming, 292
principles, 43, 45, 314
probability, 14, 92, 99, 120, 222, 298, 307
probe, 196
probiotics, 186, 360
process control, 250
producers, 2
professionals, 342

progesterone, 23, 266
progestins, 265
programmed aging, 7
pro-inflammatory, 9, 10, 53, 102, 239, 242, 243, 245, 246, 250, 279
prokaryotes, 79, 206
proliferation, 5, 20, 22, 32, 48, 79, 80, 92, 113, 138, 144, 160, 183, 234, 238, 243, 256, 259, 260, 266, 267, 293, 303, 316, 328, 343, 363, 376
proline, 33
promoter, 22, 298
propagation, 30, 145
prophylaxis, 268
proportionality, 226
prostaglandins, 157, 217, 249
prostate cancer, 270
proteasomes, 11, 120
protective factors, 202
protective mechanisms, 120, 205
protective role, 37, 62, 148, 157, 284, 353
protein family, 206, 224
protein folding, 206
protein kinase C, 21, 234, 305
protein kinases, 87, 113
protein oxidation, 20, 51, 75, 111, 146, 162, 217, 223, 302, 334, 355, 369, 374, 375
protein structure, 30, 334
protein synthesis, 2, 9, 40, 218, 227, 331
protein-protein interactions, 260
proteoglycans, 33, 34, 40, 52, 280
proteolysis, 30, 81, 147
protons, 9, 45, 216, 223, 224, 225, 226
proto-oncogene, 260, 324
psoriasis, 52, 110, 256
psoriatic arthritis, 10
psychiatric disorders, 238
psychological stress, 40, 254, 255, 257, 311, 331
psychological well-being, 268
psychosocial factors, 255
psychosocial stress, 254
puberty, 2, 268, 365
public health, 53, 56, 238
pulmonary diseases, 246
pumps, 45
pure water, 301
purpura, 67, 90
pyridoxine, 143
pyrimidine, 73, 75, 76, 77, 79, 80, 92, 97, 152, 275, 314

Q

quadriceps, 366

quality of life, 11, 209, 238, 289
quantification, 235, 337
quantum dot, 286
quantum dots, 286
Queensland, 94, 135, 335
quercetin, 150, 153, 215, 248, 311, 322
questionnaire, 158, 237
quinone, 144
quinones, 50, 109, 283

R

race, 365
Radiation, 56, 59, 68, 74, 85, 94, 169, 170, 200, 318, 362, 380
radiation damage, 61
radiation therapy, 183
radical formation, 4, 5, 11, 19, 22, 23, 43, 56, 66, 75, 83, 117, 159, 161, 167, 169, 182, 198, 222, 223, 246, 285, 297, 307
radical reactions, ix, 5, 19, 34, 43, 124, 221, 340
radio, 57
radio waves, 57
radiosensitization, 331
radiotherapy, 23, 170, 305
radon, 170
reactants, 109, 116
reactions, ix, 20, 26, 27, 28, 29, 44, 45, 56, 60, 61, 62, 74, 76, 77, 83, 88, 89, 100, 109, 115, 118, 124, 146, 149, 153, 168, 170, 183, 191, 192, 193, 205, 220, 226, 227, 233, 281, 283, 284, 285, 301, 359, 364, 369
reactivity, 19, 27, 28, 30, 63, 146, 193, 235, 286
reading, 15, 55, 89, 145, 191, 233, 253, 272, 306, 308
real time, 196
reality, 2, 23, 383
receptor sites, 290
receptors, 21, 32, 40, 89, 104, 113, 138, 149, 158, 230, 252, 264, 265, 269, 305, 353, 356, 362
recession, 3
recognition, 32, 79
recombination, 79, 119, 151, 307, 319
recommendations, 160, 247
recovery, 253, 292, 357
recreation, 57, 70, 94
recreational, 69, 94
recycling, 8, 118, 143, 182, 336, 355
red blood cells, 220
red wine, 150, 153, 229, 241, 246, 248, 296, 301, 347, 350
redistribution, 104
reducing sugars, 230, 235

redundancy, 15, 121
refractive index, 72
regenerate, 29, 77, 126, 140, 144, 145, 158, 216, 277
regeneration, 8, 46, 140, 145, 179, 184, 274, 275
regions of the world, 216, 226
regression, 239
regulations, 54
rejection, 100, 101, 244
relatives, 4
relevance, 136, 180, 324, 349
reliability, 14
relief, 84
renal failure, 230
replication, 29, 53, 77, 251, 259
repression, 131, 206
reproduction, 13, 14, 131, 211, 213, 304, 305, 306, 307, 308, 321, 340, 378
requirements, 37, 185
researchers, 14, 64, 145, 153, 209, 230, 232, 237, 239, 267, 269, 295, 296
reserves, 159
residues, 30, 60, 61, 83, 170
resilience, 33
resistance, 2, 7, 100, 148, 183, 201, 202, 203, 204, 206, 207, 208, 214, 218, 235, 287, 313, 318, 349, 351, 365, 367
resolution, 197, 242
resources, 211, 306, 307
respiration, 9, 22, 44, 46, 48, 49, 75, 80, 85, 180, 193, 200, 216, 223, 224, 225, 228, 322
respiratory rate, 224
responsiveness, 40, 157, 270
restoration, 160, 183, 203, 254
restrictions, 299
resveratrol, 151, 155, 215, 229, 272
retardation, 5, 203, 209, 211, 228
retina, 57, 131, 156
retinol, 131, 132, 138, 139, 245, 272, 273, 344, 350, 367, 379
rheumatoid arthritis, 10, 194, 238, 244, 245
rhythm, 193, 251
rhytidectomy, 293
riboflavin, 73, 88, 109, 369
ribose, 79, 119, 147, 231, 320, 329, 336
rickets, 110, 142
rings, 131, 186, 259
risk assessment, 126, 129
risk factors, 94, 95, 185, 213, 239
risks, 4, 95, 98, 110, 120, 176, 270
RNA, 73, 198, 260, 348
rodents, 101, 184, 210, 211, 212, 227, 298, 349, 369
ROOH, 117
root, 35, 322

roots, 31
ROS accompany aging, 8
rosacea, 54
roughness, 5, 110, 137, 146, 154, 274, 275
roundworms, 177
routes, 179
rubber, 231

S

safety, 54, 71, 72, 76, 77, 92, 106, 110, 126, 176, 178, 209, 285, 291, 323, 328, 341, 357, 358, 386
salmon, 149, 156
salts, 235
saturated fat, 156, 161, 239, 241, 261
saturated fatty acids, 156
saturation, 153
scaling, 138, 154, 273
scarcity, 53
scattering, 57, 59, 71, 72
scavengers, 121, 167, 183, 227, 260, 304, 348
scent, 2
science, 250, 271, 311, 327, 355, 360, 365, 370
scleroderma, 63
scope, 12, 249
scrotum, 143
sea level, 72
seafood, 239
seasonal changes, 128
seborrheic dermatitis, 143
sebum, 2, 34, 35, 161, 265, 267, 268, 279, 282, 323, 383
secondary metabolism, 149
secrete, 34, 100, 107, 243, 261, 267, 293, 304
secretion, 35, 250, 256, 257, 263, 265, 266, 269, 353
sedentary lifestyle, 185, 216
seed, 155, 278
selenium, 30, 60, 123, 140, 141, 147, 148, 220, 223, 245, 246, 272, 301, 335, 348, 372, 377
self-awareness, 97
self-destruction, 7
self-esteem, 5, 218
senescence, 3, 7, 9, 10, 12, 13, 14, 20, 21, 42, 48, 79, 80, 90, 119, 120, 147, 211, 215, 229, 234, 235, 255, 259, 260, 261, 262, 264, 268, 295, 300, 320, 333, 348, 353, 354, 355, 371, 376, 378, 386
sensation, 71
sensing, 201, 204
sensitivity, 64, 102, 133, 143, 157, 367, 369, 379
sensitization, 127, 129, 146, 285, 323
serine, 62, 346
serotonin, 253

serum, 105, 132, 133, 134, 140, 161, 194, 195, 215, 234, 245, 266, 268, 269, 314, 317, 347, 380
severe stress, 202
sex, 39, 219, 239, 264, 265, 266, 268, 323, 341, 356, 362
sex hormones, 266, 341
sex steroid, 264, 265, 268, 356, 362
shade, 287
shape, 34, 97, 247
shellfish, 239
shock, 201, 202, 203, 204, 206, 207, 208, 209, 314, 331, 366, 381
shortage, 215, 307
showing, 68, 100, 176, 202, 213
side chain, 83, 144
side effects, 110, 213, 270, 292, 300, 308, 373
signal transduction, 21, 22, 89, 113, 149, 201, 204, 264, 305, 324, 330, 338, 354, 360
signaling pathway, 20, 40, 89, 113, 132, 210, 293, 339, 378
signalling, 296
signals, 203, 215, 242, 244, 246, 247, 254, 302
signs, 1, 2, 5, 9, 11, 42, 54, 67, 90, 97, 109, 136, 145, 168, 207, 266, 273, 275, 276, 281, 289, 293, 307, 368
silver, 335
simulation, 304, 339
sister chromatid exchange, 76
skeletal muscle, 204, 210, 211, 217, 218, 230, 318, 320, 340, 350, 361, 362, 364, 365, 378, 380, 385
skeleton, 65
skin diseases, 5, 34, 37, 41, 56, 57, 101, 153, 161, 253, 256, 274, 286
sleep deprivation, 253, 254, 373
small intestine, 131
smoking, 22, 23, 28, 39, 50, 51, 52, 53, 64, 65, 66, 83, 129, 155, 170, 183, 239, 261, 289, 295, 301, 302, 303, 318, 326, 329, 336, 339, 342, 344, 347, 350, 370, 374, 378
smoking cessation, 239
smoothness, 127
social behavior, 69, 70
social class, 66
social interactions, 4
social network, 255, 301
social status, 66, 261, 321
social support, 255
society, 1, 15, 325
sodium, 208, 215, 292, 346
soleus, 366
solubility, 132, 276
solution, 5, 88, 177, 194, 214, 244, 291, 292, 296, 369
solvents, 63
somatic cell, 92, 259, 260, 306
Soviet Union, 342
speciation, 221
specter, 58
spectrophotometry, 195
spectroscopy, 377
speculation, 212
speech, 53
spending, 287
sperm, 228, 331
spin, 46, 191, 192, 196, 198, 325, 373
Sprague-Dawley rats, 384
squamous cell, 51, 91, 95, 97, 101, 256, 282
squamous cell carcinoma, 51, 91, 95, 97, 101, 256, 282
stability, 141, 203, 212, 259, 270, 277, 280, 324, 353
standardization, 278, 284
starch, 232
starvation, 202, 232, 298
state, 19, 26, 28, 30, 46, 53, 55, 56, 60, 72, 76, 77, 87, 88, 109, 113, 117, 123, 132, 147, 177, 184, 203, 206, 216, 221, 227, 228, 229, 230, 243, 247, 248, 255, 260, 261, 265, 283, 311, 325
states, 8, 10, 50, 77, 81, 83, 88, 106, 113, 152, 203, 243, 268, 274, 304, 306, 315, 321
stem cells, 81, 293, 300
steroids, 32, 109, 260, 267, 268
sterols, 32, 156, 279
stimulant, 53
storage, 61, 62, 131, 169, 185, 186, 229, 230, 342, 384
stress factors, 4, 206
stressors, 136, 201, 206, 256, 308, 324, 332, 349, 369, 382
stretching, 33, 219
stroke, 194, 218, 229
structural changes, 39
structural protein, 11, 33, 40, 229, 230, 292
structure, 3, 14, 33, 35, 63, 66, 81, 118, 131, 139, 150, 154, 160, 199, 206, 235, 278, 279, 280, 302, 319
structuring, 343
style, 69, 239, 328
subcutaneous tissue, 34, 53, 65, 265
subgroups, 150, 178
substitution, 266, 269
substitutions, 321
substrate, 27, 46, 115, 117, 124, 180, 216, 223, 227, 283, 337, 343, 352
substrates, 28, 41, 46, 222, 223, 228, 251, 339
sucrose, 234
suicide, 80, 354

Index

sulfate, 148, 150, 264, 267, 269, 280, 315
sulfur, 30, 83, 246, 253
sulphur, 26, 29
Sun, 56, 58, 67, 68, 69, 70, 91, 93, 100, 105, 108, 282, 376, 382
supervision, 110
suppression, 13, 58, 76, 92, 99, 100, 101, 111, 127, 143, 152, 182, 196, 255, 274, 277, 285, 326, 384
surface area, 31, 94, 143, 167
surface layer, 291
surface modification, 371
surface properties, 28
surgical intervention, 273
surveillance, 32, 92, 101
survival, 79, 80, 119, 153, 160, 183, 201, 203, 206, 207, 208, 209, 211, 212, 213, 214, 215, 296, 305, 306, 316, 327, 354, 378, 385
susceptibility, 2, 30, 64, 100, 101, 102, 157, 256, 282, 369, 382
sweat, 2, 33, 34, 35, 42, 50, 105, 265
Sweden, 249
sympathetic nerve fibers, 34
symptoms, 97, 106, 151, 274, 299
syndrome, 327
synergistic effect, 51, 63, 134, 139, 140, 142, 145, 148, 162, 182, 184, 192, 255, 272, 277, 295, 299, 303, 375
synovial fluid, 343
synovial tissue, 245, 373
syphilis, 143

T

T cell, 99, 237, 256, 261
tannins, 149, 221
tar, 253
target, 30, 62, 77, 81, 91, 114, 131, 138, 161, 167, 199, 231, 232, 243, 253, 260, 297, 321, 386
techniques, 191, 192, 194, 195, 196, 286, 289, 292, 301, 320, 326, 374
technologies, 290, 300
technology, 299, 360, 366
teens, 106
teeth, 34, 271, 297
telomere, 12, 15, 147, 196, 237, 255, 259, 260, 261, 262, 300, 302, 303, 307, 318, 321, 328, 348, 352, 372, 385
telomere shortening, 12, 15, 147, 259, 260, 261, 262, 300, 302, 303, 328, 352, 385
temperature, 6, 34, 50, 54, 110, 202, 204, 206, 218, 224, 226, 227, 228, 233, 298, 306, 343, 349, 352, 368, 374
tendon, 233, 234

tensile strength, 110
tension, 306, 345
terminals, 290
terpenes, 156
testing, 148, 271, 285, 341
testosterone, 263, 264, 266, 268, 269, 270
tetracycline antibiotics, 109
tetracyclines, 29
textbook, 326
texture, 2, 54, 162, 278, 280, 292
TGF, 33, 293, 354
T-helper cell, 100
therapeutic agents, 194, 353
therapeutic interventions, 1
therapy, 65, 106, 136, 137, 160, 180, 185, 187, 194, 195, 204, 260, 266, 270, 290, 292, 293, 300, 311, 320, 322, 337, 339, 344, 359, 363, 365, 368, 381
thermoregulation, 105
thinning, 3, 40, 57, 265, 273
thromboxanes, 249
thymine, 75, 76, 77, 92, 120, 133, 324
thyroid, 120, 216, 226, 263, 267
thyroid gland, 267
thyroiditis, 14
thyrotropin, 267
thyroxin, 267
tissue homeostasis, 232
titanium, 285, 371
TNF, 63, 100, 250, 279, 353
TNF-alpha, 100
TNF-α, 63, 100
tobacco, 4, 51, 52, 53, 167, 200, 253, 298, 300, 333, 350, 370, 385
tobacco smoke, 52, 53, 167, 200, 298, 300, 333, 370
tobacco smoking, 53, 350, 385
tocopherols, 128, 133, 176, 193, 200, 278, 337
total energy, 57, 304
toxic effect, 19, 221, 248, 296
toxic substances, 279
toxic waste, 46
toxicity, 29, 60, 61, 77, 113, 116, 129, 130, 143, 146, 168, 169, 183, 191, 220, 228, 285, 315, 331, 332, 337, 357, 368, 380
toxicology, 155, 345, 379
toxin, 169, 289, 290
trace elements, 185, 296
training, 4, 204, 218, 219, 312, 329, 334, 337, 340, 350, 364, 365, 373, 380
traits, 158, 304
tranquilizers, 109
transcription, 21, 29, 33, 42, 61, 77, 79, 89, 97, 99, 138, 187, 201, 205, 242, 243, 244, 246, 304, 305, 365, 370, 375, 383

transcription factors, 21, 42, 61, 89, 99, 187, 205, 242, 244, 246, 305, 370, 383
transcripts, 374
transduction, 46, 89, 201, 238, 305
transfection, 352
transferrin, 193, 221
transformation, 10, 90, 115, 185, 221
transformations, 75, 231
transforming growth factor, 33, 264, 293, 365
transition metal, 25, 27, 28, 60, 183, 194, 220, 256, 337, 341
transition metalions, 60, 220, 256
transition mutation, 76
translocation, 224
transmission, 37, 70
transplant, 101, 244
transplantation, 289
transport, 10, 19, 25, 28, 43, 44, 45, 46, 81, 110, 127, 138, 144, 161, 179, 186, 210, 216, 223, 225, 226, 228, 233, 251, 276, 293, 298, 303, 326, 342, 361, 369
trauma, 266, 292
traumatic brain injury, 215
trial, 134, 135, 136, 146, 161, 205, 311, 328, 333, 335, 338, 342, 362, 364, 375
triggers, 7, 205, 245, 249
triglycerides, 151, 156, 158, 230, 245, 346
triiodothyronine, 267
tryptophan, 88, 144, 196, 197, 232, 283, 355
TSH, 267
tumor, 63, 76, 77, 80, 90, 91, 92, 94, 97, 99, 127, 135, 137, 152, 156, 183, 237, 243, 256, 260, 298, 318, 345, 349, 352, 374, 378, 382
tumor cells, 80, 183, 260, 382
tumor development, 237, 256
tumor necrosis factor, 243
tumor progression, 256, 352
tumorigenesis, 183, 329
tumors, 72, 92, 97, 100, 101, 135, 137, 156, 183, 311, 332
turnover, 14, 33, 35, 40, 92, 136, 159, 216, 217, 227, 233, 251, 372
turtle, 307, 323, 352
twins, 64, 65, 261, 354, 360, 369
type 1 diabetes, 340
type 2 diabetes, 347, 362
tyrosine, 21, 36, 152, 170, 277, 305, 311

U

UK, 52, 71, 143, 219, 367
ulcer, 273

ultraviolet irradiation, 69, 90, 104, 273, 324, 326, 330, 367
ultraviolet-A (UVA), 141
uniform, 102
United, 95, 106, 178, 241, 285, 291, 334, 338, 350, 356, 374
United Kingdom, 95, 374
United States, 106, 178, 241, 285, 291, 334, 338, 350, 356
unstable compounds, 9
upper respiratory infection, 226
uric acid, 121, 122, 123, 162, 168, 193, 197, 382
urinary tract, 247
urinary tract infection, 247
urine, 46, 77, 191, 219, 234, 235, 256, 350, 365
US Department of Health and Human Services, 219
USA, 1, 285, 311, 312, 313, 314, 315, 324, 327, 328, 330, 331, 333, 335, 336, 337, 340, 341, 345, 346, 349, 351, 369, 370, 371, 372, 375, 381
USDA, 132, 322
UV irradiation, 30, 41, 62, 67, 69, 75, 82, 84, 89, 102, 107, 123, 124, 132, 133, 134, 140, 143, 157, 246, 252, 260, 269, 284
UV light, 2, 21, 36, 56, 58, 68, 74, 75, 83, 88, 89, 124, 134, 140, 151, 206, 208, 209, 283, 284, 317
UV radiation, 6, 9, 19, 23, 36, 37, 40, 51, 54, 56, 57, 58, 59, 62, 68, 72, 85, 87, 88, 89, 91, 95, 99, 100, 105, 107, 109, 110, 120, 127, 135, 142, 152, 154, 161, 162, 170, 183, 201, 205, 208, 253, 256, 274, 282, 283, 284, 285, 288, 297, 321, 338, 348, 373
UV spectrum, 58
UVA irradiation, 33, 88, 109, 140, 145, 162, 276, 346, 355, 364, 365
UVB irradiation, 62, 68, 81, 89, 93, 155, 157, 329, 332
UV-irradiation, 363
UV-radiation, 105, 110

V

vaccinations, 100
valence, 28, 60, 221
valine, 33
vanadium, 60, 61, 220
variables, 154, 184, 351
variations, 7, 68, 149, 363
vascular wall, 67, 90
vascularization, 68
vasculature, 265, 335
vasodilator, 219, 340
vegetable oil, 129
vegetables, 4, 120, 121, 123, 125, 147, 150, 156, 161, 171, 176, 178, 181, 184, 185, 186, 229, 236,

238, 240, 241, 243, 246, 249, 250, 261, 286, 296, 297, 298, 300, 321
vehicles, 278
vein, 240, 296
velocity, 66, 169
venules, 102
vertebrates, 131, 158, 228
vessels, 41, 100, 269
vibration, 37
victims, 331
viruses, 50, 248
vision, 131, 311
vitamin A, 52, 121, 130, 131, 133, 136, 137, 161, 175, 181, 272, 288, 311, 344, 359, 367, 374
vitamin B1, 185, 235
vitamin B12, 185
vitamin B2, 143
vitamin B3, 143, 272
vitamin B6, 53, 143, 185, 325, 346
Vitamin C, 123, 125, 127, 140, 176, 181, 245, 273, 318, 337, 342, 363, 382
vitamin D, 58, 74, 105, 110, 142, 143, 178, 185, 264, 316, 327, 334, 358, 382
vitamin E, 51, 61, 63, 122, 123, 124, 128, 129, 130, 133, 140, 141, 142, 149, 155, 157, 162, 168, 170, 176, 179, 181, 182, 183, 184, 187, 223, 243, 245, 272, 275, 277, 318, 321, 323, 328, 333, 336, 348, 351, 355, 359, 360, 368, 375, 377, 383
vitamin supplementation, 141, 181, 338
vitamins, 127, 137, 140, 141, 143, 156, 176, 178, 181, 184, 185, 193, 200, 228, 236, 239, 240, 242, 246, 271, 272, 277, 296, 297, 298, 303, 311, 319, 320, 321, 327, 335, 355, 356, 369, 373, 381, 382
vitiligo, 334

W

walking, 121, 219, 336
war, 212, 339
Washington, 324, 331, 379
waste, 13, 224, 306, 307
water diffusion, 280
wavelengths, 57, 68, 88, 109, 146, 283, 319, 368, 379
weakness, 144
wealth, 95
wear, 7, 83, 84, 287
weight control, 352
weight gain, 251
weight loss, 85, 242, 250
weight reduction, 195
well-being, 184, 218
wellness, 193
white blood cells, 196
WHO, 56, 57, 58, 59, 94, 100, 101, 186, 212, 287, 383
Wisconsin, 366
wool, 109
workers, 69, 97, 159, 177, 205, 254, 336, 342
workload, 342
World Health Organization, 58, 98, 160, 178, 212, 240
World War I, 212
worldwide, 3, 51, 151, 278, 287, 334
worms, 184, 204, 207
worry, 106
wound healing, 10, 39, 51, 148, 153, 220, 244, 249, 265, 266, 267, 270, 272, 274, 293, 304, 333, 345, 356, 366

X

xanthophyll, 131, 132

Y

yeast, 116, 144, 149, 177, 180, 182, 196, 202, 213, 246, 319, 331, 336, 342, 343, 353, 369
yield, 26, 88, 192, 227, 230, 253
young adults, 35
young people, 53
young women, 70

Z

zinc, 33, 60, 89, 146, 149, 162, 169, 179, 184, 220, 221, 222, 223, 228, 245, 246, 275, 284, 301, 351, 353, 367
ZnO, 54
zwitterions, 83